S0-ADP-091

AARP PHARMACY SERVICE

PRESCRIPTION DRUG HANDBOOK

Second Edition

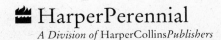

HarperPerennial

A Division of HarperCollinsPublishers

AARP PHARMACY SERVICE PRESCRIPTION
DRUG HANDBOOK *(Second Edition)*. Copyright
© 1992 by HarperCollins *Publishers*, Inc., New York,
New York and American Association of Retired Persons, Washington, D.C. All rights reserved. Printed
in the United States of America. No part of this book
may be used or reproduced in any manner whatso-
ever without written permission except in the case of
brief quotations embodied in critical articles and re-
views. For information address HarperCollins *Publishers*, Inc., 10 East 53rd Street, New York, New York
10022.

HarperCollins books may be purchased for educational, business, or sales promotional use. For information, please call or write: Special Markets
Department, HarperCollins *Publishers* Inc., 10 East
53rd Street, New York, N.Y. 10022. Telephone: (212)
207-7528; Fax: (212) 207-7222.

Library of Congress Cataloging in Publication Data

AARP pharmacy service prescription drug hand-
book—2nd ed.
    p.   cm.
   "An AARP book."
   Includes index.
   ISBN 0-06-271553-4—ISBN 0-06-277037-3
   (pbk.) (incorrect)—ISBN 0-06-263501-8 (correct)
   1. Drugs—Dictionaries. 2. Chemotherapy—
   Dictionaries.
1. American Association of Retired Persons.
RS51.A28   1992   91-58281

92 93 94 95 96 RRD 10 9 8 7 6 5 4 3 2

AARP Books is an educational and public service project of the American Association of Retired Persons, which, with a membership of more than 33 million, is the largest association of persons fifty and over in the world today. Founded in 1958, AARP provides older Americans with a wide range of membership programs and services, including legislative representation at both federal and state levels. For further information about additional association activities, write to AARP, 601 E Street, N.W., Washington, DC 20049.

CONTENTS

PREFACE

In 1982, the AARP Pharmacy Service began providing the first voluntary patient prescription drug information leaflets in the United States to AARP members. The new Medication Information Leaflets for Seniors (MILS) were and are given routinely to the Pharmacy's mail-service customers with their prescription drug orders. The leaflets were written for easy understanding, and the information was written with the assistance and cooperation of the U.S. Food and Drug Administration and carefully checked by physicians and pharmacists in geriatric medicine. The MILS have become models for health care agencies seeking to provide information for older persons to use in working with their doctors and other health care providers to manage their own health programs better.

It is a logical step for the AARP Pharmacy Service to now produce this major reference work on prescription drugs for older persons, who consume more than 30 percent of the prescription drugs sold in the United States. As the largest private, nonprofit mail-service pharmacy in the world, addressing specifically the needs of persons fifty years of age and older, the Service felt an obligation to make the information in this book available to a greater population of those who use prescription drugs and those who wish to monitor such drug use in older people they care for.

The Editorial Advisory Board members listed on the following pages provided invaluable guidance in the development and review of the manuscript for this book. Many of them are specialists in geriatric medicine, a field of medicine dealing specifically with diseases in older persons.

John R. McHugh, R.Ph., President

AARP Pharmacy Service is sponsored but not owned or controlled by AARP.

EDITORIAL ADVISORY BOARD

JERRY AVORN, MD
Associate Professor of Medicine and
   Director, Program for the Analysis of
   Clinical Strategies
Harvard Medical School
Attending Geriatrician
Brigham and Women's Hospital
Boston, Massachusetts

JEFFREY B. BLUMBERG, PhD, FACN
Associate Director
Professor of Nutrition
USDA Human Nutrition Research Center
   on Aging
Tufts University
Boston, Massachusetts

RUBIN BRESSLER, MD
Robert S. and Irene P. Flinn
Professor of Medicine and Head
   of Internal Medicine
Professor of Pharmacology
University of Arizona Health Sciences Center
Tucson, Arizona

IGOR CERNY, PharmD
Marketing Surveillance and
Enforcement Branch
U.S. Food and Drug Administration
Rockville, Maryland

FRANK E. DiBENEDETTO, PhD
Assistant Clinical Professor
Health Sciences Department
Touro College
New York, New York

ALFRED FALLAVOLLITA, JR, RPh, MS
Drug Management and Authorization Section
Investigational Drug Branch
Cancer Therapy Evaluation Program
Division of Cancer Treatment
National Cancer Institute
Bethesda, Maryland

MICHAEL L. FREEDMAN, MD
The Diane and Arthur Belfer
Professor of Geriatric Medicine,
   Director, Division of Geriatrics
New York University/Bellevue Hospital Center
New York, New York

JERRY H. GURWITZ, MD
Instructor in Medicine
Harvard Medical School
   Gerontology Division
Beth Israel Hospital
Boston, Massachusetts

MICHAEL A. JENIKE, MD
Associate Professor of Psychiatry
Harvard Medical School
Associate Chief of Psychiatry
Research Psychiatrist
Massachusetts General Hospital
Boston, Massachusetts

SARAH B. KRAMER, MD
Instructor of Clinical Medicine
New York University School of Medicine
Consulting Rheumatologist
Goldwater Hospital
New York, New York

PETER LAMY, PhD, SCD
Professor and Director
The Center for the Study of Pharmacy
   and Therapeutics for the Elderly
University of Maryland School of Pharmacy
Baltimore, Maryland

DAVID LIEBERMAN, MD
Staff Physician, Gastroenterology Section
Oregon Veterans Administration
   Medical Center
Associate Professor of Medicine
Division of Gastroenterology
Oregon Health Sciences University
Portland, Oregon

JEROME Z. LITT, MD
Assistant Clinical Professor of Dermatology
Case Western Reserve University
School of Medicine
Cleveland, Ohio

CATHERINE M. MACLEOD, MD
Director Clinical Pharmacology Unit
Rush-Presbyterian–St. Lukes Medical Center
Chicago, Illinois

WILLIAM R. MARKESBERY, MD
Professor of Pathology and Neurology
Director, Alzheimer's Disease Research Center
Sanders-Brown Research Center on Aging
University of Kentucky Medical Center
Lexington, Kentucky

MAURIE MARKMAN, MD
Vice Chairman
Department of Medicine
Memorial Sloan-Kettering Cancer Center
New York, New York

KENNETH MINAKER, MD
Associate Program Director
Beth Israel Hospital Clinical Research Center
Director, Boston/West Roxbury Veterans
Administration Geriatric Research Education
Clinical Center
Associate Professor of Medicine,
    Division on Aging
Harvard Medical School
Boston, Massachusetts

FRANK PARKER, MD
Professor and Chairman
Department of Dermatology
Oregon Health Sciences University
School of Medicine
Portland, Oregon

NEIL RESNICK, MD
Assistant Professor in Medicine
Harvard Medical School
Chief, Geriatrics and
    Director, Continence Clinic
Brigham and Women's Hospital
Boston, Massachusetts

LARRY F. RICH, MD, MS
Associate Professor of Ophthalmology
Chief, Cornea and External Disease Service
The Casey Eye Institute
Portland, Oregon

JOHN R. WALSH, MD
Chief of Gerontology Section
Veterans Administration Medical Center
Professor of Medicine
Oregon Health Sciences University
Portland, Oregon

JEANNE Y. WEI, MD, PhD
Chief, Gerontology Division
Beth Israel Hospital
Director of Claude Pepper Geriatrics
    Research and Training
Director, Division on Aging
Harvard Medical School
Boston, Massachusetts

SCOTT T. WEISS, MD, MS
Associate Professor of Medicine
Harvard Medical School
Brigham and Women's Hospital
Beth Israel Hospital
Boston, Massachusetts

LAWRENCE A. YANUZZI, MD
Vice Chairman, Department of
    Ophthalmology
Director of Retinal Services
Manhattan Eye, Ear, and Throat Hospital
Associate Clinical Professor of Ophthalmology
Columbia University Medical College
New York, New York

NANCY J. OLINS, MA
Senior Editor
Director of Program Development
and Corporate Communications
AARP Pharmacy Service
Alexandria, Virginia

AARP PHARMACY SERVICE REVIEW BOARD

Betsy Asai, RPh

Phillip L. Arends, RPh

Larry R. Bierman, RPh

Kent Blair, RPh

Jack Boylan, RPh

Diane Brown, RPh

William F. Broussard, RPh

Colleen R. Brown, RPh

Laura Carabin

Larry D. Cartier, RPh

John J. Casey, RPh

David Chan, RPh

Erin Conry, RPh

Teresa Fridley, RPh

Steve Grote, RPh

Grant Hall, RPh

Garvin Hamilton, RPh

Mary Hayward, RPh

Shirley Hopkins, RPh

Steven E. Hughes, RPh

John Iglehart, RPh

Vergilene James

Andrew Jarmer, RPh

Doris M. Kinzle, RPh

Nancy Kislowski, RPh

Paul Kwong, RPh

Rose Lang, RPh

Frederick C. Lee, RPh

Marvin Levitt, RPh

Wilfrid Lin, RPh

Richard Lukins, RPh

Michael McQuinn, RPh

William B. Martin, RPh

Beth Privratsky, RPh

Sandi Scott, PharmD

Vikki Stadick, RPh

Zana Stafford, RPh

Charles E. Thomas, RPh

Julian Williams, RPh

Soo Ping Wong, RPh

Patrick Zimmer, RPh

PUBLISHER'S NOTE:

The information contained in this book is based on research and recommendations of responsible specialists in medicine and pharmacology. It is meant to serve as a reference book and not as a substitute for the professional judgment of a doctor. Since each individual is unique and reactions to drugs vary widely, readers are urged to discuss any drug treatment with a doctor before taking a drug or discontinuing the use of a prescribed drug.

The list of brand names in each drug chart in this book may not include all such products available. Only the ones most commonly used at the time of publication are named. Since new brands are approved for patient use regularly and others become unavailable, no list can reflect all these changes. The mention of a brand name in this book does not imply endorsement, nor does absence of a name imply a problem with the brand.

OVERVIEW

As you leave your doctor's office, prescription in hand, you may not be able to decipher the handwriting indicating the name of the drug prescribed and the directions for its use. Even the label clearly typed by the pharmacist will provide you with scant information about the drug you will be swallowing or spraying, inserting or inhaling. A talk with your doctor or pharmacist may answer some of your questions, but you may later recall ones you forgot to ask, perhaps about side effects of the medicine or whether you can drink or drive while on the drug.

This book will provide you with the information you need to know about the medicines your doctor has prescribed. You will learn why a drug is being prescribed for a particular condition, what effects—both good and bad—you can expect from a drug, and how your eating habits and other aspects of your lifestyle can influence drug therapy. You will find out how a drug you are taking compares with other drugs used to treat the same condition and what other treatment options are available. In short, the information presented here will help you play a more active and positive role in maintaining your health.

As you can see from the Contents, the introductory material for this book contains five overview sections to increase your general knowledge about both prescription and over-the-counter (OTC) medicines. It is a good idea to familiarize yourself with this information before going on to read about specific products. These sections will arm you with information on proper ways to administer drugs, provide tips for remembering complicated drug schedules, and suggest appropriate questions to pose to your doctor and pharmacist. Also discussed are the use of nonprescription drugs, medicine considerations when traveling, and strategies for saving money on drugs without compromising on quality.

HOW TO USE THIS BOOK

The specific drug information is contained in thirteen chapters, each covering a group of related medical conditions (such as digestive disorders or respiratory problems). Information about each of the related medical conditions covered in the chapter appears in brief medical guides. Each medical guide offers a quick overview of the particular medical condition and discusses its causes, diagnosis, and treatment, including drug and nondrug alternatives. Following each medical guide are drug charts. These drug charts summarize, in table form, important information about the medicines that may be prescribed for the condition discussed in the medical guide.

Not every available drug for every disorder is included. Instead, this book focuses on the several hundred drugs that are most commonly prescribed for and used by people over fifty. Drugs were selected based on information gathered from the AARP Pharmacy Service, the National Diagnostic and Therapeutic Index, other government and nongovernment statistical sources, and the judgments of the members of the Editorial Advisory Board.

None of the drugs included in this book must be administered by a doctor, though most must be prescribed by a doctor. Many of the OTC drug products you may have in your home will not appear here because you don't need a doctor's prescription to purchase them. Note, however, that limited exceptions have been made to this "prescription only" rule. Drug charts for aspirin and nonaspirin pain-killers are included because of their prominent therapeutic role in treating such conditions as arthritis and mini-strokes, which are important problems in people over fifty. A drug chart is also included for calcium supplements, which are often recommended for older women. The last exception concerns vitamins and minerals. The designation of these products as "over-the-counter" or "prescription only" often depends on dosage strength; frequently used products in this category are listed, even if available without a prescription, to ensure that important vitamin combinations are included in this book.

The medical-condition index in the back of this book lists alphabetically all the medical conditions discussed in the text and can be used as a starting-off point in finding the medical guide that provides the information you want. Following the medical guides are the drug charts relevant to the condition being discussed. You might wish to look over and compare information on the various drugs available for treating your condition; you will find those charts all grouped together in one section of a chapter. The more you know about what you are taking—and what you are not—the more control you will have over your own health.

But you may be more interested in zeroing in on a specific drug than a specific illness. For example, you have been given a prescription for a medicine and want to know all about it before you take it. Or you may want to know, more specifically, if there are any special considerations for older people using this drug. To locate the appropriate drug chart, check the drug index, which appears right after the medical-condition index. The drug index lists medicines alphabetically by their generic (chemical) names (for example, tetracycline) and brand (trade) names (brand names of tetracycline, for example, include Achromycin, and Sumycin). The page numbers in boldface indicate where the drug chart appears; additional references to the drug are also listed.

To provide you with even more complete information about the drugs your doctor prescribes, a Drug Identification Section appears after page 1106. The actual-size pictures in this section are organized according to the color of the drug and listed by both brand and generic names. To locate the picture of a particular drug, see the drug identification index on pages 1094–1106, which will direct you to the correct page as well as list the color and shape of the brand-name capsule or tablet (liquids, skin patches, and suppositories are not pictured).

A Guide to the Drug Charts

The opening section of each drug chart contains the most basic information about the medicine—generic name, brand name(s), dosage forms and strengths, and, where appropriate, how much of each ingredient it contains. (See page 5 for a further explanation of this.) In some cases, not all available brands are included but the most common ones are. The number of drugs available changes regularly, with new drugs appearing on the market and others being removed. Note that the listing of dosage forms and strengths does *not* include information on how much of the drug you should take. That must be determined for you individually by your doctor and written on the prescription label.

The next section of the charts, the "Drug Profile," describes briefly what the medicine is used for and how it acts in the body.

The next section, "Before Using this Drug," alerts you to what information to give your doctor. The doctor should review your medical history and any allergic reactions or other problems you've had with similar drugs or those in a related class. Also, you should provide your doctor with a report on both prescription and OTC medicines you are currently taking. Drugs can interact in your body with other drugs, altering the effectiveness, toxicity, or side effects of either drug.

The section, "Special Restrictions While Taking this Drug," will help you get the most benefit from your medicine. It tells you, specifically, what drugs interact with your medicine and how to adjust your diet to help your medicine work more effectively. Information on medical examinations or tests you may need to take while on the drug are also outlined. In addition, any special restrictions on alcohol use, smoking, driving, sun exposure, exposure to excessive heat or cold, and exercise and exertion are discussed here. Other precautions are indicated when applicable to the particular drug.

The section on "Possible Side Effects" tells what type of side effects can be caused by the medicine and at what point to check with your doctor if you are experiencing any. Although the list of side effects is often long and can seem intimidating, keep in mind that many of the reactions are quite rare and may never happen to you.

In their concluding sections, the drug charts provide you with "Storage Instructions" for the medicine (improperly stored medicine can lose potency) and information on "Stopping or Interrupting Therapy." You may be tempted to discontinue taking the medicine when your symptoms begin to go away, but complete recovery may require longer treatment. Some drugs cannot be stopped abruptly; dosages must be diminished gradually.

Finally, the drug charts present "Special Considerations for Those over Sixty-Five." As a person ages, physical changes occur that may affect how long the drug remains in the body. This section lists side effects that are especially likely to occur in this age group and particular precautions to follow.

Although certain drugs are used to treat more than one type of medical condition, drug charts are not repeated in this book. Instead, cross-references are provided in the appropriate chapters to direct you from a particular medical condition to a relevant drug that may be listed in a different part of the book.

Drug Categories and Dosage Forms

Drugs are classified and grouped together in the drug charts in categories the Editorial Advisory Board judged to be most helpful to consumers. The "Category" listing refers to the medicines in terms that are commonly used by doctors and readily understood by patients. Where the Advisory Board concluded that drugs of a particular class were similar, the drugs appear in the same drug chart. If the judgment of the board was that certain differences outweighed similarities between products, these drugs appear in different charts.

The dosage forms (for example, capsules, suppositories, tablets) of each product are listed in alphabetical order. If the particular form of the drug has just one active ingredient, the dosage strength is given next to that form; for example: Tablet: 300 mg. However, a dosage form of a particular drug may have two or more active ingredients; this is especially common for liquids. In those cases, the drug chart lists the amounts of each of the ingredients contained in the product.

The information on dosage strengths and forms may be useful to you in a number of situations. For example, if your doctor has instructed you to take two 250-mg tablets of your medicine three times a day and the drug chart indicates that the drug also comes in a 500-mg tablet, you might ask your doctor whether one higher-strength tablet would work as well as two lower-strength tablets. Or if you have trouble swallowing tablets and the drug chart indicates that your medicine also comes in liquid form, you might want to discuss a possible switch with your doctor.

The information in these charts is presented in a concise, easy-to-understand format for quick reference. But it should not be your sole source of facts; it is designed as a supplement to information provided by your doctor, pharmacist, or other health professional. If it raises any questions or does not completely satisfy your concerns, ask a qualified health professional for clarification.

ABBREVIATIONS USED IN THIS BOOK

g = gram (there are approximately 30 grams to an ounce)

mg = milligram (one thousandth of a gram)

μg = mcg = microgram (one millionth of a gram)

ml = milliliter (one thousandth of a liter, or approximately one thousandth of a quart)

WHAT YOU SHOULD KNOW ABOUT THE DRUGS YOU TAKE

You may think you are doing all you can for your health if you go for a medical examination when you have a problem, have any prescription you are given filled by a pharmacy, and then follow the instructions on the label (as best you can) for taking the medicine. However, research has shown that people often make errors when taking prescription drugs. These errors may have serious outcomes. Not only can they undermine the effectiveness of the drug, but they may also actually cause medical harm.

Mistakes can be avoided if you ask the right questions of your doctor, pharmacist, or other health professional, but many people are reluctant to do so. They do not know what to ask, or they are afraid of taking up too much of the professional's time, or they may be concerned that they will sound mistrustful. None of these is a good reason for being uninformed—or misinformed—about the medicines you take. The potential effects on your health are too great for you to be less than fully informed.

Questions to Ask

Below is a list of questions you should ask your doctor about any medicine prescribed. Be sure to have paper and a pencil handy to jot down the answers.
• What is the drug's name? Many drugs have a brand name and a generic name. Ask about both, and write them down for your own records.

• What exactly does the drug do? At what point should you start to see an effect, and what should you do if none is apparent?

• How much medicine should you take, and how often? Ask your doctor to write on the prescription that these instructions should be included on the drug label.

• How long should you take the drug?

• What should you do if you miss taking the drug at the specified time?

• Can this drug be prescribed in a generic form, which often costs less than the brand-name version? (See pages 11–13 for more information on generic vs. brand-name medicines.)

• If you will be taking the drug for some time, could it be prescribed in a large quantity that will remain fresh at the rate you use it? This can help save you money.

• What foods, drinks, or activities and what other medicines should you avoid while on this drug?

• Should this medicine be taken with food or on an empty stomach?

• What are the common side effects and what should you do if they occur? Which ones are severe enough to warrant consulting your doctor?

• Is any written information available about this drug? Pamphlets or magazine articles can help reinforce your doctor's instructions and your own notes.

• Is there a less expensive alternative available that will have the same therapeutic effect?

• Are there effective alternatives to treatment with drugs? Some conditions can be helped by changes in diet, for example, or exercise, and you might want to explore those options first.

Your pharmacist is another valuable source of information in becoming a better informed consumer. You can raise the same types of issues mentioned above, as well as other specific concerns about your prescription:

• How much does the medicine cost?
• Is it available in a generic form?
• How should it be stored?
• Is it safe to crush a tablet or to open a capsule?
• Can this prescription be refilled?
• Can the medicine be put in a container that is easy to open?
• Is the medicine available in a more convenient or easy-to-use form?
• What does the extra labeling on the container mean?

Both your doctor and your pharmacist should be responsive to your questions and concerns about medicines, whether prescription or OTC. If you are dissatisfied with the time and attention you are receiving, consider finding a health professional who will answer your questions more fully.

Practical Pointers on Taking Drugs

Swallowing a pill may not be all there is to taking your medicine as the doctor ordered. Your medicine may come in different, less familiar forms, and you may be confused by different dosage schedules if more than one product is involved. If it is six o'clock in the evening, should you take three red tablets or two green capsules? Or is it time to get out the eye dropper or, perhaps, to change your skin patch? As medical science becomes more sophisticated, taking medicine can be more complicated.

Storage Instructions   Even the proper storage of drugs is not as simple as just lining them up in your bathroom medicine cabinet. Drugs should *not* be stored in the bathroom, where heat and moisture may affect them, but rather in a dry, cool place such as a bedroom or kitchen cabinet (*not* a cabinet above the stove). If directions call for the medicine to be refrigerated, do not place it in your freezer.

Remembering When   There are some tricks for remembering which drugs to take when. One technique involves making a list each day of the different times of day—morning, afternoon, evening, and night—and writing down next to each time the name and amount of the drug(s) you are supposed to take. Then check off the time once you have taken the appropriate medicine(s). Another memory helper is to label the compartments of a small box with the different times of day. (Make sure the box seals tightly to protect your medicines from air and moisture.) Then, fill each section with the pills you are supposed to take at that time. (You can buy a special pillbox to serve the same function.) Alternatively, you might try using vials with different-colored caps that stand for different times of day (such as blue for morning, white for afternoon, red for evening, and black for bedtime). Your pharmacist may be able to provide you with special calendars and drug-reminder charts that will jog your memory if you are faced with confusing schedules involving several drugs.

Learning How Once you have figured out *when* to take your medicine, you are still left with the problem of *how*. Pill swallowing is something most people have mastered, more or less, but what if our medicine comes in a different form, for example, a *buccal* tablet? The term *buccal* relates to the cheek and mouth, and a buccal tablet is one that should be placed in the pouch between the cheek and the gum. After taking this kind of tablet, close your mouth and let the tablet dissolve completely—do not swallow or chew it. While the tablet is dissolving, don't eat, drink, or smoke. For a *sublingual* tablet—one that is placed under the tongue while it dissolves—the recommendations and warnings are the same. Note that a *controlled-release* tablet should never be crushed or chewed.

You have probably had experience using eye, ear, and nose drops, as well as nasal sprays, but here is a brief review of safe, effective methods for administering these products.

Eye Drops

• Wash your hands with soap and water.
• Lie down (or tilt back your head) and look up at the ceiling.

• Gently pull down your lower eyelid so that a pouch is formed.
• With the dropper in your other hand, approach the eye from the side. Place the dropper close to the eye but not touching it.
• Place the prescribed number of drops into the eye pouch.
• Close your eye for a minute or two.
• Don't rub your eye. Instead, press gently with your fingers next to the bridge of your nose (on the same side as the eye into which you have inserted the drops) for about a minute. This helps prevent the eye drops from being drained from the eye.

If someone else administers the eye drops for you, have that person follow the steps outlined above, beginning with well-scrubbed hands.

Ear Drops

• Hold the bottle in your hands for a few minutes. This warms the drops to room temperature.
• Wash your hands with soap and water.
• Tilt your head or lie on your side, with the ear to be treated facing up. Gently pull the earlobe up and back.
• Place the prescribed number of drops into the ear. Do *not* insert the dropper into the ear.
• Stay in the same position for a few minutes after administering the drops.

This procedure can be done for you by somebody else, if necessary.

Nose Drops

• Blow your nose gently.

• Sit in a chair and tilt your head backward; alternatively, lie down with a pillow under your shoulders so that your head tips backward.
• Insert the nose dropper into the nostril about one third of an inch and drop the prescribed number of drops into the nose.
• Stay in the same position for several minutes.

Nasal Sprays

• Blow your nose gently.
• While sitting down, tilt your head slightly forward.
• Shake the container well.
• Insert the spray tip firmly into the nostril and point it at the back and outer side of the nose. (Close the other nostril by pressing your finger against its side.)
• Keep your mouth closed, begin to breathe in, and release one spray of the medicine.
• Remove the spray tip from the nostril and bend your head backward for a few seconds. Hold your breath for a few seconds, then breathe out through your mouth.
• If necessary, repeat the procedure for the other nostril.

Oral Inhalants

• Insert the metal canister into the mouthpiece and remove the cap.
• Shake well immediately before each use.
• Breathe out fully through the mouth, expelling as much air as possible.

• Place the mouthpiece in the mouth with the canister upright and close the lips around the mouthpiece.
• While breathing in deeply and slowly through the mouth, fully depress the canister with your index finger.
• Hold your breath as long as possible. Remove the canister from your mouth and release your finger before breathing out.
• If a second inhalation is prescribed, wait at least one to two minutes. Shake the inhaler again and repeat the above procedures.
• Cleanse the inhaler thoroughly and frequently as described in the instructions accompanying the medication.

Transdermal Patches

A relatively new method of drug delivery is transdermal, which means "through the skin." This involves placing a medicated patch on the skin, usually on a dry, nonhairy part of your body, like the stomach, back, or chest. Press the patch firmly in place for about ten to fifteen seconds, and then seal it by running your finger along its outside edge. At the prescribed time, the patch should be removed and thrown away and the next one applied.

Other Dosage Forms

caplet   A tablet that is shaped like a capsule.

controlled-release   Medicine is effective only during that period of time when the active ingredients are released and absorbed by the body at high enough rates. Dosage forms that prolong the medicine's period of effectiveness are said to have a *controlled-release* property. Other names for that property are timed-release, sustained-release, extended-release, and long-acting.

cream A semisolid preparation in which particles of medicine are combined—dissolved or undissolved—in a mixture of oil and water. Creams are applied externally; in addition to their specific medical effects, they may also soften and lubricate the areas being treated. These preparations can neither be seen nor felt after they've been applied, and they can be easily washed off with water.

elixir A liquid preparation taken orally in which particles of medicine are thoroughly dissolved in an alcohol-based solution. Elixirs may also include a sweetener or other flavoring to improve the medicine's taste. The amount of drug per dose of the medicine is measured in milligrams.

enteric-coated tablet A tablet coated with a thin outer layer that is not broken down by stomach acid but is easily dissolved by the juices of the intestines. The purpose of this outer coating is either to protect the stomach from being irritated by the medicine or to prevent the medicine from being destroyed by stomach acid.

ointment A semisolid preparation in which particles of medicine are combined—dissolved or undissolved—in a mixture of oil or animal or vegetable fats and water. Ointments have a higher oil and lower water content than do creams. They are applied externally; in addition to their specific medical effects, they may also soften and lubricate the areas being treated. These preparations can be quite greasy and are not easily washed off with water.

solution A liquid preparation taken orally in which particles of medicine are thoroughly dissolved in water or a water substitute. The amount of drug per dose of medicine is measured in milligrams.

suspension A liquid preparation taken orally in which solid particles of medicine are mixed with water or a water substitute, but are not dissolved. It is important that the particles in a suspension be evenly distributed throughout the preparation; this can be accomplished by thoroughly shaking the medication just before taking it. The amount of drug per dose of the medicine is measured in milligrams.

syrup A liquid preparation taken orally in which particles of medicine are thoroughly dissolved in water or a water substitute. A sweetener or other flavoring is added to improve the medicine's taste. The amount of drug per dose of the medicine is measured in milligrams.

SAVING MONEY ON PRESCRIPTION DRUGS

"You get what you pay for" is an axiom that has stopped many a consumer from getting bilked in the marketplace. But when it comes to medicine, price is not a reliable guide to quality. In fact, the price of the same drug can vary tenfold or more, depending on where you purchase it and under what name it is being sold.

The first key to saving money on drugs is to have some understanding of how new drugs are marketed and the difference between generic and brand names. When a new drug is being tested, it is given its *generic* name by an organization known as the United States Adopted Name Council. (This name is, in most cases, a simplified version of the product's chemical formula.) Once the drug has been approved as safe and effective by the U.S. Food and Drug Administration (FDA), it is usually marketed by just one pharmaceutical company (the innovator), which obtains a patent for the product and gives it a *brand* name. When the patent expires, other companies are free to sell the drug under its generic name or under other brand names. (The antibiotic tetracycline, for example, can be sold either under the name tetracycline or under such brand names as Achromycin and Sumycin.) An act passed by Congress in 1984 enables pharmaceutical companies to get generic drugs on the market more speedily and at lower cost than was previously possible. Savings can then be passed on to the consumer.

Most generic drugs are less expensive than brand-name versions and just as safe and effective. Therefore, when your doctor gets ready to write you a prescription for a particular medicine, inquire whether the generic form of the drug is available. Not all brand-name drugs have generic equivalents available to consumers. If your doctor prescribes by the generic name whenever possible, you will be able to save money on almost every prescription you have filled. In some states, pharmacists may substitute a generic drug for the brand-name form unless the doctor says not to.

But don't count the money you save just yet! You still have some work to do, by phone or by foot. Different pharmacies may charge very different prices for the same medicine, so be prepared to shop around. Some stores will cite their prices over the telephone, sparing you legwork. A number of states require pharmacists to post the prices of frequently prescribed drugs—another aid to the consumer. You may decide to comparison shop for each prescription. That strategy will save you the most money.

No matter what you end up paying to fill your prescription, check your medical insurance policy. Some plans pay all or part of drug costs. The time it takes for you to do the paperwork may translate into big savings on your drug bills.

You may be tempted to cut costs by not having your prescription refilled even though your doctor has instructed you to do so. That is actually a counterproductive measure that can threaten both your pocketbook and your health. Even if you feel fine, your illness may recur if you do not take your medicine for the full length of time prescribed by your doctor.

A more reasonable way to save money on drugs is to consider curtailing your OTC drugs while you are taking a prescription drug. Let your doctor decide whether the nonprescription product is necessary—or wise—for you to take at that time.

BRAND (TRADE) AND GENERIC (CHEMICAL) NAMES OF THE MOST COMMON PRESCRIPTION DRUGS

The following table will familiarize you with the generic names of over fifty brand-name drugs that, according to AARP Pharmacy Service statistics, are most commonly prescribed for persons fifty and over.

Brand (Trade) Name	Generic (Chemical) Name
Aldomet	Methyldopa
Aldoril	Methyldopa and hydrochlorothiazide
Apresoline	Hydralazine
Ativan	Lorazepam
Calan	Verapamil
Capoten	Captopril
Cardizem	Diltiazem
Catapres	Clonidine
Clinoril	Sulindac
Corgard	Nadolol
Coumadin	Warfarin
Deltasone	Prednisone
DiaBeta	Glyburide
Dilantin	Phenytoin
Dyazide	Triamterene and hydrochlorothiazide
Feldene	Piroxicam
Halcion	Triazolam
Inderal	Propranolol
Isordil	Isosorbide dinitrate
Lanoxin	Digoxin
Lasix	Furosemide
Levothroid	L-thyroxine (Levothyroxine)
Lopid	Gemfibrozil
Lopressor	Metoprolol
Lorelco	Probucol

Brand (Trade) Name	Generic (Chemical) Name
Maxzide	Triamterene and hydrochlorothiazide
Mevacor	Lovastatin
Micronase	Glyburide
Micro-K	Potassium chloride
Motrin	Ibuprofen
Naprosyn	Naproxen
Nitro-Bid	Nitroglycerin
Norpace	Disopyramide
Nolvadex	Tamoxifen
Persantine	Dipyridamole
Premarin	Conjugated estrogens
Procardia	Nifedipine
Quinidex	Quinidine sulfate
Sinemet	Levodopa and carbidopa
Synthroid	L-thyroxine (Levothyroxine)
Tagamet	Cimetidine
Timoptic	Timolol
Tenormin	Atenolol
Theo-Dur	Theophylline
Trental	Pentoxifylline
Valium	Diazepam
Vasotec	Enalapril
Ventolin	Albuterol
Voltaren	Diclofenac
Xanax	Alprazolam
Zantac	Ranitidine
Zyloprim	Allopurinol

A GUIDE TO OVER-THE-COUNTER MEDICINES

You can go into any pharmacy, buy a bottle off the shelf, and take it home with you. You do not need a doctor's prescription for it, so it must be safe. Right? Not necessarily. Although nearly everybody uses over-the-counter (OTC) medicines, often with good results, these drugs *can* cause adverse reactions. They may aggravate an already existing condition or, even worse, mask the symptoms of an underlying disease and delay proper treatment.

There are many good reasons to select OTC medicines. If your medical condition is simple enough for self-diagnosis (for example, a headache), treating it with an OTC product saves time and money. In addition, OTC medicine contains a lower amount of drug than prescription counterparts (for example, ibuprofen, corticosteroids, and antihistamines) and is therefore generally safer.

Before You Buy

To obtain the most benefit with the least risk, approach these products with caution. The elderly and anyone with a serious, long-term disorder (such as impaired liver or kidney function) should consult a doctor or pharmacist before taking a nonprescription drug. Your doctor should know about all the medicines you take, even those that may seem as harmless to you as vitamins.

Before you even buy the medicine, read the label carefully. This will tell you what symptoms the drug treats, who should *not* use the drug, the dosage, the ingredients, and possible side effects. If you decide to purchase the drug, follow the directions on the label. If you do not understand them, ask a health professional for clarification.

For the most part, OTC medicines do not cure disease but are designed to relieve its symptoms. If symptoms persist after a reasonable period of time, consult a doctor. The symptoms may not be trivial but, rather, signs of a serious condition that requires medical care.

Keep in mind, always, that nonprescription drugs are real medicines. The possibilities of overdose, serious side effects, and the interaction of one medicine with another exist. Check with your doctor or pharmacist before using an OTC product if you are on other medicines or if another nonprescription product fails to relieve your symptoms.

Drugs to Have Handy

To cut down on your trips to the pharmacy for OTC items and to be prepared for emergency situations, there are certain products you should have on hand. You should check with your doctor first to make sure these are all appropriate for you and to learn whether you should add other medicines based on your particular medical needs.

For headaches and other types of pain, you should have an *analgesic* (a pain reliever) handy, such as aspirin. If someone in your family has a "sensitive" stomach or is allergic to aspirin, a nonaspirin product like acetaminophen may be substituted. Acetaminophen would be the best choice for individuals with impaired kidney function or for persons who suffer from stomach distress with the other medicines. Be aware, also, that you should not give aspirin to children without first consulting a health professional. When given to a child with influenza or chickenpox, aspirin may induce Reye's syndrome.

For occasional heartburn or symptoms of indigestion, an *antacid* should be part of your medical supplies. If you are on a salt-restricted diet, certain antacids may be off-limits because of their high salt content; some of the newer antacids contain relatively little salt. Antacids containing aluminum hydroxide and/or calcium carbonate are not good choices for people who tend to be constipated because such drugs can aggravate this problem. An antacid containing magnesium hydroxide would be a better selection. But if you tend to suffer from diarrhea, the aluminum or calcium varieties may be more appropriate for you. Because antacids can alter bodily functions, your doctor, pharmacist, or other health professional should help to decide what type you should purchase.

Itchiness can be annoying—and an *antipruritic* can be a welcome relief if you experience prickly heat, poison ivy, or mosquito bites. Ordinary calamine lotion is generally all you will need for this. (For serious cases, low-dose corticosteroid creams and ointments are available over the counter.)

An *antiseptic* is an important item to have in your medicine supply to cleanse minor wounds. The only one that's generally necessary is rubbing alcohol, or isopropyl (70 percent) alcohol. It should be applied after the wound is washed with soap and water.

Nasal congestion is another condition you should be prepared to cope with. As a *decongestant*, keep a nasal spray or nose drops to alleviate the stuffiness that commonly accompanies a cold. However, if you have high blood pressure or an overactive thyroid gland, you may not be a candidate for these medicines. Consult your doctor or pharmacist before making your purchase.

The best way to avoid constipation is to eat a diet that is high in fiber and to drink plenty of fluids. Too many people turn to *laxatives* to deal with constipation and become laxative abusers. After many years, such abuse can actually lead to constipation by causing the bowel to lose its ability to contract and propel its contents normally. However, if you do wish to have a laxative on hand, the safest choice for frequent use is a bulk laxative, such as Metamucil or Effersyllium. (People with diabetes need to be aware that some forms of Metamucil have a high sugar content.) These products are made up of vegetable fiber and act in much the same way as fiber in the diet. If you suffer only an occasional bout of constipation, milk of magnesia is reasonable to keep on hand.

For problems with loose, frequent bowel movements, you should have an *antidiarrheal remedy* available to use when needed. Follow your doctor's advice in choosing an appropriate OTC medicine. If the condition persists, ask your doctor whether you should try a more potent medicine—and whether you should be examined.

If you suffer from hemorrhoids, you should know that nonprescription *hemorrhoidal medicines* can often be effective.

Antifungal agents are used for such conditions as jock itch and athlete's foot and should be kept on hand if you are susceptible to these. Some of these drugs were originally prescription medicines and are now available over the counter.

There are certain OTC products you should avoid. These include mercury antiseptics, such as Mercurochrome, and OTC burn ointments, which cause allergic skin reactions in some people. (Instead, use ice water or cold running water to treat minor burns.)

Appropriately stocked with the right medicines (along with such first-aid equipment as bandages and gauze pads), your medicine cabinet can give you the peace of mind that you're ready to act quickly and effectively in dealing with common medical problems and emergency situations.

TRAVELING HEALTHY

You may look forward to your trips, near or far, as a great way to lift your spirits and improve your general mental health—but don't forget to take your physical health into account as well. Discuss your itinerary with your doctor, and ask about any potential health hazards it might entail. In addition, ask for a brief summary of your significant medical history, as well as a photocopy of your most recent electrocardiogram (whether or not you have heart disease).

This is also a good time to review and update prescriptions. Ask your doctor for the generic—or chemical—names of your medicines; this will help you identify them for foreign doctors in case you need medical care abroad. Be sure to take a list of all the medicines you are currently using.

Immunizations

You should also review your past immunizations with your doctor and find out which ones you will need before your trip. You may be surprised to learn you will need any. After all, aren't "shots" for kids? Not exclusively, since many adults lose the immunity they acquired during childhood and adolescence.

If you're traveling, some health professionals advise that you be immunized against the flu, tetanus, and diphtheria. You should also be immunized against pneumococcal pneumonia if you have chronic heart and lung disease or diabetes or are undergoing cancer chemotherapy. Travelers to many parts of Asia, Africa, and South America are advised to have immunizations for yellow fever, cholera, and typhoid. In many cases, injections of gamma globulin are recommended to lower the risk of hepatitis A. Your doctor may suggest that you be vaccinated against poliomyelitis, an illness still prevalent in many areas of the world. In some older people, polio can assume a severe and often fatal form.

As yet, there is no vaccine against malaria. But the disease can usually be prevented by taking one of the chloroquine antimalarial drugs weekly starting at least two weeks before entering a malarial area and continuing for eight weeks after leaving the area. If you're traveling to eastern or central Africa, the Amazon basin, or rural areas of Southeast Asia, you may need to take a second drug, Fansidar, to combat more resistant malarial parasites.

For advice on how to avoid the scourge of adventurous tourists, traveler's diarrhea, see chapter 3 (pages 412–414).

Taking It with You

Once you're well immunized and ready to pack for your trip, make sure to leave room for a "little black bag" of medicines and supplies. You may never need these but you'll feel better having them along. This personal medical kit (which you should keep with you on the plane) should contain the following items:
• An adequate supply of all your prescription medicines (in clearly labeled, plastic bottles)
• An extra pair of eyeglasses if you use them
• A copy of your current eyeglass or contact lens prescription if you use either
• Antacids
• Analgesics (aspirin, acetaminophen, or ibuprofen)
• Motion-sickness medicine (if desired)
• Nasal decongestant
• Antihistamine
• Antidiarrheal medicine
• Calamine lotion
• Insect repellent
• Sunscreen and sunglasses
• Thermometer in a well-protected case
• Bandages and adhesive tape

If you've ever experienced serious allergies or side effects from any medicines, take along a list of those products; if those reactions are potentially life threatening, you may need to wear an identification bracelet or necklace. A traveler who has a severe illness—such as heart disease, asthma, or a bleeding disorder—should have on hand a doctor's note outlining the condition and the medicines being used to treat it.

Finding a Doctor Abroad

No matter how well equipped you are, your supplies cannot meet every possible medical emergency. You may find yourself, far from home, needing medical assistance. Again, advance planning is the key. Two organizations can provide you with listings of qualified English-speaking doctors in different parts of the world. The International Association for Medical Assistance to Travelers (IAMAT, 736 Center St., Lewiston, NY 14902; 716-754-4883) has a list covering 120 countries. There is no charge, but the organization relies on donations. You should write for the information at least eight weeks before your departure date. Intermedic (777 Third Ave., New York, NY 10017; 212-486-8900) publishes a list of competent foreign doctors whose services are available to travelers for established fees. The list is for members only; annual membership is six dollars for an individual, ten dollars for a family. In addition, if you are an American Express card holder, the company provides a service called Global Assist that allows you to phone in from wherever you may be traveling to get a medical referral.

If this strategy does not work and you need a doctor fast, call the American Consulate or American Embassy; they are prepared to respond to American tourists in emergency situations. Your next plan of action (if that one fails) would be to locate the nearest university hospital or, if your medical condition warrants it, to take a plane to a larger city. You may be a long day's journey, or more, from home, but you are unlikely to be more than a few hours away from a well-equipped medical center that can meet your health needs.

You may need to adjust dosage schedules of medicines if you will be crossing a number of time zones. For people with diabetes on insulin injections, check sugar levels and use meal time rather than clock time to determine when to take your doses. For other medicine, check with your doctor about breaking up your doses into smaller ones to take them at slightly more frequent intervals.

Those persons unaccustomed to the rigors of travel should be especially careful to follow general health precautions—eat well, do not try to do too much, and avoid extremes of either heat or cold.

Chapter 1
Disorders of the Heart and Blood Vessels

HYPERTENSION

Hypertension, or high blood pressure, is one of the most common—and insidious—medical conditions in the Western world. Hypertension becomes more frequent with age, affecting as many as 30 percent to 50 percent of people in their fifties, sixties, and seventies. But this increase in blood pressure with age is not inevitable. In many nonindustrialized societies, blood pressure does not rise with age.

Although hypertension has no symptoms, it takes a high toll in illness and death. An elevation in blood pressure is the single most important risk factor for developing serious cardiovascular disease, including stroke and heart attack, and is a leading cause of heart and kidney failure.

But the good news is that hypertension is controllable. Over the past fifteen years, deaths from stroke have decreased by 45 percent, and heart attack deaths have declined by 31 percent. This encouraging trend has been attributed mostly to better diagnosis and treatment of hypertension.

CAUSES

Hypertension refers to an increase in the force required to pump the blood through the arteries. This increase in blood pressure may stem from either a greater volume of blood or a narrowing of the arteries. Only about one in ten cases of hypertension has a clear-cut cause—usually a disorder of the kidneys or of the adrenal glands, which sit atop the kidneys. These cases of so-called secondary hypertension are often amenable to surgical correction, after which the blood pressure returns to normal.

In the majority of people with hypertension, however, no cause can be found. These people have what is known as essential, or primary, hypertension. (The word *essential* is an interesting relic of the last century, when doctors mistakenly believed that an increase in blood pressure was essential to keep blood flowing to the vital organs.) Some scientists believe that essential hypertension is caused by a defect in the body's ability to eliminate salt normally. Other explanations focus on potent hormones that raise blood pressure and on the nervous system.

Some people have the erroneous notion that hypertension is linked with emotional tension. Blood pressure does fluctuate throughout the day and can certainly rise temporarily when a person is upset. However, stress and tension do not cause high blood pressure, and a calm, peaceful existence will not cure it.

DIAGNOSIS

Because hypertension does not announce its presence with symptoms, doctors have to search for it. Hypertension is detected by measuring blood pressure with the familiar device called a sphygmomanometer, which consists of an inflatable cuff and a pressure gauge. When the blood pressure cuff is fully inflated, blood flow in the arm stops. As pressure in the cuff is gradually decreased, a health professional uses a stethoscope to listen to the sound of the blood flowing through an artery below the cuff. Several sounds are heard in sequence. The first whooshing sound represents the force of blood flow when the heart contracts, and the pressure at which this sound is heard is called the systolic blood pressure. A later, muffled sound signals blood flow between heartbeats, which marks the diastolic pressure.

Blood pressure is expressed as two numbers. If your doctor tells you that your blood pressure is, for example, 140 over 85, he or she means that your systolic blood pressure is 140 and your diastolic pressure is 85 (written as 140/85). The numbers represent millimeters of mercury, abbreviated *mm Hg*. Normal blood pressure in an adult is a diastolic pressure no higher than 90 mm Hg. This means that the odds of developing hypertension-related health problems are greater in people whose blood pressure rises above this number. It also means that treatment that reduces diastolic pressure to 90 mm Hg or less will decrease the likelihood of complications from hypertension.

After age sixty, it is not uncommon for the systolic pressure to rise without an increase in the diastolic pressure. This state is called isolated systolic hypertension. Recent studies have suggested that small doses of a diuretic may be a feasible, effective, and well-tolerated treatment for older persons who have isolated systolic hypertension. In addition, a recent study of persons aged 60 years and older with systolic hypertension showed that antihypertensive therapy reduced the risk of stroke and heart attacks.

One elevated measurement is not enough to confirm a diagnosis of hypertension. Many doctors will not treat hypertension unless readings are elevated on three separate occasions. This is because blood pressure can change with the person's situation and the time of day. In persons over age fifty, blood pressure must be measured in both a standing and a sitting position.

TREATMENT

A wide variety of medicines are effective in lowering blood pressure and reducing the complications of hypertension. In several large clinical studies, reducing high blood pressure with drugs significantly lowered the chances of illness or death from stroke or heart attack. The benefit was greatest in people over the age of sixty.

These antihypertensive drugs act by many mechanisms, so a person whose blood pressure does not respond fully to one drug may have better luck with another. Even the best drugs, however, do not cure hypertension. You most likely will have to take your medicine for life.

People who experience troublesome side effects with one drug will often have fewer or no problems when switched to another. So be sure to be honest with your doctor if the medicine he or she prescribes seems to cause problems such as fatigue, dizziness, confusion, depression, bad dreams, or loss of sexual interest.

The drug charts on pages 23–158 explain how the various blood pressure–lowering medicines work and what to expect from them.

The most important step you can take to control your hypertension is to take your medicine as your doctor prescribes. But there are other ways you can help yourself.

Your doctor will probably prescribe a moderate low-salt diet in addition to your medicine. If you are overweight, your doctor may suggest that you lose those extra pounds. For some people with hypertension, salt restriction and weight loss may bring blood pressure under control. For most people, dietary changes can at least play an important supporting role in the treatment of hypertension and may even lower your medication dose.

You can also improve your overall cardiovascular health by stopping smoking. Many doctors recommend regular exercise, such as brisk walking, to supplement drug therapy. Psychological methods for lowering blood pressure, such as relaxation and biofeedback, may have a modest effect on blood pressure but have not been shown to be strong enough to be used without drug treatment.

OUTLOOK

The dramatic reductions in stroke and heart disease that have occurred in the U.S. population as a whole have largely been brought about by better detection of high blood pressure and better treatments. You, too, can lower your risk of cardiovascular disease by having your blood pressure checked regularly. If your doctor diagnoses hypertension, you can greatly reduce the potential consequences by following the prescribed treatment. If you stick to your drug and diet treatment and your blood pressure returns to normal, your chances are better for a normal and active life.

CONDITION: **HYPERTENSION**
CATEGORY: **DIURETICS (THIAZIDES AND RELATED DRUGS)**

GENERIC (CHEMICAL) NAME	BRAND (TRADE) NAME	DOSAGE FORMS AND STRENGTHS
Chlorothiazide	DIURIL	Suspension: 250 mg per tsp Tablets: 250, 500 mg
Chlorthalidone	HYGROTON THALITONE	Tablets: 25, 50, 100 mg Tablets: 15, 25 mg
Hydrochlorothiazide	ESIDRIX HydroDIURIL ORETIC	Tablets: 25, 50, 100 mg Tablets: 25, 50, 100 mg Tablets: 25, 50 mg
Hydroflumethiazide	DIUCARDIN	Tablets: 50 mg
Methyclothiazide	AQUATENSEN ENDURON	Tablets: 5 mg Tablets: 2.5, 5 mg
Metolazone	DIULO MYKROX ZAROXOLYN	Tablets: 2.5, 5, 10 mg Tablets: 0.5 mg Tablets: 2.5, 5, 10 mg
Polythiazide	RENESE	Tablets: 1, 2, 4 mg
Trichlormethiazide	METAHYDRIN NAQUA	Tablets: 2, 4 mg Tablets: 2, 4 mg

DRUG PROFILE

Thiazide and thiazide-type diuretics are often used to help control high blood pressure. They work by increasing the amount of salt and water eliminated by the body (through urination) and by relaxing the walls of the smaller arteries so that they expand. With a smaller volume of blood (because water is eliminated) in a larger amount of space (because the artery walls are expanded), blood pressure decreases. These drugs may also be prescribed for swelling in certain parts of the body (the ankles, for example) because they help the body eliminate excess water. Thiazide diuretics are also used in the treatment of calcium stones because they decrease the amount of calcium eliminated through urination.

BEFORE USING THIS DRUG

Let your doctor know *IF*

You have ever had allergic reactions or other problems with ■ any of the thiazide or thiazide-type diuretics ■ sulfonamides (sulfa drugs).

You have ever had any of the following medical problems: ■ diabetes ■ gout ■ kidney disease ■ liver disease ■ systemic lupus erythematosus ■ disease of the pancreas ■ allergies ■ asthma.

You are taking any of the following medicines: ■ other diuretics or other medicines for high blood pressure ■ corticosteroids or corticotropin (ACTH) ■ medicine for high cholesterol ■ medicine for diabetes ■ digoxin or digitalis (heart medicines) ■ medicine for gout ■ lithium ■ methenamine (medicine to prevent urinary tract infections) ■ anticoagulants (blood thinners) ■ tetracycline ■ nonsteroidal anti-inflammatory drugs (medicine for arthritis) ■ alcohol ■ barbiturates ■ narcotics.

SPECIAL RESTRICTIONS WHILE TAKING THIS DRUG

FOOD AND DRUG INTERACTIONS

Other Drugs	Do not take any other drugs, including over-the-counter (OTC) drugs, before checking with your doctor. OTC drugs for appetite suppression, asthma, colds, cough, hay fever, or sinus problems tend to increase blood pressure.

If you are also taking cholestyramine or colestipol (medicine for high cholesterol), take your thiazide drug at least one hour before taking these medicines.

Foods and Beverages	Your doctor may prescribe a special low-salt diet, which you should follow carefully because it will help your medicine work more effectively. You may also be advised to go on a weight-reduction diet. Thiazides and related drugs may cause your body to lose large amounts of the mineral potassium. Your doctor may give you special instructions about eating or drinking foods that have a high potassium content (such as bananas and citrus fruit juices), taking a potassium supplement, or using salt substitutes. It is important that you follow your doctor's instructions exactly.

No special restrictions on alcohol use.

DAILY LIVING

Exertion and Exercise	Use caution when exercising or exerting yourself while taking this medicine because excessive sweating may cause you to become dehydrated and to feel dizzy, light-headed, or faint.
Sun Exposure/ Excessive Heat	Your skin may become more sensitive to sunlight and more likely to develop a sunburn while you are taking this medicine. It is a good idea to avoid too much sun, especially if you burn easily. Apply a sunscreen to exposed skin surfaces before going outdoors. Use caution during hot weather or when taking saunas or hot baths, since excessive sweating while taking this medicine may cause you to become dehydrated and to feel drowsy or faint.

Examinations or Tests

Many people have high blood pressure with no symptoms at all. It is important for you to keep all appointments with your doctor, even if you feel well, so that your blood pressure can be checked regularly. Blood tests at several weeks, and then again at several months, after starting therapy with this drug will probably be required.

Other Precautions

If you have diabetes, be aware that this medicine may raise blood-sugar levels. If you notice any change when testing sugar levels in your blood or urine, let your doctor know.

When first starting on this type of medicine, you may feel tired and will probably experience both greater volume and frequency of urination. Until your individual pattern of urination has been established with this medicine, it may be wise to time carefully any activity that will put you out of convenient reach of a bathroom, such as bus or car travel. In addition, taking a diuretic at bedtime will probably interfere with sleep; you should discuss your dosage schedule with your doctor.

Check with your doctor if you become ill with flulike symptoms, such as cough, fever, or body aches; lose your appetite; vomit; or have diarrhea. This may cause you to lose a great deal of fluid, making it important not to take the diuretic for one or more doses.

Following mild fluid losses, some older people are more vulnerable to symptoms of weakness or dizziness upon standing or getting up.

No special restrictions on driving or exposure to excessive cold.

POSSIBLE SIDE EFFECTS

Although this list of adverse effects may seem somewhat intimidating, keep in mind that some are quite rare. Of course, should these or any other problems arise while you are on medication, it is always a good idea to consult your doctor.

IF YOU DEVELOP	WHAT TO DO
increased skin sensitivity to sunlight (if severe) ■ dry mouth ■ increased thirst ■ dizziness or weakness upon standing or getting up ■ nausea or vomiting ■ severe stomach pain or cramps ■ joint or side pain ■ irregular heartbeat ■ weak pulse ■ difficulty in breathing ■ decreased urination ■ mood changes ■ confusion ■ muscle cramps or pain ■ tiredness or weakness	**Urgent** Get in touch with your doctor immediately.
rash or hives ■ sore throat or fever ■ bleeding or bruising ■ yellowing of eyes or skin	**May be serious** Check with your doctor as soon as possible.
diarrhea ■ loss of appetite ■ upset stomach ■ male impotence ■ clumsiness	If symptoms are disturbing or persist, let your doctor know.

STORAGE INSTRUCTIONS

Store in a cool, dark place (not in a bathroom medicine cabinet). If your medicine is in a liquid form, make sure that it does not freeze.

STOPPING OR INTERRUPTING THERAPY

Since this drug does not cure high blood pressure but only controls it, you may have to take this medicine for the rest of your life. Do not stop taking it, even if you feel better. If you miss a dose, take it as soon as possible. If it is almost time for your next dose, skip the missed dose and resume your regular schedule. Do not take two doses at the same time.

SPECIAL CONSIDERATIONS FOR THOSE OVER SIXTY-FIVE

Older people are more likely to develop such side effects as confusion, weakness, clumsiness, dizziness when getting up from a reclining or sitting position, potassium deficiency, and dehydration. Thus, it is especially important to keep all doctor's appointments as well as appointments for laboratory tests. People over sixty-five should check with a doctor if they become ill with flulike symptoms, such as cough, fever, or body aches; lose their appetite; vomit; or have diarrhea because they may then be more vulnerable to fluid losses.

CONDITION: **HYPERTENSION**

CATEGORY: **DIURETICS (POTASSIUM-SPARING)**

GENERIC (CHEMICAL) NAME	BRAND (TRADE) NAME	DOSAGE FORMS AND STRENGTHS
Triamterene	DYRENIUM	Capsules: 50, 100 mg

DRUG PROFILE

Triamterene is a potassium-sparing diuretic that is used to treat edema (swelling due to excess fluid in the body). It is usually used along with other drugs to treat high blood pressure. Triamterene increases the amount of salt and water eliminated by the body; with the resulting smaller volume of blood, blood pressure usually decreases. Potassium-sparing diuretics maintain the body's level of potassium while they work.

BEFORE USING THIS DRUG

Let your doctor know *IF*

You have ever had allergic reactions or other problems with ■ triamterene.

You have ever had any of the following medical problems: ■ diabetes ■ gout ■ heart disease ■ kidney disease, including kidney stones ■ liver disease ■ disease of the pancreas ■ alcoholism.

You are taking any of the following medicines: ■ other diuretics or medicines for high blood pressure, especially amiloride, spironolactone, or ACE inhibitors (eg, captopril, enalapril, lisinopril) ■ medicine for diabetes ■ medicine for gout ■ laxatives ■ lithium ■ potassium-containing medicines or supplements ■ aspirin, indomethacin, or other arthritis medicines (nonsteroidal anti-inflammatory drugs).

SPECIAL RESTRICTIONS WHILE TAKING THIS DRUG

FOOD AND DRUG INTERACTIONS

Other Drugs	Do not take any other drugs, including over-the-counter (OTC) drugs, before checking with your doctor. OTC drugs for appetite suppression, asthma, colds, cough, hay fever, or sinus problems tend to increase blood pressure. Also check with your doctor before using any nonsteroidal anti-inflammatory drug (such as aspirin, indomethacin, or other arthritis medicines), since these drugs combined with triamterene may affect kidney function.
Foods and Beverages	Your doctor may prescribe a special low-salt diet, which you should follow carefully because it will help your medicine work more effectively. You may also be advised to go on a weight-reduction diet. Since this medicine does not cause a loss of potassium from your body, it is not necessary to have extra potassium in your diet or take a potassium supplement; too much potassium can be harmful. Let your doctor know if you use salt substitutes; many of these products are high in potassium.

No special restrictions on alcohol use.

DAILY LIVING

Exertion and Exercise	Use caution when exercising or exerting yourself while taking this medicine because excessive sweating may cause you to become dehydrated and to feel dizzy, light-headed, or faint.
Sun Exposure/ Excessive Heat	Your skin may become more sensitive to sunlight and more likely to develop a sunburn while you are taking this medicine. It is a good idea to avoid too much sun, especially if you burn easily. Apply a sunscreen to exposed skin surfaces before going outdoors. Use caution during hot weather or while taking saunas or hot baths, since excessive sweating while taking this medicine may cause you to become dehydrated and to feel drowsy or faint.
Examinations or Tests	Many people have high blood pressure with no symptoms at all. It is important for you to keep all appointments with your doctor, even if you feel well, so that your blood pressure can be checked regularly. Periodic blood tests may be required.
Other Precautions	If you have diabetes, be aware that this medicine may raise blood-sugar levels. If you notice any change when testing sugar levels in your blood or urine, let your doctor know.
	When first starting on this type of medicine, you may feel tired and will probably experience both greater volume and frequency of urination. Until your individual pattern of urination has been established with this medicine, it may be wise to time carefully any activity that will put you out of convenient reach of a bathroom, such as bus or car travel. In addition, taking a diuretic at bedtime will probably interfere with sleep; you should discuss your dosage schedule with your doctor.

Check with your doctor if you become ill with flulike symptoms, such as cough, fever, or body aches; lose your appetite; vomit; or have diarrhea. This may cause you to lose a great deal of fluid, making it important not to take the diuretic for one or more doses.

Following mild fluid losses, some older people are more vulnerable to symptoms of weakness or dizziness upon standing or getting up.

| Helpful Hints | If this medicine upsets your stomach, taking it with milk, meals, or snacks should help. |

No special restrictions on driving or exposure to excessive cold.

POSSIBLE SIDE EFFECTS

Although this list of adverse effects may seem somewhat intimidating, keep in mind that some are quite rare. Of course, should these or any other problems arise while you are on medication, it is always a good idea to consult your doctor.

IF YOU DEVELOP	WHAT TO DO
irregular heartbeat ■ numbness or tingling in hands, feet, or lips ■ tiredness or weakness ■ confusion ■ difficulty in breathing ■ severe or continuing diarrhea ■ severe side pain ■ dry mouth ■ increased thirst ■ dizziness or weakness upon standing or getting up	**Urgent** Get in touch with your doctor immediately.
nervousness ■ heaviness of legs ■ tongue inflammation ■ cracked corners of mouth ■ rash or itching ■ sore throat or fever ■ bleeding or bruising ■ headache	**May be serious** Check with your doctor as soon as possible.

upset stomach ■ drowsiness ■ lack of energy ■ increased skin sensitivity to sunlight	If symptoms are disturbing or persist, let your doctor know.

STORAGE INSTRUCTIONS

Store in a cool, dark place (not in a bathroom medicine cabinet).

STOPPING OR INTERRUPTING THERAPY

Since this drug does not cure high blood pressure but only controls it, you may have to take this medicine for the rest of your life. Do not stop taking it, even if you feel better. If you miss a dose, take it as soon as possible. If it is almost time for your next dose, skip the missed dose and resume your regular schedule. Do not take two doses at the same time.

SPECIAL CONSIDERATIONS FOR THOSE OVER SIXTY-FIVE

Older people are more likely to develop problems caused by too much potassium in the body, such as irregular heartbeat, confusion, difficulty in breathing, and tiredness or weakness. Doctors may require regular checkups. People over sixty-five should check with a doctor if they become ill with flulike symptoms, such as cough, fever, or body aches; lose their appetite; vomit; or have diarrhea because they may then be more vulnerable to fluid losses.

CONDITION: **HYPERTENSION**

CATEGORY: **DIURETICS (POTASSIUM-SPARING)**

GENERIC (CHEMICAL) NAME	BRAND (TRADE) NAME	DOSAGE FORMS AND STRENGTHS
Spironolactone	ALDACTONE	Tablets: 25, 50, 100 mg

DRUG PROFILE

Spironolactone is a potassium-sparing diuretic that is used to treat high blood pressure, edema (swelling due to excess fluid in the body), conditions in which there is not enough potassium in the body, and certain hormonal disturbances. This drug increases the amount of salt and water eliminated by the body (through urination); with a smaller volume of blood (because water is eliminated), blood pressure usually decreases. Potassium-sparing diuretics maintain the body's level of potassium while they work.

BEFORE USING THIS DRUG

Let your doctor know *IF*

You have ever had allergic reactions or other problems with ■ spironolactone.

You have ever had any of the following medical problems: ■ diabetes ■ heart disease ■ kidney disease ■ liver disease.

You are taking any of the following medicines: ■ other diuretics or medicines for high blood pressure, especially amiloride or ACE inhibitors (eg, captopril, enalapril, lisinopril) ■ lithium ■ potassium-containing medicines or supplements ■ digoxin or digitalis (heart medicines) ■ medicine for diabetes ■ medicine containing alcohol ■ aspirin, indomethacin, or other arthritis medicines (nonsteroidal anti-inflammatory drugs).

SPECIAL RESTRICTIONS WHILE TAKING THIS DRUG

FOOD AND DRUG INTERACTIONS

Other Drugs	Do not take any other drugs, including over-the-counter (OTC) drugs, before checking with your doctor. OTC drugs for appetite suppression, asthma, colds, cough, hay fever, or sinus problems tend to increase blood pressure.
Foods and Beverages	Your doctor may prescribe a special low-salt diet, which you should follow carefully because it will help your medicine work more effectively. You may also be advised to go on a weight-reduction diet. Since

this medicine does not cause a loss of potassium from your body, it is not necessary to have extra potassium in your diet or take a potassium supplement; too much potassium can be harmful. Let your doctor know if you use salt substitutes; many of these products are high in potassium.

No special restrictions on alcohol use.

DAILY LIVING

Exertion and Exercise

Use caution when exercising or exerting yourself while taking this medicine because excessive sweating may cause you to become dehydrated and to feel dizzy, light-headed, or faint.

Sun Exposure/ Excessive Heat

Your skin may become more sensitive to sunlight and more likely to develop a sunburn while you are taking this medicine. It is a good idea to avoid too much sun, especially if you burn easily. Apply a sunscreen to exposed skin surfaces before going outdoors. Use caution during hot weather or while taking saunas or hot baths, since excessive sweating while taking this medicine may cause you to become dehydrated and to feel drowsy or faint.

Examinations or Tests

Many people have high blood pressure with no symptoms at all. It is important for you to keep all appointments with your doctor, even if you feel well, so that your blood pressure can be checked regularly.

Other Precautions

Tell any doctor or dentist you consult that you are taking this medicine, especially if you will be undergoing any type of surgery.

When first starting on this type of medicine, you may feel tired and will probably experience both greater volume and frequency of urination. Until your individual pattern of urination has been established with this medicine, it may be wise to time carefully any activity that will put you out of convenient reach of a bathroom, such as bus or car travel. In addition, taking a diuretic at bedtime will probably interfere with sleep; you should discuss your dosage schedule with your doctor.

Check with your doctor if you become ill with flulike symptoms, such as cough, fever, or body aches; lose your appetite; vomit; or have diarrhea. This may cause you to lose a great deal of fluid, making it important not to take the diuretic for one or more doses.

Following mild fluid losses, some older people are more vulnerable to symptoms of weakness or dizziness upon standing or getting up.

Helpful Hints

If this medicine upsets your stomach, taking it with milk, meals, or snacks should help.

No special restrictions on driving or exposure to excessive cold.

POSSIBLE SIDE EFFECTS

Although this list of adverse effects may seem somewhat intimidating, keep in mind that some are quite rare. Of course, should these or any other problems arise while you are on medication, it is always a good idea to consult your doctor.

IF YOU DEVELOP

irregular heartbeat ■ numbness or tingling in hands, feet, or lips ■ tiredness or weakness ■ confusion ■ difficulty in breathing ■ severe or continuing vomiting or diarrhea ■ dry mouth ■ increased thirst ■ dizziness or weakness upon standing or getting up

WHAT TO DO

Urgent Get in touch with your doctor immediately.

---

nervousness ■ heaviness of legs ■ fever ■ rash or itching ■ swelling of hands or feet	**May be serious** Check with your doctor as soon as possible.
upset stomach ■ female breast tenderness ■ male breast enlargement ■ male impotence ■ deepening voice ■ hair growth ■ clumsiness ■ headache	If symptoms are disturbing or persist, let your doctor know.

STORAGE INSTRUCTIONS

Store in a cool, dark place (not in a bathroom medicine cabinet).

STOPPING OR INTERRUPTING THERAPY

Since this drug does not cure high blood pressure but only controls it, you may have to take this medicine for the rest of your life. Do not stop taking it, even if you feel better. If you miss a dose, take it as soon as possible. If it is almost time for your next dose, skip the missed dose and resume your regular schedule. Do not take two doses at the same time.

SPECIAL CONSIDERATIONS FOR THOSE OVER SIXTY-FIVE

Older people are more likely to develop problems caused by too much potassium in the body, such as irregular heartbeat, confusion, difficulty in breathing, and tiredness or weakness. Doctors may require regular checkups. People over sixty-five should check with a doctor if they become ill with flulike symptoms, such as cough, fever, or body aches; lose their appetite; vomit; or have diarrhea because they may then be more vulnerable to fluid losses.

CONDITION: **HYPERTENSION**

CATEGORY: **DIURETICS (POTASSIUM-SPARING)**

GENERIC (CHEMICAL) NAME	BRAND (TRADE) NAME	DOSAGE FORMS AND STRENGTHS
Amiloride	MIDAMOR	Tablets: 5 mg

DRUG PROFILE

Amiloride is a potassium-sparing diuretic that is used with other drugs to treat high blood pressure or congestive heart failure. This drug decreases blood pressure by increasing the amount of salt and water eliminated by the body (through urination). Potassium-sparing diuretics maintain the body's level of potassium while they work.

BEFORE USING THIS DRUG

Let your doctor know *IF*

You have ever had allergic reactions or other problems with ■ amiloride.

You have ever had any of the following medical problems: ■ diabetes ■ heart disease ■ kidney disease ■ liver disease.

You are taking any of the following medicines: ■ other diuretics or medicines for high blood pressure, triamterene, spironolactone or ACE inhibitors (eg, captopril, enalapril, lisinopril) ■ lithium ■ potassium-containing medicines or supplements ■ salt substitutes ■ aspirin, indomethacin, or other arthritis medicines (nonsteroidal anti-inflammatory drugs).

SPECIAL RESTRICTIONS WHILE TAKING THIS DRUG

FOOD AND DRUG INTERACTIONS

Other Drugs	Do not take any other drugs, including over-the-counter (OTC) drugs, before checking with your doctor. OTC drugs for appetite suppression, asthma,

colds, cough, hay fever, or sinus problems tend to increase blood pressure.

Foods and Beverages	Your doctor may prescribe a special low-salt diet, which you should follow carefully because it will help your medicine work more effectively. You may also be advised to go on a weight-reduction diet. Since this medicine does not cause a loss of potassium from your body, it is not necessary to have extra potassium in your diet or take a potassium supplement; too much potassium can be harmful. Let your doctor know if you use salt substitutes; many of these products are high in potassium.

No special restrictions on alcohol use or smoking.

DAILY LIVING

Exertion and Exercise	Use caution when exercising or exerting yourself while taking this medicine because excessive sweating may cause you to become dehydrated and to feel dizzy, light-headed, or faint.
Excessive Heat	Use caution during hot weather or while taking saunas or hot baths, since excessive sweating while taking this medicine may cause you to become dehydrated and to feel drowsy or faint.
Examinations or Tests	Many people have high blood pressure with no symptoms at all. It is important for you to keep all appointments with your doctor, even if you feel well, so that your blood pressure can be checked regularly. Periodic blood tests are usually required.
Other Precautions	When first starting on this type of medicine, you may feel tired and will probably experience both greater volume and frequency of urination. Until your individual pattern of urination has been established with this medicine, it may be wise to time carefully any activity

that will put you out of convenient reach of a bathroom, such as bus or car travel. In addition, taking a diuretic at bedtime will probably interfere with sleep; you should discuss your dosage schedule with your doctor.

Check with your doctor if you become ill with flulike symptoms, such as cough, fever, or body aches; lose your appetite; vomit; or have diarrhea. This may cause you to lose a great deal of fluid, making it important not to take the diuretic for one or more doses.

Following mild fluid losses, some older people are more vulnerable to symptoms of weakness or dizziness upon standing or getting up.

No special restrictions on driving, sun exposure, or exposure to excessive cold.

POSSIBLE SIDE EFFECTS

Although this list of adverse effects may seem somewhat intimidating, keep in mind that some are quite rare. Of course, should these or any other problems arise while you are on medication, it is always a good idea to consult your doctor.

IF YOU DEVELOP

chest pain ■ irregular heartbeat ■ numbness or tingling in hands, feet, or lips ■ tiredness or weakness ■ confusion ■ difficulty in breathing ■ severe or continuing nausea, vomiting, or diarrhea ■ dry mouth ■ increased thirst ■ dizziness or weakness upon standing or getting up

WHAT TO DO

Urgent Get in touch with your doctor immediately.

---

heaviness of legs

May be serious Check with your doctor as soon as possible.

diarrhea ■ nausea or vomiting ■ loss of appetite ■ constipation ■ stomach pain or feeling of fullness ■ heartburn or indigestion ■ shortness of breath ■ cough ■ male impotence ■ diminished sex drive ■ muscle cramps or pain ■ tremors ■ headache ■ sleeplessness ■ drowsiness ■ depression ■ rash or itching ■ hair loss ■ taste changes ■ urinary frequency or other urinary problems

If symptoms are disturbing or persist, let your doctor know.

STORAGE INSTRUCTIONS

Store in a cool, dark place (not in a bathroom medicine cabinet).

STOPPING OR INTERRUPTING THERAPY

Since this drug does not cure high blood pressure but only controls it, you may have to take this medicine for the rest of your life. Do not stop taking it even if you feel better. If you miss a dose, take it as soon as possible. If it is almost time for your next dose, skip the missed dose and resume your regular schedule. Do not take two doses at the same time.

SPECIAL CONSIDERATIONS FOR THOSE OVER SIXTY-FIVE

Older people are more likely to develop problems caused by too much potassium in the body, such as irregular heartbeat, confusion, difficulty in breathing, and tiredness or weakness. Regular checkups may be required. All doctor's appointments should be kept. People over sixty-five should consult a doctor if they become ill with flulike symptoms such as cough, fever, or body aches; lose their appetite; vomit; or have diarrhea because they may then be more vulnerable to fluid losses.

CONDITION: **HYPERTENSION**

CATEGORY: **DIURETICS (MISCELLANEOUS)**

GENERIC (CHEMICAL) NAME	BRAND (TRADE) NAME	DOSAGE FORMS AND STRENGTHS
Indapamide	LOZOL	Tablets: 2.5 mg

DRUG PROFILE

Indapamide is a diuretic that may be used alone or in combination with other antihypertensive drugs to control high blood pressure. Like the thiazide diuretics, indapamide works by increasing the amount of salt and water you eliminate through urination. Because of this action, it is also used to treat fluid accumulation in people who have congestive heart failure.

BEFORE USING THIS DRUG

Let your doctor know *IF*

You have ever had allergic reactions or other problems with ■ indapamide ■ thiazide or thiazide-type diuretics ■ sulfonamides (sulfa drugs).

You have ever had any of the following medical problems: ■ diabetes ■ gout ■ kidney disease ■ liver disease ■ systemic lupus erythematosus ■ high cholesterol ■ thyroid disorders.

You are taking any of the following medicines: ■ other diuretics or high blood pressure medicines ■ corticosteroids or corticotropin (ACTH) ■ digoxin or digitalis (heart medicines) ■ lithium.

SPECIAL RESTRICTIONS WHILE TAKING THIS DRUG

FOOD AND DRUG INTERACTIONS

Other Drugs	Do not take any other drugs, including over-the-counter (OTC) drugs, before checking with your doctor. OTC drugs for appetite suppression, asthma, colds, cough, hay fever, or sinus problems tend to increase blood pressure. Barbiturates (sleep medicine, medicine for seizures) and narcotic pain-killers may increase risk of dizziness when sitting up or standing up.
Foods and Beverages	Your doctor may prescribe a special low-salt diet, which you should follow carefully because it will help your medicine work more effectively. You may also be advised to go on a weight-reduction diet. This medicine may cause your body to lose large amounts of the mineral potassium. Your doctor may give you special instructions about eating foods or drinking beverages that have a high potassium content (such as bananas and citrus fruit juices), taking a potassium supplement, or using salt substitutes.
Alcohol	Alcohol may increase the risk of dizziness when sitting up or standing up.

No special restrictions on smoking.

DAILY LIVING

Exertion and Exercise	Use caution when exercising or exerting yourself while taking this medicine because excessive sweating may cause you to become dehydrated and to feel dizzy, light-headed, or faint.

Excessive Heat	Use caution during hot weather or while taking saunas or hot baths, since excessive sweating while taking this medicine may cause you to become dehydrated and to feel drowsy or faint.
Examinations or Tests	Many people have high blood pressure with no symptoms at all. It is important for you to keep all appointments with your doctor, even if you feel well, so that your blood pressure can be checked regularly. Periodic blood and urine tests may be required.
Other Precautions	When first starting on this type of medicine, you may feel tired and will probably experience both greater volume and frequency of urination. Until your individual pattern of urination has been established with this medicine, it may be wise to time carefully any activity that will put you out of convenient reach of a bathroom, such as bus or car travel. In addition, taking a diuretic at bedtime will probably interfere with sleep; you should discuss your dosage schedule with your doctor.
	Check with your doctor if you become ill with flulike symptoms, such as cough, fever, or body aches; lose your appetite; vomit; or have diarrhea. This may cause you to lose a great deal of fluid, making it important not to take the diuretic for one or more doses.
	Following mild fluid losses, some older people are more vulnerable to symptoms of weakness or dizziness upon standing or getting up.

No special restrictions on driving, sun exposure, or exposure to excessive cold.

POSSIBLE SIDE EFFECTS

Although this list of adverse effects may seem somewhat intimidating, keep in mind that some are quite rare. Of course, should these or any other problems arise while you are on medication, it is always a good idea to consult your doctor.

IF YOU DEVELOP	WHAT TO DO
severe or continuing vomiting or diarrhea ■ irregular heartbeat ■ weak pulse ■ dry mouth ■ increased thirst ■ anxiety ■ agitation ■ depression ■ tiredness or weakness ■ muscle cramps or pain	**May be serious** Check with your doctor as soon as possible.
upset stomach ■ loss of appetite ■ dizziness or light-headedness, especially when getting up from a re-clining or sitting position ■ headache ■ sleep disturbances ■ blurred vision ■ changes in urination ■ constipation ■ diarrhea, nausea, or vomiting	If symptoms are disturbing or persist, let your doctor know.

STORAGE INSTRUCTIONS

Store in a cool, dark place (not in a bathroom medicine cabinet).

STOPPING OR INTERRUPTING THERAPY

Since this drug does not cure high blood pressure but only controls it, you may have to take this medicine for the rest of your life. Do not stop taking it even if you feel better. If you miss a dose, take it as soon as possible. If it is almost time for your next dose, skip the missed dose and resume your regular schedule. Do not take two doses at the same time.

SPECIAL CONSIDERATIONS FOR THOSE OVER SIXTY-FIVE

Older people are more likely to develop dizziness or light-headedness or signs of potassium loss, such as irregular heartbeat and weak pulse. Regular checkups may be required. People over sixty-five should consult a doctor if they become ill with flulike symptoms, such as cough, fever, or body aches; lose their appetite; vomit; or have diarrhea because they may then be more vulnerable to fluid losses.

CONDITION: **HYPERTENSION**

CATEGORY: **DIURETICS (COMBINATIONS)**

GENERIC (CHEMICAL) NAME	BRAND (TRADE) NAME	DOSAGE FORMS AND STRENGTHS
Triamterene and hydrochlorothiazide	DYAZIDE	Capsules: 50 mg triamterene and 25 mg hydrochlorothiazide
	MAXZIDE	Tablets: 75 mg triamterene and 50 mg hydrochlorothiazide; 37.5 mg triamterene and 25 mg hydrochlorothiazide

DRUG PROFILE

This combination of two diuretics in one tablet or capsule may be prescribed to control high blood pressure, while at the same time maintaining the body's potassium levels. Each tablet or capsule contains a thiazide diuretic as well as a potassium-sparing diuretic. This drug works by increasing the amount of salt and water eliminated through the body (through urination) and by relaxing the walls of the smaller arteries so that they expand. With a smaller volume of blood (because water is eliminated) in a larger amount of space (because the artery walls are expanded), blood pressure decreases. This drug may also be prescribed with other therapy for edema (swelling due to excess fluid in the body), because it helps the body to eliminate extra water.

BEFORE USING THIS DRUG

Let your doctor know *IF*

You have ever had allergic reactions or other problems with ■ triamterene ■ thiazide diuretics ■ sulfonamides (sulfa drugs).

You have ever had any of the following medical problems: ■ diabetes ■ gout ■ heart disease ■ kidney disease or stones ■ liver disease ■ systemic lupus erythematosus ■ disease of the pancreas.

You are taking any of the following medicines: ■ other diuretics or medicines for high blood pressure, amiloride, spironolactone, or ACE inhibitors (eg, captopril, enalapril, or lisinopril) ■ corticosteroids or corticotropin (ACTH) ■ medicine for high cholesterol ■ medicine for diabetes ■ digoxin or digitalis (heart medicines) ■ medicine for gout ■ laxatives ■ lithium ■ methenamine (medicine to prevent urinary tract infections) ■ phenobarbital ■ narcotics or other prescription pain-killers ■ anticoagulants (blood thinners) ■ aspirin, indomethacin, or other arthritis medicines (nonsteroidal anti-inflammatory drugs) ■ potassium-containing medicines or supplements ■ salt substitutes.

SPECIAL RESTRICTIONS WHILE TAKING THIS DRUG

FOOD AND DRUG INTERACTIONS

Other Drugs	Do not take any other drugs, including over-the-counter (OTC) drugs, before checking with your doctor. OTC drugs for appetite suppression, asthma, colds, cough, hay fever, or sinus problems tend to increase blood pressure.
	Check with your doctor before using any nonsteroidal anti-inflammatory drugs such as indomethacin, aspirin, or ibuprofen.
	Barbiturates (sleep medicine, medicine for seizures) and narcotic pain-killers may increase the risk of dizziness when sitting up or standing up.
Foods and Beverages	Your doctor may prescribe a special low-salt diet, which you should follow carefully because it will help your medicine work more effectively. You should continue to drink a normal amount of fluids. This medicine may either increase or decrease potassium levels in your body. Your doctor may give you special instructions about eating foods or drinking beverages that have a high potassium content (such as bananas and citrus fruit juices), taking a potassium supplement, or using salt substitutes.

Alcohol	Alcohol may increase the risk of dizziness when sitting up or standing up.

No special restrictions on smoking.

DAILY LIVING

Exertion and Exercise	Use caution when exercising or exerting yourself while taking this medicine because excessive sweating may cause you to become dehydrated and to feel dizzy, light-headed, or faint.
Sun Exposure/ Excessive Heat	Your skin may become more sensitive to sunlight and more likely to develop a sunburn while you are taking this medicine. It is a good idea to avoid too much sun, especially if you burn easily. Apply a sunscreen to exposed skin surfaces before going outdoors. Use caution during hot weather or while taking saunas or hot baths, since excessive sweating while taking this medicine may cause you to become dehydrated and to feel drowsy or faint.
Examinations or Tests	Many people have high blood pressure with no symptoms at all. It is important for you to keep all appointments with your doctor, even if you feel well, so that your blood pressure can be checked regularly. Periodic blood tests are usually required.
Other Precautions	If you have diabetes, be aware that this medicine may raise blood-sugar levels. If you notice any change when testing sugar levels in your blood or urine, let your doctor know.
	Tell any doctor or dentist you consult that you are taking this medicine, especially if you will be undergoing any type of surgery.

When first starting on this type of medicine, you may feel tired and will probably experience both greater volume and frequency of urination. Until your individual pattern of urination has been established with this medicine, it may be wise to time carefully any activity that will put you out of convenient reach of a bathroom, such as bus or car travel. In addition, taking a diuretic at bedtime will probably interfere with sleep; you should discuss your dosage schedule with your doctor.

Check with your doctor it you become ill with flulike symptoms, such as cough, fever, or body aches; lose your appetite; vomit; or have diarrhea. This may cause you to lose a great deal of fluid, making it important not to take the diuretic for one or more doses.

Following mild fluid losses, some older people are more vulnerable to symptoms of weakness or dizziness upon standing or getting up.

Your urine may appear blue, which is expected and not harmful.

No special restrictions on driving or exposure to excessive cold.

POSSIBLE SIDE EFFECTS

Although this list of adverse effects may seem somewhat intimidating, keep in mind that some are quite rare. Of course, should these or any other problems arise while you are on medication, it is always a good idea to consult your doctor.

IF YOU DEVELOP	WHAT TO DO
irregular heartbeat ■ numbness or tingling in hands, feet, or lips ■ tiredness or weakness ■ confusion ■ mood or mental changes ■ shortness of breath ■ weak pulse ■ muscle cramps or pain ■ nausea or vomiting ■ dry mouth ■ increased thirst ■ severe or continuing diarrhea	**Urgent** Get in touch with your doctor immediately.
headache ■ tongue inflammation ■ cracked corners of mouth ■ rash ■ sore throat or fever ■ bleeding or bruising ■ yellowing of eyes or skin ■ swelling of hands or feet	**May be serious** Check with your doctor as soon as possible.
upset stomach ■ loss of appetite ■ stomach cramps ■ headache ■ dizziness or light-headedness, especially when getting up from a reclining or sitting position ■ increased skin sensitivity to sunlight ■ blurred vision	If symptoms are disturbing or persist, let your doctor know.

STORAGE INSTRUCTIONS

Store in a cool, dark place (not in a bathroom medicine cabinet).

STOPPING OR INTERRUPTING THERAPY

Since this drug does not cure high blood pressure but only controls it, you may have to take this medicine for the rest of your life. Do not stop taking it, even if you feel better. If you miss a dose, take it as soon as possible. If it is almost time for your next dose, skip the missed dose and resume your regular schedule. Do not take two doses at the same time.

SPECIAL CONSIDERATIONS FOR THOSE OVER SIXTY-FIVE

Older people are more likely to develop dizziness, light-headedness, or problems caused by changing potassium levels, such as irregular heartbeat or weak pulse. People over sixty-five should consult a doctor if they become ill with flulike symptoms, such as cough, fever, or body aches; lose their appetite; vomit; or have diarrhea because they may then be more vulnerable to fluid losses.

CONDITION: **HYPERTENSION**

CATEGORY: **DIURETICS (COMBINATIONS)**

GENERIC (CHEMICAL) NAME	BRAND (TRADE) NAME	DOSAGE FORMS AND STRENGTHS
Spironolactone and hydrochlorothiazide	ALDACTAZIDE	Tablets: 25 mg spironolactone and 25 mg hydrochlorothiazide; 50 mg spironolactone and 50 mg hydrochlorothiazide

DRUG PROFILE

This combination of two diuretics in one tablet may be prescribed to control high blood pressure. Each tablet contains a thiazide diuretic as well as a potassium-sparing diuretic. This drug works by increasing the amount of salt and water eliminated by the body (through urination) and by relaxing the walls of the smaller arteries so that they expand. With a smaller volume of blood (because water is eliminated) in a larger amount of space (because the artery walls are expanded), blood pressure decreases. This drug may also be prescribed for edema (swelling due to excess fluid in the body) because it helps the body to eliminate extra water.

BEFORE USING THIS DRUG

Let your doctor know *IF*

You have ever had allergic reactions or other problems with ■ spironolactone ■ thiazide diuretics ■ sulfonamides (sulfa drugs).

You have ever had any of the following medical problems: ■ diabetes ■ gout ■ heart disease ■ liver disease ■ systemic lupus erythematosus ■ kidney disease ■ disease of the pancreas.

You are taking any of the following medicines: ■ other diuretics or medicines for high blood pressure, especially amiloride or ACE inhibitors (eg, captopril, enalapril, lisinopril) ■ corticosteroids or corticotropin (ACTH) ■ colestipol (medicine for high cholesterol) ■ medicine for diabetes ■ digoxin or digitalis (heart medicines) ■ medicine for gout ■ lithium ■ methenamine (medicine to prevent urinary tract infections) ■ anticoagulants (blood thinners) ■ aspirin ■ narcotics or other prescription pain-killers ■ potassium-containing medicines or supplements ■ salt substitutes ■ laxatives ■ phenobarbital ■ indomethacin (medicine for arthritis).

SPECIAL RESTRICTIONS WHILE TAKING THIS DRUG

FOOD AND DRUG INTERACTIONS

Other Drugs	Do not take any other drugs, including over-the-counter (OTC) drugs, before checking with your doctor. OTC drugs for appetite suppression, asthma, colds, cough, hay fever, or sinus problems tend to increase blood pressure.
Foods and Beverages	Your doctor may prescribe a special low-salt diet, which you should follow carefully because it will help your medicine work more effectively. You may also be advised to go on a weight-reduction diet. You should continue to drink normal amounts of fluids.
	This medicine may either increase or decrease potassium levels in your body. Your doctor may give you special instructions about eating foods or drinking beverages that have a high potassium content (such as bananas and citrus fruit juices), taking a potassium supplement, or using salt substitutes.

No special restrictions on alcohol use or smoking.

DAILY LIVING

Exertion and Exercise	Use caution when exercising or exerting yourself while taking this medicine because excessive sweating may cause you to become dehydrated and to feel dizzy, light-headed, or faint.

Sun Exposure/
Excessive Heat

Your skin may become more sensitive to sunlight
and more likely to develop a sunburn while you are
taking this medicine. It is a good idea to avoid too
much sun, especially if you burn easily. Apply a sunscreen to exposed skin surfaces before going outdoors. Use caution during hot weather or while taking
saunas or hot baths, since excessive sweating while
taking this medicine may cause you to become dehydrated and to feel drowsy or faint.

Examinations or Tests

Many people have high blood pressure with no
symptoms at all. It is important for you to keep all
appointments with your doctor, even if you feel well,
so that your blood pressure can be checked regularly. Periodic blood tests may be required.

Other Precautions

Tell any doctor or dentist you consult that you are
taking this medicine, especially if you will be undergoing any kind of surgery.

Although this drug has been shown to cause tumors
in rats, no relationship has been shown in humans.

When first starting on this type of medicine, you may
feel tired and will probably experience both greater
volume and frequency of urination. Until your individual pattern of urination has been established with this
medicine, it may be wise to time carefully any activity
that will put you out of convenient reach of a bathroom, such as bus or car travel. In addition, taking a
diuretic at bedtime will probably interfere with sleep;
you should discuss your dosage schedule with your
doctor.

Check with your doctor if you become ill with flulike
symptoms, such as cough, fever, or body aches; lose
your appetite; vomit; or have diarrhea. This may
cause you to lose a great deal of fluid, making it important not to take the diuretic for one or more
doses.

Following mild fluid losses, some older people are more vulnerable to symptoms of weakness or dizziness upon standing or getting up.

| Helpful Hints | If this medicine upsets your stomach, taking it with milk, meals, or snacks should help. |

No special restrictions on driving or exposure to excessive cold.

POSSIBLE SIDE EFFECTS

Although this list of adverse effects may seem somewhat intimidating, keep in mind that some are quite rare. Of course, should these or any other problems arise while you are on medication, it is always a good idea to consult your doctor.

IF YOU DEVELOP	WHAT TO DO
irregular heartbeat ■ numbness or tingling in hands, feet, or lips ■ tiredness or weakness ■ confusion ■ mood or mental changes ■ weak pulse ■ muscle cramps or pain ■ continuing nausea or vomiting ■ dry mouth ■ increased thirst ■ severe or continuing diarrhea ■ severe stomach pain	**Urgent** Get in touch with your doctor immediately.
blurred vision ■ rash ■ sore throat or fever ■ bleeding or bruising ■ yellowing of eyes or skin	**May be serious** Check with your doctor as soon as possible.
upset stomach ■ loss of appetite ■ female breast tenderness ■ male breast enlargement ■ male impotence ■ deepening voice ■ hair growth ■ clumsiness ■ headache ■ dizziness or light-headedness, especially when getting up from a reclining or sitting position ■ increased skin sensitivity to sunlight	If symptoms are disturbing or persist, let your doctor know.

STORAGE INSTRUCTIONS

Store in a cool, dark place (not in a bathroom medicine cabinet).

STOPPING OR INTERRUPTING THERAPY

Since this drug does not cure high blood pressure but only controls it, you may have to take this medicine for the rest of your life. Do not stop taking it, even if you feel better. If you miss a dose, take it as soon as possible. If it is almost time for your next dose, skip the missed dose and resume your regular schedule. Do not take two doses at the same time.

SPECIAL CONSIDERATIONS FOR THOSE OVER SIXTY-FIVE

Older people are more likely to develop dizziness, light-headedness, or problems caused by changing body potassium levels, such as irregular heartbeat or weak pulse. People over sixty-five should consult a doctor if they become ill with flulike symptoms, such as cough, fever, or body aches; lose their appetite; vomit; or have diarrhea because they may then be more vulnerable to fluid losses.

CONDITION: **HYPERTENSION**

CATEGORY: **DIURETICS (COMBINATIONS)**

GENERIC (CHEMICAL) NAME	BRAND (TRADE) NAME	DOSAGE FORMS AND STRENGTHS
Amiloride and hydrochlorothiazide	MODURETIC	Tablets: 5 mg amiloride and 50 mg hydrochlorothiazide

DRUG PROFILE

This combination of two diuretics in one tablet may be prescribed to control high blood pressure, while at the same time maintaining the body's potassium levels. Each tablet contains a thiazide diuretic as well as a potassium-sparing diuretic. This drug works by increasing the amount of salt and water eliminated through the body (through urination) and by relaxing the walls of the smaller arteries so that they expand. With a smaller volume of blood (because water is eliminated) in a larger amount of space (because the artery walls are expanded), blood pressure decreases. This drug is also used to treat fluid accumulation in people who have congestive heart failure.

BEFORE USING THIS DRUG

Let your doctor know *IF*

You have ever had allergic reactions or other problems with ■ amiloride ■ thiazide diuretics ■ sulfonamides (sulfa drugs).

You have ever had any of the following medical problems: ■ diabetes ■ gout ■ heart disease ■ kidney disease ■ liver disease ■ systemic lupus erythematosus ■ disease of the pancreas.

You are taking any of the following medicines: ■ other diuretics or medicine for high blood pressure, especially triamterene, spironolactone or ACE inhibitors (eg, captopril, enalapril, lisinopril) ■ corticosteroids or corticotropin (ACTH) ■ colestipol (medicine for high cholesterol) ■ digoxin or digitalis (heart medicines) ■ medicine for gout ■ lithium ■ methenamine (medicine to prevent urinary tract infections) ■ anticoagulants (blood thinners) ■ medicine for diabetes ■ potassium-containing medicines or supplements ■ salt substitutes ■ aspirin, indomethacin or other arthritis medicines (nonsteroidal anti-inflammatory drugs).

SPECIAL RESTRICTIONS WHILE TAKING THIS DRUG

FOOD AND DRUG INTERACTIONS

Other Drugs	Do not take any other drugs, including over-the-counter (OTC) drugs, before checking with your doctor. OTC drugs for appetite suppression, asthma, colds, cough, hay fever, or sinus problems tend to increase blood pressure.
Foods and Beverages	Your doctor may prescribe a special low-salt diet, which you should follow carefully because it will help your medicine work more effectively. You may also be advised to go on a weight-reduction diet. This medicine may either increase or decrease potassium levels in your body. Your doctor may give you special

instructions about eating foods or drinking beverages that have a high potassium content (such as bananas and citrus fruit juices), taking a potassium supplement, or using salt substitutes.

No special restrictions on alcohol use or smoking.

DAILY LIVING

Exertion and Exercise	Use caution when exercising or exerting yourself while taking this medicine because excessive sweating may cause you to become dehydrated and to feel dizzy, light-headed, or faint.
Sun Exposure/ Excessive Heat	Your skin may become more sensitive to sunlight and more likely to develop a sunburn while you are taking this medicine. It is a good idea to avoid too much sun, especially if you burn easily. Apply a sunscreen to exposed skin surfaces before going outdoors. Use caution during hot weather or while taking saunas or hot baths, since excessive sweating while taking this medicine may cause you to become dehydrated and to feel drowsy or faint.
Examinations or Tests	Many people have high blood pressure with no symptoms at all. It is important for you to keep all appointments with your doctor, even if you feel well, so that your blood pressure can be checked regularly. Periodic blood and urine tests are usually required.
Other Precautions	If you have diabetes, be aware that this medicine may raise blood-sugar levels. If you notice any change when testing sugar levels in your blood or urine, let your doctor know. When first starting on this type of medicine, you may feel tired and will probably experience both greater

volume and frequency of urination. Until your individual pattern of urination has been established with this medicine, it may be wise to time carefully any activity that will put you out of convenient reach of a bathroom, such as bus or car travel. In addition, taking a diuretic at bedtime will probably interfere with sleep; you should discuss your dosage schedule with your doctor.

Check with your doctor if you become ill with flulike symptoms, such as cough, fever, or body aches; lose your appetite; vomit; or have diarrhea. This may cause you to lose a great deal of fluid, making it important not to take the diuretic for one or more doses.

Following mild fluid losses, some older people are more vulnerable to symptoms of weakness or dizziness upon standing or getting up.

No special restrictions on driving or exposure to excessive cold.

POSSIBLE SIDE EFFECTS

Although this list of adverse effects may seem somewhat intimidating, keep in mind that some are quite rare. Of course, should these or any other problems arise while you are on medication, it is always a good idea to consult your doctor.

IF YOU DEVELOP

chest pain ■ irregular heartbeat ■ tiredness or weakness ■ numbness or tingling in hands, feet, or lips ■ confusion ■ weak pulse ■ shortness of breath ■ difficulty in breathing ■ depression ■ nervousness ■ muscle cramps or pain ■ nausea or vomiting ■ dry mouth ■ increased thirst ■ severe or continuing diarrhea

WHAT TO DO

Urgent Get in touch with your doctor immediately.

sore throat or fever ■ bleeding or bruising ■ yellowing of eyes or skin	**May be serious** Check with your doctor as soon as possible.
upset stomach ■ loss of appetite ■ constipation ■ headache ■ dizziness or light-headedness, especially when getting up from a reclining or sitting position ■ increased skin sensitivity to sunlight ■ diminished sex drive ■ male impotence ■ sleep disturbances	If symptoms are disturbing or persist, let your doctor know.

STORAGE INSTRUCTIONS

Store in a cool, dark place (not in a bathroom medicine cabinet).

STOPPING OR INTERRUPTING THERAPY

Since this drug does not cure high blood pressure but only controls it, you may have to take this medicine for the rest of your life. Do not stop taking it, even if you feel better. If you miss a dose, take it as soon as possible. If it is almost time for your next dose, skip the missed dose and resume your regular schedule. Do not take two doses at the same time.

SPECIAL CONSIDERATIONS FOR THOSE OVER SIXTY-FIVE

Older people are more likely to develop problems caused by changing body potassium levels, such as irregular heartbeat, confusion, difficulty in breathing, and tiredness or weakness. People over sixty-five should get in touch with a doctor if they develop these symptoms. All doctor's appointments should be kept.

CONDITION: **HYPERTENSION**

CATEGORY: **NONDIURETICS (BETA-BLOCKERS)**

GENERIC (CHEMICAL) NAME	BRAND (TRADE) NAME	DOSAGE FORMS AND STRENGTHS
Acebutolol	SECTRAL	Capsules: 200, 400 mg
Atenolol	TENORMIN	Tablets: 25, 50, 100 mg
Betaxolol hydrochloride	KERLONE	Tablets: 10, 20 mg
Carteolol hydrochloride	CARTROL	Tablets: 2.5, 5 mg
Labetalol hydrochloride	NORMODYNE TRANDATE	Tablets: 100, 200, 300 mg Tablets: 100, 200, 300 mg
Metoprolol tartrate	LOPRESSOR	Tablets: 50, 100 mg
Nadolol	CORGARD	Tablets: 20, 40, 80, 120, 160 mg
Penbutolol	LEVATOL	Tablets: 20 mg
Pindolol	VISKEN	Tablets: 5, 10 mg
Propranolol hydrochloride	INDERAL INDERAL LA	Tablets: 10, 20, 40, 60, 80, 90 mg Capsules: 60, 80, 120, 160 mg
Timolol maleate	BLOCADREN	Tablets: 5, 10, 20 mg

DRUG PROFILE

Beta-adrenergic blocking drugs (beta-blockers) are used to control high blood pressure. Some are used for other conditions such as angina, heart arrhythmias, migraine headaches, and hypertrophic subaortic stenosis (a disease of the heart muscle). Some have also been found to improve a person's chance of survival for several years following a heart attack. By blocking certain nerve impulses, these medicines reduce the workload of the heart and help the heart to beat more regularly.

When used in the treatment of angina, beta-blockers prevent future attacks (they are not helpful during an acute attack of chest pain). Beta-blockers differ in the duration of action and when their peak effect occurs, and it is worthwhile to discuss with your doctor precisely how to time your doses in relation to the pattern of your attacks. If you suffer a side effect, such as depression or nightmares, with one beta-blocker, your doctor may be able to prescribe a different beta-blocker that will be equally effective. Beta-blockers may be used along with other antiangina medicines.

BEFORE USING THIS DRUG

Let your doctor know *IF*

You have ever had allergic reactions or other problems with ■ any beta-blockers.

You smoke.

You have ever had any of the following medical problems: ■ history of allergy (including hay fever, hives, asthma, eczema) ■ slow heartbeat ■ bronchitis or emphysema ■ diabetes ■ any heart or blood vessel disease ■ kidney disease ■ liver disease ■ thyroid disease ■ Raynaud's syndrome (poor circulation in the fingers and toes) ■ intermittent claudication (limping) ■ glaucoma ■ myasthenia gravis ■ hypoglycemia (low blood sugar) ■ pheochromocytoma (adrenal gland tumor).

You are taking any of the following medicines: ■ any other medicine for high blood pressure ■ aminophylline, epinephrine, ephedrine, norepinephrine, isoproterenol, dyphylline, oxtriphylline, theophylline, phenylephrine (medicines for asthma or vasopressor drugs) ■ medicine for depression ■ cimetidine (medicine for ulcers) ■ heart medicine ■ medicine for glaucoma ■ aspirin, indomethacin, or phenylbutazone (medicines for arthritis) ■ medicine for diabetes ■ decongestants ■ tranquilizers ■ medicine for nausea ■ appetite suppressants.

SPECIAL RESTRICTIONS WHILE TAKING THIS DRUG

FOOD AND DRUG INTERACTIONS

Other Drugs	It is especially important to let your doctor know if you are taking any other antihypertensive drugs since the use of these drugs with a beta-blocker may cause low blood pressure, slow heartbeat, or dizziness. Also, beta-blockers may prevent asthma medicine from working effectively. Do not take any other drugs, including over-the-counter (OTC) drugs, before checking with your doctor. OTC drugs for appetite suppression, asthma, colds, cough, hay fever, or sinus problems tend to increase blood pressure. Some medicines used for pain and/or arthritis (aspirin, indomethacin, and phenylbutazone, for example) may hamper the action of beta-blockers.
Foods and Beverages	Your doctor may prescribe a special low-salt diet, which you should follow carefully because it will help your medicine work more effectively. You may also be advised to go on a weight-reduction diet.
Alcohol	Dizziness, light-headedness, or fainting may occur if you drink alcohol while taking a beta-blocker, especially labetalol. Be careful about how much alcohol you consume.
Smoking	Smoking may reduce the effect of some beta-blockers. Be sure to tell your doctor that you smoke.

DAILY LIVING

Driving	This drug may cause drowsiness. Be careful when driving, operating household appliances, or doing any other tasks that require alertness until you know how this drug affects you.
Exertion and Exercise	Since chest pain from exercise or exertion may be reduced or prevented by this medicine, you may be tempted to overwork yourself. Discuss with your doctor how much exercise is safe for you. Be especially careful when you exercise during hot weather or if you must stand for long periods of time, since this drug may cause side effects such as dizziness, light-headedness, and fainting.
Excessive Heat	Be careful during hot weather because of the possible side effects of dizziness, light-headedness, or fainting (especially with labetalol).
Excessive Cold	You may become more sensitive to cold temperatures while taking beta-blockers. Dress warmly—protecting your skin, fingers, and toes—and use caution during prolonged exposure to cold.
Examinations or Tests	*Check your pulse regularly.* If it is slower than your usual rate or less than 50 beats per minute, call your doctor. Many people have high blood pressure with no symptoms at all. It is important for you to keep all appointments with your doctor, even if you feel well, so that your blood pressure can be checked regularly. Periodic blood and urine tests may be required.
Other Precautions	Tell any doctor or dentist you consult that you are taking this medicine, especially if you will be undergoing any type of surgery.

If you have diabetes, be aware that this medicine may cause your blood-sugar level to fall. It also may mask the signs of low blood sugar (such as changes in pulse rate or increased blood pressure), leaving you unaware that your blood sugar has fallen. Your doctor may want to make adjustments in the dosage of your diabetes medicine.

Helpful Hints	If your mouth or throat feels dry, chewing sugarless gum or sucking ice chips or sugarless hard candy will help. If your eyes feel dry, you may use non-medicated or plain eyedrops for relief. If this medicine causes upset stomach, taking it with milk, meals, or snacks should help.

No special restrictions on sun exposure.

POSSIBLE SIDE EFFECTS

Although this list of adverse effects may seem somewhat intimidating, keep in mind that some are quite rare. Of course, should these or any other problems arise while you are on medication, it is always a good idea to consult your doctor.

IF YOU DEVELOP

chest pain ■ palpitations ■ irregular heartbeat ■ extremely slow heartbeat ■ swelling of face, ankles, feet, or lower legs ■ shortness of breath or coughing ■ difficulty in breathing ■ asthma or wheezing ■ restlessness, sweating, nervousness, or irritability (if you are a thyroid patient) ■ weight gain

WHAT TO DO

Urgent Get in touch with your doctor immediately.

---

dizziness, light-headedness, or fainting (especially with labetalol) ■ cold hands or feet ■ slurred speech ■ confusion ■ depression ■ fever or sore throat ■ rash or itching ■ bleeding or bruising ■ increased sweating ■ faintness or hunger ■ pale, moist skin

May be serious Check with your doctor as soon as possible.

nausea or vomiting ■ diarrhea or constipation ■ indigestion, gas, hiccups, or stomach cramps ■ dry eyes, mouth, or skin ■ hair loss ■ nail changes ■ inflammation of the nasal lining ■ visual disturbances ■ hearing problems or ringing in the ears ■ clumsiness ■ muscle or joint pain ■ numbness of fingers or toes ■ drowsiness ■ tiredness or weakness ■ anxiety, nervousness, or irritability ■ memory problems ■ male impotence ■ diminished sex drive ■ headache ■ hallucinations ■ nightmares ■ sleep disturbances ■ tingling or other abnormal skin sensations ■ urinary frequency

If symptoms are disturbing or persist, let your doctor know.

With labetalol only: taste changes

STORAGE INSTRUCTIONS

Store in a cool, dark place (not in a bathroom medicine cabinet).

STOPPING OR INTERRUPTING THERAPY

Since this drug does not cure high blood pressure but only controls it, you may have to take this medicine for the rest of your life. Do not stop taking it, even if you feel better. *Suddenly stopping your medicine may worsen your medical problem,* especially if you have angina. Your doctor can advise you on how to discontinue therapy gradually. *Always carry a supply of your medicine with you.* If you miss a dose, take the missed dose as soon as possible. If the next scheduled dose is within four hours (or within eight hours if you are taking atenolol, nadolol, labetalol, or once-a-day propranolol or metoprolol), skip the missed dose and resume your regular schedule. Do not take two doses at the same time.

SPECIAL CONSIDERATIONS FOR THOSE OVER SIXTY-FIVE

Although beta-blockers are quite effective in the treatment of cardiac disorders, older persons may suffer more adverse effects from these drugs, such as drowsiness, depression, nightmares, muscle or joint pain, cold hands or feet, and slow heartbeat. Doctors may start older persons on a lower dosage.

CONDITION: **HYPERTENSION**

CATEGORY: **NONDIURETICS (CENTRAL ALPHA-AGONISTS)**

GENERIC (CHEMICAL) NAME	BRAND (TRADE) NAME	DOSAGE FORMS AND STRENGTHS
Methyldopa	ALDOMET	Suspension: 250 mg per tsp Tablets: 125, 250, 500 mg

DRUG PROFILE

Methyldopa is used to treat high blood pressure. It acts to reduce the passage of impulses along certain nerve pathways; this relaxes the blood vessels and makes blood flow easier. Methyldopa is sometimes combined with other antihypertensive medicines, especially diuretics, for better control of hypertension.

BEFORE USING THIS DRUG

Let your doctor know *IF*

You have ever had allergic reactions or other problems with ■ methyldopa.

You have ever had any of the following medical problems: ■ angina (chest pain) ■ heart disease ■ kidney disease ■ liver disease ■ depression ■ Parkinson's disease ■ pheochromocytoma (adrenal gland tumor) ■ systemic lupus erythematosus ■ dizziness from other high blood pressure medicines.

You are taking any of the following medicines: ■ other medicine for high blood pressure ■ levodopa (medicine for Parkinson's disease) ■ medicine for depression (within the last two weeks) ■ tranquilizers ■ lithium ■ medicine for nausea.

SPECIAL RESTRICTIONS WHILE TAKING THIS DRUG

FOOD AND DRUG INTERACTIONS

Other Drugs	Do not take any other drugs, including over-the-counter (OTC) drugs, before checking with your doctor. OTC drugs for appetite suppression, asthma, colds, cough, hay fever, or sinus problems tend to increase blood pressure.
Foods and Beverages	Your doctor may prescribe a special low-salt diet, which you should follow carefully because it will help your medicine work more effectively. You may also be advised to go on a weight-reduction diet.

No special restrictions on alcohol use or smoking.

DAILY LIVING

Driving	This drug may cause drowsiness. Be careful when driving, operating household appliances, or doing any other tasks that require alertness until you know how this drug affects you.
Exertion and Exercise	Use caution when exercising, exerting yourself, or standing for long periods of time because this medicine may cause you to become dizzy, light-headed, or faint. If you feel any of these symptoms coming on, sit or lie down. It is a good idea not to get up too quickly from a reclining or sitting position.
Examinations or Tests	Many people have high blood pressure with no symptoms at all. It is important for you to keep all appointments with your doctor, even if you feel well, so that your blood pressure can be checked regularly. Periodic blood and urine tests are usually required.

Other Precautions   Tell any doctor or dentist you consult that you are taking this medicine, especially if you will be undergoing any type of surgery or if you need a blood transfusion.

No special restrictions on sun exposure or exposure to excessive heat or cold.

POSSIBLE SIDE EFFECTS

Although this list of adverse effects may seem somewhat intimidating, keep in mind that some are quite rare. Of course, should these or any other problems arise while you are on medication, it is always a good idea to consult your doctor.

IF YOU DEVELOP	WHAT TO DO
fever ■ slow or fast heartbeat ■ chest pain ■ yellowing of eyes or skin ■ dark or amber-colored urine ■ dark stools	**Urgent** Get in touch with your doctor immediately.
swelling of feet or lower legs ■ weight gain ■ sleep disturbances ■ depression ■ anxiety ■ tiredness or weakness ■ severe or continuing vomiting, diarrhea, or stomach cramps ■ pale stools ■ shakiness or unusual body movements ■ sore throat ■ bleeding or bruising ■ dizziness, light-headedness, or fainting, especially when getting up from a reclining or sitting position	**May be serious** Check with your doctor as soon as possible.
drowsiness ■ dry mouth ■ headache ■ memory problems ■ inability to concentrate ■ blurred vision ■ male impotence ■ diminished sex drive ■ upset stomach ■ constipation ■ bloating or gas ■ sore or dark tongue ■ numbness or tingling in hands or feet ■ abnormal skin sensations ■ rash ■ stuffy nose ■ female breast swelling ■ male breast enlargement	If symptoms are disturbing or persist, let your doctor know.

STORAGE INSTRUCTIONS

Store in a cool, dark place (not in a bathroom medicine cabinet). If your medicine is in a liquid form, make sure that it does not freeze.

STOPPING OR INTERRUPTING THERAPY

Since this drug does not cure high blood pressure but only controls it, you may have to take this medicine for the rest of your life. Do not stop taking it, even if you feel better. If you miss a dose, take it as soon as possible. If it is almost time for your next dose, skip the missed dose and resume your regular schedule. Do not take two doses at the same time.

SPECIAL CONSIDERATIONS FOR THOSE OVER SIXTY-FIVE

The side effects of dizziness, light-headedness, memory problems, loss of sex drive, and depression occur more frequently in older people, who may also be more prone to drowsiness and tiredness when first starting this medicine or when the dosage is increased. For these reasons, a doctor may want to start with a lower dosage.

CONDITION: **HYPERTENSION**

CATEGORY: **NONDIURETICS (CENTRAL ALPHA-AGONISTS)**

GENERIC (CHEMICAL) NAME	BRAND (TRADE) NAME	DOSAGE FORMS AND STRENGTHS
Clonidine hydrochloride	CATAPRES	Patch: 0.1, 0.2, 0.3 mg per day Tablets: 0.1, 0.2, 0.3 mg

DRUG PROFILE

Clonidine is used for treatment of high blood pressure. It acts on the central nervous system to slow your heart rate and relax your blood vessels. Clonidine is sometimes used in combination with other antihypertensive medicines, especially diuretics.

BEFORE USING THIS DRUG

Let your doctor know *IF*

You have ever had allergic reactions or other problems with ■ clonidine.

You have ever had any of the following medical problems: ■ heart or blood vessel disease ■ kidney disease ■ depression ■ Raynaud's syndrome (poor circulation in the fingers and toes).

You are taking any of the following medicines: ■ diuretics, beta-blockers (eg, propranolol, atenolol, metoprolol), or other medicines for high blood pressure ■ medicine for seizures ■ medicine for depression ■ antihistamines ■ medicine for hay fever, allergies, or colds ■ barbiturates ■ digoxin or digitalis (heart medicines) ■ medicine for Parkinson's disease ■ muscle relaxants ■ narcotics or other prescription pain-killers ■ sedatives ■ tranquilizers ■ sleep medicines.

SPECIAL RESTRICTIONS WHILE TAKING THIS DRUG

FOOD AND DRUG INTERACTIONS

Other Drugs	Do not take any other drugs, including over-the-counter (OTC) drugs, before checking with your doctor. OTC drugs for appetite suppression, asthma, colds, cough, hay fever, or sinus problems tend to increase blood pressure. Antihistamines, sleep medicines, tranquilizers, pain-killers, barbiturates, medicine for seizures, muscle relaxants, or anesthetics may worsen side effects of this drug such as dizziness, light-headedness, drowsiness, or faintness.
Foods and Beverages	Your doctor may prescribe a special low-salt diet, which you should follow carefully because it will help your medicine work more effectively. You may also be advised to go on a weight-reduction diet.
Alcohol	Drinking alcohol while taking this drug may worsen such side effects as dizziness, light-headedness, or fainting. Avoid alcohol unless your doctor has approved its use.

No special restrictions on smoking.

DAILY LIVING

Driving	This drug may cause drowsiness. Be careful when driving, operating household appliances, or doing any other tasks that require alertness until you know how this drug affects you.
Exertion and Exercise	Use caution when exercising, exerting yourself, or standing for long periods of time because this medicine may cause you to become dizzy, light-headed, or faint. If you feel any of these symptoms coming on, sit or lie down. It is a good idea not to get up too quickly from a reclining or sitting position.
Excessive Heat	Use caution during hot weather, especially when you exert yourself (see above).
Examinations or Tests	Many people have high blood pressure with no symptoms at all. It is important for you to keep all appointments with your doctor, even if you feel well, so that your blood pressure can be checked regularly. Periodic eye examinations may be required.
Other Precautions	Tell any doctor or dentist you consult that you are taking this medicine, especially if you will be undergoing any type of surgery.
Helpful Hints	If your mouth or throat feels dry, chewing sugarless gum or sucking ice chips or sugarless hard candy will help. If the patch begins to loosen, apply the adhesive overlay provided. Let your doctor know if you develop a rash or other skin problems while using the patch.

No special restrictions on exposure to excessive cold.

POSSIBLE SIDE EFFECTS

Although this list of adverse effects may seem somewhat intimidating, keep in mind that some are quite rare. Of course, should these or any other problems arise while you are on medication, it is always a good idea to consult your doctor.

IF YOU DEVELOP

difficulty in breathing ■ extreme dizziness or faintness ■ slow heartbeat ■ fast heartbeat or palpitations ■ tiredness or weakness ■ continuous vomiting

After you STOP taking this medicine: anxiety ■ chest pain ■ sleeplessness ■ nervousness ■ increased salivation ■ upset stomach ■ irregular or fast heartbeat ■ shaking of hands or fingers ■ stomach cramps ■ muscle pain ■ flushing ■ headache ■ increased sweating

WHAT TO DO

Urgent Get in touch with your doctor immediately.

swelling of feet, lower legs, or any other part of the body ■ cold fingertips or toes ■ depression ■ vivid dreams or nightmares ■ nervousness ■ hallucinations ■ fever

May be serious Check with your doctor as soon as possible.

dizziness, light-headedness, or fainting, especially when getting up from a reclining or sitting position ■ drowsiness ■ headache ■ bone pain ■ dry mouth, throat, or nasal passages ■ dry, itching, or burning eyes ■ upset stomach ■ nausea or vomiting ■ taste changes ■ weight gain ■ constipation ■ loss of appetite ■ sexual problems ■ sleep disturbances ■ tenderness of the salivary glands (around the ear) ■ paleness ■ rash, hives, itching, change in skin color, or other skin problems (especially with patch) ■ hair loss ■ urinary retention or difficulty in urination ■ need to urinate at night

If symptoms are disturbing or persist, let your doctor know.

STORAGE INSTRUCTIONS

Store in a cool, dark place (not in a bathroom medicine cabinet).

STOPPING OR INTERRUPTING THERAPY

Always make sure you have an adequate supply of clonidine on hand, especially for weekends, holidays, or if you travel. Since this drug does not cure high blood pressure but only controls it, you may have to take this medicine for the rest of your life. Do not stop taking it, even if you feel better. If you miss a dose, take it as soon as possible. Then continue on your regular schedule. If you miss two or more doses in a row, check with your doctor right away. *Abruptly stopping this medicine can cause your blood pressure to rise rapidly, which could be dangerous to your health.* Your doctor will advise you on how to reduce your dosage gradually before stopping completely.

SPECIAL CONSIDERATIONS FOR THOSE OVER SIXTY-FIVE

The side effects of drowsiness, dizziness, and fainting are more likely to occur in older patients who may be more susceptible to nervous system side effects (nightmares, difficulty sleeping, irritability) or beta-blockers.

CONDITION: **HYPERTENSION**

CATEGORY: **NONDIURETICS (CENTRAL ALPHA-AGONISTS)**

GENERIC (CHEMICAL) NAME	BRAND (TRADE) NAME	DOSAGE FORMS AND STRENGTHS
Guanabenz acetate	WYTENSIN	Tablets: 4, 8 mg

DRUG PROFILE

Guanabenz is used for treatment of high blood pressure. It acts on the central nervous system to reduce the passage of impulses along certain nerve pathways; this relaxes the blood vessels and makes blood flow easier. Guanabenz may be used in combination with other antihypertensive medicines, especially diuretics, for better control of hypertension.

BEFORE USING THIS DRUG

Let your doctor know *IF*

You have ever had allergic reactions or other problems with ■ guanabenz.

You have ever had any of the following medical problems: ■ heart or blood vessel disease ■ kidney disease ■ liver disease ■ stroke ■ significant depression.

You are taking any of the following medicines: ■ diuretics or other medicines for high blood pressure ■ medicine for seizures ■ barbiturates ■ antihistamines ■ medicine for hay fever, allergies, or colds ■ pain-killers (either prescription or over-the-counter [OTC]) ■ muscle relaxants ■ medicine for depression ■ sedatives ■ tranquilizers ■ sleep medicines.

SPECIAL RESTRICTIONS WHILE TAKING THIS DRUG

FOOD AND DRUG INTERACTIONS

Other Drugs	Do not take any other drugs, including over-the-counter (OTC) drugs, before checking with your doctor. OTC drugs for appetite suppression, asthma, colds, cough, hay fever, or sinus problems tend to increase blood pressure. Antihistamines, sleep medicines, tranquilizers, pain-killers, barbiturates, medicine for seizures, muscle relaxants, or anesthetics may worsen side effects of this drug such as dizziness, light-headedness, drowsiness, or fainting.
Foods and Beverages	Your doctor may prescribe a special low-salt diet, which you should follow carefully because it will help your medicine work more effectively. You may also be advised to go on a weight-reduction diet.
Alcohol	Drinking alcohol while taking this medicine may worsen such side effects as dizziness, light-headedness, or fainting. Avoid alcohol unless your doctor has approved its use.

No special restrictions on smoking.

DAILY LIVING

Driving	This drug often causes drowsiness. Be careful when driving, operating household appliances, or doing any other tasks that require alertness until you know how this drug affects you.
Examinations or Tests	Many people have high blood pressure with no symptoms at all. It is important for you to keep all appointments with your doctor, even if you feel well, so that your blood pressure can be checked regularly.
Other Precautions	Tell any doctor or dentist you consult that you are taking this medicine, especially if you will be undergoing any type of surgery.
Helpful Hints	If your mouth or throat feels dry, chewing sugarless gum or sucking ice chips or sugarless hard candy will help.

No special restrictions on exertion and exercise, sun exposure, or exposure to excessive heat or cold.

POSSIBLE SIDE EFFECTS

Although this list of adverse effects may seem somewhat intimidating, keep in mind that some are quite rare. Of course, should these or any other problems arise while you are on medication, it is always a good idea to consult your doctor.

IF YOU DEVELOP

severe dizziness or fainting ■ irritability ■ pinpoint pupils ■ slow heartbeat ■ tiredness or weakness ■ chest pain ■ irregular heartbeat or palpitations ■ swelling of hands and feet

WHAT TO DO

Urgent Get in touch with your doctor immediately.

After you STOP taking this medicine: anxiety ■ chest pain ■ flushing ■ headache ■ increased salivation ■ nausea or vomiting ■ shaking of hands or fingers ■ stomach cramps ■ sleep disturbances ■ increased sweating

dizziness ■ drowsiness ■ dry mouth ■ male impotence ■ headache ■ clumsiness ■ depression ■ sleep disturbances ■ blurred vision ■ difficulty in breathing ■ stuffy nose ■ ache in muscles or hands and feet ■ rash or itching ■ urinary frequency ■ male breast enlargement ■ nausea or vomiting ■ stomach pain or discomfort ■ constipation ■ taste changes

If symptoms are disturbing or persist, let your doctor know.

STORAGE INSTRUCTIONS

Store in a cool, dark place (not in a bathroom medicine cabinet).

STOPPING OR INTERRUPTING THERAPY

Since this drug does not cure high blood pressure but only controls it, you may have to take this medicine for the rest of your life. Do not stop taking it, even if you feel better. If you miss a dose, take it as soon as possible. If it is almost time for your next dose, skip the missed dose and resume your regular schedule. If you miss two or more doses in a row, check with your doctor right away. *Abruptly stopping this medicine can cause your blood pressure to rise rapidly, which could be dangerous to your health.* Your doctor will advise you on how to reduce your dosage gradually before stopping completely.

SPECIAL CONSIDERATIONS FOR THOSE OVER SIXTY-FIVE

Dizziness or fainting is more likely to occur in older people.

CONDITION: **HYPERTENSION**
CATEGORY: **NONDIURETICS (CENTRAL ALPHA-AGONISTS)**

GENERIC (CHEMICAL) NAME	BRAND (TRADE) NAME	DOSAGE FORMS AND STRENGTHS
Guanfacine hydrochloride	TENEX	Tablets: 1, 2 mg

DRUG PROFILE

Guanfacine may be used alone or in combination with a thiazide diuretic to treat high blood pressure. It acts on the central nervous system to decrease the passage of impulses along certain nerve pathways; this relaxes the blood vessels and lowers blood pressure.

BEFORE USING THIS DRUG

Let your doctor know *IF*

You have ever had allergic reactions or other problems with ■ guanfacine.

You have ever had any of the following medical problems: ■ heart attack or any other heart disease ■ stroke ■ depression ■ kidney disease ■ liver disease.

You are taking any of the following medicines: ■ medicine for seizures ■ antihistamines ■ medicine for hay fever, allergies, or colds ■ barbiturates ■ muscle relaxants ■ narcotics or other prescription pain-killers ■ sedatives ■ tranquilizers ■ sleep medicines.

SPECIAL RESTRICTIONS WHILE TAKING THIS DRUG

FOOD AND DRUG INTERACTIONS

Other Drugs	Do not take any other drugs, including over-the-counter (OTC) drugs, before checking with your doctor. OTC drugs for appetite suppression, asthma, colds, cough, hay fever, or sinus problems tend to increase blood pressure. Antihistamines, sleep medicines, tranquilizers, pain-killers, barbiturates, medicine for seizures, muscle relaxants, or anesthetics may worsen side effects of this drug such as dizziness, light-headedness, or faintness.
Foods and Beverages	Your doctor may prescribe a special low-salt diet, which you should follow carefully because it will help your medicine work more effectively. You may also be advised to go on a weight-reduction diet.
Alcohol	Drinking alcohol while taking this drug may worsen such side effects as dizziness, light-headedness, or fainting. Avoid alcohol unless your doctor has approved its use.

No special restrictions on smoking.

DAILY LIVING

Driving	This drug may cause drowsiness. Be careful when driving, operating household appliances, or doing any other tasks that require alertness until you know how this drug affects you.

Exertion and Exercise	Use caution when exercising, exerting yourself, or standing for long periods of time because this medicine may cause you to become dizzy, light-headed, or faint. If you feel any of these symptoms coming on, sit or lie down. It is a good idea not to get up too quickly from a reclining or sitting position.
Excessive Heat	Use caution during hot weather, especially when you exert yourself (see above).
Examinations or Tests	Many people have high blood pressure with no symptoms at all. It is important for you to keep all appointments with your doctor, even if you feel well, so that your blood pressure can be checked regularly.
Other Precautions	Tell any doctor or dentist you consult that you are taking this medicine, especially if you will be undergoing any type of surgery.
Helpful Hints	If your mouth or throat feels dry, chewing sugarless gum or sucking ice chips or sugarless hard candy will help. To reduce daytime drowsiness, take this medicine at bedtime. If you are taking more than one dose a day, take your last dose at bedtime.

No special restrictions on sun exposure or exposure to excessive cold.

POSSIBLE SIDE EFFECTS

Although this list of adverse effects may seem somewhat intimidating, keep in mind that some are quite rare. Of course, should these or any other problems arise while you are on medication, it is always a good idea to consult your doctor.

IF YOU DEVELOP	WHAT TO DO
shortness of breath ■ extreme drowsiness, dizziness, or fainting ■ slow heartbeat ■ palpitations ■ chest pain ■ muscle weakness ■ tiredness or weakness *After you STOP taking this medicine:* ■ chest pain ■ sleeplessness ■ nervousness ■ anxiety ■ fast or irregular heartbeat ■ shaking of hands or fingers ■ increased salivation ■ stomach cramps ■ nausea or vomiting ■ increased sweating ■ headache ■ restlessness	**Urgent** Get in touch with your doctor immediately.
depression ■ memory problems ■ confusion ■ leg cramps ■ bruising ■ rash	**May be serious** Check with your doctor as soon as possible.
dizziness, light-headedness, or fainting, especially when getting up from a reclining or sitting position ■ dry mouth ■ drowsiness ■ tiredness ■ headache ■ sleeplessness ■ nightmares ■ constipation ■ abdominal pain ■ diarrhea ■ nausea or vomiting ■ upset stomach ■ difficulty swallowing ■ decreased sex drive ■ male impotence ■ runny nose ■ taste changes ■ ringing in ears ■ vision disturbances ■ bloodshot eyes or other eye problems ■ itching or other skin problems ■ increased sweating ■ urinary incontinence ■ general ill feeling ■ tingling or burning sensations	If symptoms are disturbing or persist, let your doctor know.

STORAGE INSTRUCTIONS

Store in a cool, dark place (not in a bathroom medicine cabinet).

STOPPING OR INTERRUPTING THERAPY

Always make sure you have an adequate supply of guanfacine, especially for weekends, holidays, or if you travel. Since no drug can cure high blood pressure, but only control it, you may have to take this medicine for the rest of your life. Do not stop taking it, even if you feel better. If you miss a dose, take it as soon as possible, and then resume your regular schedule. If you miss taking guanfacine for two or more consecutive days, get in touch with your doctor.

SPECIAL CONSIDERATIONS FOR THOSE OVER SIXTY-FIVE

The side effects of drowsiness, dizziness, and fainting are more likely to occur in older people.

CONDITION: **HYPERTENSION**

CATEGORY: **NONDIURETICS (PERIPHERAL VASODILATORS)**

GENERIC (CHEMICAL) NAME	BRAND (TRADE) NAME	DOSAGE FORMS AND STRENGTHS
Hydralazine	APRESOLINE	Tablets: 10, 25, 50, 100 mg

DRUG PROFILE

Hydralazine is used to treat high blood pressure. It acts directly on the blood vessel walls to relax them. In addition, hydralazine increases the rate and output of the heart. Hydralazine is usually used in combination with other drugs.

BEFORE USING THIS DRUG

Let your doctor know *IF*

You have ever had allergic reactions or other problems with ■ hydralazine ■ tartrazine (FD&C Yellow Dye No. 5).

You have ever had any of the following medical problems: ■ heart or blood vessel disease, including stroke ■ migraine or other severe headaches ■ rheumatic mitral valve disease ■ kidney disease ■ liver disease ■ systemic lupus erythematosus.

You are taking any of the following medicines: ■ diuretics, beta-blockers (eg, propranolol, atenolol, metoprolol), or other medicines for high blood pressure ■ medicine for depression (within the last two weeks).

SPECIAL RESTRICTIONS WHILE TAKING THIS DRUG

FOOD AND DRUG INTERACTIONS

Other Drugs	Do not take any other drugs, including over-the-counter (OTC) drugs, before checking with your doctor. OTC drugs for appetite suppression, asthma, colds, cough, hay fever, or sinus problems tend to increase blood pressure.
Foods and Beverages	Your doctor may prescribe a special low-salt diet, which you should follow carefully because it will help your medicine work more effectively. You may also be advised to go on a weight-reduction diet.
Alcohol	Drinking alcohol while taking this medicine may worsen such side effects as dizziness, light-headedness, or fainting. Avoid alcohol unless your doctor has approved its use.

DAILY LIVING

Driving	This drug may cause dizziness, fainting, or weakness. Be careful when driving, operating household appliances, or doing any other tasks that require alertness until you know how this drug affects you.

Exertion and Exercise	Use caution when exercising, exerting yourself, or standing for long periods of time because this drug may cause you to become dizzy, light-headed, or faint. If you feel any of these symptoms coming on, sit or lie down. It is a good idea not to get up too quickly from a reclining or sitting position.
Excessive Heat	Use caution during hot weather, especially when you exert yourself (see above).
Examinations or Tests	Many people have high blood pressure with no symptoms at all. It is important for you to keep all appointments with your doctor, even if you feel well, so that your blood pressure can be checked regularly. Periodic blood tests are usually required.

No special restrictions on sun exposure or exposure to excessive cold.

POSSIBLE SIDE EFFECTS

Although this list of adverse effects may seem somewhat intimidating, keep in mind that some are quite rare. Of course, should these or any other problems arise while you are on medication, it is always a good idea to consult your doctor.

IF YOU DEVELOP

chest pain ■ very fast heartbeat ■ severe headache ■ severe dizziness ■ weakness ■ joint pain ■ numbness, tingling, pain, or weakness of hands or feet ■ sore throat or fever ■ chills ■ rash or itching ■ swelling of lymph glands, feet, or legs ■ weight gain ■ behavior changes

WHAT TO DO

Urgent Get in touch with your doctor immediately.

upset stomach ■ nausea or vomiting ■ headache ■ loss of appetite ■ palpitations ■ constipation or diarrhea ■ dizziness or light-headedness, especially when getting up from a reclining or sitting position ■ flushing ■ shortness of breath with exercise ■ stuffy nose ■ eye irritation ■ anxiety ■ difficulty in urination ■ muscle cramps ■ increased sweating ■ tremors ■ disorientation

If symptoms are disturbing or persist, let your doctor know.

STORAGE INSTRUCTIONS

Store in a cool, dark place (not in a bathroom medicine cabinet).

STOPPING OR INTERRUPTING THERAPY

Since this drug does not cure high blood pressure but only controls it, you may have to take this medicine for the rest of your life. Do not stop taking it, even if you feel better. If you miss a dose, take it as soon as possible. If it is almost time for your next dose, skip the missed dose and resume your regular schedule. Do not take two doses at the same time.

SPECIAL CONSIDERATIONS FOR THOSE OVER SIXTY-FIVE

Dizziness or light-headedness occurs more frequently in older people so regular checkups may be necessary.

CONDITION: **HYPERTENSION**

CATEGORY: **NONDIURETICS (PERIPHERAL VASODILATORS)**

GENERIC (CHEMICAL) NAME	BRAND (TRADE) NAME	DOSAGE FORMS AND STRENGTHS
Minoxidil	LONITEN	Tablets: 2.5, 10 mg

DRUG PROFILE

Minoxidil is used to treat severe high blood pressure that cannot be controlled by other medicines. A diuretic and a drug to slow heart rate (such as a beta-blocker or methyldopa) are usually taken along with minoxidil. Minoxidil acts by relaxing and enlarging small blood vessels to allow easier blood flow.

BEFORE USING THIS DRUG

Let your doctor know *IF*

You have ever had allergic reactions or other problems with ■ minoxidil.

You have ever had any of the following medical problems: ■ angina (chest pain) ■ heart or blood vessel disease, especially stroke or heart attack within the last month ■ kidney disease ■ pheochromocytoma (adrenal gland tumor).

You are taking any of the following medicines: ■ diuretics or other medicines for high blood pressure (especially guanethidine) ■ nitrates (medicine for chest pain) ■ calcium blockers (eg, diltiazem, nifedipine, verapamil).

SPECIAL RESTRICTIONS WHILE TAKING THIS DRUG

FOOD AND DRUG INTERACTIONS

Other Drugs	Do not take any other drugs, including over-the-counter (OTC) drugs, before checking with your doctor. OTC drugs for appetite suppression, asthma, colds, cough, hay fever, or sinus problems tend to increase blood pressure. Because this medicine causes fluid and salt retention and also rapid increases in heart rate, it is always necessary to take a diuretic and a beta-blocker or methyldopa at the same time to counteract these effects.
Foods and Beverages	Your doctor may prescribe a special low-salt diet, which you should follow carefully because it will help your medicine work more effectively. You may also be advised to go on a weight-reduction diet.

Alcohol	Drinking alcohol while taking this medicine may worsen such side effects as dizziness, light-headedness, and fainting. Avoid alcohol unless your doctor has approved its use.

DAILY LIVING

Examinations or Tests	Many people have high blood pressure with no symptoms at all. It is important for you to keep all appointments with your doctor, even if you feel well, so that your blood pressure can be checked regularly. Periodic blood and urine tests and electrocardiograms may be required.
	Your doctor may advise you to weigh yourself each morning after you get out of bed and record your weight (a weight gain of five pounds or more could indicate that the dose of your diuretic needs to be increased). Your doctor may also suggest that you monitor your blood pressure at home.
	Check your own resting pulse rate regularly, and call your doctor if it increases by twenty or more beats per minute above normal.
Helpful Hints	This drug may cause an increase in hair growth on the face, back, arms, legs, and scalp of both men and women. Shaving or using a hair remover may be helpful as a temporary measure. After treatment with this medicine has ended, the hair will stop growing, though it may take several months before the new hair growth disappears.

No special restrictions on driving, exertion and exercise, sun exposure, or exposure to excessive heat or cold.

POSSIBLE SIDE EFFECTS

Although this list of adverse effects may seem somewhat intimidating, keep in mind that some are quite rare. Of course, should these or any other problems arise while you are on medication, it is always a good idea to consult your doctor.

IF YOU DEVELOP	WHAT TO DO
irregular or fast heartbeat ■ rapid weight gain (five pounds or more) ■ chest pain ■ shortness of breath ■ dizziness, light-headedness, or fainting ■ swelling of face, hands, ankles, or stomach	**Urgent** Get in touch with your doctor immediately.
bloating ■ skin redness, itching, or rash ■ numbness, tingling, or coldness of hands, feet, or face	**May be serious** Check with your doctor as soon as possible.
increase in hair growth ■ female breast tenderness ■ male breast enlargement ■ headache ■ nausea	If symptoms are disturbing or persist, let your doctor know.

STORAGE INSTRUCTIONS

Store in a cool, dark place (not in a bathroom medicine cabinet).

STOPPING OR INTERRUPTING THERAPY

Since this drug does not cure high blood pressure but only controls it, you may have to take this medicine for the rest of your life. Do not stop taking it, even if you feel better. If you miss a dose, take it as soon as possible. If it is almost time for your next dose, skip the missed dose and resume your regular schedule. Do not take two doses at the same time.

SPECIAL CONSIDERATIONS FOR THOSE OVER SIXTY-FIVE

The side effects of dizziness, light-headedness, and fainting are more common in older people.

CONDITION: **HYPERTENSION**

CATEGORY: **NONDIURETICS (PERIPHERAL VASODILATORS)**

GENERIC (CHEMICAL) NAME	BRAND (TRADE) NAME	DOSAGE FORMS AND STRENGTHS
Prazosin hydrochloride	MINIPRESS	Capsules: 1, 2, 5 mg
Terazosin hydrochloride	HYTRIN	Tablets: 1, 2, 5, 10 mg
Doxazosin	CARDURA	Tablets: 1, 2, 4, 8 mg

DRUG PROFILE

Prazosin, terazosin and doxazosin are used for treatment of high blood pressure. They act on the blood vessel walls to relax them.

BEFORE USING THIS DRUG

Let your doctor know *IF*

You have ever had allergic reactions or other problems with ■ prazosin, terazosin or doxazosin.

You have ever had any of the following medical problems: ■ angina (chest pain) ■ heart disease ■ kidney disease.

You are taking any of the following medicines: ■ diuretics, beta-blockers (eg, propranolol, atenolol, metoprolol), calcium blockers (eg, diltiazem, nifedipine, verapamil) or other medicines for high blood pressure ■ aspirin, indomethacin or other medicine for arthritis ■ nitroglycerin or any other medicine for angina or heart problems.

SPECIAL RESTRICTIONS WHILE TAKING THIS DRUG

FOOD AND DRUG INTERACTIONS

Other Drugs	Do not take any other drugs, including over-the-counter (OTC) drugs, before checking with your doctor. OTC drugs for appetite suppression, asthma, colds, cough, hay fever, or sinus problems tend to increase blood pressure.
Foods and Beverages	Your doctor may prescribe a special low-salt diet, which you should follow carefully because it will help your medicine work more effectively. You may also be advised to go on a weight-reduction diet.
Alcohol	Drinking alcohol while taking this medicine may worsen such side effects as dizziness, light-headedness, or fainting. Avoid alcohol unless your doctor has approved its use.

No special restrictions on smoking.

DAILY LIVING

Driving	These drugs may cause dizziness or fainting, especially during the first twenty-four hours of use. Be careful when driving, operating household appliances, or doing any other tasks that require alertness until you know how this drug affects you.
Exertion and Exercise	Use caution when exercising, exerting yourself, or standing for long periods of time because this drug may cause you to become dizzy, light-headed, or faint. If you feel any of these symptoms coming on, sit or lie down. It is a good idea not to get up too quickly from a reclining or sitting position.

Excessive Heat	Use caution during hot weather, especially if you exert yourself (see above).
Examinations or Tests	Many people have high blood pressure with no symptoms at all. It is important for you to keep all appointments with your doctor, even if you feel well, so that your blood pressure can be checked regularly.
Other Precautions	You may feel light-headed or faint after the first dose of these drugs, when there has been a significant increase in your dose, or when you start taking another antihypertensive medicine. Your doctor may suggest that you take your first dose of prazosin, terazosin or doxazosin in his or her office or at bedtime after you lie down.

No special restrictions on sun exposure or exposure to excessive cold.

POSSIBLE SIDE EFFECTS

Although this list of adverse effects may seem somewhat intimidating, keep in mind that some are quite rare. Of course, should these or any other problems arise while you are on medication, it is always a good idea to consult your doctor.

IF YOU DEVELOP	WHAT TO DO
sudden fainting ■ chest pain ■ irregular heartbeat	**Urgent** Get in touch with your doctor immediately.
dizziness or light-headedness, especially when getting up from a reclining or sitting position ■ weakness ■ shortness of breath ■ swelling of legs or feet ■ weight gain ■ difficulty in urination ■ numbness or tingling in hands or feet	**May be serious** Check with your doctor as soon as possible.

drowsiness ■ lack of energy ■ headache ■ upset stomach or stomach pain ■ nausea or vomiting ■ constipation ■ diarrhea ■ rash or itching ■ hair loss ■ nervousness ■ urinary frequency or urinary incontinence ■ male impotence ■ blurred vision ■ ringing in the ears ■ red eyes ■ dry mouth ■ stuffy nose ■ increased sweating ■ joint pain ■ depression

If symptoms are disturbing or persist, let your doctor know.

STORAGE INSTRUCTIONS

Store in a cool, dark place (not in a bathroom medicine cabinet).

STOPPING OR INTERRUPTING THERAPY

Since these drugs do not cure high blood pressure but only control it, you may have to take this medicine for the rest of your life. Do not stop taking it, even if you feel better. If you miss a dose, take it as soon as possible. If it is almost time for your next dose, skip the missed dose and resume your regular schedule. Do not take two doses at the same time.

SPECIAL CONSIDERATIONS FOR THOSE OVER SIXTY-FIVE

The side effects of dizziness, light-headedness, and fainting are more common in older people.

CONDITION: **HYPERTENSION**

CATEGORY: **NONDIURETICS (SYMPATHOLYTICS)**

GENERIC (CHEMICAL) NAME	BRAND (TRADE) NAME	DOSAGE FORMS AND STRENGTHS
Reserpine	SERPASIL	Tablets: 0.1, 0.25 mg
Rauwolfia serpentina	RAUDIXIN	Tablets: 50, 100 mg

DRUG PROFILE

Reserpine and rauwolfia are used to treat high blood pressure. These medicines work by inhibiting nerves that constrict blood vessels, resulting in relaxation of blood vessels and easier blood flow. A similar action on nerves in the brain results in sedative and tranquilizing effects. These medicines may be used alone or with other antihypertensive medicines.

BEFORE USING THIS DRUG

Let your doctor know *IF*

You have ever had allergic reactions or other problems with ■ rauwolfia alkaloids ■ tartrazine (FD&C Yellow Dye No. 5).

You have ever had any of the following medical problems: ■ allergies, breathing problems, or asthma ■ breast cancer ■ epilepsy ■ gallstones ■ heart disease ■ stroke ■ kidney disease ■ depression ■ Parkinson's disease ■ pheochromocytoma (adrenal gland tumor) ■ stomach ulcer ■ ulcerative colitis.

You are taking any of the following medicines: ■ diuretics, beta-blockers (eg, propranolol, atenolol, metoprolol), or other medicine for high blood pressure ■ medicine for seizures ■ medicine for depression ■ antihistamines ■ medicine for hay fever, allergies, or colds ■ barbiturates ■ digoxin or digitalis (heart medicines) ▢ muscle relaxants ■ narcotics or other prescription pain-killers ■ any medicine containing phenylephrine.

■ quinidine (medicine for abnormal heart rhythms) ■ sedatives ■ tranquilizers ■ sleep medicines ■ levodopa (medicine for Parkinson's disease).

You are receiving electroconvulsive therapy.

SPECIAL RESTRICTIONS WHILE TAKING THIS DRUG

FOOD AND DRUG INTERACTIONS

Other Drugs	Do not take any other drugs, including over-the-counter (OTC) drugs, before checking with your doctor. OTC drugs for appetite suppression, asthma, colds, cough, hay fever, or sinus problems tend to increase blood pressure. Antihistamines, sleep medicines, tranquilizers, pain-killers, barbiturates, medicine for seizures, muscle relaxants, or anesthetics worsen such side effects of this drug as drowsiness.
Foods and Beverages	Your doctor may prescribe a special low-salt diet, which you should follow carefully because it will help your medicine work more effectively. A weight-reduction diet may also be advised.
Alcohol	Drinking alcohol while taking this medicine may worsen such side effects as dizziness or drowsiness. Avoid alcohol unless your doctor has approved its use.

No special restrictions on smoking.

DAILY LIVING

Driving	This drug may cause drowsiness, especially when you first begin to take it or when your dose is increased. Be careful when driving, operating household appliances, or doing any other tasks that require alertness until you know how this drug affects you.

Examinations or Tests	Many people have high blood pressure with no symptoms at all. It is important for you to keep all appointments with your doctor, even if you feel well, so that your blood pressure can be checked regularly.
Other Precautions	Tell any doctor or dentist you consult that you are taking this drug, especially if you will be undergoing any type of surgery.
Helpful Hints	If your mouth or throat feels dry, chewing sugarless gum or sucking ice chips or sugarless hard candy will help. Your nose may also feel dry and stuffy; check with your doctor before using nasal decongestants.
	If this medicine upsets your stomach, taking it with meals, milk, or snacks should help.

No special restrictions on exertion and exercise, sun exposure, or exposure to excessive heat or cold.

POSSIBLE SIDE EFFECTS

Although this list of adverse effects may seem somewhat intimidating, keep in mind that some are quite rare. Of course, should these or any other problems arise while you are on medication, it is always a good idea to consult your doctor.

IF YOU DEVELOP	WHAT TO DO
drowsiness or faintness ■ mood changes ■ headache ■ male impotence ■ diminished sex drive ■ lack of energy or weakness ■ depression ■ sleep disturbances or nightmares ■ nervousness or anxiety ■ seizures ■ flushing or warm feeling ■ pinpoint pupils ■ very slow pulse ■ black, tarry stools ■ vomiting, with blood *After you STOP taking reserpine or rauwolfia:* dizziness or drowsiness ■ weakness ■ irregular heartbeat ■ anxiety ■ mood changes ■ sleep disturbances ■ male impotence ■ diminished sex drive	**Urgent** Get in touch with your doctor immediately.
chest pain ■ irregular or slow heartbeat ■ shortness of breath ■ stiffness ■ leg pain ■ stomach cramps or pain ■ diarrhea ■ nausea or vomiting ■ shaking of hands or fingers ■ pain or difficulty in urination ■ rash or itching ■ bleeding (including nosebleed) or bruising ■ blurred vision or tearing ■ drooping eyelids	**May be serious** Check with your doctor as soon as possible.
upset stomach ■ dry mouth or increased salivation ■ increased appetite or loss of appetite ■ dizziness, especially when getting up from a reclining or sitting position ■ stuffy nose ■ swelling of feet or legs ■ red eyes ■ male breast enlargement ■ female breast swelling ■ hearing disturbances	If symptoms are disturbing or persist, let your doctor know.

STORAGE INSTRUCTIONS

Store in a cool, dark place (not in a bathroom medicine cabinet).

STOPPING OR INTERRUPTING THERAPY

Since this drug does not cure high blood pressure but only controls it, you may have to take this medicine for the rest of your life. Do not stop taking it, even if you feel better. If you miss a dose, skip the missed dose and resume your regular schedule. Do not take two doses at the same time.

SPECIAL CONSIDERATIONS FOR THOSE OVER SIXTY-FIVE

Side effects such as dizziness, drowsiness, and swelling from water gain are more likely to occur in older people. Also, this drug commonly causes depression, sleep disturbances, and diminished sex drive.

CONDITION: **HYPERTENSION**

CATEGORY: **NONDIURETICS (SYMPATHOLYTICS)**

GENERIC (CHEMICAL) NAME	BRAND (TRADE) NAME	DOSAGE FORMS AND STRENGTHS
Guanethidine	ISMELIN	Tablets: 10, 25 mg

DRUG PROFILE

Guanethidine is generally used for treatment of moderate or severe high blood pressure that cannot be controlled by other medicines. This medicine works by inhibiting nerves that constrict blood vessels, resulting in relaxation of blood vessels and easier blood flow. Guanethidine is usually used with other antihypertensive medicines.

BEFORE USING THIS DRUG

Let your doctor know *IF*

You have ever had allergic reactions or other problems with ■ guanethidine.

You have ever had any of the following medical problems: ■ asthma ■ diabetes ■ diarrhea ■ fever ■ heart or blood vessel disease, including heart attack, angina, or stroke ■ kidney disease ■ liver disease ■ pheochromocytoma (adrenal gland tumor) ■ stomach ulcer.

You are taking any of the following medicines: ■ diuretics or other medicines for high blood pressure ■ amphetamines ■ medicine for depression ■ barbiturates ■ digoxin or digitalis (heart medicines) ■ medicine for asthma ■ medicine for diabetes ■ narcotics or other prescription pain-killers ■ weight-reduction medicine ■ tranquilizers ■ decongestants ■ levodopa (medicine for Parkinson's disease) ■ medicine for nausea.

SPECIAL RESTRICTIONS WHILE TAKING THIS DRUG

FOOD AND DRUG INTERACTIONS

Other Drugs	Do not take any other drugs, including over-the-counter (OTC) drugs, before checking with your doctor. OTC drugs for appetite suppression, asthma, colds, cough, hay fever, or sinus problems tend to increase blood pressure. Use of reserpine or rauwolfia at the same time as guanethidine may cause fainting, slow heartbeat, and depression. The blood pressure–lowering effect of guanethidine may be reduced by amphetaminelike drugs, stimulants, antidepressants, and tranquilizers.
Foods and Beverages	Your doctor may prescribe a special low-salt diet, which you should follow carefully because it will help your medicine work more effectively. A weight-reduction diet may also be advised.
Alcohol	Drinking alcohol while taking this medicine may worsen such side effects as dizziness, light-headedness, or fainting. Avoid alcohol unless your doctor has approved its use.

No special restrictions on smoking.

DAILY LIVING

Exertion and Exercise	Use caution when exercising, exerting yourself, or standing for long periods of time because this medicine may cause you to become dizzy, light-headed, or faint. If you feel any of these symptoms coming on, sit or lie down. It is a good idea not to get up too quickly from a reclining or sitting position.
Excessive Heat	Use caution during hot weather, especially if you exert yourself (see above).

Examinations or Tests	Many people have high blood pressure with no symptoms at all. It is important for you to keep all appointments with your doctor, even if you feel well, so that your blood pressure can be checked regularly.
Other Precautions	Tell any doctor or dentist you consult that you are taking this medicine, especially if you will be undergoing any type of surgery.

No special restrictions on driving, sun exposure, or exposure to excessive cold.

POSSIBLE SIDE EFFECTS

Although this list of adverse effects may seem somewhat intimidating, keep in mind that some are quite rare. Of course, should these or any other problems arise while you are on medication, it is always a good idea to consult your doctor.

IF YOU DEVELOP	WHAT TO DO
extreme dizziness, light-headedness, or fainting, especially when getting up from a reclining or sitting position	**Urgent** Get in touch with your doctor immediately.
fever ■ swelling of feet or lower legs ■ chest pain ■ shortness of breath ■ weight gain ■ headache	**May be serious** Get in touch with your doctor as soon as possible.
diarrhea or increase in bowel movements ■ depression ■ difficulty in ejaculation (in males) ■ stuffy nose ■ weakness or tiredness ■ slow heartbeat ■ blurred vision ■ drooping eyelids ■ dry mouth ■ scalp hair loss ■ muscle pain or tremors ■ nausea or vomiting ■ loss of appetite ■ constipation ■ need to urinate at night or other urinary problems ■ rash ■ tenderness of the salivary glands (around the ear)	If symptoms are disturbing or persist, let your doctor know.

STORAGE INSTRUCTIONS

Store in a cool, dark place (not in a bathroom medicine cabinet).

STOPPING OR INTERRUPTING THERAPY

Since this drug does not cure high blood pressure but only controls it, you may have to take this medicine for the rest of your life. Do not stop taking it, even if you feel better. If you miss a dose, take it as soon as possible. If it is almost time for your next dose, skip the missed dose and resume your regular schedule. Do not take two doses at the same time.

SPECIAL CONSIDERATIONS FOR THOSE OVER SIXTY-FIVE

The side effects of dizziness, light-headedness, or fainting are more likely to occur and to be more severe in older people.

CONDITION: **HYPERTENSION**

CATEGORY: **ANGIOTENSIN-CONVERTING ENZYME (ACE) INHIBITORS**

GENERIC (CHEMICAL) NAME	BRAND (TRADE) NAME	DOSAGE FORMS AND STRENGTHS
Benazepril	LOTENSIN	Tablets: 5, 10, 20, 40 mg
Captopril	CAPOTEN	Tablets: 12.5, 25, 50, 100 mg
Enalapril	VASOTEC	Tablets: 2.5, 5, 10, 20 mg
Fosinopril	MONOPRIL	Tablets: 10, 20 mg
Lisinopril	PRINIVIL ZESTRIL	Tablets: 5, 10, 20, 40 mg Tablets: 5, 10, 20, 40 mg

Quinapril	ACCUPRIL	Tablets: 5, 10, 20 mg
Ramipril	ALTACE	Capsules: 1.25, 2.5, 5, 10 mg

DRUG PROFILE

ACE inhibitors are used to treat high blood pressure. These drugs interrupt a chain of biochemical events that lead to constriction (tightening) of the blood vessels. Blocking this process lets the blood vessels relax, lowers blood pressure, and increases the flow of blood and oxygen to the heart.

Captopril and enalapril are used to treat congestive heart failure as well. Relaxing the blood vessels reduces the congestion of blood in the lungs, lessens the load on the heart, and improves the blood flow to the kidneys, facilitating the elimination of sodium and water. Long-term use of these drugs improves exercise tolerance because blood flow to the muscle is increased.

BEFORE USING THIS DRUG

Let your doctor know *IF*

You have ever had allergic reactions or other problems with these medicines.

You have ever had any of the following medical problems: ■ kidney disease ■ systemic lupus erythematosus ■ heart or blood vessel disease ■ high blood potassium levels.

You are taking any of the following medicines: ■ diuretics or other medicines for high blood pressure ■ potassium-containing medicines or supplements ■ medicine for angina ■ corticosteroids ■ aspirin, indomethacin or other medicine for arthritis (nonsteroidal anti-inflammatory drugs) ■ lithium.

With captopril only: ■ medicine for cancer ■ medicine to prevent rejection of transplanted organs.

You are on a low-salt diet.

SPECIAL INSTRUCTIONS WHILE TAKING THIS DRUG

FOOD AND DRUG INTERACTIONS

Other Drugs	Do not take any other drugs, including over-the-counter (OTC) drugs, before checking with your doctor. Some OTC drugs for appetite suppression, asthma, colds, cough, hay fever, or sinus problems tend to increase blood pressure. If you are taking captopril or enalapril for congestive heart failure, it is especially important to let your doctor know all other drugs you are taking, especially diuretics.
Foods and Beverages	Your doctor may prescribe a special low-salt diet, which you should follow carefully because it will help your medicine work more effectively. You may also be advised to go on a weight-reduction diet. If you are taking captopril or enalapril for congestive heart failure, it is especially important to discuss your sodium intake with your doctor. These drugs may cause a build-up of the mineral potassium in your body. Let your doctor know if you are using salt substitutes because many of these products are high in potassium chloride and may increase your blood-potassium level to dangerous levels.
Helpful Hints	*For captopril only:* This medicine should be taken one hour before meals.

No special restrictions on alcohol use or smoking.

DAILY LIVING

Exertion and Exercise	These drugs increase your risk of becoming dehydrated. Be careful during strenuous exercise; make

sure you drink plenty of liquids to make up for water loss by perspiration.

If you are taking captopril or enalapril for congestive heart failure, avoid a sudden increase in physical activity, even if you feel better.

Sun Exposure/ Excessive Heat	Use caution during hot weather, especially when you are exercising or exerting yourself (see above). While taking captopril, your skin may become more sensitive to sunlight and more likely to develop a sunburn. It is a good idea to avoid too much sun, especially if you burn easily. Apply a sunscreen to exposed skin surfaces before going outdoors.
Examinations or Tests	Many people have high blood pressure with no symptoms at all. Whether you are being treated for heart failure or for high blood pressure, it is important for you to keep all appointments with your doctor so that your progress can be checked. Periodic blood and urine tests may be required before and during therapy.
Other Precautions	Tell any doctor or dentist you consult that you are taking this medicine, especially if you will be undergoing any type of surgery.

If you should become sick and have severe or prolonged vomiting or diarrhea, let your doctor know, as you may be at risk of becoming dehydrated.

If you feel light-headed while taking this medicine, let your doctor know. If you actually faint, stop taking the medicine until you have checked with your doctor.

If you are taking captopril, check with your doctor if you become ill with flulike symptoms, such as cough, fever, or body aches; lose your appetite; vomit; or have diarrhea, especially if you are also taking a diuretic. This may cause you to lose a great deal of fluid. |

No special restrictions on driving or exposure to excessive cold.

POSSIBLE SIDE EFFECTS

Although this list of adverse effects may seem somewhat intimidating, keep in mind that some are quite rare. Of course, should these or any other problems arise while you are on medication, it is always a good idea to consult your doctor.

IF YOU DEVELOP

sore throat or fever ■ cough ■ severe dizziness or light-headedness ■ swelling of face, mouth, vocal cords, fingers, ankles, or feet ■ hoarseness ■ fainting (if you faint, stop taking the drug until you have checked with your doctor)

WHAT TO DO

Urgent Get in touch with your doctor immediately.

---

irregular heartbeat ■ chest pain

With captopril only: rapid heartbeat ■ cold fingers or toes ■ flushing or paleness

May be serious Check with your doctor as soon as possible.

---

light-headedness or faintness, especially when getting up from a reclining or sitting position ■ rash or itching ■ headache ■ dizziness ■ nausea ■ increased sweating ■ sleeplessness ■ nervousness ■ drowsiness ■ tingling sensation ■ stomach pain ■ tiredness or weakness ■ diarrhea

With captopril only: increased skin sensitivity to sunlight ■ taste changes ■ loss of appetite ■ weight loss ■ hair loss ■ constipation ■ mouth sores ■ vomiting

With enalapril only: indigestion ■ muscle cramps ■ male impotence

If symptoms are disturbing or persist, let your doctor know.

STORAGE INSTRUCTIONS

Store in a cool, dark place (not in a bathroom medicine cabinet).

STOPPING OR INTERRUPTING THERAPY

Do not stop taking the drug prescribed for you, even if you feel better. If you are being treated for hypertension, you may have to take it for the rest of your life, as these drugs do not cure high blood pressure but only control it. If you miss a dose, take it as soon as possible. If it is almost time for your next dose, skip the missed dose and resume your regular schedule. Do not take two doses at the same time.

SPECIAL CONSIDERATIONS FOR THOSE OVER SIXTY-FIVE

None.

CONDITION: **HYPERTENSION**

CATEGORY: **CALCIUM BLOCKERS**

GENERIC (CHEMICAL) NAME	BRAND (TRADE) NAME	DOSAGE FORMS AND STRENGTHS
Bepridil	VASCOR	Tablets: 200, 300, 400 mg
Diltiazem	CARDIZEM SR	Sustained-release capsules: 60, 90, 120 mg
Felodipine	PLENDIL	Sustained-release tablets: 5, 10 mg
Isradipine	DYNACIRC	Capsules: 2.5, 5 mg
Nicardipine	CARDENE	Capsules: 20, 30 mg

Nifedipine	PROCARDIA XL	Extended-release tablets: 30, 60, 90 mg
Verapamil	CALAN	Tablets: 40, 80, 120 mg
	CALAN SR	Controlled-release tablets: 120, 180, 240 mg
	ISOPTIN	Tablets: 40, 80, 120 mg
	ISOPTIN SR	Controlled-release tablets: 180, 240 mg
	VERELAN	Sustained-release capsules: 120, 240 mg

DRUG PROFILE

The calcium blockers are used to relieve and control angina pectoris (chest pain) and to treat high blood pressure. Calcium is needed for muscle cells to contract; by decreasing the passage of calcium into the muscle cells, these drugs relax the blood vessels and heart muscle. This increases the supply of blood and oxygen to the heart, reduces its workload, and prevents spasms of the blood vessels of the heart. Other antianginal drugs can be used along with a calcium blocker, if necessary. Calcium blockers lower blood pressure; if you are taking another antihypertensive agent, its dosage may need to be lowered.

For complete information on these drugs, see pages 169–189.

CONDITION: **HYPERTENSION**

CATEGORY: **DIURETIC-NONDIURETIC COMBINATIONS**

GENERIC (CHEMICAL) NAME	BRAND (TRADE) NAME	DOSAGE FORMS AND STRENGTHS
Atenolol and chlorthalidone	TENORETIC	Tablets: 50 mg atenolol and 25 mg chlorthalidone; 100 mg atenolol and 25 mg chlorthalidone

Labetalol hydrochloride and hydrochlorothiazide	NORMOZIDE TRANDATE HCT	Tablets: 100 mg labetalol hydrochloride and 25 mg hydrochlorothiazide; 200 mg labetalol and 25 mg hydrochlorothiazide; 300 mg labetalol and 25 mg hydrochlorothiazide
Metoprolol tartrate and hydrochlorothiazide	LOPRESSOR HCT	Tablets: 50 mg metoprolol tartrate and 25 mg hydrochlorothiazide; 100 mg metoprolol tartrate and 25 mg hydrochlorothiazide; 100 mg metoprolol tartrate and 50 mg hydrochlorothiazide
Nadolol and bendroflumethiazide	CORZIDE	Tablets: 40 mg nadolol and 5 mg bendroflumethiazide; 80 mg nadolol and 5 mg bendroflumethiazide
Propranolol hydrochloride and hydrochlorothiazide	INDERIDE	Tablets: 40 mg propranolol hydrochloride and 25 mg hydrochlorothiazide; 80 mg propranolol hydrochloride and 25 mg hydrochlorothiazide

	INDERIDE LA	Capsules (long-acting): 80 mg propranolol hydrochloride and 50 mg hydrochloro- thiazide; 120 mg propranolol hydrochloride and 50 mg hydrochlorothiazide; 160 mg propranolol hydrochloride and 50 mg hydrochloro- thiazide
Timolol maleate and hydrochlorothiazide	TIMOLIDE	Tablets: 10 mg timolol maleate and 25 mg hydrochlorothiazide

DRUG PROFILE

This medicine is a combination of two kinds of drugs that lower blood pressure, and is used for maintenance therapy after your doctor has adjusted the level of your blood pressure with other medications. By blocking certain nerve impulses, beta-blockers relax blood vessels, increase the supply of blood and oxygen to the heart, and reduce the workload and pumping rate of the heart (see Beta-blockers, pages 59–64). Thiazide diuretics work by increasing the amount of salt and water you eliminate through urination (see Thiazide Diuretics on pages 23–28). Other drugs that lower blood pressure may be added to this combination drug if necessary.

BEFORE USING THIS DRUG

Let your doctor know *IF*

You have ever had allergic reactions or other problems with ■ any of the thiazide or thiazide-type diuretics ■ beta-blockers ■ sulfonamides (sulfa drugs).

You have ever had any of the following medical problems: ■ allergies ■ hay fever, hives, asthma, or eczema ■ bronchitis or emphysema ■ slow heartbeat ■ diabetes ■ any heart or blood vessel disease ■ kidney disease ■ liver disease ■ thyroid disease ■ Raynaud's syndrome (poor circulation in the fingers and toes) ■ glaucoma ■ myasthenia gravis ■ hypoglycemia (low blood sugar) ■ pheochromocytoma (adrenal gland tumor) ■ gout ■ systemic lupus erythematosus ■ disease of the pancreas.

You are taking any of the following medicines; ■ any other medicines for high blood pressure ■ medicine for asthma ■ aminophylline, epinephrine, ephedrine, norepinephrine, isoproterenol, dyphylline, oxtriphylline, theophylline, or phenylephrine (vasopressor drugs) ■ calcium blockers (eg, diltiazem, nifedipine, verapamil) ■ medicine for depression ■ cimetidine (medicine for ulcers) ■ heart medicine ■ medicine for abnormal heart rhythm ■ medicine for glaucoma ■ aspirin, indomethacin, or other arthritis medicines (nonsteroidal anti-inflammatory drugs) ■ medicine for diabetes ■ decongestants ■ medicine for colds ■ medicine for nausea ■ tranquilizers ■ corticosteroids or corticotropin (ACTH) ■ medicine for high cholesterol ■ medicine for gout ■ lithium (medicine for manic-depression) ■ methenamine (medicine to prevent urinary tract infections) ■ anticoagulants (blood thinners) ■ tetracycline ■ calcium-containing medicine or supplements ■ barbiturates ■ sodium bicarbonate.

SPECIAL RESTRICTIONS WHILE TAKING THIS DRUG

FOOD AND DRUG INTERACTIONS

Other Drugs	Do not take any other drugs, including over-the-counter (OTC) drugs, before checking with your doctor. OTC drugs for appetite suppression, asthma, colds, cough, hay fever, or sinus problems tend to increase blood pressure.
	Some medicines used for pain and/or arthritis (aspirin, indomethacin, and phenylbutazone, for example) may hamper the action of the beta-blocker-thiazide combination.
	If you are also taking cholestyramine or colestipol (medicine for high cholesterol), take your beta-blocker-thiazide drug at least one hour before taking these medicines.
Foods and Beverages	Your doctor may prescribe a special low-salt diet, which you should follow carefully because it will help your medicine work more effectively.

This medicine may cause your body to lose large amounts of the mineral potassium. Your doctor may give you special instructions about eating foods or drinking beverages that have a high potassium content (such as bananas, dates, and figs, citrus fruit juices), taking a potassium supplement, or using salt substitutes.

Alcohol	Alcohol may worsen side effects of this medicine such as dizziness, light-headedness, or fainting. Be careful about how much alcohol you consume.

No special restrictions on smoking.

DAILY LIVING

Driving	This drug may cause drowsiness. Be careful when driving, operating household appliances, or doing any other tasks that require alertness until you know how this drug affects you.
Exertion and Exercise	Since chest pain from exercise or exertion may be reduced or prevented by this medicine, you may be tempted to overwork yourself. Discuss with your doctor how much exercise is safe for you. Be especially careful when you exercise during hot weather or if you must stand for long periods of time, since this drug may cause side effects such as dizziness, light-headedness, and fainting.
Sun Exposure/ Excessive Heat	Your skin may become more sensitive to sunlight and more likely to develop a sunburn while you are taking this medicine. It is a good idea to avoid too much sun, especially if you burn easily. Apply a sunscreen to exposed skin surfaces before going outdoors. Use caution during hot weather or while taking

saunas or hot baths, since excessive sweating while taking this medicine may cause you to become dehydrated and to feel drowsy or faint.

Excessive Cold	You may become more sensitive to cold temperatures while taking this medicine. Dress warmly—protecting your skin, fingers, and toes—and use caution during prolonged exposure to cold.
Examinations or Tests	*Check your pulse regularly.* If it is much slower than your usual rate or less than 50 beats per minute, call your doctor. Many people have high blood pressure with no symptoms at all. It is important for you to keep all appointments with your doctor, even if you feel well, so that your blood pressure can be checked regularly. Periodic blood and urine tests may be required.
Other Precautions	If you have diabetes, be aware that this medicine may raise blood-sugar levels. If you notice any change in the sugar levels in your blood or urine, let your doctor know.

Tell any doctor or dentist you consult that you are taking this medicine, especially if you will be undergoing any type of surgery.

When first starting on this type of medicine, you may feel tired and will probably experience both greater volume and frequency of urination. Until your individual pattern of urination has been established with the medicine, it may be wise to carefully time any activity that will put you out of convenient reach of a bathroom, such as bus or car travel. In addition, taking a diuretic at bedtime will probably interfere with sleep; you should discuss your dosage schedule with your doctor.

Check with your doctor if you become ill with flulike symptoms, such as cough, fever, or body aches; lose your appetite; vomit; or have diarrhea. This may cause you to lose a great deal of fluid, making it important not to take this medicine for one or more doses.

Following mild fluid losses, some older people may feel weak or dizzy when standing or getting up.

Helpful Hints	Swallow the controlled-release tablets or capsules whole—do not break, crush, or chew them.

POSSIBLE SIDE EFFECTS

Although this list of adverse effects may seem somewhat intimidating, keep in mind that some are quite rare. Of course, should these or any other problems arise while you are on medication, it is always a good idea to consult your doctor.

IF YOU DEVELOP

chest pain ∎ palpitations ∎ irregular heartbeat ∎ extremely slow heartbeat ∎ swelling of face, ankles, feet, or lower legs ∎ difficulty in breathing, shortness of breath, or coughing ∎ asthma or wheezing ∎ restlessness, sweating, nervousness, and irritability (if you are a thyroid patient) ∎ weight gain ∎ severe or continuing vomiting or diarrhea ∎ confusion ∎ depression ∎ severe stomach pain or cramps ∎ joint or side pain ∎ weak pulse ∎ decreased urination ∎ extreme weakness ∎ sore throat or fever ∎ rash or hives ∎ bleeding or bruising ∎ yellowing of eyes or skin

After you STOP taking this medicine: ∎ chest pain ∎ fast or irregular heartbeat ∎ general ill feeling ∎ headache ∎ shortness of breath ∎ shaking of hands or fingers ∎ increased sweating

WHAT TO DO

Urgent Get in touch with your doctor immediately.

dizziness, light-headedness, or confusion upon getting up from a reclining or sitting position ■ cold hands or feet ■ dry mouth ■ increased thirst ■ muscle cramps or pain ■ severe skin sensitivity to light	**May be serious** Check with your doctor as soon as possible.
diarrhea or constipation ■ upset stomach, gas or bloating ■ taste changes (with labetalol) ■ nausea or vomiting ■ change in appetite ■ drowsiness ■ difficulty in concentrating ■ dry skin or eyes ■ hair loss ■ abnormal vision ■ eye problems ■ yellowing of vision ■ numbness or tingling in fingers or toes ■ leg cramps ■ urinary problems ■ anxiety ■ disorientation ■ impotence or diminished sex drive ■ hallucinations ■ nightmares or vivid dreams ■ sleep disturbances ■ headache ■ earache ■ ringing in ears ■ behavior change ■ slurred speech ■ cough ■ hoarseness ■ tenderness of salivary glands	If symptoms are disturbing or persist, let your doctor know.

STORAGE INSTRUCTIONS

Store in a cool, dark place (not in a bathroom medicine cabinet).

STOPPING OR INTERRUPTING THERAPY

Since this drug does not cure high blood pressure but only controls it, you may have to take this medicine for the rest of your life. Do not stop taking it, even if you feel better. *Suddenly stopping your medicine may worsen your medical problem.* Your doctor can advise you on how to discontinue therapy gradually. *Always carry a supply of your medicine with you.* Also, make sure you have a supply to last over holiday periods. If you miss a dose, take the missed dose as soon as possible. If the next scheduled dose is within four hours (or within eight hours if you are taking atenolol and chlorothalidone, labetalol and hydrochlorothiazide, nadolol and bendroflumethiazide, or extended-release propranolol and hydrochlorothiazide), skip the missed dose and resume your regular schedule. Do not take two doses at the same time.

SPECIAL CONSIDERATIONS FOR THOSE OVER SIXTY-FIVE

Older people may be especially prone to such side effects as confusion, weakness, clumsiness, or dizziness when getting up from a reclining or sitting position, especially when first starting on this drug. Those who develop such symptoms should get in touch with a doctor, who may want to measure the amount of medicine that is reaching the bloodstream.

CONDITION: **HYPERTENSION**

CATEGORY: **DIURETIC-NONDIURETIC COMBINATIONS**

GENERIC (CHEMICAL) NAME	BRAND (TRADE) NAME	DOSAGE FORMS AND STRENGTHS
Captopril and hydrochlorothiazide	CAPOZIDE	Tablets: 25 mg captopril and 15 mg hydrochlorothiazide; 25 mg captopril and 25 mg hydrochlorothiazide; 50 mg captopril and 15 mg hydrochlorothiazide; 50 mg captopril and 25 mg hydrochlorothiazide
Enalapril maleate and hydrochlorothiazide	VASERETIC	Tablets: 10 mg enalapril maleate and 25 mg hydrochlorothiazide
Lisinopril and hydrochlorothiazide	PRINZIDE	Tablets: 20 mg lisinopril and 12.5 mg hydrochlorothiazide; 20 mg lisinopril and 25 mg hydrochlorothiazide
	ZESTORETIC	Tablets: 20 mg lisinopril and 12.5 mg hydrochlorothiazide; 20 mg lisinopril and 25 mg hydrochlorothiazide

DRUG PROFILE

These medicines are a combination of two kinds of drugs that lower blood pressure. Captopril, enalapril, and lisinopril work by relaxing the blood vessels, which increases the flow of blood and oxygen to the heart (see Captopril, Enalapril, and Lisinopril on pages 98–103). Hydrochlorothiazide is a thiazide diuretic that increases the amount of salt and water you eliminate through urination (see Thiazide Diuretics on pages 23–28).

BEFORE USING THIS DRUG

Let your doctor know *IF*

You have ever had allergic reactions or other problems with ■ captopril ■ enalapril ■ lisinopril ■ any of the thiazide diuretics ■ sulfonamides (sulfa drugs).

You have ever had any of the following medical problems: ■ kidney disease ■ liver disease ■ systemic lupus erythematosus ■ heart or blood vessel disease ■ high blood-potassium levels ■ diabetes ■ gout ■ disease of the pancreas ■ allergies ■ asthma ■ high blood-calcium levels ■ bone marrow problems ■ stroke.

You are taking any of the following medicines: ■ aspirin, indomethacin or other medicine for arthritis ■ medicine for gout ■ corticosteroids or corticotropin (ACTH) ■ potassium-containing medicine or supplements ■ medicine for angina ■ medicine for high cholesterol ■ medicine for diabetes ■ digoxin or digitalis (heart medicines) ■ lithium (medicine for manic-depression) ■ diuretics ■ medicine for high blood pressure ■ methenamine (medicine to prevent urinary tract infections) ■ anticoagulants (blood thinners) ■ tetracycline ■ estrogens (female hormones) ■ amiodarone (medicine for abnormal heart rhythms) ■ calcium-containing medicine or supplements ■ medicine for seizures ■ sleep medicines ■ narcotics or other prescription pain-killers ■ tranquilizers ■ barbiturates ■ muscle relaxants ■ salt substitutes.

With captopril-hydrochlorothiazide only: ■ medicine for cancer ■ medicine to prevent rejection of transplanted organs.

You are on a low-salt diet.

SPECIAL RESTRICTIONS WHILE TAKING THIS DRUG

FOOD AND DRUG INTERACTIONS

Other Drugs	Do not take any other drugs, including over-the-counter (OTC) drugs, before checking with your doctor. Some OTC drugs for appetite suppression, asthma, colds, cough, hay fever, or sinus problems tend to increase blood pressure. If you are also taking cholestyramine or colestipol (medicine for high cholesterol), take these combination preparations at least one hour before taking these medicines.
Foods and Beverages	Your doctor may prescribe a special low-salt diet, which you should follow carefully because it will help your medicine work more effectively. You may also be advised to go on a weight-reduction diet.
Alcohol	Drinking alcohol while taking this medicine may worsen such side effects as dizziness, light-headedness, or fainting. Avoid alcohol unless your doctor has approved its use.

No special restrictions on smoking.

DAILY LIVING

Exertion and Exercise	Use caution when exercising or exerting yourself while taking this medicine because excessive sweating may cause you to become dehydrated and to feel dizzy, light-headed, or faint. Make sure you drink plenty of liquids to make up for water loss.

Sun Exposure/ Excessive Heat	Use caution during hot weather, especially when you are exercising or exerting yourself (see above). While taking these drugs, your skin may become more sensitive to sunlight and more likely to develop a sunburn. When you first begin taking this medicine, it is a good idea to avoid too much sun, especially if you burn easily. Apply a sunscreen to exposed skin surfaces before going out of doors.
Examinations or Tests	Many people have high blood pressure with no symptoms at all. It is important for you to keep all appointments with your doctor so that your progress can be checked. Periodic blood and urine tests may be required before and during therapy.
Other Precautions	Tell any doctor or dentist you consult that you are taking this medicine, especially if you will be undergoing any type of surgery.
	If you have diabetes, be aware that this medicine may raise blood-sugar levels. If you notice any change when testing sugar levels in your blood or urine, let your doctor know.
	When first starting on this type of medicine, you may feel tired and will probably experience both greater volume and frequency of urination. Until your individual pattern of urination has been established with this medicine, it may be wise to time carefully any activity that will put you out of convenient reach of a bathroom, such as bus or car travel. In addition, taking a diuretic at bedtime will probably interfere with your sleep; you should discuss your dosage schedule with your doctor.
	Check with your doctor if you become ill with flulike symptoms, such as cough, fever, or body aches; lose your appetite; vomit; or have diarrhea. This may cause you to lose a great deal of fluid.

Following mild fluid losses, some older people are more vulnerable to symptoms of weakness or dizziness upon standing up or getting out of bed.

No special restrictions on driving or exposure to excessive cold.

Helpful Hints   Captopril-containing medicines should be taken one hour before meals.

POSSIBLE SIDE EFFECTS

Although this list of adverse effects may seem somewhat intimidating, keep in mind that some are quite rare. Of course, should these or any other problems arise while you are on medication, it is always a good idea to consult your doctor.

IF YOU DEVELOP

difficulty in breathing ■ shortness of breath ■ swelling of face, mouth, vocal cords, fingers, ankles, or feet ■ fever or chills ■ sore throat ■ hoarseness ■ severe dizziness or light-headedness ■ nausea or vomiting ■ severe stomach pain or cramps ■ joint or side pain ■ irregular heartbeat ■ weak pulse ■ tingling sensation in hands, feet, or lips ■ weakness or heaviness in legs ■ decreased urination ■ mood changes ■ confusion ■ muscle cramps or pain ■ tiredness or weakness ■ cough ■ painful breathing ■ fainting (if you faint, stop taking the drug until you have checked with your doctor)

WHAT TO DO

Urgent Get in touch with your doctor immediately.

increased skin sensitivity to sunlight (if severe) ■ dry mouth ■ increased thirst ■ mouth sores ■ rash or hives ■ bleeding or bruising ■ chest pain ■ yellowing of eyes or skin ■ yellowing of vision ■ flushing or paleness

May be serious Check with your doctor as soon as possible.

diarrhea ■ loss of appetite ■ stomach pain ■ upset stomach ■ male impotence ■ clumsiness ■ itching ■ headache ■ light-headedness or faintness, especially when getting up from a reclining or sitting position ■ drowsiness ■ lack of energy ■ increased skin sensitivity to sunlight ■ dizziness ■ increased sweating ■ sleeplessness ■ nervousness ■ tingling sensation ■ tiredness or weakness ■ constipation ■ muscle spasms ■ blurred vision ■ taste changes ■ weight loss

If symptoms are disturbing or persist, let your doctor know.

STORAGE INSTRUCTIONS

Store in a cool, dark place (not in a bathroom medicine cabinet).

STOPPING OR INTERRUPTING THERAPY

Since these drugs do not cure high blood pressure, but only control it, you may have to take this medicine for the rest of your life. *Do not stop taking it, even if you feel better.* If you miss a dose, take it as soon as possible. If it is almost time for your next dose, skip the missed dose and resume your regular schedule. Do not take two doses at the same time.

SPECIAL CONSIDERATIONS FOR THOSE OVER SIXTY-FIVE

Older people are more likely to develop symptoms of low blood-potassium levels such as dizziness, light-headedness, fainting, or weakness. If these symptoms are troublesome, let your doctor know.

CONDITION: **HYPERTENSION**

CATEGORY: **DIURETIC-NONDIURETIC COMBINATIONS**

GENERIC (CHEMICAL) NAME	BRAND (TRADE) NAME	DOSAGE FORMS AND STRENGTHS
Methyldopa and hydrochlorothiazide	ALDORIL	Tablets: 250 mg methyldopa and 15 mg hydrochlorothiazide; 250 mg methyldopa and 25 mg hydrochlorothiazide; 500 mg methyldopa and 30 mg hydrochlorothiazide; 500 mg methyldopa and 50 mg hydrochlorothiazide

DRUG PROFILE

This combination of an antihypertensive agent (methyldopa) and a thiazide diuretic (hydrochlorothiazide) is used to lower high blood pressure. Methyldopa reduces transmission along certain nerve pathways, resulting in the relaxation of blood vessels and a lowering of blood pressure. Hydrochlorothiazide's main action is to increase the amount of salt and water eliminated by the body through urination. (See Methyldopa on pages 65–68 and Thiazide Diuretics on pages 23–28.)

BEFORE USING THIS DRUG

Let your doctor know *IF*

You have ever had allergic reactions or other problems with ■ methyldopa or hydrochlorothiazide, alone or combined ■ any of the thiazide or thiazide-type drugs ■ sulfonamides (sulfa drugs).

You have ever had any of the following medical problems: ■ diabetes ■ chest pain ■ heart disease ■ gout ■ liver disease ■ kidney disease ■ systemic lupus erythematosus ■ depression ■ disease of the pancreas ■ Parkinson's disease ■ pheochromocytoma (adrenal gland tumor).

You are taking any of the following medicines: ■ diuretics or any other medicines for high blood pressure ■ corticosteroids or corticotropin (ACTH) ■ medicine for high cholesterol ■ medicine for diabetes ■ digoxin or digitalis (heart medicines) ■ levodopa (medicine for Parkinson's disease) ■ methenamine (medicine to prevent urinary tract infections) ■ anticoagulants (blood thinners) ■ tranquilizers ■ medicine for depression ■ medicine for gout.

SPECIAL RESTRICTIONS WHILE TAKING THIS DRUG

FOOD AND DRUG INTERACTIONS

Other Drugs	Do not take any other drugs, including over-the-counter (OTC) drugs, before checking with your doctor. OTC drugs for appetite suppression, asthma, colds, cough, hay fever, or sinus problems tend to increase blood pressure.
Foods and Beverages	Your doctor may prescribe a special low-salt diet, which you should follow carefully because it will help your medicine work more effectively. You may also be advised to go on a weight-reduction diet. This drug may cause your body to lose large amounts of the mineral potassium. Your doctor may give you special instructions about eating foods or drinking beverages that have a high potassium content (such as bananas and citrus fruit juices), taking a potassium supplement, or using salt substitutes.
Alcohol	Be careful about the amount of alcohol you drink while taking this medicine. Drinking alcohol may worsen such side effects as dizziness, light-headedness, or fainting. Avoid alcohol unless your doctor has approved its use.

No special restrictions on smoking.

DAILY LIVING

Driving	This drug may cause drowsiness. Be careful when driving, operating household appliances, or doing any other tasks that require alertness until you know how this drug affects you.
Exertion and Exercise	Use caution when exercising or exerting yourself or if you must stand for long periods of time; this drug may cause side effects such as dizziness, light-headedness, or fainting. If you feel any of these symptoms coming on, sit or lie down. It is a good idea not to get up too quickly from a reclining or sitting position.
Sun Exposure/ Excessive Heat	Your skin may become more sensitive to sunlight and heat and more likely to develop a sunburn while you are taking this medicine. It is a good idea to avoid too much sun, especially if you burn easily. Use caution during hot weather or while taking saunas or hot baths, as excessive sweating while taking this medicine may cause you to become dehydrated and to feel drowsy or faint.
Examinations or Tests	Many people have high blood pressure with no symptoms at all. It is important for you to keep all appointments with your doctor, even if you feel well, so that your blood pressure can be checked regularly.
Other Precautions	If you have diabetes, be aware that this medicine may raise blood-sugar levels. If you notice any change when testing sugar levels in your blood or urine, let your doctor know. Tell any doctor or dentist you consult that you are taking this medicine, especially if you will be undergoing any type of surgery.

No special restrictions on exposure to excessive cold.

POSSIBLE SIDE EFFECTS

Although this list of adverse effects may seem somewhat intimidating, keep in mind that some are quite rare. Of course, should these or any other problems arise while you are on medication, it is always a good idea to consult your doctor.

IF YOU DEVELOP	WHAT TO DO
fever ■ very slow or fast heartbeat ■ chest pain ■ yellowing of eyes or skin ■ dark or amber-colored urine ■ change in stool color ■ dry mouth ■ increased thirst ■ nausea or vomiting ■ diarrhea or stomach cramps ■ joint or side pain ■ irregular heartbeat ■ weak pulse ■ difficulty in breathing ■ muscle cramps or pain ■ tiredness or weakness ■ depression ■ anxiety	**Urgent** Get in touch with your doctor immediately.
rash or hives ■ sore throat ■ bleeding or bruising ■ chills ■ sleeplessness ■ nightmares or vivid dreams ■ swelling of feet or lower legs ■ shakiness or unusual body movements ■ frequent urination or need to urinate at night	**May be serious** Check with your doctor as soon as possible.
dizziness or light-headedness, especially when getting up from a reclining or sitting position ■ drowsiness ■ headache ■ memory problems ■ inability to concentrate ■ male impotence ■ diminished sex drive ■ fainting ■ increased skin sensitivity to sunlight ■ loss of appetite ■ upset stomach ■ constipation ■ bloating or gas ■ sore or dark tongue ■ numbness, tingling, pain, or weakness in hands or feet ■ female breast swelling ■ male breast enlargement ■ blurred vision	If symptoms are disturbing or persist, let your doctor know.

STORAGE INSTRUCTIONS

Store in a cool, dark place (not in a bathroom medicine cabinet).

STOPPING OR INTERRUPTING THERAPY

Since this drug does not cure high blood pressure but only controls it, you may have to take this medicine for the rest of your life. Do not stop taking it, even if you feel better. If you miss a dose, take it as soon as possible. If it is almost time for your next dose, skip the missed dose and resume your regular schedule. Do not take two doses at the same time.

SPECIAL CONSIDERATIONS FOR THOSE OVER SIXTY-FIVE

Older people are more likely to develop depression, dizziness, or light-headedness. They are also more likely to develop signs of dehydration, such as weakness or dizziness, when getting up from a reclining or sitting position. In addition, signs of potassium loss such as irregular heartbeat, weak pulse, and tiredness or weakness are more likely to develop in older people. Such people should get in touch with a doctor if they develop any of these symptoms. All doctor's appointments should be kept.

CONDITION: **HYPERTENSION**

CATEGORY: **DIURETIC-NONDIURETIC COMBINATIONS**

GENERIC (CHEMICAL) NAME	BRAND (TRADE) NAME	DOSAGE FORMS AND STRENGTHS
Reserpine, hydralazine hydrochloride, and hydrochlorothiazide	SER-AP-ES	Tablets: 0.1 mg reserpine, 25 mg hydralazine hydrochloride, and 15 mg hydrochlorothiazide

DRUG PROFILE

This combination of two different antihypertensive agents (reserpine and hydralazine) plus a thiazide diuretic (hydrochlorothiazide) is used to lower high blood pressure. Reserpine and hydralazine act together to relax the muscles of the blood vessel walls so that the blood can flow more freely. In addition, reserpine has sedative and tranquilizing effects, and hydralazine increases the rate and output of the heart. The thiazides' main action is to increase the amount of salt and water eliminated by the body through urination. (See Rauwolfia serpentina/Reserpine on pages 91–95, Hydralazine on pages 80–83, and Thiazide and Thiazide-type Diuretics on pages 23–28.)

BEFORE USING THIS DRUG

Let your doctor know *IF*

You have ever had allergic reactions or other problems with ■ hydralazine ■ thiazide diuretics ■ rauwolfia alkaloids ■ sulfonamides (sulfa drugs).

You have ever had any of the following medical problems: ■ allergies, breathing problems, or asthma ■ angina (chest pain) ■ diabetes ■ epilepsy or other seizure disorders ■ gout ■ stomach ulcer ■ ulcerative colitis ■ disease of the heart or blood vessels, including rheumatic mitral valve disease and stroke ■ systemic lupus erythematosus ■ kidney disease ■ liver disease ■ depression ■ disease of the pancreas.

You are taking any of the following medicines: ■ diuretics or other medicines for high blood pressure ■ corticosteroids or corticotropin (ACTH) ■ anticoagulants (blood thinners) ■ medicine for seizures ■ medicine for depression (within the last two weeks) ■ antihistamines ■ medicine for hay fever, allergies, or colds ■ barbiturates ■ medicine for high cholesterol ■ medicine for diabetes ■ digoxin or digitalis (heart medicines) ■ medicine for asthma ■ quinidine (medicine for abnormal heart rhythms) ■ sedatives ■ tranquilizers ■ sleep medicines ■ levodopa (medicine for Parkinson's disease) ■ muscle relaxants ■ narcotics or other prescription pain-killers ■ decongestants ■ potassium-containing medicines or supplements ■ lithium ■ indomethacin or other medicine for arthritis.

SPECIAL RESTRICTIONS WHILE TAKING THIS DRUG

FOOD AND DRUG INTERACTIONS

Other Drugs	Do not take any other drugs, including over-the-counter (OTC) drugs, before checking with your doctor. OTC drugs for appetite suppression, asthma, colds, cough, hay fever, or sinus problems tend to

increase blood pressure. Antihistamines, sleep medicines, tranquilizers, pain-killers, barbiturates, medicine for seizures, muscle relaxants, or anesthetics may worsen such side effects as light-headedness, drowsiness, or fainting.

Foods and Beverages	Your doctor may prescribe a special low-salt diet, which you should follow carefully because it will help your medicine work more effectively. You may also be advised to go on a weight-reduction diet. This drug may cause your body to lose large amounts of the mineral potassium. Your doctor may give you special instructions about eating foods or drinking beverages that have a high potassium content (such as bananas and citrus fruit juices), taking a potassium supplement, or using salt substitutes.
Alcohol	Drinking alcohol while taking this medicine may worsen such side effects as dizziness and drowsiness. Avoid alcohol unless your doctor has approved its use.

No special restrictions on smoking.

DAILY LIVING

Driving	This drug may cause drowsiness. Be careful when driving, operating household appliances, or doing any other tasks that require alertness until you know how this drug affects you.
Exertion and Exercise	Use caution when exercising, exerting yourself, or standing for long periods of time because this drug may cause you to become dizzy, light-headed, or faint. If you feel any of these symptoms coming on, sit or lie down. It is a good idea not to get up too quickly from a reclining or sitting position.

Sun Exposure/ Excessive Heat	Your skin may become more sensitive to sunlight and more likely to develop a sunburn while you are taking this medicine. It is a good idea to avoid too much sun, especially if you burn easily. Apply a sunscreen to exposed skin surfaces before going outdoors. Use caution during hot weather or while taking saunas or hot baths, since excessive sweating while taking this medicine may cause you to become dehydrated and to feel drowsy or faint.
Examinations or Tests	Many people have high blood pressure with no symptoms at all. It is important for you to keep all appointments with your doctor, even if you feel well, so that your blood pressure can be checked regularly. Periodic blood and urine tests may be required.
Other Precautions	If you have diabetes, be aware that this medicine may raise blood-sugar levels. If you notice any change in the sugar levels in your blood or urine, let your doctor know.
	Tell any doctor or dentist you consult that you are taking this medicine, especially if you will be undergoing any type of surgery.
	When first starting on this type of medicine, you may feel tired and will probably experience both greater volume and frequency of urination. Until your individual pattern of urination has been established with this medicine, it may be wise to time carefully any activity that will put you out of convenient reach of a bathroom, such as bus or car travel. In addition, taking a diuretic at bedtime will probably interfere with sleep; you should discuss your dosage schedule with your doctor.
	Check with your doctor if you become ill with flulike symptoms, such as cough, fever, or body aches; lose your appetite; vomit; or have diarrhea. This may

cause you to lose a great deal of fluid, making it important not to take this medicine for one or more doses.

Following mild fluid losses, some older people are more vulnerable to symptoms of weakness or dizziness upon standing or getting up.

Helpful Hints

If your mouth or throat feels dry, chewing sugarless gum or sucking ice chips or sugarless hard candy will help. Your nose may also feel dry or stuffy; check with your doctor before using nasal decongestants.

If this medicine upsets your stomach, taking it with milk, meals, or snacks should help.

No special restrictions on exposure to excessive cold.

POSSIBLE SIDE EFFECTS

Although this list of adverse effects may seem somewhat intimidating, keep in mind that some are quite rare. Of course, should these or any other problems arise while you are on medication, it is always a good idea to consult your doctor.

IF YOU DEVELOP

general body discomfort or weakness, drowsiness, or faintness ■ headache ■ mood changes, depression, or inability to concentrate ■ anxiety or nervousness ■ disorientation ■ early-morning sleeplessness, vivid dreams, or nightmares ■ male impotence ■ diminished sex drive ■ seizures ■ dry mouth ■ flushing ■ increased thirst ■ muscle cramps or pain ■ nausea or vomiting ■ pinpoint pupils ■ changes in heart rate ■ black, tarry stools ■ vomiting, with blood ■ chest pain ■ irregular heartbeat ■ joint or side pain ■ shortness of breath ■ severe stomach pain ■ numbness, tingling, pain, or weakness in hands or feet

(If any of these side effects occur after you STOP taking this medicine, let your doctor know immediately.)

WHAT TO DO

Urgent Get in touch with your doctor immediately.

---

diarrhea ■ sore throat or fever ■ rash or itching ■ stiffness ■ leg pain ■ swelling of lymph glands ■ shaking of hands and fingers ■ swelling of fingers or ankles ■ pain or difficulty in urination ■ chills ■ bleeding (including nosebleed) or bruising ■ yellowing of eyes or skin ■ blurred vision or tearing ■ drooping eyelids ■ weight gain

May be serious Check with your doctor as soon as possible.

---

constipation ■ upset stomach ■ dizziness, especially when getting up from a reclining or sitting position ■ loss of appetite ■ stuffy nose ■ red eyes ■ male breast enlargement ■ female breast swelling ■ hearing disturbances ■ increased skin sensitivity to sunlight ■ increased sweating ■ increased salivation

If symptoms are disturbing or persist, let your doctor know.

STORAGE INSTRUCTIONS

Store in a cool, dark place (not in a bathroom medicine cabinet).

STOPPING OR INTERRUPTING THERAPY

Since this drug does not cure high blood pressure but only controls it, you may have to take this medicine for the rest of your life. Do not stop taking it, even if you feel better. If you miss a dose, take it as soon as possible. If it is almost time for your next dose, skip the missed dose and resume your regular schedule. Do not take two doses at the same time.

SPECIAL CONSIDERATIONS FOR THOSE OVER SIXTY-FIVE

Dizziness or faintness is more likely to occur in older people. Thus, doctors may require regular checkups. People over sixty-five should consult a doctor if they become ill with flulike symptoms, such as cough, fever, or body aches; lose their appetite; vomit; or have diarrhea, since they may then be more vulnerable to fluid losses.

CONDITION: **HYPERTENSION**

CATEGORY: **DIURETIC-NONDIURETIC COMBINATIONS**

GENERIC (CHEMICAL) NAME	BRAND (TRADE) NAME	DOSAGE FORMS AND STRENGTHS
Atenolol and chlorthalidone	TENORETIC	Tablets: 50 mg atenolol and 25 mg chlorthalidone; 100 mg atenolol and 25 mg chlorthalidone

DRUG PROFILE

This medicine is a combination of two kinds of drugs that lower blood pressure. By blocking certain nerve impulses, the beta-blocker atenolol relaxes blood vessels, increases the supply of blood and oxygen to the heart, and reduces the workload and pumping rate of the heart (see Beta-blockers, pages 59–64). Chlorthalidone is a thiazide diuretic that increases the amount of salt and water you eliminate through urination (see Thiazide and Thiazide-type Diuretics on pages 23–28). Other drugs that lower blood pressure may be added to this combination drug if necessary.

BEFORE USING THIS DRUG

Let your doctor know *IF*

You have ever had allergic reactions or other problems with ■ any of the thiazide or thiazide-type diuretics ■ beta-blockers ■ sulfonamides (sulfa drugs).

You have ever had any of the following medical problems: ■ allergies ■ hay fever, hives, asthma, or eczema ■ bronchitis or emphysema ■ slow heartbeat ■ diabetes ■ any heart or blood vessel disease ■ kidney disease ■ liver disease ■ thyroid disease ■ Raynaud's syndrome (poor circulation in the fingers and toes) ■ glaucoma ■ myasthenia gravis ■ hypoglycemia (low blood sugar) ■ pheochromocytoma (adrenal gland tumor) ■ gout ■ systemic lupus erythematosus ■ disease of the pancreas.

You are taking any of the following medicines: ■ any other medicines for high blood pressure ■ medicine for asthma ■ aminophylline, epinephrine, ephedrine, norepinephrine, isoproterenol, dyphylline, oxtriphylline, theophylline, or phenylephrine (vasopressor drugs) ■ calcium blockers (eg, diltiazem, nifedipine, verapamil) ■ medicine for depression ■ cimetidine (medicine for ulcers) ■ heart medicine ■ medicine for glaucoma ■ aspirin, indomethacin, or phenylbutazone (medicine for arthritis) ■ medicine for diabetes ■ decongestants ■ medicine for colds ■ medicine for nausea ■ tranquilizers ■ corticosteroids or corticotropin (ACTH) ■ medicine for high cholesterol ■ medicine for gout ■ lithium ■ methenamine (medicine to prevent urinary tract infections) ■ anticoagulants (blood thinners) ■ tetracycline.

SPECIAL RESTRICTIONS WHILE TAKING THIS DRUG

FOOD AND DRUG INTERACTIONS

Other Drugs	Do not take any other drugs, including over-the-counter (OTC) drugs, before checking with your doctor. OTC drugs for appetite suppression, asthma, colds, cough, hay fever, or sinus problems tend to increase blood pressure.
Foods and Beverages	Your doctor may prescribe a special low-salt diet, which you should follow carefully because it will help your medicine work more effectively.

This medicine may cause your body to lose large amounts of the mineral potassium. Your doctor may give you special instructions about eating foods or drinking beverages that have a high potassium content (such as bananas and citrus fruit juices), taking a potassium supplement, or using salt substitutes.

Alcohol	Alcohol may worsen side effects of this medicine such as dizziness, light-headedness, or fainting. Be careful about how much alcohol you consume.

No special restrictions on smoking.

DAILY LIVING

Driving	This drug may cause drowsiness. Be careful when driving, operating household appliances, or doing any other tasks that require alertness until you know how this drug affects you.
Sun Exposure/ Excessive Heat	Your skin may become more sensitive to sunlight and more likely to develop a sunburn while you are taking this medicine. It is a good idea to avoid too much sun, especially if you burn easily. Apply a sunscreen to exposed skin surfaces before going outdoors. Use caution during hot weather or while taking saunas or hot baths, since excessive sweating while taking this medicine may cause you to become dehydrated and to feel drowsy or faint.
Excessive Cold	You may become more sensitive to cold temperatures while taking this medicine. Dress warmly—protecting your skin, fingers, and toes—and use caution during prolonged exposure to cold.
Examinations and Tests	Check your pulse regularly. If it is slower than your usual rate or less than fifty beats per minute, call your doctor. Many people have high blood pressure

with no symptoms at all. It is important for you to keep all appointments with your doctor, even if you feel well, so that your blood pressure can be checked regularly. Periodic blood and urine tests may be required.

Other Precautions

Be sure to tell any doctor or dentist you consult that you are taking this medicine, especially if you will be undergoing any type of surgery.

If you have diabetes, be aware that this medicine may cause your blood-sugar level to fall. It may also mask the signs of low blood sugar (such as changes in pulse rate or increased blood pressure) leaving you unaware that your blood sugar has fallen. Your doctor may want to make changes in the dosage of your diabetes medicine.

When first starting on this type of medicine, you may feel tired and will probably experience both greater volume and frequency of urination. Until your individual pattern of urination has been established with this medicine, it may be wise to time carefully any activity that will put you out of convenient reach of a bathroom, such as bus or car travel. In addition, taking a diuretic at bedtime will probably interfere with sleep; you should discuss your dosage schedule with your doctor.

Check with your doctor if you become ill with flulike symptoms, such as cough, fever, or body aches; lose your appetite; vomit; or have diarrhea. This may cause you to lose a great deal of fluid, making it important not to take this drug for one or more doses.

Helpful Hints

If your mouth or throat feels dry, chewing sugarless gum or sucking ice chips or sugarless hard candy will help. If your eyes feel dry, you may use nonmedicated or plain eyedrops for relief.

No special restrictions on exertion and exercise.

POSSIBLE SIDE EFFECTS

Although this list of adverse effects may seem somewhat intimidating, keep in mind that some are quite rare. Of course, should these or any other problems arise while you are on medication, it is always a good idea to consult your doctor.

IF YOU DEVELOP

increased skin sensitivity to sunlight ■ chest pain ■ palpitations ■ irregular heartbeat ■ extremely slow heartbeat ■ swelling of face, ankles, feet, or lower legs ■ difficulty in breathing, shortness of breath, or coughing ■ asthma or wheezing ■ restlessness, sweating, nervousness, and irritability (if you are a thyroid patient) ■ weight gain ■ severe or continuing vomiting or diarrhea ■ confusion ■ depression ■ severe stomach pain or cramps ■ joint or side pain ■ weak pulse ■ decreased urination ■ dry mouth ■ increased thirst ■ muscle cramps or pain ■ weakness

WHAT TO DO

Urgent Get in touch with your doctor immediately.

---

dizziness, light-headedness, or confusion upon getting up from a reclining or sitting position ■ cold hands or feet ■ sore throat or fever ■ rash or hives ■ bleeding or bruising ■ yellowing of eyes or skin

May be serious Check with your doctor as soon as possible.

---

diarrhea ■ upset stomach ■ nausea or vomiting ■ loss of appetite ■ drowsiness ■ dry skin or eyes ■ numbness or tingling in fingers or toes ■ anxiety ■ male impotence ■ diminished sex drive ■ hallucinations ■ nightmares or vivid dreams ■ sleep disturbances ■ headache ■ clumsiness

If symptoms are disturbing or persist, let your doctor know.

STORAGE INSTRUCTIONS

Store in a cool, dark place (not in a bathroom medicine cabinet).

STOPPING OR INTERRUPTING THERAPY

Since this drug does not cure high blood pressure but only controls it, you may have to take this medicine for the rest of your life. Do not stop taking it, even if you feel better. If you miss a dose, take it as soon as possible. If it is almost time for your next dose, skip the missed dose and resume your regular schedule. Do not take two doses at the same time.

SPECIAL CONSIDERATIONS FOR THOSE OVER SIXTY-FIVE

Older people may be especially prone to such side effects as confusion, weakness, clumsiness, or dizziness when getting up from a reclining or sitting position, especially when first starting on this drug. Those who develop such symptoms should get in touch with a doctor, who may want to measure the amount of medicine that reaches the bloodstream.

CONDITION: **HYPERTENSION**

CATEGORY: **DIURETIC-NONDIURETIC COMBINATIONS**

GENERIC (CHEMICAL) NAME	BRAND (TRADE) NAME	DOSAGE FORMS AND STRENGTHS
Reserpine and hydroflumethiazide	SALUTENSIN	Tablets: 0.125 mg reserpine and 50 mg hydroflumethiazide
	SALUTENSIN-Demi	Tablets: 0.125 mg reserpine and 25 mg hydroflumethiazide

Reserpine and hydrochlorothiazide	HYDROPRES	Tablets: 0.125 mg reserpine and 25 mg hydrochlorothiazide; 0.125 mg reserpine and 50 mg hydrochlorothiazide
	SERPASIL-ESIDRIX	Tablets: 0.1 mg reserpine and 25 mg hydrochlorothiazide; 0.1 mg reserpine and 50 mg hydrochlorothiazide
Reserpine and chlorthalidone	REGROTON	Tablets: 0.25 mg reserpine and 50 mg chlorthalidone
	DEMI-REGROTON	Tablets: 0.125 mg reserpine and 25 mg chlorthalidone
Reserpine and chlorothiazide	DIUPRES	Tablets: 0.125 mg reserpine and 250 mg chlorothiazide; 0.125 mg reserpine and 500 mg chlorothiazide
Deserpidine and methychlothiazide	ENDURONYL	Tablets: 0.25 mg deserpidine and 5 mg methyclothiazide
	ENDURONYL Forte	Tablets: 0.5 mg deserpidine and 5 mg methyclothiazide

DRUG PROFILE

This combination of an antihypertensive agent (a rauwolfia alkaloid) and a thiazide diuretic is used to lower high blood pressure. The rauwolfia alkaloids (reserpine, deserpidine, rauwolfia serpentina) cause the muscles of the blood vessels to relax, so the blood can flow more freely. The rauwolfia alkaloids also have sedative and tranquilizing effects. The thiazides' main action is to increase the amount of salt and water eliminated by the body through urination. (See Rauwolfia serpentina/ Reserpine on pages 91–95 and Thiazide and Thiazide-type Diuretics on pages 23–28.)

BEFORE USING THIS DRUG

Let your doctor know *IF*

You have ever had allergic reactions or other problems with ■ rauwolfia alkaloids ■ thiazide or thiazide-type diuretics ■ tartrazine (FD&C Yellow Dye No. 5) ■ sulfonamides (sulfa drugs).

You have ever had any of the following medical problems: ■ allergies, breathing problems, or asthma ■ diabetes ■ epilepsy ■ gallstones ■ stomach ulcer ■ ulcerative colitis ■ gout ■ disease of the heart or blood vessels, including stroke ■ kidney disease ■ liver disease ■ systemic lupus erythematosus ■ depression ■ disease of the pancreas ■ Parkinson's disease ■ breast cancer ■ pheochromocytoma (adrenal gland tumor).

You are taking any of the following medicines: ■ diuretics, beta-blockers (eg, propranolol, atenolol, metoprolol), or other medicines for high blood pressure ■ corticosteroids or corticotropin (ACTH) ■ anticoagulants (blood thinners) ■ medicine for seizures ■ medicine for depression (within the last two weeks) ■ antihistamines ■ medicine for hay fever, allergies, or colds ■ barbiturates ■ sedatives ■ tranquilizers ■ sleep medicines ■ medicine for high cholesterol ■ medicine for diabetes ■ digoxin or digitalis (heart medicines) ■ medicine for gout ■ levodopa (medicine for Parkinson's disease) ■ lithium ■ methenamine (medicine to prevent urinary tract infections) ■ muscle relaxants ■ narcotics or other prescription pain-killers ■ decongestants ■ medicine for asthma ■ quinidine (medicine for abnormal heart rhythms).

You are receiving electroconvulsive therapy.

You have ever undergone sympathectomy.

SPECIAL RESTRICTIONS WHILE TAKING THIS DRUG

FOOD AND DRUG INTERACTIONS

Other Drugs	Do not take any other drugs, including over-the-counter (OTC) drugs, before checking with your doctor. OTC drugs for appetite suppression, asthma, cough, hay fever, or sinus problems tend to increase blood pressure. Antihistamines, sleep medicines, tranquilizers, pain-killers, barbiturates, medicine for

seizures, muscle relaxants, or anesthetics may
worsen such side effects as dizziness, light-
headedness, drowsiness, or fainting.

Foods and Beverages

Your doctor may prescribe a special low-salt diet,
which you should follow carefully because it will help
your medicine work more effectively. You may also
be advised to go on a weight-reduction diet. This
drug may cause your body to lose large amounts of
the mineral potassium. Your doctor may give you
special instructions about eating foods or drinking
beverages that have a high potassium content (such
as bananas and citrus fruit juices), taking a potassium supplement, or using salt substitutes.

Alcohol

Drinking alcohol while taking this medicine may
worsen such side effects as dizziness and drowsiness. Avoid alcohol unless your doctor has approved
its use.

No special restrictions on smoking.

DAILY LIVING

Driving

This drug may cause drowsiness. Be careful when
driving, operating household appliances, or doing any
other tasks that require alertness until you know how
this drug affects you.

Exertion and Exercise

Use caution when exercising or exerting yourself
while taking this medicine because excessive sweating may cause you to become dehydrated and to feel
dizzy, light-headed, or faint.

**Sun Exposure/
Excessive Heat**

Your skin may become more sensitive to sunlight
and more likely to develop a sunburn while you are
taking this medicine. It is a good idea to avoid too

much sun, especially if you burn easily. Apply a sunscreen to exposed skin surfaces before going outdoors. Use caution during hot weather or while taking saunas or hot baths, since excessive sweating while taking this medicine may cause you to become dehydrated and to feel drowsy or faint.

Examinations or Tests	Many people have high blood pressure with no symptoms at all. It is important for you to keep all appointments with your doctor, even if you feel well, so that your blood pressure can be checked regularly. Periodic blood and urine tests may be required.
Other Precautions	Tell any doctor or dentist you consult that you are taking this medicine, especially if you will be undergoing any type of surgery.

If you have diabetes, be aware that this medicine may raise blood-sugar levels. If you notice any change when testing sugar levels in your blood or urine, let your doctor know.

When first starting on this type of medicine, you may feel tired and will probably experience both greater volume and frequency of urination. Until your individual pattern of urination has been established with this medicine, it may be wise to time carefully any activity that will put you out of convenient reach of a bathroom, such as bus or car travel. In addition, taking a diuretic at bedtime will probably interfere with sleep; you should discuss your dosage schedule with your doctor.

Check with your doctor if you become ill with flulike symptoms, such as cough, fever, or body aches; lose your appetite; vomit; or have diarrhea. This may cause you to lose a great deal of fluid, making it important not to take this drug for one or more doses.

Helpful Hints	If this medicine upsets your stomach, taking it with milk, meals, or snacks should help.
	If your mouth or throat feels dry, chewing sugarless gum or sucking ice chips or sugarless hard candy will help.

No special restrictions on exposure to excessive cold.

POSSIBLE SIDE EFFECTS

Although this list of adverse effects may seem somewhat intimidating, keep in mind that some are quite rare. Of course, should these or any other problems arise while you are on medication, it is always a good idea to consult your doctor.

IF YOU DEVELOP

severe dizziness or drowsiness ■ dry mouth ■ flushing ■ increased thirst ■ muscle cramps or pain ■ nausea or vomiting ■ pinpoint pupils ■ changes in heart rate ■ weakness ■ headache ■ mood changes ■ depression ■ inability to concentrate ■ nervousness or anxiety ■ early-morning sleeplessness ■ vivid dreams or nightmares ■ male impotence ■ diminished sex drive ■ seizures ■ black, tarry stools ■ vomiting, with blood ■ shortness of breath ■ joint or side pain

After you STOP taking this medicine: dizziness, drowsiness, or fainting ■ weakness ■ male impotence ■ diminished sex drive ■ irregular heart-beat ■ mood changes ■ depression ■ inability to concentrate ■ anxiety ■ sleep disturbances

WHAT TO DO

Urgent Get in touch with your doctor immediately.

diarrhea ■ weight gain ■ chills ■ stiffness ■ shaking of hands or fingers ■ fever or sore throat ■ rash, hives, or itching ■ pain or difficulty in urination ■ stomach cramps or pain ■ bleeding (including nosebleed) or bruising ■ yellowing of eyes or skin ■ blurred vision or tearing ■ drooping eyelids

May be serious Check with your doctor as soon as possible.

loss of appetite or increased appetite ■ increased salivation ■ upset stomach ■ stuffy nose ■ dizziness, especially when getting up from a reclining or sitting position ■ breast enlargement ■ hearing disturbances ■ increased skin sensitivity to sunlight	If symptoms are disturbing or persist, let your doctor know.

STORAGE INSTRUCTIONS

Store in a cool, dark place (not in a bathroom medicine cabinet).

STOPPING OR INTERRUPTING THERAPY

Since this drug does not cure high blood pressure but only controls it, you may have to take this medicine for the rest of your life. Do not stop taking it, even if you feel better. If you miss a dose, take it as soon as possible. If it is almost time for your next dose, skip the missed dose and resume your regular schedule. Do not take two doses at the same time.

SPECIAL CONSIDERATIONS FOR THOSE OVER SIXTY-FIVE

Older people are more likely to develop dizziness, light-headedness, fainting, and weakness. Thus, doctors may require regular checkups.

CONDITION: **HYPERTENSION**

CATEGORY: **DIURETIC-NONDIURETIC COMBINATIONS**

GENERIC (CHEMICAL) NAME	BRAND (TRADE) NAME	DOSAGE FORMS AND STRENGTHS
Hydralazine and hydrochlorothiazide	APRESAZIDE	Capsules: 25 mg hydralazine and 25 mg hydrochlorothiazide; 50 mg hydralazine and 50 mg hydrochlorothiazide; 100 mg hydralazine and 50 mg hydrochlorothiazide

DRUG PROFILE

This medicine is a combination of two kinds of drugs that lower blood pressure. Hydralazine relaxes the blood vessel walls so that the blood can flow more freely; this drug also increases the rate and output of the heart. Hydrochlorothiazide is a thiazide diuretic that increases the amount of salt and water eliminated by the body through urination. (See Hydralazine on pages 80–83 and Thiazide and Thiazide-type Diuretics on pages 23–28).

BEFORE USING THIS DRUG

Let your doctor know *IF*

You have ever had allergic reactions or other problems with ■ hydralazine ■ thiazide or thiazide-type diuretics ■ sulfonamides (sulfa drugs).

You have ever had any of the following medical problems: ■ allergies ■ asthma ■ diabetes ■ gout ■ heart or blood vessel disease, including stroke and rheumatic mitral valve disease ■ kidney disease ■ liver disease ■ systemic lupus erythematosus ■ disease of the pancreas.

You are taking any of the following medicines: ■ diuretics or other medicines for high blood pressure ■ corticosteroids or corticotropin (ACTH) ■ anticoagulants (blood thinners) ■ medicine for depression ■ medicine for high cholesterol ■ medicine for diabetes ■ digoxin or digitalis (heart medicines) ■ medicine for gout ■ lithium ■ methenamine (medicine to prevent urinary tract infections) ■ barbiturates ■ muscle relaxants ■ narcotics or other prescription pain-killers.

You have ever undergone sympathectomy.

SPECIAL RESTRICTIONS WHILE TAKING THIS DRUG

FOOD AND DRUG INTERACTIONS

Other Drugs	Do not take any other drugs, including over-the-counter (OTC) drugs, before checking with your doctor. OTC drugs for appetite suppression, asthma, colds, cough, hay fever, or sinus problems tend to increase blood pressure.

Foods and Beverages	Your doctor may prescribe a special low-salt diet, which you should follow carefully because it will help your medicine work more effectively. You may also be advised to go on a weight-reduction diet. This drug may cause your body to lose large amounts of the mineral potassium. Your doctor may give you special instructions about eating foods or drinking beverages that have a high potassium content (such as bananas and citrus fruit juices), taking a potassium supplement, or using salt substitutes.
Alcohol	Avoid alcohol unless your doctor has approved its use. Drinking alcohol while taking this medicine may worsen such side effects as dizziness or drowsiness.

No special restrictions on smoking.

DAILY LIVING

Driving	This drug may cause drowsiness. Be careful when driving, operating household appliances, or doing any other tasks that require alertness until you know how this drug affects you.
Exertion and Exercise	Use caution when exercising, exerting yourself, or standing for long periods of time because this medicine may cause you to become dizzy, light-headed, or faint. If you feel any of these symptoms coming on, sit or lie down. It is a good idea not to get up too quickly from a reclining or sitting position.
Sun Exposure/ Excessive Heat	Your skin may become more sensitive to sunlight and more likely to develop a sunburn while you are taking this medicine. It is a good idea to avoid too much sun, especially if you burn easily. Apply a sunscreen to exposed skin surfaces before going outdoors. Use caution during hot weather or while taking

saunas or hot baths, since excessive sweating while taking this medicine may cause you to become dehydrated and to feel drowsy or faint.

Examinations or Tests

Many people have high blood pressure with no symptoms at all. It is important for you to keep all appointments with your doctor, even if you feel well, so that your blood pressure can be checked regularly. Periodic blood tests are usually required.

Other Precautions

If you have diabetes, be aware that this medicine may raise blood-sugar levels. If you notice any change when testing sugar levels in your blood or urine, let your doctor know.

When first starting on this type of medicine, you may feel tired and will probably experience both greater volume and frequency of urination. Until your individual pattern of urination has been established with this medicine, it may be wise to time carefully any activity that will put you out of convenient reach of a bathroom, such as bus or car travel. In addition, taking a diuretic at bedtime will probably interfere with sleep; you should discuss your dosage schedule with your doctor.

Check with your doctor if you become ill with flulike symptoms, such as cough, fever, or body aches; lose your appetite; vomit; or have diarrhea. This may cause you to lose a great deal of fluid, making it important not to take this medicine for one or more doses.

No special restrictions on exposure to excessive cold.

POSSIBLE SIDE EFFECTS

Although this list of adverse effects may seem somewhat intimidating, keep in mind that some are quite rare. Of course, should these or any other problems arise while you are on medication, it is always a good idea to consult your doctor.

IF YOU DEVELOP	WHAT TO DO
severe nausea or vomiting ■ dry mouth ■ increased thirst ■ irregular heartbeat ■ mood changes ■ muscle cramps or pain ■ weak pulse ■ chest pain ■ tiredness or weakness ■ joint pain ■ numbness ■ tingling, pain, or weakness in hands or feet ■ severe stomach pain or cramps ■ difficulty in breathing	**Urgent** Get in touch with your doctor immediately.
chills ■ rash or itching ■ sore throat or fever ■ swollen lymph glands ■ bleeding or bruising ■ yellowing of eyes or skin ■ weight gain	**May be serious** Check with your doctor as soon as possible.
upset stomach ■ diarrhea, nausea or vomiting ■ loss of appetite ■ constipation ■ headache ■ changes in heart rate ■ dizziness or light-headedness, especially when getting up from a reclining or sitting position ■ increased skin sensitivity to sunlight ■ flushing ■ shortness of breath with exercise ■ stuffy nose ■ eye irritation ■ depression ■ anxiety ■ disorientation ■ difficulty in urination ■ increased sweating ■ tremors	If symptoms are disturbing or persist, let your doctor know.

STORAGE INSTRUCTIONS

Store in a cool, dark place (not in a bathroom medicine cabinet).

STOPPING OR INTERRUPTING THERAPY

Since this drug does not cure high blood pressure but only controls it, you may have to take this medicine for the rest of your life. Do not stop taking it, even if you feel better. If you miss a dose, take it as soon as possible. If it is almost time for your next dose, skip the missed dose and resume your regular schedule. Do not take two doses at the same time.

SPECIAL CONSIDERATIONS FOR THOSE OVER SIXTY-FIVE

Older people are more likely to develop dizziness; light-headedness; fainting; and signs of potassium loss, such as irregular heartbeat, weak pulse, and tiredness or weakness. Thus, doctors may require regular checkups.

CONDITION: **HYPERTENSION**

CATEGORY: **DIURETIC-NONDIURETIC COMBINATIONS**

GENERIC (CHEMICAL) NAME	BRAND (TRADE) NAME	DOSAGE FORMS AND STRENGTHS
Clonidine and chlorthalidone	COMBIPRES	Tablets: 0.1, 0.2, or 0.3 mg clonidine and 15 mg chlorthalidone

DRUG PROFILE

This combination of an antihypertensive agent (clonidine) and a thiazide diuretic (chlorthalidone) is used to lower high blood pressure. Clonidine slows the heart rate and relaxes the muscles of the blood vessels so that the blood can flow more freely. The thiazides' main action is to increase the amount of salt and water eliminated by the body through urination. (See Clonidine on pages 68–72 and Thiazide and Thiazide-type Diuretics on pages 23–28.)

BEFORE USING THIS DRUG

Let your doctor know *IF*

You have ever had allergic reactions or other problems with ■ clonidine ■ thiazide or thiazide-type diuretics ■ sulfonamides (sulfa drugs).

You have ever had any of the following medical problems: ■ diabetes ■ gout ■ heart or blood vessel disease ■ problems with your veins ■ kidney disease ■ liver disease ■ systemic lupus erythematosus ■ depression ■ disease of the pancreas ■ Raynaud's syndrome (poor circulation in the fingers and toes).

You are taking any of the following medicines: ■ diuretics or other medicines for high blood pressure, especially beta-blockers (eg, propranolol, atenolol, metoprolol) ■ corticosteroids or corticotropin (ACTH) ■ medicine for seizures ■ anticoagulants (blood thinners) ■ medicine for depression ■ lithium ■ antihistamines ■ medicine for hay fever, allergies, sinus problems, or colds ■ barbiturates ■ sedatives

■ tranquilizers ■ sleep medicines ■ medicine for gout ■ muscle relaxants ■ narcotics or other prescription pain-killers ■ methenamine or nalidixic acid (medicines to prevent urinary tract infections) ■ medicine for Parkinson's disease ■ digoxin or digitalis (heart medicines) ■ medicine for arthritis ■ fenfluramine (appetite suppressant) ■ methoxsalen or trioxsalen (medicines for vitiligo and psoriasis) ■ medicine for high cholesterol.

SPECIAL RESTRICTIONS WHILE TAKING THIS DRUG

FOOD AND DRUG INTERACTIONS

Other Drugs	Do not take any other drugs, including over-the-counter (OTC) drugs, before checking with your doctor. OTC drugs for appetite suppression, asthma, colds, cough, hay fever, or sinus problems tend to increase blood pressure. Antihistamines, sleep medicines, tranquilizers, pain-killers, barbiturates, medicine for seizures, muscle relaxants, or anesthetics may worsen side effects of this drug such as dizziness, light-headedness, drowsiness, or fainting.
Foods and Beverages	Your doctor may prescribe a special low-salt diet, which you should follow carefully because it will help your medicine work more effectively. A weight-reduction diet may also be advised. This drug may cause your body to lose large amounts of the mineral potassium. Your doctor may give you special instructions about eating foods or drinking beverages that have a high potassium content (such as bananas and citrus fruit juices), taking a potassium supplement, or using salt substitutes.
Alcohol	Drinking alcohol while taking this medicine may worsen such side effects as dizziness or drowsiness. Avoid alcohol unless your doctor has approved its use.

No special restrictions on smoking.

DAILY LIVING

Driving	This drug may cause drowsiness. Be careful when driving, operating household appliances, or doing any other tasks that require alertness until you know how this drug affects you.
Exertion and Exercise	Use caution when exercising, exerting yourself, or standing for long periods of time because this drug may cause you to become dizzy, light-headed, or faint. If you feel any of these symptoms coming on, sit or lie down. It is a good idea not to get up too quickly from a reclining or sitting position.
Sun Exposure/ Excessive Heat	Your skin may become more sensitive to sunlight and more likely to develop a sunburn while you are taking this medicine. It is a good idea to avoid too much sun, especially if you burn easily. Apply a sunscreen to exposed skin surfaces before going outdoors. Use caution during hot weather or while taking saunas or hot baths, since excessive sweating while taking this medicine may cause you to become dehydrated and to feel drowsy or faint.
Examinations or Tests	Many people have high blood pressure with no symptoms at all. It is important for you to keep all appointments with your doctor, even if you feel well, so that your blood pressure can be checked regularly. Periodic blood, urine, and eye tests may be required.
Other Precautions	If you have diabetes, be aware that this medicine may raise blood-sugar levels. If you notice any change when testing sugar levels in your blood or urine, let your doctor know.

Tell any doctor or dentist you consult that you are taking this medicine, especially if you will be undergoing any type of surgery.

When first starting on this type of medicine, you may feel tired and will probably experience both greater volume and frequency of urination. Until your individual pattern of urination has been established with this medicine, it may be wise to time carefully any activity that will put you out of convenient reach of a bathroom, such as bus or car travel. In addition, taking a diuretic at bedtime will probably interfere with sleep; you should discuss your dosage schedule with your doctor.

Check with your doctor if you become ill with flulike symptoms, such as cough, fever, or body aches; lose your appetite; vomit; or have diarrhea. This may cause you to lose a great deal of fluid, making it important not to take this drug for one or more doses.

No special restrictions on exposure to excessive cold.

POSSIBLE SIDE EFFECTS

Although this list of adverse effects may seem somewhat intimidating, keep in mind that some are quite rare. Of course, should these or any other problems arise while you are on medication, it is always a good idea to consult your doctor.

IF YOU DEVELOP

difficulty in breathing ■ extreme dizziness or fainting ■ irregular or slow heartbeat ■ palpitations ■ vomiting ■ tiredness or weakness ■ depression ■ nervousness ■ severe diarrhea ■ severe stomach pain or cramps ■ dry mouth ■ increased thirst ■ mood or mental changes ■ muscle cramps or pain ■ weak pulse ■ joint or side pain ■ decreased urination ■ pain in urination

After you STOP taking this medicine: anxiety ■ chest pain ■ sleep disturbances ■ nervousness ■ flushing ■ headache ■ increased salivation ■ upset stomach ■ stomach cramps ■ irregular or fast heartbeat ■ shaking of hands or fingers ■ increased sweating ■ muscle pain

WHAT TO DO

Urgent Get in touch with your doctor immediately.

---

swelling of feet or lower legs ■ cold fingertips or toes ■ rash or itching ■ sore throat or fever ■ bleeding or bruising ■ vivid dreams or nightmares ■ yellowing of eyes or skin ■ changes in vision ■ hallucinations

May be serious Check with your doctor as soon as possible.

---

constipation ■ diarrhea ■ drowsiness ■ sexual problems ■ sleep disturbances ■ dizziness, light-headedness, or fainting, especially when getting up from a reclining or sitting position ■ upset stomach ■ nausea or vomiting ■ ear pain ■ headache ■ taste changes ■ increased skin sensitivity to sunlight ■ loss of appetite ■ weight gain ■ paleness ■ hair loss ■ dry nasal passages ■ dry, itching, or burning eyes ■ bone pain ■ tenderness of the salivary glands (around the ear) ■ urinary retention or difficulty in urination ■ need to urinate at night

If symptoms are disturbing or persist, let your doctor know.

STORAGE INSTRUCTIONS

Store in a cool, dark place (not in a bathroom medicine cabinet).

STOPPING OR INTERRUPTING THERAPY

Since this drug does not cure high blood pressure but only controls it, you may have to take this medicine for the rest of your life. *Do not stop taking it, even if you feel better.* If you miss a dose, take it as soon as possible. Then continue on your regular schedule. If you miss two doses in a row, check with your doctor right away. *Abruptly stopping this medicine can cause your blood pressure to rise rapidly, which could be dangerous to your health.* Your doctor will advise you on how to reduce your dosage gradually before stopping completely. Always make sure you have an adequate supply of this drug on hand.

SPECIAL CONSIDERATIONS FOR THOSE OVER SIXTY-FIVE

The side effects of drowsiness, dizziness, or fainting are more likely to occur in older people.

CONDITION: **HYPERTENSION**

CATEGORY: **DIURETIC-NONDIURETIC COMBINATIONS**

GENERIC (CHEMICAL) NAME	BRAND (TRADE) NAME	DOSAGE FORMS AND STRENGTHS
Guanethidine and hydrochlorothiazide	ESIMIL	Tablets: 10 mg guanethidine and 25 mg hydrochlorothiazide

DRUG PROFILE

This medicine is a combination of two kinds of drugs that lower blood pressure—an antihypertensive agent (guanethidine) and a thiazide diuretic (hydrochlorothiazide). Guanethidine causes the muscles of the blood vessels to relax so that the blood can flow more freely. The thiazides' main action is to increase the amount of salt and water eliminated by the body through urination. (See Guanethidine on pages 95–98 and Thiazide and Thiazide-type Diuretics on pages 23–28.)

BEFORE USING THIS DRUG

Let your doctor know *IF*

You have ever had allergic reactions or other problems with ■ guanethidine
■ thiazide or thiazide-type diuretics ■ sulfonamides (sulfa drugs).

You have ever had any of the following medical problems: ■ allergies ■ asthma
■ diabetes ■ diarrhea ■ fever ■ gout ■ heart or blood vessel disease, especially a
recent heart attack, stroke or angina ■ systemic lupus erythematosus ■ kidney
disease ■ liver disease ■ disease of the pancreas ■ pheochromocytoma (adrenal
gland tumor) ■ stomach ulcer.

You are taking any of the following medicines: ■ diuretics or any other medicines for
high blood pressure ■ corticosteroids or corticotropin (ACTH) ■ amphetamines
■ anticoagulants (blood thinners) ■ medicine for depression ■ medicine for high
cholesterol ■ digoxin or digitalis (heart medicines) ■ diltiazem, nicardipine,
nifedipine, or verapamil (calcium blockers) ■ nitrates (medicine for chest pain)
■ barbiturates ■ medicine for diabetes ■ medicine for gout ■ lithium ■ tranquilizers
■ medicine for nausea ■ ephedrine (medicine for asthma or bronchitis) ■ decongestants ■ medicine for narcolepsy ■ narcotics or other prescription pain-killers
■ weight-reduction medicines ■ methenamine (medicine to prevent urinary tract
infections) ■ levodopa (medicine for Parkinson's disease) ■ tetracycline.

You have ever undergone sympathectomy.

SPECIAL RESTRICTIONS WHILE TAKING THIS DRUG

FOOD AND DRUG INTERACTIONS

Other Drugs	Do not take any other drugs, including over-the-counter (OTC) drugs, before checking with your doctor. OTC drugs for appetite suppression, asthma, colds, cough, hay fever, or sinus problems tend to increase blood pressure.
	Use of reserpine or rauwolfia at the same time as guanethidine may cause fainting, slow heartbeat, and depression.

Stimulants, antidepressants, and tranquilizers may reduce the antihypertensive effectiveness of guanethidine.

Barbiturates and narcotic pain-killers may worsen the side effects of dizziness and faintness.

Foods and Beverages	Your doctor may prescribe a special low-salt diet, which you should follow carefully because it will help your medicine work more effectively. You may also be advised to go on a weight-reduction diet. This drug may cause your body to lose large amounts of the mineral potassium. Your doctor may give you special instructions about eating foods or drinking beverages that have a high potassium content (such as bananas and citrus fruit juices), taking a potassium supplement, or using salt substitutes.
Alcohol	Drinking alcohol while taking this medicine may worsen such side effects as dizziness or drowsiness. Avoid alcohol unless your doctor has approved its use.

No special restrictions on smoking.

DAILY LIVING

Exertion and Exercise	Use caution when exercising or standing for long periods of time because this drug may cause you to become dizzy, light-headed, or faint. If you feel any of these symptoms coming on, sit or lie down.
Sun Exposure/ Excessive Heat	Your skin may become more sensitive to sunlight and more likely to develop a sunburn while you are taking this medicine. It is a good idea to avoid too much sun, especially if you burn easily. Apply a sunscreen to exposed skin surfaces before going outdoors. Use caution during hot weather or while taking

saunas or hot baths, since excessive sweating while taking this medicine may cause you to become dehydrated and to feel drowsy or faint.

Examinations or Tests

Many people have high blood pressure with no symptoms at all. It is important for you to keep all appointments with your doctor, even if you feel well, so that your blood pressure can be checked regularly. Periodic blood and urine tests may be required.

Other Precautions

If you have diabetes, be aware that this medicine may raise blood-sugar levels. If you notice any change when testing sugar levels in your blood or urine, let your doctor know.

Tell any doctor or dentist you consult that you are taking this medicine, especially if you will be undergoing any type of surgery.

When first starting on this type of medicine, you may feel tired and will probably experience both greater volume and frequency of urination. Until your individual pattern of urination has been established with this medicine, it may be wise to time carefully any activity that will put you out of convenient reach of a bathroom, such as bus or car travel. In addition, taking a diuretic at bedtime will probably interfere with sleep; you should discuss your dosage schedule with your doctor.

Check with your doctor if you become ill with flulike symptoms, such as cough, fever, or body aches; lose your appetite; vomit; or have diarrhea. This may cause you to lose a great deal of fluid, making it important not to take this drug for one or more doses.

No special restrictions on driving or exposure to excessive cold.

POSSIBLE SIDE EFFECTS

Although this list of adverse effects may seem somewhat intimidating, keep in mind that some are quite rare. Of course, should these or any other problems arise while you are on medication, it is always a good idea to consult your doctor.

IF YOU DEVELOP

WHAT TO DO

severe vomiting or diarrhea ■ dry mouth ■ increased thirst ■ irregular heartbeat ■ confusion ■ depression ■ muscle cramps or pain ■ weak pulse ■ tiredness or weakness ■ chest pain ■ severe stomach pain or cramps ■ joint or side pain ■ difficulty in breathing ■ decreased urination

Urgent Get in touch with your doctor immediately.

sore throat or fever ■ headache ■ rash or hives ■ bleeding or bruising ■ yellowing of eyes or skin ■ weight gain ■ swelling of feet or lower legs

May be serious Check with your doctor as soon as possible.

diarrhea or increased bowel movements ■ dizziness, light-headedness, or fainting, especially when getting up from a reclining or sitting position ■ difficulty in ejaculation (in males) ■ stuffy nose ■ slow heartbeat ■ blurred vision ■ drooping eyelids ■ increased skin sensitivity to sunlight ■ loss of appetite ■ upset stomach ■ hair loss ■ need to urinate at night or other urinary problems ■ tenderness of the salivary glands (around the ear)

If symptoms are disturbing or persist, let your doctor know.

STORAGE INSTRUCTIONS

Store in a cool, dark place (not in a bathroom medicine cabinet).

STOPPING OR INTERRUPTING THERAPY

Since this drug does not cure high blood pressure but only controls it, you may have to take this medicine for the rest of your life. Do not stop taking it, even if you feel better. If you miss a dose, take it as soon as possible. If it is almost time for your next dose, skip the missed dose and resume your regular schedule. Do not take two doses at the same time.

SPECIAL CONSIDERATIONS FOR THOSE OVER SIXTY-FIVE

Older people are more likely to develop dizziness; light-headedness; fainting; and signs of potassium loss, such as irregular heartbeat, weak pulse, and tiredness or weakness.

CONDITION: **HYPERTENSION**

CATEGORY: **DIURETIC-NONDIURETIC COMBINATIONS**

GENERIC (CHEMICAL) NAME	BRAND (TRADE) NAME	DOSAGE FORMS AND STRENGTHS
Prazosin and polythiazide	MINIZIDE	Capsules: 1, 2, 5 mg prazosin and 0.5 mg polythiazide

DRUG PROFILE

This combination of an antihypertensive agent (prazosin) and a thiazide diuretic (polythiazide) is used to lower high blood pressure. Prazosin relaxes the muscles of the blood vessels so that the blood can flow more freely. The thiazides' main action is to increase the amount of salt and water eliminated by the body through urination. (See Prazosin on pages 87–90 and Thiazide and Thiazide-type Diuretics on pages 23–28.)

BEFORE USING THIS DRUG

Let your doctor know *IF*

You have ever had allergic reactions or other problems with ■ prazosin ■ thiazide or thiazide-type diuretics ■ sulfonamides (sulfa drugs).

You have ever had any of the following medical problems: ■ allergy ■ asthma ■ angina (chest pain) ■ diabetes ■ gout ■ heart disease ■ kidney disease ■ liver disease ■ systemic lupus erythematosus ■ disease of the pancreas.

You are taking any of the following medicines: ■ diuretics or other medicine for high blood pressure, especially beta-blockers (eg, propranolol, atenolol, metoprolol) ■ corticosteroids or corticotropin (ACTH) ■ medicine for diabetes ■ medicine for gout ■ lithium ■ muscle relaxants ■ tetracycline ■ medicine for high cholesterol ■ digoxin or digitalis (heart medicines) ■ anticoagulants (blood thinners) ■ methenamine (medicine to prevent urinary tract infections) ■ indomethacin or other medicine for arthritis.

You have ever undergone sympathectomy.

SPECIAL RESTRICTIONS WHILE TAKING THIS DRUG

FOOD AND DRUG INTERACTIONS

Other Drugs	Do not take any other drugs, including over-the-counter (OTC) drugs, before checking with your doctor. OTC drugs for appetite suppression, asthma, colds, cough, hay fever, or sinus problems tend to increase blood pressure. Barbiturates or narcotic pain-killers may worsen the side effect of dizziness.
Foods and Beverages	Your doctor may prescribe a special low-salt diet, which you should follow carefully because it will help your medicine work more effectively. You may also be advised to go on a weight-reduction diet. This drug may cause your body to lose large amounts of the mineral potassium. Your doctor may give you special instructions about eating foods or drinking beverages that have a high potassium content (such as bananas and citrus fruit juices), taking a potassium supplement, or using salt substitutes.
Alcohol	Drinking alcohol while you are taking this medicine may worsen such side effects as dizziness or drowsiness. Avoid alcohol unless your doctor has approved its use.

No special restrictions on smoking.

DAILY LIVING

Driving	This drug may make you dizzy. Use caution when driving, operating household appliances, or doing any other tasks that require alertness until you know how this drug affects you.
Exertion and Exercise	Use caution when exercising, exerting yourself, or standing for long periods of time because this medicine may cause you to become dizzy, light-headed, or faint. If you feel any of these symptoms coming on, sit or lie down. It is a good idea not to get up too quickly from a reclining or sitting position.
Sun Exposure/ Excessive Heat	Your skin may become more sensitive to sunlight and more likely to develop a sunburn while you are taking this medicine. It is a good idea to avoid too much sun, especially if you burn easily. Apply a sunscreen to exposed skin surfaces before going outdoors. Use caution during hot weather or while taking saunas or hot baths, since excessive sweating while taking this medicine may cause you to become dehydrated and to feel drowsy or faint.
Examinations or Tests	Many people have high blood pressure with no symptoms at all. It is important for you to keep all appointments with your doctor, even if you feel well, so that your blood pressure can be checked regularly. Periodic blood and urine tests may be required.
Other Precautions	You may feel faint or actually lose consciousness after taking the first dose of this drug or if there has been a significant increase in your dose. Your doctor may suggest that you take your first dose in his or her office.

If you have diabetes, be aware that this medicine may raise blood-sugar levels. If you notice any |

change when testing sugar levels in your blood or urine, let your doctor know.

Tell any doctor or dentist you consult that you are taking this medicine, especially if you will be undergoing any type of surgery.

When first starting on this type of medicine, you may feel tired and will probably experience both greater volume and frequency of urination. Until your individual pattern of urination has been established with this medicine, it may be wise to time carefully any activity that will put you out of convenient reach of a bathroom, such as bus or car travel. In addition, taking a diuretic at bedtime will probably interfere with sleep; you should discuss your dosage schedule with your doctor.

Check with your doctor if you become ill with flulike symptoms, such as cough, fever, or body aches; lose your appetite; vomit; or have diarrhea. This may cause you to lose a great deal of fluid, making it important not to take this drug for one or more doses.

No special restrictions on exposure to excessive cold.

POSSIBLE SIDE EFFECTS

Although this list of adverse effects may seem somewhat intimidating, keep in mind that some are quite rare. Of course, should these or any other problems arise while you are on medication, it is always a good idea to consult your doctor.

IF YOU DEVELOP

severe nausea or vomiting ■ dry mouth ■ increased thirst ■ irregular heartbeat ■ palpitations ■ mood or mental changes ■ muscle cramps or pain ■ weak pulse ■ weakness ■ chest pain ■ shortness of breath

WHAT TO DO

Urgent Get in touch with your doctor immediately.

dizziness or light-headedness, especially when getting up from a reclining or sitting position ■ fainting ■ swelling of feet or lower legs ■ weight gain ■ difficulty in urination ■ joint, stomach, or side pain ■ numbness or tingling in hands or feet ■ rash or hives ■ sore throat or fever ■ bleeding or bruising ■ yellowing of eyes or skin	**May be serious** Check with your doctor as soon as possible.
diarrhea ■ constipation ■ vomiting ■ headache ■ loss of appetite ■ increased skin sensitivity to sunlight ■ tiredness ■ upset stomach ■ hair loss ■ nervousness ■ male impotence ■ blurred vision ■ ringing in ears ■ red eyes ■ stuffy nose ■ increased sweating	If symptoms are disturbing or persist, let your doctor know.

STORAGE INSTRUCTIONS

Store in a cool, dark place (not in a bathroom medicine cabinet).

STOPPING OR INTERRUPTING THERAPY

Since this drug does not cure high blood pressure but only controls it, you may have to take this medicine for the rest of your life. Do not stop taking it, even if you feel better. If you miss a dose, take it as soon as possible. If it is almost time for your next dose, skip the missed dose and resume your regular schedule. Do not take two doses at the same time.

SPECIAL CONSIDERATIONS FOR THOSE OVER SIXTY-FIVE

Older people are more likely to develop dizziness; light-headedness; fainting; and signs of potassium loss, such as irregular heartbeat, weak pulse, and tiredness or weakness. Thus, doctors may require regular checkups.

ANGINA

You probably saw the treatment before you even heard of the disease. A character in a movie, looking pained, furtively slips a pill under his tongue. One scene later, he is laid up in the hospital with a cardiac condition signaled by the pain of angina.

CAUSES

In real life, angina doesn't have to land you in the hospital, but the pain associated with it is all too real. Angina actually is a temporary, recurring pain or tightness in the chest, often radiating to the arms, neck, jaw, or back. It is usually caused by either a spasm or a blockage of the coronary arteries—the large blood vessels that carry oxygen to the heart—or both. As people grow older, their coronary arteries tend to accumulate fatty deposits known as plaques, which may cause narrowings in the arteries and can ultimately prevent an adequate supply of blood (and, consequently, oxygen) from reaching the heart. This lack of oxygen may cause the pain of angina. (Sometimes chest pain does not occur, even when the heart is not being supplied with enough oxygen. This condition, called silent ischemia, is more common in people with diabetes and in older people.)

About 6 percent of men and 3 percent of women over fifty have angina. Although the condition can be both frightening and debilitating, several forms of treatment are available to bring it under control. Before prescribing treatment, however, your doctor must determine what type of angina you have by learning as much as possible about your symptoms and by performing diagnostic tests.

TYPES OF ANGINA

Chest pain, although the hallmark of angina, is not its only symptom. Angina can also be associated with shortness of breath, dizziness, indigestion, and numbness in the arms and hands. In general, all these symptoms usually follow one of three patterns:

• Classic angina is brought on by physical exertion, emotional stress, or any other factor that causes the heart to work harder than usual. This most common type of angina is always caused by coronary artery disease.

• Variant angina flares up during rest or moderate, unstressful activity and appears to be caused by a spasm in a coronary artery rather than by coronary artery disease.

• Unstable angina, the most serious form of angina, occurs when a patient with classic angina begins to suffer from more serious symptoms, for example, if the attacks occur more frequently, last longer, are more severe, or occur when the patient is sedentary or asleep.

Heart attacks are more common in people with unstable angina, so this form of angina requires especially prompt treatment, often including hospitalization until the episodes are under control.

DIAGNOSIS

If you visit your doctor because of chest pain, one of the first things he or she will do is hook you up to an electrocardiogram (ECG) machine, which will record the pattern of electrical activity in your heart. This test will help determine whether you have had a heart attack or are experiencing episodes of angina. However, it is important to know that the ECG is often normal between anginal attacks, and sometimes even during an attack. In the meantime, other possible causes of angina symptoms will be ruled out. Arthritis and certain digestive disorders, for example, can mimic angina, as can muscle disorders and infections. It's important to remember that not all chest pain is a signal of heart disease.

After the initial ECG, the doctor may ask you to take an exercise stress test. In this test, you will exercise on a treadmill while hooked up to an ECG machine. If the ECG shows abnormalities, further tests may be needed.

One of these tests, a radionuclide stress evaluation, helps the doctor see where your coronary arteries may be obstructed. This test involves injecting a radioactive substance into a vein immediately following exercise, then obtaining an image of the heart with a special machine. By tracking the radioactive material through the image, the doctor can pinpoint obstructions in the arteries.

A more complicated test called a coronary angiogram can also help locate constricted areas in the arteries, as well as determine the severity of the blockage. In this procedure, the doctor injects dye into the coronary arteries through a catheter that is inserted into an artery in the leg or arm. Through electronic images of the heart, it is possible to see the movement of the dye through the arteries.

TREATMENT

Drug treatment usually begins as soon as noncardiac causes of chest pain are ruled out. For detailed information on the most common treatments for angina—the nitrates, the beta-blockers, the calcium blockers, aspirin, and dipyridamole—see the charts on pages 162–192.

If your angina does not improve with drug treatment, your doctor may recommend angioplasty or bypass surgery. These procedures are commonly used to relieve angina and improve the underlying heart disease. In coronary angioplasty, the doctor passes a balloon into a coronary artery and inflates the balloon, expanding the artery. In coronary artery bypass surgery, the doctor uses a vein graft removed from a leg or an arterial graft from the chest to bypass a blockage in a coronary artery. Both techniques have been used with success in older people.

OUTLOOK

With or without surgery, your doctor will probably recommend that, in addition to taking medicine, you try to lose any excess weight. Some people may also benefit from a medically supervised exercise program. You should also stop smoking. It is important to avoid stressful situations that may provoke attacks. Most people with angina can be effectively treated through a combination of drugs and lifestyle changes.

CONDITION: **ANGINA**

CATEGORY: **NITRATES**

GENERIC (CHEMICAL) NAME	BRAND (TRADE) NAME	DOSAGE FORMS AND STRENGTHS
Isosorbide dinitrate	DILATRATE-SR	Controlled-release capsules: 40 mg
	ISORDIL	Controlled-release tablets: 40 mg
		Sublingual tablets: 2.5, 5, 10 mg
		Tablets: 5, 10, 20, 30, 40 mg
	SORBITRATE	Chewable tablets: 5, 10 mg
		Controlled-release tablets: 40 mg
		Sublingual tablets: 2.5, 5, 10 mg
		Tablets: 5, 10, 20, 30, 40 mg
Nitroglycerin	DEPONIT	Skin patch: 0.2, 0.4 mg per hour
	NITRO-BID	Controlled-release capsules: 2.5, 6.5, 9 mg
		Ointment: 2%
	NITRODISC	Disc: 0.2, 0.3, 0.4 mg per hour
	NITRO-DUR	Skin patch: 0.1, 0.2, 0.3, 0.4, 0.6 mg per hour
	NITROGARD	Controlled-release, buccal tablets: 1, 2, 3 mg
	NITROL	Ointment: 2%
	NITROLINGUAL	Spray: 0.4 mg/spray

| NITROSTAT | Sublingual tablets: 0.15, 0.3, 0.4, 0.6 mg |
| TRANSDERM-NITRO | Skin patch: 0.1, 0.2, 0.4, 0.6 mg per hour |

DRUG PROFILE

Nitrates are used to treat angina pectoris (chest pain) and to prevent angina attacks. These drugs relax the blood vessels and increase the supply of blood and oxygen to the heart. At the same time, they reduce the workload and oxygen demands of the heart. The nitrates are available in a number of dosage forms. Fast-acting nitrates— sublingual (under the tongue), buccal (in the cheek or under the lip), chewable tablets, or spray—are used both to relieve an ongoing angina attack and to prevent angina. The slower-acting dosage forms (controlled-release capsules or tablets that are swallowed, skin ointments, or patches) are taken only to prevent angina. If needed, a fast-acting nitrate may be used to supplement a longer-acting one.

BEFORE USING THIS DRUG

Let your doctor know *IF*

You have ever had allergic reactions or other problems with ■ nitrates or nitrites.

You have ever had any of the following medical problems: ■ anemia ■ overactive thyroid ■ recent heart attack ■ stroke ■ head trauma (such as a blow to the head) ■ migraine or other vascular headaches ■ congestive heart failure ■ glaucoma ■ low blood pressure ■ diarrhea, loose stools, or other intestinal problems.

You are taking any of the following medicines: ■ diuretics or other medicines for high blood pressure ■ any other heart medicine, including nitrates and nitrites ■ medicine for asthma ■ medicine for colds, hay fever, or sinus problems ■ tranquilizers ■ medicine for nausea ■ appetite suppressants ■ calcium blockers (eg, diltiazem, nifedipine, verapamil) ■ narcotics or other prescription pain-killers.

You are often exposed to organic nitrates (eg, you work in a plant that processes organic nitrates).

SPECIAL RESTRICTIONS WHILE TAKING THIS DRUG

FOOD AND DRUG INTERACTIONS

Other Drugs	Diuretics and other medicines for high blood pressure, calcium blockers (medicine for high blood pressure or angina), phenothiazines (tranquilizers), and narcotics and prescription pain-killers may increase the side effects of dizziness or faintness when taken with nitrates.
Foods and Beverages	Angina may be provoked by eating a meal that is too heavy.
Alcohol	Drinking alcohol while taking nitrate medicine may worsen such side effects as dizziness, light-headedness, or fainting. Avoid alcohol unless your doctor has approved its use.
Smoking	Smoking increases your chance of having an angina attack. If you smoke, try to stop or at least cut down.

DAILY LIVING

Exertion and Exercise	Use caution when exercising or if you must stand for long periods of time because this type of medicine may cause dizziness, light-headedness, or weakness. To prevent exercise-induced angina, take a chewable or sublingual tablet ten minutes before beginning exercise.
Excessive Heat	Use caution during hot weather, especially if you exert yourself, as this drug may cause dizziness, weakness, or light-headedness.

Excessive Cold	Use caution during cold weather, since excessive cold may provoke an angina attack. Your doctor may recommend that you take a chewable sublingual tablet before exposure to excessive cold.
Examinations or Tests	It is important for you to keep all appointments with your doctor, even if you feel well, so that your progress can be checked.
Other Precautions	Emotional stress may trigger an angina attack. If you are taking nitrate tablets and notice partially dissolved tablets in your stool, let your doctor know; you may not be receiving the correct amount of your medicine.
Helpful Hints	*Capsules and tablets to be swallowed.* Take with a full glass of water on an empty stomach. Do not break, crush, or chew tablets or capsules. *Chewable tablets.* Chew well and hold in your mouth for about two minutes. For relief of an angina attack, you may take up to three tablets over a thirty-minute period. If you still have chest pain, call your doctor or get to a hospital emergency room immediately, as you may be experiencing a heart attack. *Sublingual tablets.* Do not eat, drink, or smoke while a tablet is dissolving. For relief of an angina attack, you may take up to three tablets over a fifteen-minute period. If you still have chest pain, call your doctor or get to a hospital emergency room immediately. *Buccal tablets.* Allow the tablet to dissolve slowly between the cheek and gum or lower lip and gum. If you eat or drink, transfer the tablet to between the upper lip and gum. If you still feel chest pain after five minutes, call your doctor.

Ointment. Before applying a new dose, clean off any ointment remaining from the previous dose. Apply ointment in a thin, even layer to a clean area of the skin; do not massage in. To prevent irritation, apply ointment to a different area each time. Your doctor may instruct you to use an occlusive wrapping; follow instructions carefully.

Skin patch. Apply the patch to a clean, dry, hairless area of skin (not near hands or feet). If a patch becomes loose or falls off, apply a new one. If you miss a dose, apply it as soon as possible, and then go back to your regular schedule.

Spray. Sit down if possible, holding the canister upright and the spray opening as close to the mouth as possible. Press the grooved button firmly to release the spray onto or under the tongue, and close your mouth immediately. Do not inhale for five to ten seconds and hold the vapor in your mouth for thirty to sixty seconds before swallowing. If you are taking this medicine for an attack and the chest pain persists, call your doctor or get to a hospital emergency room immediately.

For relief of angina attack. Sit down before you take your fast-acting medicine. If you feel dizzy or faint after taking the medicine, bend forward, put your head between your knees, and breathe deeply. You should feel relief from angina pain within one to five minutes.

To prevent angina attack: Factors that trigger angina include emotional stress, eating a heavy meal, smoking, and cold weather (see "Food and Drug Interactions" and "Daily Living"). If you anticipate being in a trigger situation, take a chewable or sublingual tablet five to ten minutes beforehand.

Headaches. You may experience either mild or severe headache with nitrate medicines, which should decrease in frequency and severity with continued therapy. If aspirin, acetaminophen, or ibuprofen does not control your headache, your doctor may be able to decrease your nitrate dose. If you are using an oral form, it may help to take your medicine with meals.

No special restrictions on driving or sun exposure.

POSSIBLE SIDE EFFECTS

Although this list of adverse effects may seem somewhat intimidating, keep in mind that some are quite rare. Of course, should these or any other problems arise while you are on medication, it is always a good idea to consult your doctor.

IF YOU DEVELOP	WHAT TO DO
collapse ■ blurred vision ■ cold sweat ■ inability to control urination or bowel movements ■ confusion (that persists even after fifteen minutes of lying down)	**Urgent** Get in touch with your doctor immediately.
rash ■ dry mouth ■ swelling of hands, feet, or ankles	**May be serious** Check with your doctor as soon as possible.
dizziness, light-headedness, or fainting, especially when getting up from a reclining or sitting position ■ headache ■ flushing of face, neck, and chest ■ upset stomach ■ nausea or vomiting ■ fast heartbeat ■ restlessness ■ weakness ■ paleness	If symptoms are disturbing or persist, let your doctor know.

STORAGE INSTRUCTIONS

Store in a cool, dark place (not in a bathroom medicine cabinet). For sublingual tablets, remove the cotton plug that comes with the bottle and keep the medicine in its original container. Pick up only the tablet you are about to take, and replace the bottle cap quickly and tightly.

Doctors generally recommend that you keep a small supply of nitroglycerin tablets with you at all times in case of an emergency. Specially designed containers are available for this purpose so that you can avoid handling the original bottle too often, since this may destroy the potency of its contents before the expiration date.

INTERRUPTING OR STOPPING THERAPY

If you are taking this medicine on a regular schedule, abruptly stopping can bring on angina attacks. Your doctor will advise you on how to reduce your dose gradually before stopping completely. If you miss a dose, take it as soon as possible unless your next scheduled dose is within two hours (chewable tablets) or six hours (controlled-release capsules or tablets). In that case, return to your regular schedule. Do not take two doses at the same time.

SPECIAL CONSIDERATIONS FOR THOSE OVER SIXTY-FIVE

The side effects of dizziness and light-headedness, especially when getting up from a reclining or sitting position, are more likely to occur in older people.

CONDITION: **ANGINA**

CATEGORY: **BETA-BLOCKERS**

GENERIC (CHEMICAL) NAME	BRAND (TRADE) NAME	DOSAGE FORMS AND STRENGTHS
Atenolol	TENORMIN	Tablets: 25, 50, 100 mg
Metoprolol tartrate	LOPRESSOR	Tablets: 50, 100 mg
Nadolol	CORGARD	Tablets: 20, 40, 80, 120, 160 mg
Propranolol hydrochloride	INDERAL	Tablets: 10, 20, 40, 60, 80, 90 mg
	INDERAL LA	Capsules: 60, 80, 120, 160 mg

DRUG PROFILE

Beta-adrenergic blocking drugs (beta-blockers) are used to control high blood pressure. Some are used for other conditions such as angina, heart arrhythmias, migraine headaches, and hypertrophic subaortic stenosis (a disease of the heart muscle). Some have also been found to improve a person's chance of survival for several years following a heart attack. By blocking certain nerve impulses, these medicines reduce the workload of the heart and help the heart to beat more regularly.

When used in the treatment of angina, beta-blockers prevent future attacks (they are not helpful during an acute attack of chest pain). Beta-blockers differ in the duration of action and when their peak effect occurs, and it is worthwhile to discuss with your doctor precisely how to time your doses in relation to the pattern of your attacks. If you suffer a side effect, such as depression or nightmares, with one beta-blocker, your doctor may be able to prescribe a different beta-blocker that will be equally effective. Beta-blockers may be used along with other antiangina medicines.

For complete information on these drugs, see pages 59–64.

CONDITION: **ANGINA**

CATEGORY: **CALCIUM BLOCKERS**

GENERIC (CHEMICAL) NAME	BRAND (TRADE) NAME	DOSAGE FORMS AND STRENGTHS
Bepridil	VASCOR	Tablets: 200, 300, 400 mg

DRUG PROFILE

The calcium blockers are used to relieve and control angina pectoris (chest pain). Calcium is needed for muscle cells to contract. By decreasing the passage of calcium into the muscle cells, these drugs relax the blood vessels and heart muscle. This increases the supply of blood and oxygen to the heart, reduces its workload, and prevents spasms of the blood vessels of the heart. Other antianginal drugs can be used along with a calcium blocker, if necessary. Calcium blockers tend to lower blood pressure. If you are also taking an antihypertensive agent, its dosage may need to be lowered. Bepridil is used to treat angina in patients who are not satisfactorily treated with other antianginal agents.

BEFORE USING THIS DRUG

Let your doctor know *IF*

You have ever had allergic reactions or other problems with ■ bepridil ■ other calcium blockers.

You have ever had any of the following medical problems: ■ other heart or blood vessel disease including problems with irregular heartbeat ■ low blood pressure ■ recent heart attack (in the past 3 months) ■ kidney disease ■ liver disease.

You are taking any of the following medicines: ■ other medicines for angina ■ beta-blockers (eg, propranolol, atenolol, metoprolol, etc.) ■ medicine for high blood pressure ■ diuretics ■ aspirin or aspirinlike medicine ■ digoxin or digitalis (heart medicine) ■ medicine for irregular heart rhythm, including quinidine, procainamide and others ■ antidepressants.

SPECIAL INSTRUCTIONS WHILE TAKING THIS DRUG

FOOD AND DRUG INTERACTIONS

Food and Beverages	Remember that angina may be provoked by eating a meal that is too heavy.
Alcohol	Drinking alcohol while taking calcium blockers may worsen such side effects as dizziness, light-headedness, or fainting. Avoid alcohol unless your doctor has approved its use.
Smoking	Smoking increases your chance of an angina attack. If you smoke, try to stop or at least cut down.

DAILY LIVING

Exertion and Exercise	Since this medicine may reduce or prevent chest pain associated with exercise, you may be tempted to become overactive. You should discuss with your doctor how much exercise is safe for you.
Excessive Cold	Use caution during cold weather, as excessive cold may provoke an angina attack.
Examinations or Tests	It is important for you to keep all appointments with your doctor, even if you feel well, so that your progress can be monitored and your blood pressure checked. Periodic blood and urine tests may be required.
Other Precautions	Check your pulse regularly, and call your doctor if it falls below fifty beats per minute.
	Tell any doctor or dentist you consult that you are taking this medicine, especially if you will be undergoing any type of surgery.
	Remember that emotional stress may trigger an angina attack.
Helpful Hints	If bepridil causes nausea or an upset stomach, taking it with meals or at bedtime may help.
	If your doctor has prescribed potassium supplements or potassium-sparing diuretics, it is important to take them as directed. Low potassium levels can increase the side effects of this medicine.
	You may have headaches after taking this medicine. Headaches usually stop with continued use of the medicine; if they do not, or if they are particularly severe, call your doctor.

No special restrictions on sun exposure, driving, or exposure to excessive heat.

POSSIBLE SIDE EFFECTS

Although this list of adverse effects may seem somewhat intimidating, keep in mind that some are quite rare. Of course, should these or any other problems arise while you are on medication, it is always a good idea to consult your doctor.

IF YOU DEVELOP	WHAT TO DO
irregular, fast, or slow heartbeat ■ palpitations ■ difficulty in breathing ■ wheezing ■ swelling of the ankles, feet, or lower legs ■ fainting ■ hallucinations ■ severe dizziness ■ difficulty in balance	**Urgent** Get in touch with your doctor immediately.
changes in behavior ■ rash ■ sore throat, fever, chills ■ unusual tiredness or weakness ■ depression ■ coughing ■ chest congestion ■ blurred vision or other visual problems ■ numbness or tingling of the hands or feet	**May be serious** Check with your doctor as soon as possible.
dizziness or light-headedness ■ drowsiness ■ nervousness ■ headache ■ tiredness ■ weakness ■ sleeplessness ■ ringing in the ears ■ nausea ■ diarrhea ■ constipation ■ stomach cramps ■ upset stomach ■ dry mouth ■ gas ■ loss of appetite ■ tremor ■ stuffy nose ■ anxiety ■ taste changes ■ "flu" symptoms ■ weight gain ■ sexual problems	If symptoms are disturbing or persist, let your doctor know.

STORAGE INSTRUCTIONS

Store in a cool, dark place (not in a bathroom medicine cabinet).

STOPPING OR INTERRUPTING THERAPY

Take this medicine exactly as directed, even if you do not feel chest pain. Do not take more of the medicine or take it more frequently than prescribed by your doctor. Suddenly stopping your medicine may worsen your medical problem. Your doctor will advise you on how to discontinue therapy gradually before stopping completely. If you miss a dose, take it as soon as possible; if it is almost time for your next dose, skip the missed dose and resume your regular schedule. Do not take two doses at the same time.

SPECIAL CONSIDERATIONS FOR THOSE OVER SIXTY-FIVE

Dizziness, light-headedness, and fainting, especially when getting up from a reclining or sitting position, are more likely to occur in older people, who may be advised to take their first dose in a situation in which they will be able to lie down, if necessary. Such people may also be more susceptible to constipation as a side effect.

Also, older people tend not to eliminate the calcium blockers as readily as young adults; thus, the drug may reach higher concentrations and remain in the bloodstream for a longer time. Doctors may require checkups to make sure that the proper dosage is being administered and that too much drug is not accumulating in the body.

CONDITION: **ANGINA**

CATEGORY: **CALCIUM BLOCKERS**

GENERIC (CHEMICAL) NAME	BRAND (TRADE) NAME	DOSAGE FORMS AND STRENGTHS
Diltiazem	CARDIZEM	Tablets: 30, 60, 90, 120 mg

DRUG PROFILE

The calcium blockers are used to relieve and control angina pectoris (chest pain). Calcium is needed for muscle cells to contract; by decreasing the passage of calcium into the muscle cells, these drugs relax the blood vessels and heart muscle. This increases the supply of blood and oxygen to the heart, reduces its workload, and prevents spasms of the blood vessels of the heart. Other antianginal drugs can be used along with a calcium blocker, if necessary. Calcium blockers tend to lower blood pressure; if you are also taking an antihypertensive medicine, its dosage may need to be lowered. Diltiazem can also be prescribed for hypertension.

BEFORE USING THIS DRUG

Let your doctor know *IF*

You have ever had allergic reactions or other problems with ■ diltiazem ■ other calcium blockers.

You have ever had any of the following medical problems: ■ other heart or blood vessel disease ■ kidney disease ■ liver disease ■ low blood pressure.

You are taking any of the following medicines: ■ beta-blockers (eg, propranolol, atenolol, metoprolol) or other medicines for high blood pressure or angina ■ anticoagulants (blood thinners) ■ aspirin or aspirinlike medicine ■ sulfonamides (sulfa drugs) ■ cimetidine (medicine for ulcers) ■ digoxin or digitalis (heart medicines) ■ disopyramide or quinidine (medicine for abnormal heart rhythms) ■ medicine for seizures ■ medicine for malaria ■ theophylline (medicine to improve breathing) ■ cyclosporine.

SPECIAL RESTRICTIONS WHILE TAKING THIS DRUG

FOOD AND DRUG INTERACTIONS

Foods and Beverages	Remember that angina may be provoked by eating a meal that is too heavy.
Alcohol	Drinking alcohol while taking calcium blockers may worsen such side effects as dizziness, light-headedness, or fainting. Avoid alcohol unless your doctor has approved its use.
Smoking	Smoking increases your chance of an angina attack. If you smoke, try to stop or at least cut down.

DAILY LIVING

Exertion and Exercise	Since this medicine is taken before exercise to reduce or prevent associated chest pain, you may be tempted to become overactive. You should discuss with your doctor how much exercise is safe for you.

Sun Exposure	While taking this medicine, your eyes may become more sensitive to light; wearing dark glasses when exposed to the sun should help.
Excessive Cold	Use caution during cold weather, since excessive cold may provoke an angina attack.
Examinations or Tests	It is important for you to keep all appointments with your doctor, even if you feel well, so that your progress can be monitored and your blood pressure checked. Periodic blood and urine tests may be required.
Other Precautions	Check your pulse regularly, and call your doctor if it falls below fifty beats per minute. Tell any doctor or dentist you consult that you are taking this medicine, especially if you will be undergoing any type of surgery. Remember that emotional stress may trigger an angina attack.
Helpful Hints	For best effects, take this medicine one hour before or two hours after meals. You may have headaches after taking this medicine. Headaches usually stop with continued use of the medicine; if they do not, or if they are particularly severe, call your doctor.

No special restrictions on driving or exposure to excessive heat.

POSSIBLE SIDE EFFECTS

Although this list of adverse effects may seem somewhat intimidating, keep in mind that some are quite rare. Of course, should these or any other problems arise while you are on medication, it is always a good idea to consult your doctor.

IF YOU DEVELOP	WHAT TO DO
difficulty in breathing ■ coughing or wheezing ■ chest congestion ■ irregular or slow heartbeat ■ palpitations ■ rash, hives, or itching ■ swelling of ankles, feet, or lower legs ■ fainting ■ sore throat ■ blurred vision ■ difficulty in balance ■ fever ■ chills ■ increased sweating ■ hallucinations	**May be serious** Check with your doctor as soon as possible.
flushing or feeling of warmth ■ headache ■ dizziness or light-headedness, especially when getting up from a reclining or sitting position ■ tiredness or weakness ■ drowsiness ■ depression ■ confusion ■ sleepless-ness ■ giddiness ■ anxiety ■ mood changes ■ gas ■ constipation ■ nausea or vomiting ■ stomach cramps or upset stomach ■ loss of appetite ■ diarrhea ■ heartburn ■ stuffy nose ■ increased eye sensitivity to sunlight ■ muscle cramps ■ joint stiff-ness or swelling ■ gum problems ■ increased urina-tion ■ need to urinate at night	If symptoms are disturbing or persist, let your doctor know.

STORAGE INSTRUCTIONS

Store in a cool, dark place (not in a bathroom medicine cabinet).

STOPPING OR INTERRUPTING THERAPY

Take this medicine exactly as directed, even if you do not feel chest pain. Do not take more of the medicine or take it more frequently than prescribed by your doctor. Suddenly stopping your medicine may worsen your medical problem. Your doctor will advise you on how to discontinue therapy gradually before stopping completely. If you miss a dose, take it as soon as possible. If it is almost time for your next dose, skip the missed dose and resume your regular schedule. Do not take two doses at the same time.

SPECIAL CONSIDERATIONS FOR THOSE OVER SIXTY-FIVE

Dizziness, light-headedness, and fainting, especially when getting up from a reclining or sitting position, are more likely to occur in older people, who may be advised to take their first dose in a situation in which they will be able to lie down, if necessary.

Also, older people tend not to eliminate the calcium blockers as readily as young adults; thus, the drug may reach high concentrations and remain in the bloodstream for a longer time. Doctors may require regular checkups to make sure that the proper dosage is being administered and that too much drug is not accumulating in the body.

CONDITION: **ANGINA**
CATEGORY: **CALCIUM BLOCKERS**

GENERIC (CHEMICAL) NAME	BRAND (TRADE) NAME	DOSAGE FORMS AND STRENGTHS
Nifedipine	ADALAT	Capsules: 10, 20 mg
	PROCARDIA	Capsules: 10, 20 mg
	PROCARDIA XL	Extended-release tablets: 30, 60, 90 mg

DRUG PROFILE

The calcium blockers are used to relieve and control angina pectoris (chest pain). Calcium is needed for muscle cells to contract; by decreasing the passage of calcium into the muscle cells, these drugs relax the blood vessels and heart muscle. This increases the supply of blood and oxygen to the heart, reduces its workload, and prevents spasms of the blood vessels of the heart. Other antianginal drugs can be used along with a calcium blocker, if necessary. Calcium blockers tend to lower blood pressure; if you are also taking an antihypertensive medicine, its dosage may need to be lowered.

BEFORE USING THIS DRUG

Let your doctor know *IF*

You have ever had allergic reactions or other problems with ■ nifedipine ■ other calcium blockers.

You have ever had any of the following medical problems: ■ other heart or blood vessel disease ■ kidney disease ■ liver disease ■ low blood pressure.

You are taking any of the following medicines: ■ beta-blockers (eg, propranolol, atenolol, metoprolol) or other medicines for high blood pressure or angina ■ anticoagulants (blood thinners) ■ aspirin or aspirinlike medicine ■ sulfonamides (sulfa drugs) ■ cimetidine (medicine for ulcers) ■ quinidine (medicine for abnormal heart rhythms) ■ medicine for seizures ■ medicine for malaria ■ theophylline (medicine to improve breathing) ■ cyclosporine.

SPECIAL INSTRUCTIONS WHILE TAKING THIS DRUG

FOOD AND DRUG INTERACTIONS

Foods and Beverages	Remember that angina may be provoked by eating a meal that is too heavy.
Alcohol	Drinking alcohol while taking calcium blockers may worsen such side effects as dizziness, light-headedness, or fainting. Avoid alcohol unless your doctor has approved its use.
Smoking	Smoking increases your chance of an angina attack. If you smoke, try to stop or at least cut down.

DAILY LIVING

Exertion and Exercise	Since this medicine is taken before exercise to reduce or prevent associated chest pain, you may be tempted to become overactive. You should discuss with your doctor how much exercise is safe for you.

Sun Exposure	While taking this medicine, your eyes may become more sensitive to light; wearing dark glasses when exposed to the sun should help.
Excessive Cold	Use caution during cold weather, as excessive cold may provoke an angina attack.
Examinations or Tests	It is important for you to keep all appointments with your doctor, even if you feel well, so that your progress can be monitored and your blood pressure checked. Periodic blood and urine tests may be required.
Other Precautions	Tell any doctor or dentist you consult that you are taking this medicine, especially if you will be undergoing any type of surgery. Remember that emotional stress may trigger an angina attack.
Helpful Hints	For best effects, take this medicine one hour before or two hours after meals. You may have headaches after taking this medicine. Headaches usually stop with continued use of the medicine; if they do not, or if they are particularly severe, call your doctor.

No special restrictions on driving or excessive heat.

POSSIBLE SIDE EFFECTS

Although this list of adverse effects may seem somewhat intimidating, keep in mind that some are quite rare. Of course, should these or any other problems arise while you are on medication, it is always a good idea to consult your doctor.

IF YOU DEVELOP

difficulty in breathing ■ coughing or wheezing ■ chest congestion ■ irregular heartbeat or palpitations ■ rash, hives, or itching ■ swelling of ankles, feet, or lower legs ■ fainting ■ sore throat ■ blurred vision ■ difficulty in balance ■ fever ■ chills ■ increased sweating ■ hallucinations

WHAT TO DO

May be serious Check with your doctor as soon as possible.

---

flushing or feeling of warmth ■ headache ■ dizziness or light-headedness, especially when getting up from a reclining or sitting position ■ tiredness or weakness ■ drowsiness ■ depression ■ confusion ■ sleeplessness ■ giddiness ■ anxiety ■ mood changes ■ gas ■ constipation ■ nausea or vomiting ■ stomach cramps or upset stomach ■ loss of appetite ■ diarrhea ■ heartburn ■ stuffy nose ■ increased eye sensitivity to sunlight ■ muscle cramps ■ joint stiffness or swelling ■ gum problems ■ sexual problems

If symptoms are disturbing or persist, let your doctor know.

STORAGE INSTRUCTIONS

Store in a cool, dark place (not in a bathroom medicine cabinet).

STOPPING OR INTERRUPTING THERAPY

Take this medicine exactly as directed, even if you do not feel chest pain. Do not take more of the medicine or take it more frequently than prescribed by your doctor. Suddenly stopping your medicine may worsen your medical problem. Your doctor will advise you on how to discontinue therapy gradually before stopping completely. If you miss a dose, take it as soon as possible. If it is almost time for your next dose, skip the missed dose and resume your regular schedule. Do not take two doses at the same time.

SPECIAL CONSIDERATIONS FOR THOSE OVER SIXTY-FIVE

Dizziness, light-headedness, and fainting, especially when getting up from a reclining or sitting position, are more likely to occur in older people, who may be advised to take their first dose in a situation in which they will be able to lie down, if necessary.

Also, older people tend not to eliminate the calcium blockers as rapidly as young adults; thus, the drug may reach higher concentrations and remain in the bloodstream for a longer time. Doctors may require regular checkups to make sure that the proper dosage is being administered and that too much drug is not accumulating in the body.

CONDITION: **ANGINA**

CATEGORY: **CALCIUM BLOCKERS**

GENERIC (CHEMICAL) NAME	BRAND (TRADE) NAME	DOSAGE FORMS AND STRENGTHS
Nicardipine hydrochloride	CARDENE	Capsules: 20, 30 mg

DRUG PROFILE

The calcium blockers are used to relieve and control angina pectoris (chest pain); some are used to control high blood pressure as well. Calcium is needed for muscle cells to contract; by decreasing the passage of calcium into the muscle cells, these drugs relax the blood vessels and heart muscle. This increases the supply of blood and oxygen to the heart, reduces its workload, and prevents spasms of the blood vessels of the heart. Other antianginal drugs (nitrates, beta-blockers) can be used along with a calcium blocker if necessary. Calcium blockers tend to lower blood pressure; if you are also taking an antihypertensive agent, its dosage may need to be lowered.

BEFORE USING THIS DRUG

Let your doctor know *IF*

You have ever had allergic reactions or other problems with ■ nicardipine ■ other calcium blockers.

You have ever had any of the following medical problems: ■ other heart or blood vessel disease ■ kidney disease ■ liver disease ■ low blood pressure ■ stroke.

You are taking any of the following medicines: ■ beta-blockers (eg, propranolol, atenolol, metoprolol) or other medicine for high blood pressure ■ cimetidine (medicine for ulcers) ■ digoxin or digitalis (heart medicine) ■ cyclosporine ■ theophylline (medicine to improve breathing).

SPECIAL RESTRICTIONS WHILE TAKING THIS DRUG

FOOD AND DRUG INTERACTIONS

Other Drugs	If you are being treated for hypertension, do not take any other drugs, including over-the-counter (OTC) drugs, before checking with your doctor. OTC drugs for appetite suppression, asthma, cough, colds, hay fever, or sinus problems tend to increase blood pressure.
Foods and Beverages	If you are being treated for angina, remember that your condition can be provoked by eating a meal that is too heavy. If you are being treated for hypertension, your doctor may prescribe a special low-salt diet, which you should follow carefully because it will help your medicine work more effectively.
Alcohol	Drinking alcohol while taking calcium blockers may worsen such side effects as dizziness, light-headedness, or fainting. Avoid alcohol unless your doctor has approved its use.

Smoking	If you are being treated for angina, remember that smoking increases your chance of an attack. If you smoke, try to stop or at least cut down.

DAILY LIVING

Exertion and Exercise	Since chest pain from exercise or exertion may be reduced or prevented with this medicine, you may be tempted to overwork yourself. Discuss with your doctor how much exercise is safe for you.
Excessive Cold	If you are being treated for angina, use caution during cold weather, as excessive cold may provoke an attack.
Examinations or Tests	It is important for you to keep all appointments with your doctor, even if you feel well, so that your progress can be monitored and your blood pressure checked. Periodic blood and urine tests may be required.
Other Precautions	Tell any doctor or dentist you consult that you are taking this medicine, especially if you will be undergoing any type of surgery. If you are being treated for angina, remember that emotional stress may trigger an attack.

No special restrictions on driving, sun exposure, or excessive heat.

POSSIBLE SIDE EFFECTS

Although this list of adverse effects may seem somewhat intimidating, keep in mind that some are quite rare. Of course, should these or any other problems arise while you are on medication, it is always a good idea to consult your doctor.

IF YOU DEVELOP	**WHAT TO DO**
Signs of overdose: ■ slow heartbeat with severe dizziness or fainting ■ drowsiness ■ confusion ■ slurred speech ■ chest pain	**Urgent** Get in touch with your doctor immediately.
difficulty in breathing ■ rapid heartbeat ■ palpitations ■ swelling of feet or any other swelling ■ flushing ■ fainting	**May be serious** Check with your doctor as soon as possible.
dizziness ■ headache ■ weakness ■ drowsiness ■ nausea or vomiting ■ indigestion ■ dry mouth ■ rash ■ general ill feeling ■ nervousness ■ shaking ■ tingling or burning sensations ■ muscle cramps ■ constipation ■ sleeplessness ■ abnormal dreams ■ hot flashes ■ hyperactivity ■ male impotence ■ depression ■ confusion ■ anxiety ■ dizziness or light-headedness when getting up from a reclining or sitting position ■ cold hands and feet ■ sore throat ■ sinus problems ■ runny nose ■ blurred vision ■ increased urination ■ need to urinate at night ■ aching joints ■ ringing in ears	If symptoms are disturbing or persist, let your doctor know.

STORAGE INSTRUCTIONS

Store in a cool, dark place (not in a bathroom medicine cabinet).

STOPPING OR INTERRUPTING THERAPY

Take this medicine exactly as directed, even if you feel well. Suddenly stopping your medicine may worsen your medical problem. If you miss a dose, take it as soon as possible. If it is almost time for your next dose, skip the missed dose and resume your regular schedule. Do not take two doses at the same time.

SPECIAL CONSIDERATIONS FOR THOSE OVER SIXTY-FIVE

Older people may be more likely to experience dizziness, lightheadedness, or faintness when getting up from a reclining position. When getting up from a sitting or lying position, get up slowly to allow your body to adjust to your changing postural position.

CONDITION: **ANGINA**

CATEGORY: **CALCIUM BLOCKERS**

GENERIC (CHEMICAL) NAME	BRAND (TRADE) NAME	DOSAGE FORMS AND STRENGTHS
Verapamil	CALAN	Tablets: 40, 80, 120 mg
	ISOPTIN	Tablets: 40, 80, 120 mg

DRUG PROFILE

The calcium blockers are used to relieve and control angina pectoris (chest pain). Calcium is needed for muscle cells to contract; by decreasing the passage of calcium into the muscle cells, these drugs relax the blood vessels and heart muscle. This increases the supply of blood and oxygen to the heart, reduces its workload, and prevents spasms of the blood vessels of the heart. Other antianginal drugs can be used along with a calcium blocker, if necessary. Calcium blockers tend to lower blood pressure; if you are also taking an antihypertensive agent, its dosage may need to be lowered. Verapamil can also be prescribed to treat high blood pressure.

BEFORE USING THIS DRUG

Let your doctor know *IF*

You have ever had allergic reactions or other problems with ■ verapamil ■ other calcium blockers.

You have ever had any of the following medical problems: ■ other heart or blood vessel disease ■ kidney disease ■ liver disease.

You are taking any of the following medicines: ■ beta-blockers (eg, propranolol, atenolol, metoprolol) or other medicines for high blood pressure or angina ■ anticoagulants (blood thinners) ■ aspirin or aspirinlike medicine ■ sulfonamides (sulfa drugs) ■ cimetidine (medicine for ulcers) ■ digoxin or digitalis (heart medicines) ■ disopyramide, flecainide or quinidine (medicine for abnormal heart rhythms) ■ phenobarbital or carbamazepine (medicine for seizures) ■ medicine for malaria ■ lithium ■ rifampin ■ cyclosporine.

SPECIAL INSTRUCTIONS WHILE TAKING THIS DRUG

FOOD AND DRUG INTERACTIONS

Foods and Beverages	Remember that angina may be provoked by eating a meal that is too heavy.
Alcohol	Drinking alcohol while taking calcium blockers may worsen such side effects as dizziness, light-headedness, or fainting. Avoid alcohol unless your doctor has approved its use.
Smoking	Smoking increases your chance of an angina attack. If you smoke, try to stop or at least cut down.

DAILY LIVING

Exertion and Exercise	Since this medicine is taken before exercise to reduce or prevent associated chest pain, you may be tempted to become overactive. You should discuss with your doctor how much exercise is safe for you.
Sun Exposure	While taking this medicine, your eyes may become more sensitive to light; wearing dark glasses when exposed to the sun should help.
Excessive Cold	Use caution during cold weather, as excessive cold may provoke an angina attack.

Examinations or Tests	It is important for you to keep all appointments with your doctor, even if you feel well, so that your progress can be monitored and your blood pressure checked. Periodic blood and urine tests may be required.
Other Precautions	Check your pulse regularly, and call your doctor if it falls below fifty beats per minute.
	Tell any doctor or dentist you consult that you are taking this medicine, especially if you will be undergoing any type of surgery.
	Remember that emotional stress may trigger an angina attack.
Helpful Hints	You may have headaches after taking this medicine. Headaches usually stop with continued use of the medicine; if they do not, or if they are particularly severe, call your doctor.
	The controlled-release tablets may be broken in half, but should not be crushed or chewed. Take the controlled-release tablets with food.

No special restrictions on driving or exposure to excessive heat.

POSSIBLE SIDE EFFECTS

Although this list of adverse effects may seem somewhat intimidating, keep in mind that some are quite rare. Of course, should these or any other problems arise while you are on medication, it is always a good idea to consult your doctor.

IF YOU DEVELOP	WHAT TO DO
difficulty in breathing ■ coughing or wheezing ■ chest congestion ■ irregular or slow heartbeat ■ palpitations ■ rash, hives, or itching ■ swelling of ankles, feet, or lower legs ■ fainting ■ sore throat or fever ■ blurred vision ■ difficulty in balance ■ chills ■ increased sweating ■ hallucinations	**May be serious** Check with your doctor as soon as possible.
constipation ■ flushing or feeling of warmth ■ headache ■ dizziness or light-headedness, especially when getting up from a reclining or sitting position ■ tiredness or weakness ■ drowsiness ■ depression ■ confusion ■ sleeplessness ■ giddiness ■ anxiety ■ mood changes ■ gas ■ nausea or vomiting ■ stomach cramps or upset stomach ■ loss of appetite ■ diarrhea ■ heartburn ■ stuffy nose ■ increased eye sensitivity to sunlight ■ muscle cramps ■ joint stiffness or swelling ■ gum problems ■ sexual problems	If symptoms are disturbing or persist, let your doctor know.

STORAGE INSTRUCTIONS

Store in a cool, dark place (not in a bathroom medicine cabinet).

STOPPING OR INTERRUPTING THERAPY

Take this medicine exactly as directed, even if you do not feel chest pain. Do not take more of the medicine or take it more frequently than prescribed by your doctor. Suddenly stopping your medicine may worsen your medical problem. Your doctor will advise you on how to discontinue therapy gradually before stopping completely. If you miss a dose, take it as soon as possible. If it is almost time for your next dose, skip the missed dose and resume your regular schedule. Do not take two doses at the same time.

SPECIAL CONSIDERATIONS FOR THOSE OVER SIXTY-FIVE

Dizziness, light-headedness, and fainting, especially when getting up from a reclining or sitting position, are more likely to occur in older people, who may be advised to take their first dose in a situation in which they will be able to lie down, if necessary. Such people may also be more susceptible to constipation as a side effect.

Also, older people tend not to eliminate the calcium blockers as readily as young adults; thus, the drug may reach higher concentrations and remain in the bloodstream for a longer time. Doctors may require checkups to make sure that the proper dosage is being administered and that too much drug is not accumulating in the body.

CONDITION: **ANGINA**

CATEGORY: **ANTIANGINAL AGENTS (MISCELLANEOUS)**

GENERIC (CHEMICAL) NAME	BRAND (TRADE) NAME	DOSAGE FORMS AND STRENGTHS
Dipyridamole	PERSANTINE	Tablets: 25, 50, 75 mg

DRUG PROFILE

Dipyridamole is used, along with another drug, to prevent angina attacks. However, the Food and Drug Administration has not approved the use of dipyridamole for angina. You should discuss its use with your doctor. Dipyridamole is also prescribed, together with an anticoagulant drug, to prevent blood clots in people who have artificial heart valves.

BEFORE USING THIS DRUG

Let your doctor know *IF*

You have ever had allergic reactions or other problems with ■ dipyridamole.

You have ever had any of the following medical problems: ■ low blood pressure ■ congestive heart failure.

You are taking any of the following medicines: ■ medicine for high blood pressure ■ anticoagulants (blood thinners) ■ aspirin or aspirinlike medicine.

SPECIAL RESTRICTIONS WHILE TAKING THIS DRUG

FOOD AND DRUG INTERACTIONS

Other Drugs	Diuretics and other medicine for high blood pressure may increase the effects of dizziness, light-headedness, or fainting when taken together with dipyridamole.
Foods and Beverages	Remember that angina may be provoked by eating a meal that is too heavy.
Alcohol	Drinking alcohol while taking this medicine may worsen such side effects as dizziness, light-headedness, or fainting. Avoid alcohol unless your doctor has approved its use.
Smoking	Smoking increases your chance of an angina attack. If you smoke, try to stop or at least cut down.

DAILY LIVING

Exertion and Exercise	Since this medicine reduces or prevents chest pain from exercise, you may be tempted to become over-active. You should discuss with your doctor how much exercise is safe for you.
Excessive Cold	Use caution during cold weather, as excessive cold may provoke an angina attack.
Examinations or Tests	It is important for you to keep all appointments with your doctor, even if you feel well, so that your progress can be monitored and your blood pressure checked. Periodic blood and urine tests may be required.

Other Precautions	Remember that emotional stress may trigger an angina attack.
	Dipyridamole is used to *prevent* angina and is not effective once an angina attack has already started. Check with your doctor if you feel you need a fast-acting drug such as nitroglycerin that will relieve the pain of an actual attack.
Helpful Hints	Swallow the tablets whole (do not chew). For best effects, take this medicine with a full glass of water at least one hour before meals.

No special restrictions on driving, sun exposure, or exposure to excessive heat.

POSSIBLE SIDE EFFECTS

Although this list of adverse effects may seem somewhat intimidating, keep in mind that some are quite rare. Of course, should these or any other problems arise while you are on medication, it is always a good idea to consult your doctor.

IF YOU DEVELOP	WHAT TO DO
chest pain or tightness	**May be serious** Check with your doctor as soon as possible.
dizziness, light-headedness, or fainting, especially when getting up from a reclining or sitting position ■ flushing ■ headache ■ nausea or vomiting ■ diarrhea ■ upset stomach or stomach cramps ■ rash ■ weakness ■ itching	If symptoms are disturbing or persist, let your doctor know.

STORAGE INSTRUCTIONS

Store in a cool, dark place (not in a bathroom medicine cabinet).

STOPPING OR INTERRUPTING THERAPY

Take this medicine exactly as prescribed by your doctor. It may take two or three months before you notice beneficial effects. Do not stop taking it if you feel it is not working; check with your doctor instead. If you miss a dose, take it as soon as possible, unless it is within four hours of your next scheduled dose. In that case, skip the missed dose and resume your regular schedule. Do not take two doses at the same time.

SPECIAL CONSIDERATIONS FOR THOSE OVER SIXTY-FIVE

The side effects of light-headedness, dizziness, and fainting are more likely to occur in older people.

CONGESTIVE HEART FAILURE

Although most heart conditions are becoming less common, congestive heart failure is on the increase. In 1989, well over one million people over the age of 65 were treated in the hospital with congestive heart failure. This condition is six times more common in those sixty-five to seventy-five years of age than in those forty-five to fifty-four years of age.

CAUSES

Congestive heart failure is not actually a single disease but rather a condition that can develop from a number of underlying disorders. It occurs when the heart loses its ability to keep up with the body's demand for oxygen-rich blood. If you have congestive heart failure, it means that your heart may be pumping too weakly either to supply adequate blood to the rest of your body or to keep up with the return of oxygen-depleted blood once it has passed through the circulatory system. Or it may mean that the ability of your heart to fill with blood is impaired.

The condition may occur in the left or the right side of the heart. Left-sided heart failure is the most common variety. It is usually caused by dysfunction of the heart muscle, heart valve disease, or circulatory obstruction in the heart. If failure in the left side of the heart goes unchecked, the right side of the heart will also be affected, as blood backs up from the left chambers to the right. Various lung diseases can also cause right-sided heart failure. In addition, certain conditions outside the cardiovascular system—such as thyroid disease, severe anemia, and severe malnutrition—can lead to congestive heart failure.

DIAGNOSIS

The symptoms of congestive heart failure vary, depending on the part of the heart that is affected. Because the condition is often marked by low cardiac output—the inability of the heart to pump sufficient blood to meet the body's needs—you may feel tired and have trouble performing even routine physical tasks. If you have left-sided heart failure, you may also find breathing difficult (this can occur when you are lying flat as well as during activity). If the heart failure has extended to the right side, you may also notice edema, which is swelling of the arms or legs (particularly the ankles) caused by fluid retention.

In severe congestive heart failure, organs other than the heart may be damaged. Left-sided heart failure can lead to a kidney disease called pre-renal azotemia. Occasionally, in right-sided heart failure fluid will accumulate in the abdomen and fill the liver and intestines, causing nausea, loss of appetite, abdominal pain, and an inability to absorb nutrients.

Older people sometimes assume that the symptoms of congestive heart failure are normal changes of aging;

they may think that fatigue and shortness of breath are to be expected with advancing years. Similarly, they may misinterpret abdominal discomfort resulting from fluid accumulation as a simple touch of the flu. If you have any of these symptoms and they persist, you should consult a doctor. Your doctor will look for signs of congestive heart failure such as abnormal heart sounds or lung sounds, distension of the jugular veins (important blood vessels leading from the brain to the heart), and edema of the legs.

If these signs and symptoms lead your doctor to suspect congestive heart failure, the next step will be to take an X ray of the chest to look for enlargement of the heart and fluid in the lungs, and an echocardiogram to look for evidence of underlying heart disease. An echocardiogram is an image of the heart electronically composed from sound waves bounced off the chest. One other test, a radionuclide ventriculogram (angiogram), may also be performed to determine the degree of heart failure. In this test, the doctor injects a small amount of radioactive material into a vein and films the treated blood as it moves through the heart.

Both the echocardiogram and the ventriculogram (angiogram) help determine a figure known as the heart's "ejection fraction"—the amount of blood the heart pumps out with each contraction. If you have an ejection fraction of 40 percent or less, it may mean that congestive heart failure has developed. Some people develop symptoms of congestive heart failure with normal ejection fractions, while other people with very low ejection fractions may not have any symptoms.

TREATMENT

Congestive heart failure may be the result of a treatable underlying condition, such as valvular disease. Your therapy will be aimed at both relieving the heart failure and eliminating its cause. The drugs discussed in the charts on pages 195–208, including digoxin, diuretics like furosemide or bumetanide, and so-called ACE inhibitors (like captopril, enalapril, and lisinopril), are the mainstays of treatment for congestive heart failure. Surgery may be recommended for treating the valve disease. Once such underlying causes are removed, congestive heart failure may no longer be a problem.

OUTLOOK

Many patients, however, will have to continue treatment even after their symptoms go away. Your doctor will probably recommend a low-salt diet to decrease your retention of fluids; in addition, you will need to have regular checkups to make sure your medicine is working properly. If you follow these recommendations, your heart condition should not unduly affect your way of life.

CONDITION: **CONGESTIVE HEART FAILURE**

CATEGORY: **LOOP DIURETICS**

GENERIC (CHEMICAL) NAME	BRAND (TRADE) NAME	DOSAGE FORMS AND STRENGTHS
Furosemide	LASIX	Solution: 10 mg per ml Tablets: 20, 40, 80 mg

DRUG PROFILE

Furosemide is a diuretic that is used to treat the edema (fluid accumulation) that may be a result of congestive heart failure, kidney disease, or liver disease. It is also sometimes prescribed to lower high blood pressure. Furosemide is known as a "loop" diuretic because it acts on a part of the kidney called the loop of Henle. This drug helps the kidneys eliminate excess salt and water through urination. This not only relieves edema but also decreases the volume of blood flowing through the blood vessels, which results in lower blood pressure.

BEFORE USING THIS DRUG

Let your doctor know *IF*

You have ever had allergic reactions or other problems with ■ furosemide ■ thiazide or thiazide-type diuretics ■ tartrazine (FD&C Yellow Dye No. 5) ■ aspirin ■ sulfonamides (sulfa drugs).

You have ever had any of the following medical problems: ■ diabetes ■ kidney disease ■ liver disease ■ systemic lupus erythematosus ■ gout ■ disease of the pancreas ■ heart disease ■ hearing problems ■ diarrhea.

You are taking any of the following medicines: ■ diuretics or other medicines for high blood pressure ■ corticosteroids ■ large doses of aspirin or aspirinlike medicine ■ clofibrate (medicine for high cholesterol) ■ medicine for diabetes ■ barbiturates ■ digoxin or digitalis (heart medicines) ■ medicine for gout ■ medicine for arthritis, including indomethacin ■ lithium ■ narcotics or other prescription pain-killers

■ sleep medicines ■ aminoglycoside antibiotics ■ medicine for seizures
■ methenamine (medicine to prevent urinary tract infections).

You are or have recently been on a low-salt diet.

SPECIAL RESTRICTIONS WHILE TAKING THIS DRUG

FOOD AND DRUG INTERACTIONS

Other Drugs	If you are taking this medicine for high blood pressure, do not take any other drugs, including over-the-counter (OTC) drugs, before checking with your doctor. Some OTC drugs for appetite suppression, asthma, colds, cough, hay fever, or sinus problems tend to increase blood pressure. Your doctor will probably reduce the dose of or discontinue other medicines you may be taking for high blood pressure when you start taking furosemide.
Foods and Beverages	Your doctor may prescribe a special low-salt diet, which you should follow carefully because it will help your medicine work more effectively. You may also be advised to go on a weight-reduction diet. Continue to drink a normal amount of fluids. This drug may cause your body to lose large amounts of the mineral potassium. Your doctor may give you special instructions about eating foods or drinking beverages that have a high potassium content (such as bananas and citrus fruit juices), taking a potassium supplement, or using salt substitutes.
Alcohol	Drinking alcohol may worsen such side effects as dizziness or drowsiness. Avoid alcohol unless your doctor has approved its use.

No special restrictions on smoking.

DAILY LIVING

Exertion and Exercise	Use caution when exercising or standing for long periods of time because this medicine may cause you to become dehydrated and dizzy, light-headed, or faint.
Sun Exposure/ Excessive Heat	Your skin may become more sensitive to sunlight and more likely to develop a sunburn while you are taking this medicine. It is a good idea to avoid too much sun, especially if you burn easily. Apply a sunscreen to exposed skin surfaces before going outdoors. Use caution during hot weather or while taking saunas or hot baths, since excessive sweating while taking this medicine may cause you to become dehydrated and to feel drowsy or faint.
Examinations or Tests	Many people have high blood pressure with no symptoms at all. It is important for you to keep all appointments with your doctor, even if you feel well, so that your blood pressure can be checked regularly. Periodic blood and urine tests may be required.
Other Precautions	If you have diabetes, be aware that this medicine may raise blood-sugar levels. If you notice any change when testing sugar levels in your blood or urine, let your doctor know.
	Tell any doctor or dentist you consult that you are taking this medicine, especially if you will be undergoing any type of surgery.
	When first starting on this type of medicine, you will probably experience both greater volume and frequency of urination. Until your individual pattern of urination has been established with this medicine, it may be wise to time carefully any activity that will put you out of convenient reach of a bathroom, such as

bus or car travel. In addition, taking a diuretic at bed-time will probably interfere with sleep; you should discuss your dosage schedule with your doctor.

Check with your doctor if you become ill with flulike symptoms, such as cough, fever, or body aches; lose your appetite; vomit; or have diarrhea. This may cause you to lose a great deal of fluid, making it important not to take the diuretic for one or more doses.

Following mild fluid losses, some older people are more vulnerable to symptoms of weakness or dizziness upon standing or getting up.

Helpful Hints

If your mouth or throat feels dry, chewing sugarless gum or sucking ice chips or sugarless hard candy will help.

When you first begin to take this medicine, you may feel tired and notice that you urinate more frequently. These effects should lessen with time.

No special restrictions on driving or exposure to excessive cold.

POSSIBLE SIDE EFFECTS

Although this list of adverse effects may seem somewhat intimidating, keep in mind that some are quite rare. Of course, should these or any other problems arise while you are on medication, it is always a good idea to consult your doctor.

IF YOU DEVELOP	WHAT TO DO
tiredness or weakness ■ irregular or fast heartbeat ■ confusion ■ mood or mental changes ■ numbness or tingling of fingers or toes ■ severe or continuing nausea, vomiting, or diarrhea ■ dry mouth ■ increased thirst ■ weak pulse ■ muscle cramps or pain ■ bladder spasms ■ stomach pain or cramps	**Urgent** Get in touch with your doctor immediately.
joint pain ■ hearing disturbances ■ rash or hives ■ sore throat or fever ■ bleeding or bruising ■ yellowing of eyes or skin ■ swelling of hands or feet ■ blurred or yellow vision ■ headache ■ flulike symptoms, such as cough, fever, or body aches, with nausea, vomiting, and diarrhea.	**May be serious** Check with your doctor as soon as possible.
dizziness or light-headedness, especially when getting up from a reclining or sitting position ■ nausea or vomiting ■ upset stomach ■ loss of appetite ■ diarrhea ■ constipation ■ increased skin sensitivity to sunlight ■ increased sweating ■ restlessness	If symptoms are disturbing or persist, let your doctor know.

STORAGE INSTRUCTIONS

Store in a cool, dark place (not in a bathroom medicine cabinet). If your medicine is in a liquid form, make sure that it does not freeze.

STOPPING OR INTERRUPTING THERAPY

If you are taking furosemide for hypertension, you may have to take it for the rest of your life, as this drug does not cure high blood pressure but only controls it. Do not stop taking it, even if you feel better. If you miss a dose, take it as soon as possible. If it is almost time for your next dose, skip the missed dose and resume your regular schedule. Do not take two doses at the same time.

SPECIAL CONSIDERATIONS FOR THOSE OVER SIXTY-FIVE

The side effects of dizziness and light-headedness are more likely to occur in older people, who should be especially careful to follow doctor's instructions on how much of the drug to take. Too much furosemide can cause dehydration, which could have serious effects on one's health. Also, people over sixty-five who are not eating a well-balanced diet will be more prone to potassium deficiency and other problems. Such persons should check with a doctor if they become ill with flulike symptoms, such as cough, fever, or body aches; lose their appetite; vomit; or have diarrhea because they may then be more vulnerable to fluid losses.

CONDITION: **CONGESTIVE HEART FAILURE**

CATEGORY: **LOOP DIURETICS**

GENERIC (CHEMICAL) NAME	BRAND (TRADE) NAME	DOSAGE FORMS AND STRENGTHS
Bumetanide	BUMEX	Tablets: 0.5, 1, 2 mg

DRUG PROFILE

Bumetanide is a diuretic that is used to treat edema (fluid accumulation) that may be a byproduct of congestive heart failure, kidney disease, or liver disease. Bumetanide is known as a "loop" diuretic because it acts on a part of the kidney called the loop of Henle. This drug helps the kidneys eliminate excess salt and water through urination. It tends to act more quickly and for a shorter period of time than furosemide, another loop diuretic.

BEFORE USING THIS DRUG

Let your doctor know *IF*

You have ever had allergic reactions or other problems with ■ bumetanide ■ thiazide or thiazide-type diuretics ■ sulfonamides (sulfa drugs).

You have ever had any of the following medical problems: ■ diabetes ■ abnormal heart rhythms ■ gout ■ diarrhea (recent or current) ■ kidney disease ■ liver disease.

You are taking any of the following medicines: ■ other diuretics or medicines for high blood pressure ■ antibiotics ■ medicine for cancer ■ digoxin or digitalis (heart medicines) ■ aspirin, indomethacin or other medicine for arthritis ■ probenecid (medicine for gout) ■ lithium ■ corticosteroids or corticotropin (ACTH) ■ medicine for malaria ■ tetracycline.

SPECIAL INSTRUCTIONS WHILE TAKING THIS DRUG

FOOD AND DRUG INTERACTIONS

Foods and Beverages	This drug may cause your body to lose large amounts of the mineral potassium. Your doctor may give you special instructions about eating foods or drinking beverages that have a high potassium content (such as bananas and citrus fruit juices), taking a potassium supplement, or using salt substitutes.

No special restrictions on alcohol use or smoking.

DAILY LIVING

Exertion and Exercise	Use caution when exercising or exerting yourself, since excessive sweating while taking this medicine may cause you to become dehydrated.
Excessive Heat	Use caution during hot weather, since excessive sweating while taking this medicine may cause you to become dehydrated.
Examinations or Tests	It is important for you to keep all appointments with your doctor so that you can be checked regularly. Periodic blood and urine tests may be required.
Other Precautions	If you have diabetes, be aware that this medicine may raise blood-sugar levels. If you notice any change when testing sugar levels in your blood or urine, let your doctor know.

Tell any doctor or dentist you consult that you are taking this medicine, especially if you will be undergoing any type of surgery.

When first starting on this type of medicine you will probably experience both greater volume and frequency of urination. Until your individual pattern of urination has been established with this medicine, it may be wise to time carefully any activity that will put you out of convenient reach of a bathroom, such as bus or car travel. In addition, taking a diuretic at bedtime will probably interfere with sleep; you should discuss your dosage schedule with your doctor.

Check with your doctor if you become ill with flulike symptoms, such as cough, fever, or body aches; lose your appetite; vomit; or have diarrhea. This may cause you to lose a great deal of fluid, making it important not to take the diuretic for one or more doses.

Following mild fluid losses, some older people are more vulnerable to symptoms of weakness or dizziness upon standing or getting up.

Helpful Hints

If your mouth or throat feels dry, chewing sugarless gum or sucking ice chips or sugarless hard candy will help.

When you first begin to take this medicine, you may feel tired and notice that you urinate more frequently. These effects should lessen with time.

No special restrictions on driving, sun exposure, or exposure to excessive cold.

POSSIBLE SIDE EFFECTS

Although this list of adverse effects may seem somewhat intimidating, keep in mind that some are quite rare. Of course, should these or any other problems arise while you are on medication, it is always a good idea to consult your doctor.

IF YOU DEVELOP	WHAT TO DO
tiredness or weakness ■ confusion ■ mood or mental changes ■ irregular heartbeat ■ tingling sensation in fingers or toes	**Urgent** Get in touch with your doctor immediately.
chest pain ■ nausea or vomiting ■ diarrhea ■ uncontrollable movements ■ dizziness ■ light-headedness ■ headache ■ loss of appetite ■ dry mouth ■ increased thirst ■ weak pulse ■ muscle cramps or pain ■ hearing disturbances ■ rash, itching, or hives ■ bleeding or bruising ■ difficulty in breathing	**May be serious** Check with your doctor as soon as possible.
stomach cramps or pain ■ upset stomach ■ male impotence ■ premature ejaculation (in males) ■ nipple tenderness ■ joint pain ■ increased sweating	If symptoms are disturbing or persist, let your doctor know.

STORAGE INSTRUCTIONS

Store in a cool, dark place (not in a bathroom medicine cabinet).

STOPPING OR INTERRUPTING THERAPY

Your doctor may prescribe a special schedule for you, whereby you take this drug on some days and do not take it on other days. Follow your doctor's instructions exactly. If you miss a dose, take it as soon as possible. If it is almost time for your next dose, skip the missed dose and resume your regular schedule. Do not take two doses at the same time.

SPECIAL CONSIDERATIONS FOR THOSE OVER SIXTY-FIVE

The side effects of dizziness and light-headedness are more likely to occur in older people. They should be especially careful to follow doctor's instructions on how much of the drug to take. Too much bumetanide can cause dehydration, which could have serious effects on one's health. People over sixty-five should check with a doctor if they become ill with flulike symptoms, such as cough, fever, or body aches; lose their appetite; vomit; or have diarrhea because they may then be more vulnerable to fluid losses.

CONDITION: **CONGESTIVE HEART FAILURE**

CATEGORY: **INOTROPIC DRUGS**

GENERIC (CHEMICAL) NAME	BRAND (TRADE) NAME	DOSAGE FORMS AND STRENGTHS
Digoxin	LANOXICAPS	Capsules: 0.05, 0.1, 0.2 mg
	LANOXIN	Tablets: 0.125, 0.25, 0.5 mg

DRUG PROFILE

The cardiac glycosides, extracted from the leaves of the digitalis plant (foxglove), are used to treat heart failure or abnormal heart rhythms. These medicines, called inotropic drugs, act directly on the heart to increase the force and efficiency of each heartbeat and control the rhythm of the beats. This improves blood circulation, helps the body rid itself of excess fluid, and results in easier breathing and greater overall strength.

BEFORE USING THIS DRUG

Let your doctor know *IF*

You have ever had allergic reactions or other problems with ■ digoxin ■ any other digitalis medicines.

You have ever had any of the following medical problems: ■ any heart disease ■ heart attack ■ rheumatic fever ■ asthma or other lung disease ■ high or low calcium blood levels ■ low potassium or magnesium blood levels ■ kidney disease ■ liver disease ■ thyroid disease ■ prolonged diarrhea ■ congestive heart failure.

You are taking any of the following medicines: ■ diuretics or other medicines for high blood pressure ■ antacids ■ antibiotics ■ medicine for cancer ■ medicine for asthma or hay fever ■ beta-blockers (eg, propranolol, atenolol, metoprolol) ■ cholestyramine (medicine for high cholesterol) ■ medicine for cough or cold ■ appetite suppressants ■ decongestants ■ medicine for diarrhea ■ laxatives ■ medicine for stomach pain or cramps ■ medicine for ulcers ■ medicine for glaucoma ■ aspirin or aspirinlike medicine ■ medicine for nausea.

You have taken any of the following within the last two weeks: digitalis, quinidine, or other heart medicines ■ corticosteroids or corticotropin (ACTH) ■ calcium blockers (eg, diltiazem, nifedipine, verapamil) ■ sleep medicines ■ tranquilizers ■ medicine for seizures ■ potassium-containing medicines or supplements ■ medicine for thyroid disorders.

SPECIAL INSTRUCTIONS WHILE TAKING THIS DRUG

FOOD AND DRUG INTERACTIONS

Other Drugs	Do not take any other drugs, including over-the-counter (OTC) drugs, before checking with your doctor. Some OTC drugs, such as those used for appetite suppression, asthma, colds, cough, hay fever, diarrhea, constipation, and acid indigestion (ie, antacids), may react adversely with the cardiac glycosides. Taking digoxin with quinidine or verapamil may result in dangerously high blood levels of digoxin. It is especially important to let your doctor know if you are taking either of these drugs.
Foods and Beverages	Tell your doctor if you are on a high-fiber diet. In general, try to maintain a well-balanced diet. If these drugs are taken with a meal high in bran fiber, absorption of medicine into the body may be reduced. If you are deficient in potassium or magnesium (as may occur if you are taking a diuretic or not eating properly), these drugs may not work correctly. Ask your doctor for diet suggestions.

Smoking	Nicotine may precipitate abnormal heart rhythms. If you smoke, try to stop or at least cut down.

No special restrictions on alcohol use.

DAILY LIVING

Examinations or Tests	It is important for you to keep all appointments with your doctor, even if you feel well, so that your progress can be checked. Periodic blood and urine tests may be required. While you are taking digitalis, you should check your pulse regularly and tell your doctor if you notice any changes in rhythm, rate, or force.
Other Precautions	Tell any doctor or dentist you consult that you are taking this medicine, especially if you will be undergoing any type of surgery. The effective level of this medicine is very close to the toxic level; you should immediately report any signs of overdose (listed below as "Urgent").
Helpful Hints	During the first one to two days of therapy, you may urinate more frequently than usual. This effect should disappear as you continue to take your medicine.

No special restrictions on driving, exertion and exercise, sun exposure, or exposure to excessive heat or cold.

POSSIBLE SIDE EFFECTS

Although this list of adverse effects may seem somewhat intimidating, keep in mind that some are quite rare. Of course, should these or any other problems arise while you are on medication, it is always a good idea to consult your doctor.

IF YOU DEVELOP	WHAT TO DO
loss of appetite ■ stomach pain ■ nausea or vomiting ■ diarrhea ■ mouth watering ■ difficulty in swallowing ■ hiccups ■ bloating ■ irregular heartbeat, palpitations, or a marked increase or decrease in your heart rate ■ headache ■ tiredness or weakness ■ drowsiness ■ general ill feeling ■ dizziness ■ fainting ■ excitement, restlessness, or nervousness ■ sleeplessness ■ euphoria ■ irritability ■ seizures ■ pain around the face or any other pain ■ tremors ■ memory problems ■ personality changes ■ nightmares ■ delirium ■ depression ■ confusion ■ hallucinations ■ blurred vision ■ changes in color vision or other visual disturbances ■ increased eye sensitivity to light	**Urgent** Get in touch with your doctor immediately.
rash, hives, itching, or other skin problems	**May be serious** Check with your doctor as soon as possible.
female breast tenderness ■ male breast enlargement	If symptoms are disturbing or persist, let your doctor know.

STORAGE INSTRUCTIONS

Store in a cool, dark place (not in a bathroom medicine cabinet).

STOPPING OR INTERRUPTING THERAPY

It is important to continue taking this medicine, even if you feel well. Suddenly stopping this medicine may seriously worsen your medical condition; follow your doctor's instructions carefully. If you miss a dose of this medicine, skip the missed dose and resume your regular schedule. Do not take two doses at the same time. If you miss doses for two or more days, check with your doctor.

SPECIAL CONSIDERATIONS FOR THOSE OVER SIXTY-FIVE

Older people may be more sensitive to the side effects of this drug and may accumulate toxic blood levels of the drug at lower doses. Such people should get in touch with a doctor if they develop any of the symptoms listed under "Possible Side Effects."

CONDITION: **CONGESTIVE HEART FAILURE**

CATEGORY: **ANGIOTENSIN-CONVERTING ENZYME INHIBITORS**

GENERIC (CHEMICAL) NAME	BRAND (TRADE) NAME	DOSAGE FORMS AND STRENGTHS
Captopril	CAPOTEN	Tablets: 12.5, 25, 50, 100 mg
Enalapril maleate	VASOTEC	Tablets: 2.5, 5, 10, 20 mg

DRUG PROFILE

Captopril and enalapril are used to treat high blood pressure and congestive heart failure. These drugs interrupt a chain of biochemical events that lead to constriction (tightening) of the blood vessels. Blocking this process lets blood vessels relax, lowers blood pressure, and increases flow of blood and oxygen to the heart. Relaxing the blood vessels reduces the congestion of blood in the lungs, lessens the load on the heart, and improves the blood flow to the kidneys, facilitating the elimination of sodium and water. Long-term use of this drug improves exercise tolerance because blood flow to the heart muscle is increased.

For complete information on this drug, see pages 98–103.

ABNORMAL HEART RHYTHMS

A steady, measured beat is one of the hallmarks of a healthy heart. This rhythm is the result of a finely tuned electrical current that originates in the sinus node, a group of pacemaker cells in the heart's upper right side. The current then darts through the atria, the heart's upper chambers, toward the atrioventricular node, a group of conductor cells located between the heart's upper and lower chambers. Finally, the impulse travels to the ventricles, the lower chambers of the heart.

If you've been told you have an arrhythmia, the term for abnormal heart rhythms, this indicates that the heart's circuitry has been thrown awry. This can happen as the result of heart diseases and other illnesses, or effects of medicines and nonmedicinal drugs such as caffeine, alcohol, and tobacco. Arrhythmias are most common among older people, with some forms affecting more than 10 percent of the over-sixty-five population.

CAUSES

Different types of disruptions cause different disorders in the heart's rhythm. If the sinus node malfunctions, the resulting pattern of arrhythmias is known as the sick sinus syndrome. This syndrome can cause an abnormally slow rate (fewer than sixty beats per minute) or both an abnormally fast rate (over one hundred beats per minute) and an abnormally slow heart rate.

Another possible disruption known as heart block occurs when the conduction system malfunctions. Though heart block itself sometimes does not create noticeable problems, it can lead to a loss of conduction to the ventricles. When this happens, the upper and lower heart chambers no longer contract in the pattern needed to prevent serious symptoms of arrhythmias.

Occasionally, the electrical impulse begins outside the heart's normal conduction system, producing another type of arrhythmia. If the impulse begins in the atrium, the resulting arrythmia is called premature atrial contraction; if it begins in the ventricle, it is called premature ventricular contraction. You may have heard your doctor refer to these arrhythmias as PACs and PVCs. (Occasional PACs or PVCs are common among people over sixty-five, often without noticeable symptoms.)

Sometimes, the conduction system becomes disorganized and the electrical current travels in circles. If this malfunction occurs in the atrium, it is called atrial fibrillation, or flutter; in the ventricle, it is called ventricular tachycardia, or ventricular fibrillation.

DIAGNOSIS

The symptoms of arrythmias stem from two factors: the regularity of contractions and the heart rate. When contractions are irregular, you experience a sensation of missed beats, irregular pulse, or palpitations. With a fast heart rate, you may feel dizzy, light-headed, or short of breath or notice a feeling of fullness and fluttering in the chest. With a slow heart rate, you may actually faint.

Most serious arrhythmias are detected through an electrocardiogram (ECG), a device that graphs the pattern of electrical activity in your heart over a period of several minutes. In some instances, the ECG will not show evidence of an arrhythmia, even though symptoms point to one. Therefore, the doctor may want you to wear a Holter monitor for an extended period as you go about your daily activities. The Holter monitor records the heart's electrical activity for up to twenty-four hours. While you wear the monitor, your doctor may want you to write down your heart signs and symptoms as well as your activities. Your record will be compared with that of the Holter monitor so your doctor can see any changes in heart rhythm that occurred when you were experiencing symptoms.

TREATMENT

When an abnormally slow heart rate develops from sick sinus syndrome or heart block, the doctor may recommend a pacemaker, an electronic device implanted beneath the skin near the heart or elsewhere in the chest. The pacemaker will supply the current to appropriately pace the heart in people with these conditions. In rare instances, surgery is required for frequent PVCs to remove the tissue that is generating an abnormal current.

The drugs discussed in the charts on pages 211–241—including quinidine, digoxin, procainamide, disopyramide, tocainide, and mexiletine—are used both to correct abnormal heart rhythms and to prevent their occurrence. In some instances, the doctor will want to check a drug's effectiveness by having you wear a Holter monitor during treatment.

OUTLOOK

Many people with arrhythmias may need to continue their medicine indefinitely. To make the medicine more effective, you should avoid stimulants such as caffeine, as well as alcohol and tobacco. Finally, you should have regular checkups to make sure that the medicine is working properly.

CONDITION: **ABNORMAL HEART RHYTHMS**

CATEGORY: **ANTIARRHYTHMICS**

GENERIC (CHEMICAL) NAME	BRAND (TRADE) NAME	DOSAGE FORMS AND STRENGTHS
Quinidine gluconate	QUINAGLUTE	Controlled-release tablets: 324 mg
Quinidine sulfate	QUINIDEX	Controlled-release tablets: 300 mg
Quinidine sulfate		Tablets: 200, 300 mg

This drug is available under a variety of brand names.

DRUG PROFILE

This drug helps normalize irregular heartbeats and also slows down the heart if it is beating too rapidly. Quinidine works directly on the heart itself, as well as on the nerves that lead to the heart muscles.

BEFORE USING THIS DRUG

Let your doctor know *IF*

You have ever had allergic reactions or other problems with ■ quinidine ■ quinine.

You have ever had any of the following medical problems: ■ asthma or other lung disease ■ high or low blood pressure ■ congestive heart failure or other heart problems ■ liver disease ■ kidney disease ■ muscle weakness ■ myasthenia gravis ■ thyroid disorder ■ blood disease ■ recent infection ■ psoriasis.

You are taking any of the following medicines: ■ other medicine for abnormal heart rhythms ■ phenobarbital, phenytoin, or other medicine for seizures ■ medicine for

Parkinson's disease ■ medicine for urinary retention ■ medicine for ulcers or irritable bowel syndrome ■ cimetidine ■ anticoagulants (blood thinners) ■ digoxin or digitalis (heart medicines) ■ diuretics ■ antacids ■ Bicitra, Polycitra (medicine to make the urine less acidic) ■ phenothiazines or other tranquilizers ■ sinus medicines ■ medicine for nausea ■ muscle relaxants ■ medicine for myasthenia gravis ■ medicine for glaucoma ■ antibiotics ■ sleep medicines ■ potassium-containing medicines or supplements.

SPECIAL INSTRUCTIONS WHILE TAKING THIS DRUG

FOOD AND DRUG INTERACTIONS

Other Drugs	Use of this drug with digoxin may result in dangerously high blood levels of digoxin. It is especially important to let your doctor know if you are taking digoxin.
Alcohol	Drinking alcohol while taking this medicine may worsen such side effects as drowsiness, light-headedness, or dizziness. Avoid alcohol unless your doctor has approved its use.
Smoking	Smoking may aggravate cardiac arrhythmias. If you smoke, try to stop or at least cut down.

No special restrictions on foods and beverages.

DAILY LIVING

Examinations or Tests	It is important for you to keep all appointments with your doctor so that your progress and reactions to therapy can be checked. Periodic electrocardiograms and blood tests may be required.

Other Precautions	Tell any doctor or dentist you consult that you are taking this medicine, especially if you will be undergoing any type of surgery.

Occasionally, patients experience blurred vision or loss of consciousness with their first dose. If this happens, contact your doctor immediately.

Helpful Hints	Quinidine is usually taken on an empty stomach— one hour before or two hours after meals—with a full glass of water. However, if this medicine upsets your stomach, ask your doctor if you may take it with food or milk.

Swallow the controlled-release tablets whole—do not break, crush, or chew them.

No special restrictions on exertion and exercise, driving, sun exposure, or exposure to excessive heat or cold.

POSSIBLE SIDE EFFECTS

Although this list of adverse effects may seem somewhat intimidating, keep in mind that some are quite rare. Of course, should these or any other problems arise while you are on medication, it is always a good idea to consult your doctor.

IF YOU DEVELOP

difficulty in breathing ■ visual disturbances ■ dizziness ■ headache ■ ringing in the ears ■ hearing loss ■ faintness or light-headedness ■ fever ■ rash ■ bleeding or bruising ■ very fast heartbeat ■ irregular heartbeat ■ tremors ■ nausea or vomiting ■ blurred vision or fainting after the first dose

WHAT TO DO

Urgent Get in touch with your doctor immediately.

nervousness ■ excitement ■ confusion ■ personality changes ■ cold sweat ■ delirium ■ yellowing of eyes or skin ■ diarrhea ■ slow heart rate ■ low blood pressure	**May be serious** Check with your doctor as soon as possible.
bitter taste ■ loss of appetite ■ stomach pain or cramps ■ flushed skin with itching ■ joint pain ■ increased eye sensitivity to light	If symptoms are disturbing or persist, let your doctor know.

STORAGE INSTRUCTIONS

Store in a cool, dark place (not in a bathroom medicine cabinet).

STOPPING OR INTERRUPTING THERAPY

Take this drug exactly as instructed. Check with your doctor on what to do should you miss a dose.

SPECIAL CONSIDERATIONS FOR THOSE OVER SIXTY-FIVE

Older people sometimes metabolize quinidine more slowly, which may allow the drug to reach higher concentrations and accumulate in the body. Doctors will adjust the dosage accordingly.

CONDITION: **ABNORMAL HEART RHYTHMS**

CATEGORY: **ANTIARRHYTHMICS**

GENERIC (CHEMICAL) NAME	BRAND (TRADE) NAME	DOSAGE FORMS AND STRENGTHS
Disopyramide phosphate	NORPACE NORPACE CR	Capsules: 100, 150 mg Controlled-release capsules: 100, 150 mg

DRUG PROFILE

This drug helps normalize irregular heartbeats and also slows down the heart if it is beating too rapidly. Disopyramide works directly on the heart itself, as well as on the nerves that lead to the heart muscles.

BEFORE USING THIS DRUG

Let your doctor know *IF*

You have ever had allergic reactions or other problems with ■ disopyramide.

You have ever had any of the following medical problems: ■ congestive heart failure or any other heart problems ■ low blood pressure ■ diabetes ■ hypoglycemia (low blood sugar) ■ high or low blood-potassium levels ■ urinary retention ■ enlarged prostate ■ glaucoma or a family history of glaucoma ■ liver disease ■ kidney disease ■ myasthenia gravis ■ malnutrition.

You are taking any of the following medicines: ■ other medicine for abnormal heart rhythms ■ anticoagulants (blood thinners) ■ medicine for diabetes ■ medicine for high blood pressure, including beta-blockers ■ medicine for angina or other heart problems ■ sleep medicines ■ phenobarbital, phenytoin, or other medicine for seizures ■ potassium-containing medicines or supplements ■ rifampin (medicine for tuberculosis) ■ medicine for glaucoma.

SPECIAL RESTRICTIONS WHILE TAKING THIS DRUG

FOOD AND DRUG INTERACTIONS

Other Drugs	Do not take any other drugs, including over-the-counter (OTC) drugs, before checking with your doctor. OTC drugs for appetite suppression, coughs, colds, asthma, allergies, or sinus problems may aggravate your heart problems.
Foods and Beverages	Your doctor may give you special instructions about eating foods or drinking beverages that have a high potassium content (such as bananas and citrus fruit juices), taking a potassium supplement, or using salt substitutes.

| Alcohol | Drinking alcohol while taking this medicine may worsen such side effects as hypoglycemia (low blood sugar) or dizziness. Avoid alcohol unless your doctor has approved its use. |
| Smoking | Smoking may aggravate cardiac arrhythmias. If you smoke, try to stop or at least cut down. |

DAILY LIVING

Driving	This drug may cause drowsiness. Be careful when driving, operating household appliances, or doing any other tasks that require alertness until you know how this drug affects you.
Exertion and Exercise	This medicine may cause you to sweat less than normally. Sweating is your body's natural way of cooling down, and not sweating enough can be dangerous. Use caution not to become overheated when you exercise or exert yourself.
Excessive Heat	Use caution during hot weather, especially if you exert yourself (see above).
Examinations or Tests	It is important for you to keep all appointments with your doctor, even if you feel well, so that your progress can be checked. Periodic blood or urine tests may be required.
Other Precautions	If you experience symptoms of low blood sugar (see list of symptoms in "Possible Side Effects"), eat or drink something containing sugar and contact your doctor immediately.

Helpful Hints	For best results, take this medicine on an empty stomach—either one hour before or two hours after meals.
	Swallow the controlled-release capsules whole—do not break, crush, or chew them.
	If your mouth or throat feels dry, chewing sugarless gum or sucking ice chips or sugarless hard candy will help. Your nose may also feel dry or stuffy; check with your doctor before using nasal decongestants.

No special restrictions on sun exposure or exposure to excessive cold.

POSSIBLE SIDE EFFECTS

Although this list of adverse effects may seem somewhat intimidating, keep in mind that some are quite rare. Of course, should these or any other problems arise while you are on medication, it is always a good idea to consult your doctor.

IF YOU DEVELOP	WHAT TO DO
shortness of breath ■ urinary retention ■ difficult urination	**Urgent** Get in touch with your doctor immediately.

urinary urgency or frequency ■ chest pain
■ dizziness, light-headedness, or fainting, especially
when getting up from a reclining or sitting position
■ confusion ■ depression ■ muscle weakness
■ swelling of feet or lower legs ■ numbness or tingling ■ very rapid or irregular heartbeat ■ rapid
weight gain ■ eye pain ■ sore throat or fever
■ yellowing of eyes or skin ■ nausea or vomiting
■ diarrhea ■ stomach pain ■ rash, itching, or other
skin problems ■ personality changes ■ tiredness
■ headache ■ general ill feeling

Signs of low blood sugar: anxiety, chills, pale skin,
headache, hunger, nausea, shakiness, increased
sweating, tiredness

May be serious Check with
your doctor as soon as
possible.

dry mouth, eyes, nose, and throat ■ bloating or gas
■ blurred vision ■ constipation ■ loss of appetite
■ male impotence ■ sleep disturbances
■ male breast enlargement ■ aches and pains

If symptoms are disturbing
or persist, let your doctor
know.

STORAGE INSTRUCTIONS

Store in a cool, dark place (not in a bathroom medicine cabinet).

STOPPING OR INTERRUPTING THERAPY

It is very important to continue taking this medicine, even if you feel better. Suddenly
stopping this medicine may seriously worsen your medical condition. Follow your
doctor's instructions carefully. If you miss a dose of this medicine, take it as soon as
possible unless your next regular dose will be within the next four hours. If so, skip
the missed dose and resume your regular schedule. Do not take two doses at the
same time.

SPECIAL CONSIDERATIONS FOR THOSE OVER SIXTY-FIVE

Dizziness and light-headedness are more likely to occur in older people. The side
effects of constipation, blurred vision, and urinary retention or difficult urination can
also be particularly troublesome. In addition, this drug lessens the effectiveness of
glaucoma treatment.

CONDITION: **ABNORMAL HEART RHYTHMS**

CATEGORY: **ANTIARRHYTHMICS**

GENERIC (CHEMICAL) NAME	BRAND (TRADE) NAME	DOSAGE FORMS AND STRENGTHS
Procainamide hydrochloride	PROCAN SR	Controlled-release tablets: 250, 500, 750, 1000 mg
	PRONESTYL	Capsules: 250, 375, 500 mg Tablets: 250, 375, 500 mg
	PRONESTYL-SR	Controlled-release tablets: 500 mg

DRUG PROFILE

This drug helps normalize irregular heartbeats and also slows down the heart if it is beating too rapidly. Procainamide works directly on the heart itself, as well as on the nerves that lead to the heart muscles.

BEFORE USING THIS DRUG

Let your doctor know *IF*

You have ever had allergic reactions or other problems with ■ procainamide ■ procaine or any other "caine-type" medicines ■ aspirin ■ tartrazine (FD&C Yellow Dye No. 5) (contained in Pronestyl tablets).

You have ever had any of the following medical problems: ■ any heart disease ■ asthma ■ kidney disease ■ liver disease ■ systemic lupus erythematosus ■ high or low blood-potassium levels ■ high blood pressure ■ myasthenia gravis.

You are taking any of the following medicines: ■ other medicine for heart disease, including medicine for abnormal heart rhythms ■ antibiotics ■ medicine for high blood pressure ■ medicine for myasthenia gravis ■ cimetidine (medicine for ulcers) ■ medicine for Parkinson's disease ■ medicine for urinary retention ■ medicine for irritable bowel syndrome.

SPECIAL RESTRICTIONS WHILE TAKING THIS DRUG

FOOD AND DRUG INTERACTIONS

Alcohol	Drinking alcohol while taking this medicine may worsen such side effects as drowsiness, light-headedness, or dizziness. Avoid alcohol unless your doctor has approved its use.
Smoking	Smoking may aggravate cardiac arrhythmias. If you smoke, try to stop or at least cut down.

No special restrictions on foods and beverages.

DAILY LIVING

Driving	This drug may cause light-headedness or dizziness. Be careful when driving, operating household appliances, or doing any other tasks that require alertness until you know how this drug affects you.
Examinations or Tests	It is important for you to keep all appointments with your doctor, even if you feel well, so that your progress can be checked. Periodic blood and urine tests may be required.
Other Precautions	Tell any doctor or dentist you consult that you are taking this medicine, especially if you will be undergoing any type of surgery.
Helpful Hints	For best results, take this medicine at the exact intervals indicated, on an empty stomach—either one hour before or two hours after meals. However, if this drug upsets your stomach, ask your doctor if you can take it with food or milk.

Swallow the controlled-release capsules whole—do not break, crush, or chew them. Do not be concerned if you notice the remains of the controlled-release tablets in your stool; your body has already absorbed the medicine that was in the tablet.

No special restrictions on exertion and exercise, sun exposure, or exposure to excessive heat or cold.

POSSIBLE SIDE EFFECTS

Although this list of adverse effects may seem somewhat intimidating, keep in mind that some are quite rare. Of course, should these or any other problems arise while you are on medication, it is always a good idea to consult your doctor.

IF YOU DEVELOP	WHAT TO DO
severe dizziness or fainting ■ seizures ■ irregular or fast heartbeat	**Urgent** Get in touch with your doctor immediately.
fever or chills ■ general ill feeling ■ decreased or dark urination ■ drowsiness ■ nausea or vomiting ■ rash, hives, or itching ■ joint pain or swelling ■ pain or difficulty in breathing ■ confusion ■ depression ■ personality changes ■ hallucinations ■ sore mouth, gums, or throat ■ bleeding or bruising ■ tiredness or weakness ■ muscle pain ■ headache	**May be serious** Check with your doctor as soon as possible.
diarrhea ■ stomach pain ■ bitter taste ■ loss of appetite ■ dizziness or light-headedness	If symptoms are disturbing or persist, let your doctor know.

STORAGE INSTRUCTIONS

Store in a cool, dark place (not in a bathroom medicine cabinet).

STOPPING OR INTERRUPTING THERAPY

It is very important to continue taking this medicine exactly as prescribed, even if you feel well. Suddenly stopping this medicine may seriously worsen your medical condition. Your doctor will advise you on how to reduce the dosage gradually when you no longer need this drug. If you miss a dose, take it as soon as possible, unless it is within two hours (regular dosage forms) or four hours (controlled-release dosage forms) of your next scheduled dose. In that case, skip the missed dose and resume your regular schedule. Do not take two doses at the same time.

SPECIAL CONSIDERATIONS FOR THOSE OVER SIXTY-FIVE

The side effects of dizziness, light-headedness, and fainting are more likely to occur in older people, who should take care to avoid falling.

CONDITION: **ABNORMAL HEART RHYTHMS**

CATEGORY: **ANTIARRHYTHMICS**

GENERIC (CHEMICAL) NAME	BRAND (TRADE) NAME	DOSAGE FORMS AND STRENGTHS
Mexiletine hydrochloride	MEXITIL	Capsules: 150, 200, 250 mg

DRUG PROFILE

This drug helps normalize irregular heartbeats and also slows down the heart if it is beating too rapidly. Mexiletine acts directly on the heart itself.

BEFORE USING THIS DRUG

Let your doctor know *IF*

You have ever had allergic reactions or other problems with ■ mexiletine.

You have ever had any of the following medical problems: ■ liver disease ■ heart disease.

You are taking any of the following medicines: ■ other medicine for abnormal heart rhythms ■ medicine to make the urine more acidic ■ narcotics or other prescription pain-killers ■ phenobarbital ■ cimetidine (medicine for ulcers) ■ magnesium aluminum hydroxide (antacid) ■ metoclopramide (medicine for nausea or vomiting) ■ phenytoin (medicine for seizures) ■ rifampin (antibiotic) ■ any medicine containing atropine ■ theophylline (medicine for asthma).

SPECIAL INSTRUCTIONS WHILE TAKING THIS DRUG

FOOD AND DRUG INTERACTIONS

Smoking	Smoking may aggravate cardiac arrhythmias. If you smoke, try to stop or at least cut down.

No special restrictions on other drugs, food and beverages, or alcohol use.

DAILY LIVING

Exertion and Exercise	Physical exertion may worsen some kinds of arrhythmias. Ask your doctor to recommend a safe exercise program.
Examinations or Tests	It is important for you to keep all appointments with your doctor, even if you feel well, so that your progress can be checked. Periodic tests and electrocardiograms may be required.
Helpful Hints	Take this medicine with food, milk, or an antacid to reduce upset stomach.

No special restrictions on driving, sun exposure, or exposure to excessive heat or cold.

POSSIBLE SIDE EFFECTS

Although the list of adverse effects may seem somewhat intimidating, keep in mind that some are quite rare. Of course, should these or any other problems arise while you are on medication, it is always a good idea to consult your doctor.

IF YOU DEVELOP	WHAT TO DO
irregular heartbeat ■ seizures ■ chest pain ■ fainting ■ difficulty in breathing ■ coma	**Urgent** Get in touch with your doctor immediately.
chills, fever, or sore throat ■ bleeding or bruising ■ tremors ■ difficulty in coordination ■ tiredness or weakness ■ drowsiness ■ swelling of hands or feet ■ hot flashes ■ nervousness ■ confusion ■ difficulty in speech ■ numbness or tingling in hands or feet ■ ringing in ears ■ depression ■ memory problems ■ hallucinations ■ behavior or mood changes ■ blurred vision or other visual disturbances ■ decreased urination ■ rash ■ painful joints ■ hoarseness ■ taste changes ■ general ill feeling	**May be serious** Check with your doctor as soon as possible.
upset stomach ■ heartburn ■ nausea or vomiting ■ diarrhea ■ constipation ■ stomach pain or discomfort ■ change in appetite ■ difficulty in swallowing ■ hiccups ■ dizziness or light-headedness ■ sleep disturbances ■ headache ■ male impotence ■ diminished sex drive ■ dry mouth or other mouth changes ■ dry skin ■ increased sweating ■ hair loss	If symptoms are disturbing or persist, let your doctor know.

STORAGE INSTRUCTIONS

Store in a cool, dark place (not in a bathroom medicine cabinet).

STOPPING OR INTERRUPTING THERAPY

Take this drug exactly as instructed. Check with your doctor on what to do should you miss a dose.

SPECIAL CONSIDERATIONS FOR THOSE OVER SIXTY-FIVE

Older people may be more susceptible to such side effects as drowsiness, dizziness, and light-headedness. They should get in touch with their doctor if they develop any of these symptoms.

CONDITION: **ABNORMAL HEART RHYTHMS**

CATEGORY: **ANTIARRHYTHMICS**

GENERIC (CHEMICAL) NAME	BRAND (TRADE) NAME	DOSAGE FORMS AND STRENGTHS
Tocainide hydrochloride	TONOCARD	Tablets: 400, 600 mg

DRUG PROFILE

This drug helps normalize irregular heartbeats and also slows down the heart if it is beating too rapidly. Tocainide acts directly on the heart itself.

BEFORE USING THIS DRUG

Let your doctor know *IF*

You have ever had allergic reactions or other problems with ■ tocainide ■ local anesthetics, such as lidocaine.

You have ever had any of the following medical problems: ■ heart disease, including congestive heart failure ■ high blood pressure ■ kidney disease ■ liver disease ■ asthma or other respiratory disease.

You are taking any of the following medicines: ■ other medicine for abnormal heart rhythms ■ beta-blockers (eg, propranolol, atenolol, metoprolol) ■ anticoagulants (blood thinners) ■ diuretics ■ digoxin or digitalis (heart medicines) ■ theophylline.

SPECIAL RESTRICTIONS WHILE TAKING THIS DRUG

FOOD AND DRUG INTERACTIONS

Smoking	Smoking may aggravate cardiac arrhythmias. If you smoke, try to stop or at least cut down.

No special restrictions on other drugs, foods and beverages, or alcohol use.

DAILY LIVING

Driving	This drug may cause dizziness, light-headedness, or loss of alertness. Be careful when driving, operating household appliances, or doing any other tasks that require alertness until you know how this drug affects you.
Examinations and Tests	It is important for you to keep all appointments with your doctor, even if you feel well, so that your progress can be checked. Periodic blood tests, especially during the first three months of therapy, and electrocardiograms may be required.
Other Precautions	Tell any doctor or dentist you consult that you are taking this drug, especially if you will be undergoing any type of surgery.
Helpful Hints	Taking this drug with meals or a snack may help prevent the side effects of nausea, dizziness, and light-headedness.

No special restrictions on exertion and exercise, sun exposure, or exposure to excessive heat or cold.

POSSIBLE SIDE EFFECTS

Although this list of adverse effects may seem somewhat intimidating, keep in mind that some are quite rare. Of course, should these or any other problems arise while you are on medication, it is always a good idea to consult your doctor.

IF YOU DEVELOP

severe dizziness or fainting ■ seizures ■ irregular or fast heartbeat ■ chest pain ■ coma ■ convulsions ■ confusion ■ disorientation ■ hallucinations ■ difficulty in breathing ■ coughing or wheezing ■ bleeding or bruising ■ fever, chills, or sore throat ■ mouth soreness or ulcers

slow heartbeat ■ swelling of hands or feet ■ tremors ■ shakiness ■ loss of coordination ■ clumsiness ■ difficulty in balance ■ disturbances in walking ■ anxiety ■ double vision or other visual disturbances ■ ringing in ears, earache, or other ear problems ■ tiredness ■ drowsiness ■ depression ■ behavior changes ■ changes in taste or smell ■ inability to concentrate or memory problems ■ speech problems ■ sleeplessness ■ increased thirst ■ muscle weakness ■ muscle twitch or spasm ■ rash, itching, or other skin problems ■ muscle or joint pain ■ chilliness ■ clammy skin ■ night sweats ■ hot flashes ■ increased urination ■ urinary retention ■ general ill feeling ■ strange taste in mouth ■ neck pain ■ unusual paleness or flushing ■ pressure on shoulder ■ yawning ■ yellowing of eyes or skin ■ numbness, tingling, pain, or cold in fingers or toes

WHAT TO DO

Urgent Get in touch with your doctor immediately.

May be serious Check with your doctor as soon as possible.

light-headedness or dizziness ■ leg cramps
■ nervousness ■ agitation ■ headache ■ blurred vision ■ nausea or vomiting ■ diarrhea ■ loss of appetite ■ indigestion ■ stomach pain ■ constipation
■ difficulty in swallowing ■ dry mouth ■ hiccups ■ hair loss

If symptoms are disturbing or persist, let your doctor know.

STORAGE INSTRUCTIONS

Store in a cool, dark place (not in a bathroom medicine cabinet).

STOPPING OR INTERRUPTING THERAPY

Take this drug exactly as instructed. Check with your doctor on what to do should you miss a dose.

SPECIAL CONSIDERATIONS FOR THOSE OVER SIXTY-FIVE

Older people may be more susceptible to such side effects as drowsiness, dizziness, and light-headedness.

CONDITION: **ABNORMAL HEART RHYTHMS**

CATEGORY: **ANTIARRHYTHMICS**

GENERIC (CHEMICAL) NAME	BRAND (TRADE) NAME	DOSAGE FORMS AND STRENGTHS
Amiodarone	CORDARONE	Tablets: 200 mg

DRUG PROFILE

This drug helps normalize irregular heartbeats by working directly on the heart muscle cells. Amiodarone is reserved for cases where the patient is unable to take other antiarrhythmic drugs or where other therapies have proved ineffective.

BEFORE USING THIS DRUG

Let your doctor know *IF*

You have ever had allergic reactions or other problems with ■ amiodarone.

You have ever had any of the following medical problems: ■ heart disease ■ liver disease ■ thyroid disease ■ low blood-potassium or magnesium levels ■ lung disease.

You are taking any of the following medicines: ■ other medicine for abnormal heart rhythms ■ thyroid medicine ■ phenytoin (medicine for seizures) ■ digoxin or digitalis (heart medicine) ■ anticoagulants (blood thinners) ■ diuretics ■ beta-blockers (eg, propranolol, atenolol, metoprolol) ■ calcium blockers (eg, diltiazem, nifedipine, verapamil) ■ barbiturates.

SPECIAL RESTRICTIONS WHILE TAKING THIS DRUG

FOOD AND DRUG INTERACTION

Other drugs	Do not take any other drugs, including over-the-counter (OTC) drugs, before checking with your doctor. OTC drugs for appetite suppression, coughs, colds, asthma, allergies, or sinus problems may aggravate your heart problems.
Smoking	Smoking may aggravate cardiac arrhythmias. If you smoke, try to stop or at least cut down.

No special restrictions on foods and beverages or alcohol.

DAILY LIVING

Sun Exposure	You may find that your skin becomes more sensitive to light while you are taking amiodarone. Your skin may also develop blue-gray discolorations after exposure to the sun. Try to minimize sun exposure. It is a good idea to apply a sunscreen to exposed skin surfaces before going outdoors.

Exams or Tests	It is important for you to keep all appointments with your doctor, even if you feel well, so that your progress can be checked. Periodic blood tests may be required.
Other Precautions	Tell any doctor or dentist you consult that you are taking this medicine, especially if you will be undergoing any type of surgery.

No special restrictions on driving, exertion and exercise, or exposure to heat or cold.

POSSIBLE SIDE EFFECTS

Although this list of adverse effects may seem somewhat intimidating, keep in mind that some are quite rare. Of course, should these or any other problems arise while you are on medication, it is always a good idea to consult your doctor.

IF YOU DEVELOP

cough ■ shortness of breath ■ painful breathing ■ fast or irregular heatbeat ■ slow heartbeat ■ yellowing of eyes or skin

WHAT TO DO

Urgent Get in touch with your doctor immediately.

swelling of feet or lower legs ■ blurred vision, halos, or any other visual disturbance ■ dry eyes ■ fever ■ tiredness ■ general ill feeling ■ difficulty in coordination ■ disturbances in walking ■ trembling or shaking ■ jerky, uncontrollable movements ■ numbness or tingling in fingers or toes ■ weakness in arms and legs ■ sensitivity to light ■ rash ■ blue-gray skin discoloration ■ pain and swelling in scrotum

May be serious Check with your doctor as soon as possible.

Signs of hypothyroidism: ■ coldness ■ dry, puffy skin
■ weight gain ■ tiredness

Signs of hyperthyroidism: ■ nervousness
■ sensitivity to heat ■ sweating ■ sleeplessness
■ weight loss

After you STOP taking this medicine: ■ cough ■ fever
■ shortness of breath ■ painful breathing

---

flushing ■ nausea or vomiting ■ loss of appetite
■ constipation ■ stomach pain ■ dizziness ■ tingling
or burning sensations ■ abnormal taste ■ decreased
sex drive ■ headache ■ sleep disturbances ■ hair
loss

If symptoms are disturbing
or persist, let your doctor
know.

STORAGE INSTRUCTIONS

Store in a cool, dark place (not in a bathroom medicine cabinet).

STOPPING OR INTERRUPTING THERAPY

It is very important to continue taking this medicine exactly as prescribed, even if you
feel well. Suddenly stopping this medicine may seriously worsen your medical condition. Your doctor will advise you on how to reduce the dosage gradually when you no
longer need this drug. If you miss a dose, do not take the missed dose, but continue
on your regular schedule. If you miss two or more doses, contact your doctor.

SPECIAL CONSIDERATIONS FOR THOSE OVER SIXTY-FIVE

Older people may be more susceptible to such side effects as coordination difficulties. If this becomes a problem, let your doctor know.

CONDITION: **ABNORMAL HEART RHYTHMS**

CATEGORY: **ANTIARRHYTHMICS**

GENERIC (CHEMICAL) NAME	BRAND (TRADE) NAME	DOSAGE FORMS AND STRENGTHS
Propafenone	RYTHMOL	Tablets: 150, 300 mg

DRUG PROFILE

Propafenone produces its effect by slowing the electrical impulses in the heart and making the heart tissue less sensitive.

BEFORE USING THIS DRUG

Let your doctor know *IF*

You have ever had allergic problems with ■ propafenone.

You have had any of the following medical problems: ■ asthma ■ bronchitis ■ emphysema ■ slow heart rate or any problems with heart rhythm ■ heart failure ■ kidney disease ■ liver disease ■ recent heart attack ■ are using a pacemaker.

You are taking any of the following medicines: ■ digoxin ■ warfarin (blood thinner) ■ beta-blockers (propranolol, atenolol, metoprolol) ■ quinidine ■ cimetidine.

SPECIAL RESTRICTIONS WHILE TAKING THIS DRUG

FOOD AND DRUG INTERACTIONS

Smoking	Smoking may aggravate cardiac arrhythmias. If you smoke, try to stop or at least cut down.

No special restrictions on other drugs or foods and beverages.

DAILY LIVING

Driving

This drug may cause dizziness or lightheadedness. Be careful when driving or operating household appliances or doing any other tasks that require alertness until you know how this drug affects you.

Examinations and Tests

Your doctor may require periodic blood tests, especially during the first three months of therapy; an electrocardiogram may also be required. It is important to keep all appointments with your doctor so that your progress can be checked and to also prevent the occurrence of unwanted side effects.

Other Precautions

Tell any doctor or dentist you consult that you are taking this medicine, especially if you are undergoing any type of surgery or diagnostic testing. Your doctor may want you to carry a medical identification bracelet stating that you are using this medicine.

No special restrictions on exertion and exercise, sun exposure, or exposure to excessive heat or cold.

POSSIBLE SIDE EFFECTS

Although this list of adverse effects may seem somewhat intimidating, keep in mind that some are quite rare. Of course, should these or any other problems arise while you are on this medication, it is always a good idea to consult your doctor.

IF YOU DEVELOP

fast or irregular heart beats ■ chest pain ■ shortness of breath ■ swelling of feet or lower legs ■ fever or chills ■ joint pain ■ slow heartbeat ■ trembling or shaking ■ faintness

taste changes ■ dizziness ■ blurred vision ■ constipation or diarrhea ■ dryness of mouth ■ headache ■ nausea or vomiting ■ rash ■ unusual tiredness or weakness ■ anxiety ■ loss of appetite ■ upset stomach ■ gas ■ sleeplessness ■ sweating ■ loss of balance

WHAT TO DO

May be serious Check with your doctor immediately.

If symptoms are disturbing or persist, let your doctor know.

STORAGE INSTRUCTIONS

Store in a cool, dark place (not in a bathroom medicine cabinet).

STOPPING OR INTERRUPTING THERAPY

Take this medicine exactly as prescribed by your doctor. Do not suddenly discontinue taking this medicine. If you miss a dose, take it as soon as possible. If it is almost time for your next dose, skip the missed dose and resume your regular schedule. Do not take two doses at the same time.

SPECIAL CONSIDERATIONS FOR THOSE OVER SIXTY FIVE

None.

CONDITION: **ABNORMAL HEART RHYTHM**

CATEGORY: **ANTIARRHYTHMICS**

GENERIC (CHEMICAL) NAME	BRAND (TRADE) NAME	DOSAGE FORMS AND STRENGTHS
Moricizine	ETHMOZINE	Tablets: 200, 250, 300 mg

DRUG PROFILE

Moricizine produces its effect by slowing the electrical impulses in the heart and making the heart tissue less sensitive.

BEFORE USING THIS DRUG

Let your doctor know *IF*

You have ever had allergic problems with moricizine.

You have had any of the following medical problems: ■ asthma ■ bronchitis ■ emphysema ■ slow heart rate ■ heart failure ■ kidney failure ■ liver disease ■ recent heart attack ■ are using a pacemaker.

You are taking any of the following medicines: ■ digoxin ■ cimetidine (medicine for ulcers) ■ beta-blockers (eg, propranolol, atenolol, metoprolol) ■ theophylline.

SPECIAL RESTRICTIONS WHILE TAKING THIS DRUG

FOOD AND DRUG INTERACTIONS

Smoking	Smoking may aggravate cardiac arrhythmias. If you smoke, try to stop or at least cut down.

No special restrictions on other drugs, foods and beverages.

DAILY LIVING

Driving	This drug may cause dizziness or light-headedness. Be careful when driving or operating household appliances or doing any other tasks that require alertness until you know how this drug affects you.
Examinations and Tests	Your doctor may require periodic blood tests, especially during the first three months of therapy; an electrocardiogram may also be required. It is important to keep all appointments with your doctor so that your progress can be checked and to also prevent the occurrence of unwanted side effects.
Other Precautions	Tell any doctor or dentist you consult that you are taking this medicine, especially if you are undergoing any type of surgery or diagnostic testing. Your doctor may want you to carry a medical identification bracelet stating that you are using this medicine.

No special restrictions on exertion and exercise, sun exposure, or exposure to excessive heat or cold.

POSSIBLE SIDE EFFECTS

Although this list of adverse effects may seem somewhat intimidating, keep in mind that some are quite rare. Of course, should these or any other problems arise while you are on this medication, it is always a good idea to consult your doctor.

IF YOU DEVELOP	WHAT TO DO
fast or irregular heartbeat ■ chest pain ■ slow heart-beat ■ shortness of breath ■ swelling of feet or lower legs ■ seizures	**Urgent** Get in touch with your doctor immediately.
trembling or shaking ■ vomiting ■ dizziness ■ tiredness or weakness ■ fever or chills ■ joint pain ■ muscle aches and pains ■ yellowing of eyes ■ fainting ■ increased or decreased urination ■ increased sensitivity to heat or cold ■ loss of coordination ■ difficulty in sleeping ■ ringing in ears ■ speech problems ■ double vision ■ increased sensitivity to pain ■ swelling of lips or tongue ■ difficulty swallowing ■ loss of consciousness	**May be serious** Check with your doctor immediately.
bitter taste ■ blurred vision ■ constipation or diarrhea ■ dryness of mouth ■ headache ■ loss of appetite ■ rash ■ eye pain ■ unusual tiredness or weakness ■ nervousness ■ forgetfulness ■ light-headedness	If symptoms are disturbing or persist, let your doctor know.

STORAGE INSTRUCTIONS

Store in a cool, dark place (not in a bathroom medicine cabinet).

STOPPING OR INTERRUPTING THERAPY

Take this medicine as prescribed by your doctor. Do not suddenly discontinue taking this medicine. If you miss a dose, take it as soon as possible. If it is almost time for your next dose, skip the missed dose and resume your regular schedule. Do not take two doses at the same time.

SPECIAL CONSIDERATIONS FOR THOSE OVER SIXTY-FIVE

None.

CONDITION: **ABNORMAL HEART RHYTHMS**

CATEGORY: **ANTIARRHYTHMICS**

GENERIC (CHEMICAL) NAME	BRAND (TRADE) NAME	DOSAGE FORMS AND STRENGTHS
Flecainide acetate	TAMBOCOR	Tablets: 50, 100, 150 mg

DRUG PROFILE

Flecainide helps normalize irregular heartbeats by working directly on the heart muscle cells. Flecainide is reserved for very severe arrhythmias.

BEFORE USING THIS DRUG

Let your doctor know *IF*

You have ever had allergic reactions or other problems with ■ flecainide ■ local anesthetics, such as lidocaine.

You have ever had any of the following medical problems: ■ heart attack, congestive heart failure, or any other heart disease ■ liver disease ■ kidney disease ■ high or low blood-potassium levels.

You are taking any of the following medicines: ■ other medicine for abnormal heart rhythms ■ cimetidine (medicine for ulcers) ■ potassium-containing medicines or supplements ■ diuretics ■ beta-blockers (eg, propranolol, atenolol, metoprolol) ■ calcium blockers (eg, diltiazem, nifedipine, or verapamil) ■ sleep medicines ■ medicine for seizures ■ digoxin or digitalis (heart medicines) ■ captopril (medicine for hypertension and heart failure).

SPECIAL RESTRICTIONS WHILE TAKING THIS DRUG

FOOD AND DRUG INTERACTIONS

Other Drugs	Do not take any other drugs, including over-the-counter (OTC) drugs, before checking with your doctor. OTC drugs for appetite suppression, coughs, colds, asthma, allergies, or sinus problems may aggravate your heart problem.
Alcohol	Drinking alcohol while taking this medicine may worsen such side effects as drowsiness, light-headedness, or dizziness. Avoid alcohol unless your doctor has approved its use.
Smoking	Smoking may aggravate cardiac arrhythmias. If you smoke, try to stop or at least cut down.
Foods and Beverages	If you are a strict vegetarian, be sure to tell your doctor. This type of diet can increase the quantity of drug in your body by slowing the amount removed by the kidneys.

DAILY LIVING

Driving	This drug may cause light-headedness or dizziness. Be careful when driving, operating household appliances, or doing any other tasks that require alertness until you know how this drug affects you.
Examinations or Tests	It is important for you to keep all appointments with your doctor, even if you feel well, so that your progress can be checked. Periodic blood tests may be required.

Other Precautions

Tell any doctor or dentist you consult that you are taking this medicine, especially if you will be undergoing any type of surgery.

This drug may cause bleeding from the gums. If this happens, your doctor will give you special instructions for oral hygiene.

No special restrictions on exertion and exercise, sun exposure, or exposure to excessive heat or cold.

POSSIBLE SIDE EFFECTS

Although this list of adverse effects may seem somewhat intimidating, keep in mind that some are quite rare. Of course, should these or any other problems arise while you are on medication, it is always a good idea to consult your doctor.

IF YOU DEVELOP	WHAT TO DO
abnormally slow heartbeat ■ severe dizziness or fainting ■ shortness of breath ■ chest pain ■ irregular heartbeat ■ yellowing of eyes or skin	**Urgent** Get in touch with your doctor immediately.
swelling of feet or lower legs ■ trembling or shaking ■ fever or chills ■ unusual bleeding or bruising	**May be serious** Check with your doctor as soon as possible.
blurred or double vision or other visual disturbances ■ dizziness, light-headedness, faintness, or unsteadiness ■ headache ■ tiredness or weakness ■ ringing in the ears ■ drowsiness ■ anxiety ■ depression ■ difficulty in coordination ■ flushing ■ sweating ■ general ill feeling ■ nausea or vomiting ■ stomach pain ■ indigestion ■ loss of appetite ■ constipation ■ diarrhea ■ rash ■ abnormal sensations such as tingling, burning, or numbness	If symptoms are disturbing or persist, let your doctor know.

STORAGE INSTRUCTIONS

Store in a cool, dark place (not in a bathroom medicine cabinet).

STOPPING OR INTERRUPTING THERAPY

It is very important to continue taking this medicine exactly as prescribed, even if you feel well. Suddenly stopping this medicine may seriously worsen your medical condition. Your doctor will advise you on how to reduce the dosage gradually when you no longer need this drug. If you miss a dose, take it as soon as possible if you remember within six hours. If more than six hours have passed, skip the missed dose and resume your regular schedule. Do not take two doses at the same time.

SPECIAL CONSIDERATIONS FOR THOSE OVER SIXTY-FIVE

Older people may be more susceptible to such side effects as drowsiness, light-headedness, and dizziness. They should get in touch with their doctor if they develop any of these symptoms.

TRANSIENT ISCHEMIC ATTACKS

Most doctors view transient ischemic attacks (TIAs) not as an illness but as a warning. These short episodes of blurred vision, slurred speech, or dizziness are signals that a person may be heading for a serious stroke. Fortunately, it is a warning that can be heeded with good medical care.

CAUSES

TIAs are not uncommon; it is estimated that up to 10 percent of people over the age of sixty-five experience these attacks. Often called ministrokes, TIAs result from a temporary reduction in the blood supply to specific portions of the brain. Several different contributing factors may be involved, the most common of which is blockage of a blood vessel due to atherosclerosis—the buildup of fatty deposits on the blood vessel walls. Small blood clots or clumps of platelets (blood cells that are instrumental in clotting) may also lead to TIAs. Undetected or uncontrolled high blood pressure may be another important underlying cause (see guide to hypertension on pages 20–22).

DIAGNOSIS

In addition to the symptoms noted above, TIAs may cause temporary blindness, confusion, numbness or paralysis in the arms or legs, and twitching, or difficulty in performing routine tasks. These problems may last anywhere from a few seconds to up to twenty-four hours; in most people they clear in less than an hour. Unlike true strokes, TIAs do not leave residual problems, such as continued paralysis or weakness in the limbs or brain damage.

The symptoms themselves are the best clues that doctors have in diagnosing TIAs. The type and frequency of these episodes provide important information and may even pinpoint the areas of the brain that are affected.

TREATMENT

Once a firm diagnosis of a TIA is made, your doctor can choose from a range of medical or surgical treatment options (see drug charts on pages 244–248). Anticoagulant drugs are often prescribed to prevent the formation of clots in the blood vessels that feed the brain. These drugs will not dissolve existing blood clots, but they can limit their growth and help prevent new ones.

If you're taking anticoagulant drugs, your doctor will order a test called prothrombin time or protime to see how long it takes for your blood to clot. The results will help determine how much of the drug you can take safely.

Aspirin is another drug that is often used to prevent TIAs. Recent studies have found that aspirin interferes with platelet function and may therefore help to forestall the development of clots.

The most common type of surgery for TIAs involves removal of fatty deposits from the carotid arteries, which are located on the sides of the neck and are the major blood vessels carrying blood to the brain. Two recent studies indicate that such surgery *may* be beneficial in preventing future strokes in *some* patients who have suffered TIAs or have had a previous stroke.

OUTLOOK

Although experiencing TIAs may be frightening, they actually serve a positive function—they signal that a stroke may be impending and that medical help should be sought. If you follow your doctor's treatment plan carefully, there's a good chance that these ministrokes will become part of your medical past—and that a full-blown stroke will *not* await you in the future.

Caution: Some drugs in this section may affect pregnancy or fetal development. Check with your doctor if this concerns you.

CONDITION: **TRANSIENT ISCHEMIC ATTACKS**

CATEGORY: **ANTICOAGULANTS**

GENERIC (CHEMICAL) NAME	BRAND (TRADE) NAME	DOSAGE FORMS AND STRENGTHS
Warfarin	COUMADIN	Tablets: 1, 2, 2.5, 5, 7.5, 10 mg
	PANWARFIN	Tablets: 2, 2.5, 5, 7.5, 10 mg

DRUG PROFILE

Warfarin is an anticoagulant—a drug that slows the clotting of the blood and prevents harmful clots from forming and blocking the blood vessels. This type of drug interferes with the action of vitamin K, which is involved in the production of four different clotting factors. An anticoagulant is often used to treat certain heart and blood vessel conditions that make a person more likely to develop blood clots. This medicine cannot dissolve a blood clot that has already formed but can prevent an existing clot from getting larger.

BEFORE USING THIS DRUG

Let your doctor know *IF*

You have ever had allergic reactions or other problems with ■ anticoagulants ■ tartrazine (FD&C Yellow Dye No. 5) (contained in Panwarfin 7.5 mg tablets).

Any member of your family has had problems taking anticoagulant drugs.

You have ever had any of the following medical problems: ■ any heart or blood vessel disease, including stroke or transient ischemic attacks ■ severe allergies ■ asthma or other lung disease ■ diabetes ■ kidney disease ■ liver disease ■ high blood pressure ■ high cholesterol ■ congestive heart failure ■ infectious disease, such as hepatitis ■ seizures ■ ulcers ■ bleeding problems ■ any fall or blow to body or head ■ recent fever lasting longer than a few days ■ malnutrition or vitamin deficiency ■ jaundice ■ severe or continuing diarrhea ■ recent medical or dental surgery ■ gallbladder disease ■ collagen disorders ■ swelling of hands, feet, or ankles ■ thyroid disease ■ arthritis ■ mental illness ■ alcoholism ■ cancer.

You are taking any of the following medicines: ■ any other medicine for heart or blood vessel disease ■ aspirin ■ medicine for arthritis ■ medicine for gout ■ narcotics or other prescription pain-killers ■ medicine for fungal infection ■ antibiotics ■ medicine for seizures ■ sleep medicines ■ thyroid hormones ■ male or female hormones ■ medicine for high cholesterol ■ medicine for high blood pressure ■ vitamins C, E, or K ■ corticosteroids or corticotropin (ACTH) ■ medicine for ulcers ■ tranquilizers ■ muscle relaxants ■ medicine for diabetes ■ medicine for tuberculosis or malaria ■ medicine for abnormal heart rhythms ■ medicine for cancer ■ antacids ■ medicine for nausea ■ medicine for colds or sinus problems ■ medicine for depression or other mental illness ■ vaccines ■ mineral oil ■ any other medicine, including over-the-counter (OTC) drugs.

You are on a weight-reduction diet.

You are undergoing radiation therapy.

SPECIAL RESTRICTIONS WHILE TAKING THIS DRUG

FOOD AND DRUG INTERACTIONS

Other Drugs	Many drugs affect or are affected by warfarin. Tell your doctor *all* other medicines you are taking, including over-the-counter (OTC) drugs, before starting treatment with warfarin or any other anticoagulant. In addition, *do not stop* taking any other medicines before checking with your doctor.
Foods and Beverages	Eat a well-balanced diet; check with your doctor before going on any weight-reduction diet. Do not begin taking vitamins or other supplements without checking with your doctor. Vitamin K may interfere with the action of warfarin. Do not eat large amounts of foods that contain vitamin K (fish, liver, onions, spinach, kale, cauliflower, and cabbage).

Alcohol	Alcohol interferes with the effectiveness of warfarin. Do not drink regularly while taking this medicine. If you do drink, do not have more than one or two drinks at a time.

No special restrictions on smoking.

DAILY LIVING

Exertion and Exercise	Because bleeding, either external or internal, may be dangerous while you are taking this medicine, try to avoid sports or activities (such as moving heavy objects) that may cause injury.
Excessive Heat	Hot weather may make this medicine less effective.
Examinations or Tests	It is very important for you to keep all appointments with your doctor, even if you feel well, so that your progress can be checked. Periodic blood and urine tests may be required.
Other Precautions	Wear protective gloves when working in a situation in which you may cut or injure yourself. When you brush your teeth, use a soft toothbrush; floss gently. When shaving, use an electric shaver instead of a blade. If you do suffer a cut or injury, call your doctor immediately. Continue these precautions after stopping therapy, as it will take about five days before clotting returns to normal.

No special restrictions on driving, sun exposure, or exposure to excessive cold.

POSSIBLE SIDE EFFECTS

Although this list of adverse effects may seem somewhat intimidating, keep in mind that some are quite rare. Of course, should these or any other problems arise while you are on medication, it is always a good idea to consult your doctor.

IF YOU DEVELOP	WHAT TO DO
sore throat, fever, or chills ■ sores in mouth or throat ■ any change in urination ■ weight gain ■ swelling of feet or lower legs ■ tiredness ■ yellowing of eyes or skin ■ pain or color changes (to blue or purple) in toes ■ heavy bleeding or oozing from cuts or wounds ■ nosebleeds ■ bleeding from gums after brushing teeth ■ bruises or other skin marks ■ vomiting or coughing blood or material that looks like coffee grounds ■ bloody or black, tarry stools ■ constipation ■ blood in urine ■ pain or swelling of abdomen, back, joints, or stomach ■ severe headache ■ dizziness	**Urgent** Get in touch with your doctor immediately.
diarrhea ■ nausea or vomiting ■ rash, hives, or itching	**May be serious** Check with your doctor as soon as possible.
bloating or gas ■ visual problems ■ loss of appetite ■ hair loss	If symptoms are disturbing or persist, let your doctor know.

STORAGE INSTRUCTIONS

Store in a cool, dark place (not in a bathroom medicine cabinet).

STOPPING OR INTERRUPTING THERAPY

Take this medicine for exactly the time prescribed. Do not stop taking it abruptly; your doctor will advise you on how to gradually reduce your dosage. When you stop taking this medicine, it usually takes about five days before your clotting ability returns to normal. If you miss a dose of this medicine, take it as soon as possible. If it is almost time for your next dose, skip the missed dose and resume your regular schedule. Do not take two doses at the same time.

SPECIAL CONSIDERATIONS FOR THOSE OVER SIXTY-FIVE

None.

CONDITION: **TRANSIENT ISCHEMIC ATTACKS**
CATEGORY: **ANTIPLATELET DRUGS**

GENERIC (CHEMICAL) NAME	BRAND (TRADE) NAME	DOSAGE FORMS AND STRENGTHS
Aspirin and other salicylate drugs		

Aspirin and other salicylate drugs are available over the counter under a variety of brand names, dosage forms, and strengths. Some of these preparations have a special coating or contain ingredients (buffers) to help protect the lining of the stomach against possible irritation. Because of the importance of salicylate drugs in the treatment of chronic pain, even though they are most often nonprescription drugs, they are included in this book for reader reference.

DRUG PROFILE

Aspirin and other drugs in the salicylate family are used to relieve pain, inflammation, and fever. Large doses are used to treat symptoms of arthritis and rheumatism such as swelling, stiffness, and joint pain. Aspirin and other salicylates are thought to control pain and swelling by blocking the production of naturally occurring triggers of pain and inflammation, called prostaglandins. These drugs relieve fever by resetting the body's thermostat to its normal temperature.

Because aspirin helps prevent the blood cells, called platelets, from clumping together, it is also sometimes prescribed to reduce the risk of recurrent ministrokes (transient ischemic attacks, or TIAs) and stroke. The benefits of aspirin in ministrokes have to date been proven only in men—but not in women. Aspirin may also help prevent another heart attack in people who have survived a heart attack or who have the extremely severe type of chest pain known as unstable angina. Aspirin is also sometimes prescribed to prevent blood clots in people who are susceptible to this problem.

For complete information on these drugs, see pages 471–475.

HYPERLIPIDEMIA

Hyperlipidemia is usually a silent problem. For most people, the first indication is a blood test showing high levels of cholesterol or triglycerides—fatty substances known as lipids. If you have a family history of either coronary artery disease or premature atherosclerosis, your doctor will probably want to order such a blood test.

CAUSES

Our bodies need small amounts of cholesterol in order to make certain hormones and to keep the nerve fibers healthy. But if there is too much cholesterol in the blood, it tends to accumulate in the walls of the blood vessels. This can lead to atherosclerosis, the narrowing of vital blood vessels that is a major cause of heart attacks and strokes.

Some triglycerides are burned for energy, while the remainder are stored as body fat. For many years, doctors believed that an excess of triglycerides in the blood could lead to heart disease, but today they are not so sure. What is known, however, is that a very high level of triglycerides can cause stomach pain and inflammation of the pancreas (acute pancreatitis).

DIAGNOSIS

When your doctor told you that you had hyperlipidemia, he or she probably mentioned some numbers. Lipids are measured in milligrams (mg) per deciliter (dl) of blood (for example, 200 mg/dl). This is often shortened to 200 mg or simply given as a number (for example, 200). Blood tests not only measure triglycerides and total cholesterol but fractions or types of cholesterol as well. This is important information, since each type of cholesterol plays a different role in the body and may require a different treatment.

A blood test for lipids will give your doctor four numbers: one expresses the triglyceride level and the others stand for three types of cholesterol:

- LDL (low-density lipoprotein) cholesterol. This is the so-called bad cholesterol that seems to be a culprit in the development of atherosclerosis and is associated with a high risk of heart disease.

- HDL (high-density lipoprotein) cholesterol. This is the "good" cholesterol; it helps clear lipids from the bloodstream and appears to protect against heart disease.

- VLDL (very low density lipoprotein) cholesterol. An excess of this type of cholesterol in the blood is linked to high triglyceride levels and also contributes to the production of LDL cholesterol.

Ideally, your HDL level should be at least one-fourth of your total blood cholesterol. Thus, if your total cholesterol count is 200 mg, your HDL level should be at least 50.

Normally, your body manufactures all the cholesterol it needs. Additional cholesterol comes from dietary sources, such as red meat, egg yolk, butter, lard, whole milk, and hard cheese. However, the body's ability to clear cholesterol from the blood varies widely from one individual to another. For this reason, some people who conscientiously follow a low-cholesterol diet may still have high blood-cholesterol levels, while others who are not so careful about what they eat may maintain relatively low cholesterol counts.

High triglyceride levels are usually related to lifestyle habits. A rich, high-calorie diet can send triglyceride levels soaring; so can large amounts of alcohol, being overweight, cigarette smoking, and a lack of physical activity. In addition, chronic illnesses, such as diabetes and kidney disease, and certain drugs, such as beta-blockers and thiazide diuretics, may cause a problem with triglycerides.

TREATMENT

According to the American Heart Association (AHA), the ideal total cholesterol level for adults is under 200 mg. When the cholesterol level exceeds 220, the AHA recommends a change in diet. This means reducing your intake of the above-mentioned foods, which are high in cholesterol and saturated fat, and replacing them with skinless poultry, veal, seafood, margarine, vegetable oils, and skimmed or low-fat milk products. Certain types of fiber found in apples, carrots, soybeans, dried beans and peas, and oatmeal are believed to lower the cholesterol level. The use of psyllium (eg, Metamucil, Fiberall, etc.) has also been shown to be effective in reducing cholesterol levels in combination with a low-cholesterol diet. Fish oils, especially those from "fatty" fish like salmon, trout, and mackerel, also seem to have a cholesterol-lowering effect. Regular, moderate exercise (like a daily walking program) is often recommended as an accompaniment to dietary changes. Although exercise by itself will not lower total cholesterol, it does seem to boost the level of HDL ("good") cholesterol in the blood.

When a blood test reports a cholesterol level of 265 or more, diet and exercise changes may not be enough. At this point, your doctor may choose to prescribe one or more drugs to bring your cholesterol level down. A number of factors may influence this decision. If, for example, you are overweight, smoke cigarettes, or have high blood pressure or a family history of early heart disease, the doctor may be more likely to start you on lipid-lowering drugs right away.

Triglyceride levels seem to rise naturally as we grow older. However, if they exceed 200 mg, it may be time for diet or drug therapy. As a first step, doctors sometimes suggest a low-fat diet. If, after a trial period of several weeks, your triglyceride level stays high, medicine may be necessary to bring it under control. In cases in which the triglyceride count is abnormally high (over 300) or is causing severe stomach pain, doctors often start off by prescribing medicine.

OUTLOOK

Drugs that lower triglyceride and cholesterol levels will not completely cure the problem, but they do help to interrupt the body's manufacture and storage of excess lipids. Don't expect immediate results. It usually takes several weeks of regular use before these drugs have a noticeable effect, and the prescription may have to be continued for months or even years to get cholesterol or triglycerides down to healthy levels. At that point, your doctor may taper off the drugs to see if diet and other changes (increased exercise, stopping smoking, losing weight) will keep your lipid levels under control. It is very important that this medicine be taken as directed by your doctor to effectively lower your cholesterol. For some people, it may be necessary to continue the medicine indefinitely. (See charts on pages 252–267.)

To lower particularly high or stubborn lipid levels, your doctor may prescribe two or more of these drugs together. Such combinations may also be used when both triglyceride and LDL cholesterol levels are high.

In people whose high triglyceride levels are causing severe stomach pain, drug treatment will probably produce welcome relief within a few days. However, treatment for hyperlipidemia will not make an obvious difference in the way most people feel from day to day. But in the following months, their blood tests may well show a gradual decline in lipid levels. And, as the cholesterol count falls, so does the risk of heart disease. A recent major study sponsored by the National Institutes of Health demonstrated that for every 1 percent reduction in blood cholesterol level, there was a 2 percent decrease in the risk of heart attack. Other studies indicate that a combination of the lipid-lowering drug cholestyramine and dietary modification may slow or possibly even reverse the process of atherosclerosis—an encouraging sign that effective treatment of hyperlipidemia can help prevent heart disease and stroke.

Caution: Some drugs in this section may affect pregnancy or fetal development. Check with your doctor if this concerns you.

CONDITION: **HYPERLIPIDEMIA**

CATEGORY: **LIPID-LOWERING AGENTS**

GENERIC (CHEMICAL) NAME	BRAND (TRADE) NAME	DOSAGE FORMS AND STRENGTHS
Clofibrate	ATROMID-S	Capsules: 500 mg

DRUG PROFILE

Clofibrate lowers excess amounts of triglycerides (fatty substances) in the blood. This may help guard against atherosclerosis ("hardening" of the arteries caused by deposits of fat) and lower your risk of developing heart disease.

BEFORE USING THIS DRUG

Let your doctor know *IF*

You have ever had allergic reactions or other problems with ■ clofibrate.

You have ever had any of the following medical problems: ■ gallstones ■ heart disease ■ kidney disease ■ liver disease, including jaundice ■ stomach or intestinal ulcer ■ underactive thyroid ■ diabetes ■ angina (chest pain).

You are taking any of the following medicines: ■ cholestyramine (medicine for high cholesterol) ■ anticoagulants (blood thinners) ■ furosemide (diuretic) ■ medicine for diabetes ■ phenytoin (medicine for seizures) ■ probenecid.

This drug may increase your risk for tumors, liver disease, inflammation of the pancreas, and gallstones. Be sure to discuss these possible risks with your doctor before taking clofibrate.

SPECIAL INSTRUCTIONS WHILE TAKING THIS DRUG

FOOD AND DRUG INTERACTIONS

Other Drugs	It is especially important to let your doctor know if you are taking an anticoagulant (blood thinner) because clofibrate can exaggerate the effect of the anticoagulant.
Foods and Beverages	Your doctor may prescribe a special diet for you that is low in fats and/or cholesterol, which you should follow carefully. If you are overweight, a weight-reduction diet may be recommended.
Alcohol	Alcohol may be a cause of high cholesterol. Your doctor will probably suggest that you reduce your intake of alcoholic beverages.

No special restrictions on smoking.

DAILY LIVING

Examinations or Tests	It is important for you to keep all appointments with your doctor, even if you feel well, so that your progress can be checked. Periodic blood tests may be required.
Helpful Hints	To lessen the chance of upset stomach, take this medicine with or immediately after a meal.

No special restrictions on driving, exertion and exercise, sun exposure, or exposure to excessive heat or cold.

POSSIBLE SIDE EFFECTS

Although this list of adverse effects may seem somewhat intimidating, keep in mind that some are quite rare. Of course, should these or any other problems arise while you are on medication, it is always a good idea to consult your doctor.

IF YOU DEVELOP	WHAT TO DO
chest pain ■ irregular heartbeat ■ severe stomach pain with nausea and vomiting ■ shortness of breath	**Urgent** Get in touch with your doctor immediately.
blood in urine ■ decreased urination ■ swelling of feet or lower legs ■ fever, chills, or sore throat	**May be serious** Check with your doctor as soon as possible.
diarrhea ■ nausea or vomiting ■ increased appetite or weight gain ■ sores in the mouth or on the lips ■ stomach pain ■ gas or bloating ■ heartburn ■ aching or cramped muscles ■ tiredness or weakness ■ male impotence ■ diminished sex drive ■ headache ■ dizziness ■ drowsiness ■ male breast tenderness ■ rash, hives, or itching ■ dry skin or hair ■ hair loss ■ pain or difficulty in urination	If symptoms are disturbing or persist, let your doctor know.

STORAGE INSTRUCTIONS

Store in a cool, dark place (not in a bathroom medicine cabinet).

STOPPING OR INTERRUPTING THERAPY

Take this medicine exactly as directed by your doctor and do not stop taking it without checking with your doctor. If you miss a dose, take it as soon as possible; if it is almost time for your next dose, skip the missed dose and resume your regular schedule. Do not take two doses at the same time.

SPECIAL CONSIDERATIONS FOR THOSE OVER SIXTY-FIVE

Older people may be more troubled by such side effects as nausea. They should let their doctors know if such problems are particularly bothersome.

CONDITION: **HYPERLIPIDEMIA**

CATEGORY: **LIPID-LOWERING AGENTS**

GENERIC (CHEMICAL) NAME	BRAND (TRADE) NAME	DOSAGE FORMS AND STRENGTHS
Gemfibrozil	LOPID	Tablets: 600 mg

DRUG PROFILE

Gemfibrozil is used to lower high levels of triglycerides (fatty substances) in the blood. Lowering these substances is important because the buildup of these substances along the walls of the blood vessels can lead to such serious conditions as angina, heart attack, or stroke.

BEFORE USING THIS DRUG

Let your doctor know *IF*

You have ever had allergic reactions or other problems with ■ gemfibrozil.

You have ever had any of the following medical problems: ■ gallbladder disease, including gallstones ■ heart disease ■ kidney disease ■ liver disease ■ underactive thyroid ■ diabetes.

You are taking: ■ anticoagulants (blood thinners) ■ lovastatin.

This drug may increase your risk for tumors, liver disease, inflammation of the pancreas, and gallstones. Be sure to discuss these possible risks with your doctor before taking gemfibrozil.

SPECIAL INSTRUCTIONS WHILE TAKING THIS DRUG

FOOD AND DRUG INTERACTIONS

Other Drugs	It is especially important to let your doctor know if you are taking an anticoagulant (blood thinner), because gemfibrozil can exaggerate the effect of the anticoagulant.
Foods and Beverages	Your doctor may suggest a diet low in fats and/or cholesterol. If you are overweight, a weight-reduction diet may be recommended.
Alcohol	Alcohol may be a cause of high cholesterol. Your doctor will probably suggest that you reduce your intake of alcoholic beverages.

No special restrictions on smoking.

DAILY LIVING

Exertion or Exercise	To get the maximum benefit from this medicine, follow both a proper diet and a regular exercise program.
Examinations or Tests	It is important for you to keep all appointments with your doctor, even if you feel well, so that your progress can be checked. Periodic blood tests may be required.
Other Precautions	Although there have been no reports of major problems from gemfibrozil, this drug is very similar to clofibrate, which has been found to increase the risk of gallstones (see clofibrate chart, pages 252–254).

If you have diabetes, be aware that this medicine may raise blood-sugar levels. If you notice any change when testing sugar levels in your blood or urine, let your doctor know.

No special restrictions on driving, sun exposure, or exposure to excessive heat or cold.

POSSIBLE SIDE EFFECTS

Although this list of adverse effects may seem somewhat intimidating, keep in mind that some are quite rare. Of course, should these or any other problems arise while you are on medication, it is always a good idea to consult your doctor.

IF YOU DEVELOP	WHAT TO DO
fever, chills, or sore throat ■ severe stomach pain with nausea and vomiting ■ irregular heartbeat	**Urgent** Get in touch with your doctor immediately.
diarrhea ■ nausea and vomiting ■ stomach pain ■ gas ■ heartburn ■ rash, hives, or itching ■ muscle or bone pain ■ blurred vision ■ headache ■ dizziness	**May be serious** Check with your doctor as soon as possible.

STORAGE INSTRUCTIONS

Store in a cool, dark place (not in a bathroom medicine cabinet).

STOPPING OR INTERRUPTING THERAPY

If you miss a dose of this medicine, take it as soon as possible. If it is almost time for your next dose, skip the missed dose and resume your regular schedule. Do not take two doses at the same time.

SPECIAL CONSIDERATIONS FOR THOSE OVER SIXTY-FIVE

None.

CONDITION: **HYPERLIPIDEMIA**

CATEGORY: **LIPID-LOWERING AGENTS**

GENERIC (CHEMICAL) NAME	BRAND (TRADE) NAME	DOSAGE FORMS AND STRENGTHS
Probucol	LORELCO	Tablets: 250, 500 mg

DRUG PROFILE

Probucol is used to treat high levels of cholesterol in the blood. Lowering high cholesterol is important because the buildup of cholesterol along the walls of the blood vessels can lead to such serious conditions as angina, heart attack, or stroke.

BEFORE USING THIS DRUG

Let your doctor know *IF*

You have ever had allergic reactions or other problems with ■ probucol.

You have ever had any of the following medical problems: ■ gallbladder disease or gallstones ■ heart disease, especially heart attack or abnormal heart rhythms ■ liver disease ■ underactive thyroid ■ diabetes ■ fainting spells.

You are taking any of the following medicines: ■ clofibrate (medicine for high cholesterol) ■ tricyclic antidepressants ■ medicine for heart rhythm ■ beta-blockers (eg, propranolol, atenolol, metoprolol) ■ digoxin (medicine for heart failure) ■ medicine for emotional disorders (eg, chlorpromazine, prochlorperazine).

SPECIAL INSTRUCTIONS WHILE TAKING THIS DRUG

FOOD AND DRUG INTERACTIONS

Foods and Beverages	Your doctor may suggest a diet low in fats and/or cholesterol. If you are overweight, a weight-reduction diet may be recommended.

Alcohol	Alcohol may be a cause of high cholesterol. Your doctor will probably suggest that you reduce your intake of alcoholic beverages.

No special restrictions on other drugs or smoking.

DAILY LIVING

Exertion and Exercise	To get the maximum benefit from this medicine, follow both a proper diet and a regular exercise program.
Examinations or Tests	It is important for you to keep all appointments with your doctor, even if you feel well, so that your progress can be checked. Periodic blood tests may be required. Your doctor may also want to take an electrocardiogram before and during therapy.
Other Precautions	Occasionally, there may be a reaction at the beginning of therapy that consists of fainting or dizziness, irregular heartbeat, nausea, vomiting, and sometimes chest pain as well. If this should occur, call your doctor at once.
Helpful Hints	This medicine works best when taken with meals.

No special restrictions on driving, sun exposure, or exposure to excessive heat or cold.

POSSIBLE SIDE EFFECTS

Although this list of adverse effects may seem somewhat intimidating, keep in mind that some are quite rare. Of course, should these or any other problems arise while you are on medication, it is always a good idea to consult your doctor.

IF YOU DEVELOP	WHAT TO DO
When beginning therapy: fainting ■ dizziness ■ irregular heartbeat ■ nausea or vomiting	**Urgent** Get in touch with your doctor immediately.
swelling of face, hands, feet, or inside of mouth ■ irregular heartbeat ■ chest pain ■ fainting ■ dizziness	**May be serious:** Check with your doctor as soon as possible.
diarrhea or loose stools ■ nausea or vomiting ■ indigestion ■ stomach pain ■ gas ■ headache ■ numbness or tingling in fingers, toes, or face ■ diminished sense of taste or smell ■ blurred vision ■ tearing ■ red or itching eyes ■ ringing in the ears ■ increased or decreased appetite ■ sleeplessness ■ rash or hives ■ need to urinate at night ■ male sexual problems ■ increased sweating or foul-smelling sweat	If symptoms are disturbing or persist, let your doctor know.

STORAGE INSTRUCTIONS

Store in a cool, dark place (not in a bathroom medicine cabinet).

STOPPING OR INTERRUPTING THERAPY

Because this medicine only controls and does not cure high cholesterol, you may have to take it for a long period of time. Suddenly stopping this medicine may raise your cholesterol level. Your doctor will advise you on how to gradually decrease your medicine when you no longer need it. If you miss a dose, take it as soon as possible. If it is almost time for your next dose, skip the missed dose and resume your regular schedule. Do not take two doses at the same time.

SPECIAL CONSIDERATIONS FOR THOSE OVER SIXTY-FIVE

None.

CONDITION: **HYPERLIPIDEMIA**

CATEGORY: **LIPID-LOWERING AGENTS**

GENERIC (CHEMICAL) NAME	BRAND (TRADE) NAME	DOSAGE FORMS AND STRENGTHS
Cholestyramine	QUESTRAN	Powder: 4 g of anhydrous cholestyramine resin in 9 g of powder per packet or scoopful
	CHOLYBAR	Bar: 4 g of anhydrous cholestyramine resin in a 9 g chewable bar

DRUG PROFILE

Cholestyramine is used to lower blood levels of cholesterol. Lowering high choles-terol is important because the buildup of cholesterol along the walls of the blood vessels can lead to such serious conditions as angina, heart attack, or stroke. Cholestyramine is also used to relieve severe itching caused by high levels of bile acids in the blood of people whose bile ducts are obstructed. This drug is not actu-ally absorbed into the body but works by remaining in the digestive tract and attack-ing certain substances in the intestine.

BEFORE USING THIS DRUG

Let your doctor know *IF*

You have ever had allergic reactions or other problems with ■ cholestyramine
  ■ tartrazine (FD&C Yellow Dye No. 5) ■ aspirin.

You have ever had any of the following medical problems: ■ heart or blood vessel disease ■ liver disease ■ bleeding problems ■ gallstones ■ obstruction of the gallbladder or bile ducts ■ kidney disease ■ stomach ulcer ■ constipation ■ hemorrhoids ■ underactive thyroid ■ diabetes ■ osteoporosis.

You are taking any of the following medicines: ■ anticoagulants (blood thinners) digoxin or digitalis (heart medicines) ■ thyroid medicine ■ vitamins ■ medicine for arthritis or gout ■ diuretics ■ tetracycline ■ penicillin ■ medicine for seizures ■ sleep medicines ■ medicine for gallstones.

SPECIAL RESTRICTIONS WHILE TAKING THIS DRUG

FOOD AND DRUG INTERACTIONS

Other Drugs	Do not take other medicine at the same time you take cholestyramine. Other drugs should be taken one hour before or four to six hours after taking a dose of cholestyramine. In addition, if you have been taking both cholestyramine and digitalis and suddenly stop taking cholestyramine, concentrations of digitalis in the blood can rise to dangerous levels.
Foods and Beverages	Your doctor may suggest a diet low in fats and/or cholesterol. If you are overweight, a weight-reduction diet may be recommended. It is important to drink plenty of fluids while taking this medicine. This drug may interfere with your absorption of certain vitamins. If you develop a vitamin deficiency, your doctor may give you special vitamin supplements.

No special restrictions on smoking or alcohol use.

DAILY LIVING

Exertion and Exercise	To get the most benefit from this medicine, follow both a proper diet and a regular exercise program.

Examinations or Tests	It is important for you to keep all appointments with your doctor, even if you feel well, so that your progress can be checked. Periodic blood tests are usually required.

Helpful Hints	Do not take the powder in dry form. Mix one scoopful or packetful with at least two to six fluid ounces of water, fruit juice, milk, or any other noncarbonated beverage. Let the powder sit, without stirring, for a minute or two, and then stir until it is completely mixed; it will not dissolve. After drinking, add a little more liquid to the glass and drink it to make sure you have swallowed all the medicine.
	Mild constipation is a common side effect of this drug and can usually be relieved by laxatives or stool softeners. Let your doctor know if constipation continues or is severe.

No special restrictions on driving, sun exposure, or exposure to excessive heat or cold.

POSSIBLE SIDE EFFECTS

Although this list of adverse effects may seem somewhat intimidating, keep in mind that some are quite rare. Of course, should these or any other problems arise while you are on medication, it is always a good idea to consult your doctor.

IF YOU DEVELOP	WHAT TO DO
black, tarry stools ■ severe stomach pain with nausea and vomiting	**Urgent** Get in touch with your doctor immediately.
constipation ■ weight loss ■ aggravation of hemorrhoids	**May be serious** Check with your doctor as soon as possible.

heartburn ■ indigestion ■ diarrhea ■ nausea or vomiting ■ loss of appetite ■ stomach pain ■ belching, bloating, or gas ■ rash or soreness of skin, tongue, or anal tissues

If symptoms are disturbing or persist, let your doctor know.

STORAGE INSTRUCTIONS

Store in a cool, dark place (not in a bathroom medicine cabinet).

STOPPING OR INTERRUPTING THERAPY

Because this medicine controls but does not cure high cholesterol, you may have to take it for an extended period of time. If you miss a dose, take it as soon as possible. If it is almost time for your next dose, skip the missed dose and resume your regular dosing schedule. Do not take two doses at the same time.

SPECIAL CONSIDERATIONS FOR THOSE OVER SIXTY-FIVE

Older people may be more prone to the side effect of constipation. Also, this drug may worsen osteoporosis because it causes loss of calcium, an important component of bone.

CONDITION: **HYPERLIPIDEMIA**

CATEGORY: **LIPID-LOWERING AGENTS**

GENERIC (CHEMICAL) NAME	BRAND (TRADE) NAME	DOSAGE FORMS AND STRENGTHS
Lovastatin	MEVACOR	Tablets: 10, 20, 40 mg

DRUG PROFILE

Lovastatin is used to treat high levels of cholesterol in the blood. Lowering high cholesterol is important because the buildup of cholesterol in the walls of the blood vessels can lead to such serious conditions as angina, heart attack, or stroke.

BEFORE USING THIS DRUG

Let your doctor know *IF*

You have ever had allergic reactions or other problems with ■ lovastatin.

You have ever had any of the following medical problems: ■ liver disease ■ kidney, heart, or liver transplant ■ alcoholism ■ seizures.

You are taking any of the following medicines: ■ other medicine for high cholesterol (eg, niacin, gemfibrozil) ■ medicine to prevent rejection of transplanted organs ■ cyclosporine ■ anticoagulants (blood thinners) ■ erythromycin.

SPECIAL RESTRICTIONS WHILE TAKING THIS DRUG

FOOD AND DRUG INTERACTIONS

Foods and Beverages	Your doctor may prescribe a special diet for you that is low in fats and/or cholesterol, which you should follow carefully. If you are overweight, a weight-reduction diet may be recommended.
Alcohol	Alcohol may be a cause of high cholesterol. Your doctor will probably suggest that you reduce your intake of alcoholic beverages.

No special restrictions on smoking.

DAILY LIVING

Examinations or Tests	It is important for you to keep all appointments with your doctor, even if you feel well, so that your progress can be checked. Periodic blood, liver, and eye tests may be required.
Other Precautions	Tell any doctor or dentist you consult that you are taking this medicine, especially if you will be undergoing any type of surgery.

| Helpful Hints | This medicine should be taken with food. |

No special restrictions on exertion and exercise, driving, sun exposure, or exposure to excessive heat or cold.

POSSIBLE SIDE EFFECTS

Although this list of adverse effects may seem somewhat intimidating, keep in mind that some are quite rare. Of course, should these or any other problems arise while you are on medication, it is always a good idea to consult your doctor.

IF YOU DEVELOP	WHAT TO DO
yellow eyes or skin	**Urgent** Get in touch with your doctor immediately.
aching, tender or cramping muscles ■ muscle weakness ■ blurred vision ■ fever ■ tiredness or weakness ■ general ill feeling	**May be serious** Check with your doctor as soon as possible.
constipation ■ nausea ■ diarrhea ■ gas ■ heartburn ■ stomach pain or cramps ■ dizziness ■ headache ■ rash ■ itching ■ taste changes ■ vision problems	If symptoms are disturbing or persist, let your doctor know.

STORAGE INSTRUCTIONS

Store in a cool, dark place (not in a bathroom medicine cabinet).

STOPPING OR INTERRUPTING THERAPY

If you miss a dose, take it as soon as possible. If it is almost time for your next dose, skip the missed dose and resume your regular schedule. Do not take two doses at the same time.

SPECIAL CONSIDERATION FOR THOSE OVER SIXTY-FIVE

None.

CONDITION: **HYPERLIPIDEMIA**

CATEGORY: **LIPID-LOWERING AGENTS**

GENERIC (CHEMICAL) NAME	BRAND (TRADE) NAME	DOSAGE FORMS AND STRENGTHS
Niacin	NICOBID	Controlled-release capsules: 125, 250, 500 mg

This drug is available both by prescription and over the counter under a variety of brand names and dosage forms.

DRUG PROFILE

Niacin helps the body break down food so that it can be used for energy. This type of supplement is used to prevent or treat niacin deficiency, or pellagra. Niacin is also used to lower blood levels of fats and cholesterol.

For complete information on this drug, see pages 660–662.

INTERMITTENT CLAUDICATION

Intermittent claudication, which literally means "limping that comes and goes," is the name of a condition that affects the legs. Cramping leg pain during walking or exercise or very tired legs are its most common symptoms. It is usually the first sign of chronic peripheral atherosclerotic disease, a type of atherosclerosis—or "hardening of the arteries"—that affects the arteries in the legs and arms.

CAUSES

In atherosclerosis, a fatty plaque partially or completely blocks the artery. The amount of blood that can get through a partially blocked artery may be sufficient at rest, but an active muscle demands more circulating blood than a resting one; if no more blood can pass through the artery, intermittent claudication results.

People who smoke; are obese; or have diabetes, hypertension, or high blood-cholesterol levels face the greatest risk for developing intermittent claudication. This condition affects men almost twice as often as women and becomes increasingly common with age. In fact, one out of every one hundred people between the ages of sixty-five and seventy-four has intermittent claudication.

DIAGNOSIS

The pain associated with intermittent claudication is usually in the calf, but some people have pain in the foot, thigh, hip, buttock, or even the lower back. Usually one leg is involved. The symptom is quite consistent, occurring after the same amount of exercise each time. Some people suffer from weakness and fatigue rather than pain. Relief comes two to five minutes after stopping the activity.

If the blockage in the artery worsens, intermittent claudication progresses to leg pain even at rest. In this advanced stage, other symptoms that you may develop include numbness, burning, changes in skin color (to pale or red), loss of hair on the leg, bluish nails, and ulcers. Permanent damage to the leg, including gangrene, can occur.

To find out if you have this condition, your doctor will probably use a blood pressure cuff to check your ankle pulse; this pulse is faint or even absent in intermittent claudication. Doppler ultrasound may be used to measure blood flow. This measurement is taken by moving a transducer over the skin to direct sound waves into the blood vessels. The sonic echoes reflected back measure the amount of blood flow with great accuracy, in addition to locating the blockage.

If you haven't had a physical examination in some time, your doctor may decide to test for conditions that can be associated with intermittent claudication. Your examination might then include a glucose tolerance test for diabetes and a blood test for elevated cholesterol.

TREATMENT

The most important part of treatment involves steps—both literally and otherwise—you can take on your own. Walking is ideal for anyone who has intermittent claudication. It should be done every day for at least thirty to sixty minutes. When discomfort occurs, stop and wait until it subsides; then continue walking. Although exercise may set off an attack, regular exercise will actually help develop new blood vessels and improve your tolerance.

Tobacco in all forms must be avoided because it aggravates this condition. Diabetes, elevated cholesterol, and high blood pressure should be carefully controlled by diet and by any drugs that are prescribed. If you are overweight, ask your doctor to recommend a diet and an exercise program. Weight loss can make a big difference in how much exertion you can tolerate.

Give your feet tender, loving care. Reduced circulation may have made your feet less sensitive, so a daily inspection for injuries is mandatory. Your shoes should fit correctly, and your feet should be kept clean and dry. Clip your toenails regularly, cutting straight across and taking care not to injure your toes. Because even minor injuries pose the danger of infection, seek the services of a podiatrist for treatment of corns, calluses, and ingrown toenails.

Surgery is seldom necessary for mild or moderate intermittent claudication. However, if the condition worsens and becomes advanced, a graft to bypass the blockage (arterial bypass surgery) may be done.

There are several different drugs that can be prescribed to treat intermittent claudication. For detailed information on these drugs, see the charts on pages 270–277.

OUTLOOK

A diagnosis of intermittent claudication may be the first indication that you have atherosclerosis. Although atherosclerosis cannot be cured, the chances of further complications can be reduced. Most of the success in controlling peripheral atherosclerotic disease will come from your own efforts. By working with your doctor and taking the prescribed medicines, you may find that you are living a healthier life than before.

CONDITION: **INTERMITTENT CLAUDICATION**

CATEGORY: **HEMORHEOLOGIC DRUGS**

GENERIC (CHEMICAL) NAME	BRAND (TRADE) NAME	DOSAGE FORMS AND STRENGTHS
Pentoxifylline	TRENTAL	Controlled-release tablets: 400 mg

DRUG PROFILE

Pentoxifylline is used to treat intermittent claudication. It is a hemorheologic drug, which means that it works by making the red blood cells more flexible. This allows the blood to flow more easily, especially through the smaller blood vessels in the limbs.

BEFORE USING THIS DRUG

Let your doctor know *IF*

You have ever had allergic reactions or other problems with ■ pentoxifylline ■ caffeine ■ aminophylline, oxtriphylline, or theophylline (medicine for asthma).

You have ever had any of the following medical problems: ■ high or low blood pressure ■ angina (chest pain) ■ abnormal heart rhythm ■ stroke or other disease of the blood vessels ■ heart disease ■ kidney disease ■ stomach ulcers ■ recent surgery.

You are taking any of the following medicines: ■ medicine for high blood pressure ■ anticoagulants (blood thinners).

SPECIAL INSTRUCTIONS WHILE TAKING THIS DRUG

FOOD AND DRUG INTERACTIONS

Smoking	Smoking may worsen your medical condition. If you smoke, try to stop or at least cut down.

No special restrictions on other drugs, foods and beverages, or alcohol use.

DAILY LIVING

Examinations or Tests	It is important for you to keep all appointments with your doctor so that your progress can be checked.
Helpful Hints	To avoid upset stomach, take this medicine with meals or a snack. Swallow the controlled-release tablets whole—do not break, chew, or crush them.

No special restrictions on driving, exertion and exercise, sun exposure, or exposure to excessive heat or cold.

POSSIBLE SIDE EFFECTS

Although this list of adverse effects may seem somewhat intimidating, keep in mind that some are quite rare. Of course, should these or any other problems arise while you are on medication, it is always a good idea to consult your doctor.

IF YOU DEVELOP	WHAT TO DO
drowsiness ■ flushing ■ fainting ■ excitement ■ fever ■ seizures ■ chest pain	**Urgent** Get in touch with your doctor immediately.

irregular or fast heartbeat ■ nervousness ■ agitation ■ sleeplessness ■ difficulty breathing	**May be serious** Check with your doctor as soon as possible.
dizziness ■ headache ■ tremors ■ nausea or vomiting ■ upset stomach ■ loss of appetite ■ belching ■ bloating or gas ■ skin rash ■ itching	If symptoms are disturbing or persist, let your doctor know.

STORAGE INSTRUCTIONS

Store in a cool, dark place (not in a bathroom medicine cabinet).

STOPPING OR INTERRUPTING THERAPY

It may take several weeks before you feel any beneficial effects from this medicine. Do not stop taking this drug without checking with your doctor. If you miss a dose, take it as soon as possible. If it is almost time for your next dose, skip the missed dose and resume your regular schedule. Do not take two doses at the same time.

SPECIAL CONSIDERATIONS FOR THOSE OVER SIXTY-FIVE

None.

CONDITION: **INTERMITTENT CLAUDICATION**

CATEGORY: **PERIPHERAL VASODILATORS**

GENERIC (CHEMICAL) NAME	BRAND (TRADE) NAME	DOSAGE FORMS AND STRENGTHS
Nylidrin hydrochloride	ARLIDIN	Tablets: 6, 12 mg

DRUG PROFILE

Nylidrin plays a supporting role in the treatment of conditions caused by poor circulation, such as diabetic vascular disease, Raynaud's syndrome, phlebitis, frostbite, inner ear disturbances, cerebral vascular disease, and atherosclerosis. The National Academy of Sciences, the National Research Council, and the Food and Drug Administration have classified this drug as "possibly" effective and recommended that it be reevaluated. You should discuss its use with your doctor.

BEFORE USING THIS DRUG

Let your doctor know *IF*

You have ever had allergic reactions or other problems with ■ nylidrin.

You have ever had any of the following medical problems: ■ angina (chest pain) ■ heart disease, including recent heart attack ■ fast or irregular heartbeat ■ stomach ulcer ■ overactive thyroid.

SPECIAL RESTRICTIONS WHILE TAKING THIS DRUG

FOOD AND DRUG INTERACTIONS

Smoking	Smoking may reduce the beneficial effects of this drug. If you smoke, try to stop or at least cut down.

No special restrictions on other drugs, foods and beverages, or alcohol use.

DAILY LIVING

Helpful Hints	Because this drug can cause fast or pounding heartbeat, do not take your last dose just before bedtime, since it may disturb your sleep. Discuss with your doctor the best dosage schedule for you.

No special restrictions on exertion and exercise, sun exposure, or exposure to excessive heat or cold.

POSSIBLE SIDE EFFECTS

Although this list of adverse effects may seem somewhat intimidating, keep in mind that some are quite rare. Of course, should these or any other problems arise while you are on medication, it is always a good idea to consult your doctor.

IF YOU DEVELOP	WHAT TO DO
chest pain ■ decreased urination or inability to urinate ■ fever ■ blurred vision ■ metallic taste	**Urgent** Get in touch with your doctor immediately.
irregular or fast heartbeat ■ dizziness, faintness, or light-headedness, especially when getting up from a reclining or sitting position ■ tiredness or weakness	**May be serious** Check with your doctor as soon as possible.
nausea or vomiting ■ headache ■ tremors ■ nervousness ■ flushing ■ chilliness	If symptoms are disturbing or persist, let your doctor know.

STORAGE INSTRUCTIONS

Store in a cool, dark place (not in a bathroom medicine cabinet).

STOPPING OR INTERRUPTING THERAPY

Do not stop taking this medicine, even if you see no difference in your condition, without consulting your doctor. If you miss a dose of this medicine, take it as soon as possible. If it is almost time for your next dose, skip the missed dose and resume your regular schedule. Do not take two doses at the same time.

SPECIAL CONSIDERATIONS FOR THOSE OVER SIXTY-FIVE

None.

CONDITION: **INTERMITTENT CLAUDICATION**

CATEGORY: **PERIPHERAL VASODILATORS**

GENERIC (CHEMICAL) NAME	BRAND (TRADE) NAME	DOSAGE FORMS AND STRENGTHS
Cyclandelate	CYCLOSPASMOL	Capsules: 200, 400 mg

DRUG PROFILE

Cyclandelate plays a supporting role in the treatment of conditions caused by poor circulation, such as diabetic vascular disease, Raynaud's syndrome, phlebitis, intermittent claudication, night leg cramps, and atherosclerosis. The National Academy of Sciences, the National Research Council, and the Food and Drug Administration have classified this drug as "possibly" effective and recommended that it be reevaluated. You should discuss its use with your doctor.

BEFORE USING THIS DRUG

Let your doctor know *IF*

You have ever had allergic reactions or other problems with ■ cyclandelate.

You have ever had any of the following medical problems: ■ angina (chest pain) ■ recent heart attack or stroke ■ glaucoma ■ bleeding problems.

SPECIAL INSTRUCTIONS WHILE TAKING THIS DRUG

FOOD AND DRUG INTERACTIONS

Smoking	Smoking may reduce the benefits of this drug. If you smoke, try to stop or at least cut down.

No special restrictions on other drugs, foods and beverages, or alcohol use.

DAILY LIVING

Other Precautions	This drug may cause dizziness; use caution when getting up from a reclining or sitting position or when climbing stairs, and let your doctor know if the dizziness becomes a problem. You also may experience flushing, headache, weakness, or fast heartbeat, especially during the first few weeks of therapy.
Helpful Hints	If this medicine upsets your stomach, taking it with milk, meals, snacks, or an antacid should help.

No special restrictions on driving, exertion and exercise, sun exposure, or exposure to excessive heat or cold.

POSSIBLE SIDE EFFECTS

Although this list of adverse effects may seem somewhat intimidating, keep in mind that some are quite rare. Of course, should these or any other problems arise while you are on medication, it is always a good idea to consult your doctor.

IF YOU DEVELOP

fast heartbeat ■ dizziness, especially when getting up from a reclining or sitting position ■ tiredness or weakness ■ headache ■ flushing ■ tingling in face, fingers, or toes ■ increased sweating ■ gas ■ heartburn ■ nausea ■ stomach pain or discomfort

WHAT TO DO

If symptoms are disturbing or persist, let your doctor know.

STORAGE INSTRUCTIONS

Store in a cool, dark place (not in a bathroom medicine cabinet).

STOPPING OR INTERRUPTING THERAPY

It may take several weeks before you feel any beneficial effects from this medicine. Do not stop taking this medicine without checking with your doctor. If you miss a dose, take it as soon as possible. If it is almost time for your next dose, skip the missed dose and resume your regular schedule. Do not take two doses at the same time.

SPECIAL CONSIDERATIONS FOR THOSE OVER SIXTY-FIVE

Older people may be more prone to the side effect of dizziness, especially when getting up from a reclining or sitting position.

Chapter 2
Disorders of the Brain and Nervous System

MEMORY DISORDERS

Perhaps the greatest fear many of us have about growing older is that we will lose part of ourselves—our memory. We forget a name, and we are convinced we are on a one-way road to "senility." But occasional forgetfulness is not a sign of mental decline. Nor is "senility" an inevitable part of growing older.

Severe memory loss, however, does occur in some older people. It may be coupled with confusion and other changes in personality and behavior. There are a number of causes for this, many of which respond to prompt treatment. (These reversible conditions include, for example, a minor head injury, a high fever, vitamin deficiency, or an adverse reaction to a drug.) In other instances, treatment can help to reduce symptoms but not restore lost brain function. Therefore, it is important to find out the source of the symptoms.

CAUSES

Alzheimer's Disease The most common cause of memory loss that is as yet incurable is Alzheimer's disease, a condition that afflicts up to 10 percent of the population aged sixty-five and older. The severe intellectual impairments it produces—serious confusion, memory lapses, and loss of recognition of family and friends—stem from abnormal changes in the cerebral cortex (the outer layer of the brain), as well as from deeper structures in the brain. A number of theories have been advanced as to the underlying cause of Alzheimer's, but none has yet been confirmed.

The first sign of Alzheimer's disease is usually the inability to recall recent events. These memory lapses are minor at first, and are sometimes blamed on physical illness or emotional upsets. Eventually, these memory lapses and the failure to recognize friends and family interfere with work and social life. Personality changes, trouble with language, and difficulty with routines of daily living, such as brushing teeth, are other early symptoms.

As the disease progresses, victims of Alzheimer's disease lose the ability to handle finances and to carry out such routine tasks as marketing or traveling to familiar places. Frequently they develop crying spells and admit to a sense of shame about their memory problems. The disease may develop gradually, with these earlier stages lasting many years.

With further progression, people with Alzheimer's reach the point at which they can no longer dress or bathe themselves without help. They may become agitated, and delusions can set in. Symptoms may accelerate so rapidly that home care is no longer possible. In the final stages of the disease, individuals can no longer care for themselves at all. They lose the ability to speak intelligibly and become bedridden.

Multi-Infarct Dementia The second most common cause of mental impairment in older people is multi-infarct dementia. In this condition, a series of minor strokes results in widespread death of brain tissue and the progressive loss of mental functioning.

The combination of Alzheimer's disease and multi-infarct dementia is probably the third most common cause of dementia.

Emotional Problems Memory loss sometimes accompanies such emotional problems as depression (including loss of self-esteem) and anxiety. These problems may be mistakenly confused with irreversible brain disease, and a depressed individual labeled "senile." This will lead to inappropriate treatment.

DIAGNOSIS

To rule out the possibility of a treatable disease, people with severe memory loss and mental confusion should have a comprehensive workup, including thorough physical, psychological, and neurological evaluations. Laboratory studies of the blood and computed axial tomography (CAT) scans of the brain are often important in differentiating Alzheimer's disease from other conditions causing similar symptoms. However, it should be emphasized that there is not a single definitive test for Alzheimer's disease. Genetic markers for Alzheimer's disease are being studied, and it is possible that these discoveries may eventually provide the basis for a diagnostic test.

If other disorders are ruled out, the diagnosis of Alzheimer's disease can be made on the basis of the person's current symptoms, laboratory data, and the way in which the illness has progressed. A relative or close friend may be called in to help piece together past events, giving the doctor an accurate picture of the person's medical history.

Testing does not come to an end once the diagnosis is made. Many doctors perform periodic neurological examinations and psychological tests to evaluate the progress of the disease and its response to therapy.

TREATMENT

Serious memory loss is sometimes treated by cerebral vasodilators, such as ergoloid mesylates, isoxsuprine, and papaverine. These medicines act by relaxing and dilating the blood vessels in the brain, allowing more oxygen to reach the brain. The efficacy of these drugs, however, has not been established; the Food and Drug Administration considers isoxsuprine and papaverine to be lacking in substantial evidence of effectiveness. Hydergine, a combination of ergoloid mesylates, is the only FDA-approved medication for the treatment of Alzheimer's disease. However, a recent study showed this treatment to be ineffective as well. More information on these products appears in the drug charts on pages 283–291.

So far, there is no known cure or prevention for Alzheimer's disease. However, some of the troubling symptoms can be alleviated through proper medical care. Antidepressant medicines help control the depression seen in the early stages of the illness, and tranquilizers can lessen the agitation and anxiety associated with more advanced stages. Appropriate medicine can also help improve sleeping patterns. Some researchers are testing drugs that raise brain levels of the chemical acetylcholine in an effort to make up for the deficiency of that nerve signal transmitter, which is characteristic of Alzheimer's disease patients.

OUTLOOK

Family members and friends can provide a great deal of help for people who have multi-infarct dementia and those who have Alzheimer's disease. It's important to keep activities as close to normal as possible and to encourage physical activities and social contacts. Memory aids—such as calendars, lists of chores, and written reminders of safety measures—often help in the early stages. Although people with these illnesses may not be able to undertake shopping trips, or go to movies, go on hikes, or go to ball games or other athletic activities alone, they can still participate in them with a friend or family member as company.

Victims of Alzheimer's disease are often cared for at home during the early stages. When this becomes impossible, a day-care center may answer the need for supervised care. During later stages, however, a full-time care facility usually becomes necessary.

Self-help and support groups for relatives of people with Alzheimer's disease and similar illnesses are forming throughout the country. These groups are an important source of information and a place to share experiences with others. For the location of a group in your area, contact the Alzheimer's Disease and Related Disorders Association, 360 North Michigan Avenue, Chicago, IL 60601.

CONDITION: **MEMORY DISORDERS, ALZHEIMER'S DISEASE, AND VASCULAR DEMENTIA**

CATEGORY: **CEREBRAL VASODILATORS**

GENERIC (CHEMICAL) NAME	BRAND (TRADE) NAME	DOSAGE FORMS AND STRENGTHS
Ergoloid mesylates	HYDERGINE	Liquid: 1 mg per ml Oral tablets: 1 mg Sublingual tablets: 0.5 or 1 mg
	HYDERGINE LC	Capsules: 1 mg

DRUG PROFILE

Ergoloid mesylates are used to improve mental function by enhancing the circulation of blood to the brain. This medicine is used to treat changes in mood and memory as well as depression.

BEFORE USING THIS DRUG

Let your doctor know *IF*

You have ever had allergic reactions or other problems with ■ ergoloid mesylates ■ ergotamine.

You have ever had any of the following medical problems: ■ mental illness ■ slow pulse ■ low blood pressure ■ liver disease.

You are taking any of the following medicines: ■ ergotamine or methysergide (medicine for migraine headaches) ■ medicine for depression or other mental illness.

SPECIAL RESTRICTIONS WHILE TAKING THIS DRUG

FOOD AND DRUG INTERACTIONS

Other Drugs	Do not take any other drugs, including over-the-counter (OTC) drugs, before checking with your doctor.
Smoking	Smoking may reduce the beneficial effects of this drug. Let your doctor know if you smoke.

No special restrictions on foods and beverages or alcohol use.

DAILY LIVING

Excessive Cold	Avoid long periods of exposure to cold, since this medicine may interfere with your body's ability to adjust to cold temperatures.
Examinations or Tests	It is important for you to keep all appointments with your doctor so that your progress can be checked.
Other Precautions	Take this medicine exactly as directed by your doctor; do not take more of it or take it for a longer time than prescribed.
Helpful Hints	The sublingual tablets should not be chewed or swallowed; instead, dissolve them under your tongue. Do not eat, drink, or smoke while taking them.

No special restrictions on driving, exertion and exercise, sun exposure, or exposure to excessive heat.

POSSIBLE SIDE EFFECTS

Although this list of adverse effects may seem somewhat intimidating, keep in mind that some are quite rare. Of course, should these or any other problems arise while you are on medication, it is always a good idea to consult your doctor.

IF YOU DEVELOP

nausea or vomiting ■ stomach cramps ■ loss of appetite ■ dizziness or light-headedness, especially when getting up from a reclining or sitting position ■ drowsiness ■ slow pulse ■ blurred vision ■ headache ■ flushing ■ stuffy nose ■ runny nose ■ rash

With sublingual tablets: soreness under the tongue

WHAT TO DO

If symptoms are disturbing or persist, let your doctor know.

STORAGE INSTRUCTIONS

Store in a cool, dark place (not in a bathroom medicine cabinet). If your medicine is in a liquid form, make sure that it does not freeze.

STOPPING OR INTERRUPTING THERAPY

Some people do not show improvement with this medicine; let your doctor know if your symptoms have not improved after several weeks. If you miss a dose, take it as soon as possible. If it is almost time for your next dose, skip the missed dose and resume your regular schedule. Do not take two doses at the same time.

SPECIAL CONSIDERATIONS FOR THOSE OVER SIXTY-FIVE

None.

CONDITION: **MEMORY DISORDERS, ALZHEIMER'S DISEASE, AND VASCULAR DEMENTIA**

CATEGORY: **CEREBRAL VASODILATORS**

GENERIC (CHEMICAL) NAME	BRAND (TRADE) NAME	DOSAGE FORMS AND STRENGTHS
Isoxsuprine hydrochloride	VASODILAN	Tablets: 10, 20 mg

DRUG PROFILE

Isoxsuprine is prescribed for problems that are caused by poor circulation of blood to the head (cerebral vascular insufficiency) and to the extremities, such as the tip of the nose (Buerger's disease, Raynaud's syndrome). It is also prescribed for arteriosclerosis obliterans, a condition in which some of the arteries in the body narrow so much that blood cannot pass through them. The Food and Drug Administration has ruled that this drug lacks substantial evidence of effectiveness. You should discuss with your doctor why you are being treated with it and what you can expect from therapy with this drug.

BEFORE USING THIS DRUG

Let your doctor know *IF*

You have ever had allergic reactions or other problems with ∎ isoxsuprine.

You have ever had any of the following medical problems: ∎ hardening of the arteries ∎ recent heart attack or stroke ∎ angina (chest pain) ∎ bleeding problems ∎ glaucoma.

SPECIAL RESTRICTIONS WHILE TAKING THIS DRUG

FOOD AND DRUG INTERACTIONS

Other Drugs	Do not take any other drugs, including over-the-counter (OTC) drugs, before checking with your doctor.

Smoking	Smoking may reduce the beneficial effects of this drug. Let your doctor know if you smoke.

No special restrictions on foods and beverages or alcohol use.

DAILY LIVING

Driving	This drug may cause dizziness or light-headedness. Be careful when driving, operating household appliances, or doing any other tasks that require alertness until you know how this drug affects you.
Examinations or Tests	It is important for you to keep all appointments with your doctor so that your progress can be checked.
Helpful Hints	If this drug upsets your stomach, taking it with meals, milk, snacks, or an antacid should help. Dizziness or light-headedness may occur, especially when you get up from a reclining or sitting position. Getting up slowly may help prevent this.

No special restrictions on exertion and exercise, sun exposure, or exposure to excessive heat or cold.

POSSIBLE SIDE EFFECTS

Although this list of adverse effects may seem somewhat intimidating, keep in mind that some are quite rare. Of course, should these or any other problems arise while you are on medication, it is always a good idea to consult your doctor.

IF YOU DEVELOP	**WHAT TO DO**
chest pain ■ irregular or fast heartbeat	**Urgent** Get in touch with your doctor immediately.

rash ■ dizziness or fainting, especially when getting up from a reclining or sitting position ■ tremors ■ nervousness ■ weakness ■ flushing	**May be serious** Check with your doctor as soon as possible.
nausea or vomiting ■ stomach discomfort	If symptoms are disturbing or persist, let your doctor know.

STORAGE INSTRUCTIONS

Store in a cool, dark place (not in a bathroom medicine cabinet).

STOPPING OR INTERRUPTING THERAPY

If you miss a dose of this medicine, take it as soon as possible. If it is almost time for your next dose, skip the missed dose and resume your regular schedule. Do not take two doses at the same time.

SPECIAL CONSIDERATIONS FOR THOSE OVER SIXTY-FIVE

None.

CONDITION: **MEMORY DISORDERS, ALZHEIMER'S DISEASE, AND VASCULAR DEMENTIA**

CATEGORY: **CEREBRAL VASODILATORS**

GENERIC (CHEMICAL) NAME	BRAND (TRADE) NAME	DOSAGE FORMS AND STRENGTHS
Papaverine hydrochloride	PAVABID	Controlled-release capsules: 150 mg
	PAVABID HP	Tablets: 300 mg

DRUG PROFILE

Papaverine is used to treat conditions that are caused by poor circulation of blood to the head (cerebral vascular insufficiency), limbs (peripheral vascular insufficiency), and heart (angina). This drug works by relaxing and enlarging the blood vessels. The Food and Drug Administration has ruled that this drug lacks substantial evidence of effectiveness. You should discuss with your doctor why you are being treated with it and what you can expect from therapy with this drug.

BEFORE USING THIS DRUG

Let your doctor know *IF*

You have ever had allergic reactions or other problems with ■ papaverine.

You have ever had any of the following medical problems: ■ angina (chest pain) ■ heart or blood vessel disease, including recent heart attack or stroke ■ glaucoma.

You are taking any of the following medicines: ■ levodopa (medicine for Parkinson's disease) ■ narcotics or other prescription pain-killers ■ sleep medicines ■ medicine for seizures.

SPECIAL INSTRUCTIONS WHILE TAKING THIS DRUG

FOOD AND DRUG INTERACTIONS

Other Drugs	Do not take any other drugs, including over-the-counter (OTC) drugs, before checking with your doctor.
Alcohol	The action of this medicine may be affected by alcohol. Avoid alcohol unless your doctor has approved its use.
Smoking	Smoking may reduce the beneficial effects of this drug. Let your doctor know if you smoke.

No special restrictions on foods and beverages.

DAILY LIVING

Driving	This drug may cause dizziness or light-headedness. Be careful when driving, operating household appliances, or doing any other tasks that require alertness until you know how this drug affects you.
Examinations or Tests	It is important for you to keep all appointments with your doctor so that your progress can be checked.
Helpful Hints	If this drug upsets your stomach, taking it with meals, milk, snacks, or antacids should help.
	Do not crush or chew the capsules; instead, swallow them whole. If the capsule is too large for you, you can mix the contents with a spoonful of jam and swallow it without chewing.
	If your mouth or throat feels dry, chewing sugarless gum or sucking ice chips or sugarless hard candy will help.

No special restrictions on exertion or exercise, sun exposure, or exposure to excessive heat or cold.

POSSIBLE SIDE EFFECTS

Although this list of adverse effects may seem somewhat intimidating, keep in mind that some are quite rare. Of course, should these or any other problems arise while you are on medication, it is always a good idea to consult your doctor.

IF YOU DEVELOP	WHAT TO DO
blurred or double vision ■ drowsiness ■ weakness ■ rash or itching ■ depression ■ yellowing of eyes or skin	**May be serious** Check with your doctor as soon as possible.
deep breathing ■ dizziness, especially when getting up from a reclining or sitting position ■ headache ■ nausea or vomiting ■ loss of appetite ■ constipation ■ diarrhea ■ stomach discomfort ■ general ill feeling ■ flushing ■ increased sweating ■ dry mouth or throat	If symptoms are disturbing or persist, let your doctor know.

STORAGE INSTRUCTIONS

Store in a cool, dark place (not in a bathroom medicine cabinet).

STOPPING OR INTERRUPTING THERAPY

This medicine may take a while to produce noticeable results. Do not stop taking it, even if you see no difference in your condition, without consulting your doctor. If you miss a dose, take it as soon as possible. If it is almost time for your next dose, skip the missed dose and resume your regular schedule. Do not take two doses at the same time.

SPECIAL CONSIDERATIONS FOR THOSE OVER SIXTY-FIVE

None.

DIZZINESS/VERTIGO

Nearly everyone has experienced dizziness or vertigo at some point in their lives. The sensation of vertigo is an uncomfortable one—the feeling that you are spinning or that the room is whirling around you, or that you are about to fall down. At the same time, you might become nauseated or even vomit.

An attack of vertigo can last for only a few seconds or go on for hours. It can affect people at any age and for many reasons. Finding and treating the cause in older people can be particularly difficult if other medical problems are present.

CAUSES

You may have heard that your sense of balance, or equilibrium, is maintained by structures in your inner ear in an area behind your eardrum. Therefore, a disease or disturbance in your inner ear could be the reason for your vertigo. This is thought to be what happens in people who suffer from motion sickness—the swaying of the vehicle disrupts the equilibrium center of the inner ear, causing the sensation of dizziness.

But other organs and systems also play a part. For instance, you may feel dizzy if you cannot see clearly, or if things are moving too fast for your eyes to keep up with them. Glaucoma, in which there is too much pressure inside the eye, can cause dizziness too. (See pages 976–977 for a detailed discussion of glaucoma.)

You may also feel dizzy if you have low blood pressure or if your heart is not pumping enough blood to your brain. Your body normally sends messages to your brain about balance and position; dizziness can occur when arthritis or a neck injury causes pressure on the nerves that transmit those messages or when certain diseases damage the nerves.

DIAGNOSIS

To help determine the underlying reason for your vertigo, your doctor will ask you when your dizzy spells occur, what seems to bring them on, how long they last, and what other symptoms accompany them. A thorough medical history may also provide a clue to your problem. You may wonder about questions regarding your consumption of coffee, aspirin, alcohol, and cigarettes. The reason for such questions is that all of these ordinary things can cause dizziness.

Dizziness is sometimes caused by a sudden drop in blood pressure, which often happens in older people when they stand up. Therefore, your doctor will probably check your pressure when you are lying down, when you sit up, and again when you stand. At the same time, the doctor will be checking your pulse to see whether your heart rate changes the way it should as you move.

The way your eyes move when you get dizzy can also suggest some causes, so your doctor might observe your eyes as you turn your head sharply from side to side. You may be asked to walk in heel-to-toe fashion, with your eyes open and with your eyes closed, as another part of the exam.

After all this activity, you may be referred to a specialist for further evaluation, or the source of your problem may be apparent and quite simply managed. For example, you might have a buildup of wax in your outer ear, which is pressing against your eardrum and causing problems in your inner ear. Or the cause of the vertigo could be an infection that is treatable with antibiotics.

If your dizzy spells only occur when you move your head—and nothing else seems to be wrong with you—your doctor might say you have "benign positional vertigo." This is a temporary condition that will eventually go away by itself without causing any damage. It is the most frequent cause of dizziness in adults.

TREATMENT

For some people, just knowing that the vertigo is not a sign of a serious problem is enough to make the epi-sodes bearable. Others may need drugs to relieve their symptoms. If you fall into this category, your doctor may prescribe certain antihistamines, described in detail in the drug charts on pages 294–296, to control the nausea, vomiting, and dizziness caused by a benign disturbance in the inner ear.

If your doctor finds that your vertigo is caused by a problem of the heart or circulatory system, a reaction to other medicine, or a visual or neurological disturbance, treatment will focus on the underlying problem.

OUTLOOK

Vertigo is a serious symptom and should be paid attention to. However, that whirling, giddy, or unsteady feeling does not have to keep you from enjoying life. Even if the medical evaluation of your vertigo takes time—and perhaps visits to more than one doctor—quick symptomatic relief might be available through prescription medicine. Then, with correct diagnosis and treatment of the underlying problem, you may find that you can once again get on with your daily activities.

CONDITION: **VERTIGO**

CATEGORY: **ANTIHISTAMINES**

GENERIC (CHEMICAL) NAME	BRAND (TRADE) NAME	DOSAGE FORMS AND STRENGTHS
Meclizine hydrochloride	ANTIVERT	Chewable tablets: 25 mg Tablets: 12.5, 25, 50 mg

DRUG PROFILE

Meclizine, which belongs to the category of drugs called antihistamines, is used to prevent the nausea, vomiting, and dizziness that are associated with motion sickness. This medicine also is used to treat dizziness resulting from inner-ear disturbances. Meclizine works by reducing the sensitivity of the nerves in the inner ear that control balance; it also blocks the nerve pathways to the part of the brain that controls vomiting.

BEFORE USING THIS DRUG

Let your doctor know *IF*

You have ever had allergic reactions or other problems with ■ meclizine ■ other antihistamines.

You have ever had any of the following medical problems: ■ asthma or other lung disease ■ enlarged prostate ■ urinary problems, including difficulty in urination ■ glaucoma ■ epilepsy or other seizure disorders ■ intestinal blockage ■ stomach ulcer.

You are taking any of the following medicines: ■ medicine for nausea ■ antihistamines ■ medicine for Parkinson's disease ■ tranquilizers ■ medicine for depression ■ cimetidine or ranitidine (medicine for ulcers) ■ medicine for stomach pain or cramps ■ medicine for spasmodic conditions of the digestive or urinary tract ■ medicine for asthma or bronchitis.

SPECIAL RESTRICTIONS WHILE TAKING THIS DRUG

FOOD AND DRUG INTERACTIONS

Other Drugs	Do not take any other drugs, including over-the-counter (OTC) drugs, before checking with your doctor. This drug increases the effects of drugs that depress the central nervous system—such as antihistamines; medicine for hay fever, allergies, or colds; sleep medicines; tranquilizers; medicine for depression; narcotics or other prescription painkillers; muscle relaxants; and medicine for seizures. This drug may mask ringing in the ears caused by aspirin. Let your doctor know if you are taking aspirin or aspirinlike medicine.
Alcohol	Drinking alcohol while taking this medicine may increase the risk of such side effects as dizziness, light-headedness, or drowsiness. Avoid alcohol unless your doctor has approved its use.

No special restrictions on foods and beverages or smoking.

DAILY LIVING

Driving	This drug may cause drowsiness or blurred vision. Be careful when driving, operating household appliances, or doing any other tasks that require alertness until you know how this drug affects you.
Other Precautions	Because this drug controls nausea and vomiting, it can mask some of the symptoms of appendicitis. If you develop sharp pains in your stomach or lower abdomen, be sure to let your doctor know at once.
	If you are going to be tested for allergies, let the doctor in charge know that you are taking this drug, since it affects the results of allergy tests.

Helpful Hints

If this drug upsets your stomach, taking it with meals, milk, snacks, or water should help.

If your mouth or throat feels dry, chewing sugarless gum or sucking ice chips or sugarless hard candy will help.

No special restrictions on exertion and exercise, sun exposure, or exposure to excessive heat or cold.

POSSIBLE SIDE EFFECTS

Although this list of adverse effects may seem somewhat intimidating, keep in mind that some are quite rare. Of course, should these or any other problems arise while you are on medication, it is always a good idea to consult your doctor.

IF YOU DEVELOP

drowsiness ■ tiredness ■ irregular or fast heartbeat ■ headache ■ blurred vision ■ nervousness or restlessness ■ sleep disturbances ■ loss of appetite ■ upset stomach ■ dry mouth, nose, or throat ■ pain or difficulty in urination ■ rash

WHAT TO DO

If symptoms are disturbing or persist, let your doctor know.

STORAGE INSTRUCTIONS

Store in a cool, dark place (not in a bathroom medicine cabinet).

STOPPING OR INTERRUPTING THERAPY

If you are taking this medicine regularly and you miss a dose, take it as soon as possible. If it is almost time for your next dose, skip the missed dose and resume your regular schedule. Do not take two doses at the same time.

SPECIAL CONSIDERATIONS FOR THOSE OVER SIXTY-FIVE

None.

PARKINSON'S DISEASE

Parkinson's disease occurs in one out of every one hundred individuals over the age of sixty-five. It begins so gradually and its early symptoms are so mild that many people do not even suspect they have it. They might just feel more tired than usual or notice a slight, occasional tremor in a finger, which may gradually affect the hand and arm as well. Or the first sign might be stiffness of a hand or leg, a slouching posture, or difficulty in rising from a chair. A family member or friend might be the first to observe that the person is slowing down, limping a little, or talking in a monotonous tone of voice.

Eventually almost all patients will experience the three major features of Parkinson's disease: tremor, rigidity, and akinesia. Tremor is a continual shaking of the limbs and may be an upsetting symptom to patients because it is very visible. Rigidity is a stiffness of the muscles and may lead to postural deformities of the body or the limbs. Akinesia is a slowness in carrying out ordinary movements such as eating, bathing, and dressing. Akinesia may be the most disabling feature of Parkinson's disease.

CAUSES

The causes of Parkinson's disease are not known; however, at the root of the disease is a deficiency of dopamine, which is an important chemical messenger in the brain and nervous system. Not enough dopamine means a slowdown in the transmission of messages from the nerve cells in the brain to the nerve cells in the muscles of the arms, legs, and face. Therefore, a person with Parkinson's disease cannot always control his or her movements.

EXERCISE, PHYSICAL THERAPY, AND COPING

Keeping active is especially important for people with Parkinson's disease, to keep already rigid muscles in the arms and legs from growing stiffer. Your doctor may recommend stretching exercises to keep your muscles flexible as well as exercises to improve your balance. If your symptoms are interfering with your daily routine, your doctor may refer you to a physical therapist for help in planning strategies for overcoming these practical problems. Some helpful tips are outlined below.

Walking
• Wear leather-soled shoes rather than rubber or crepe soles, which grip the floor and can cause you to fall forward.
• Try consciously to take steps as large as possible, raising your toes up when you step forward and hitting the ground on your heel.
• Keep your feet nine to fifteen inches apart and your posture straight, arms swinging at your sides. Practice swinging your right arm with your

left leg and your left arm with your right leg.

• Look straight ahead, not at the floor.

• In cases of "freezing," relax back on your heels, toes raised. To start moving again, tap the leg that you want to move or shift your weight from side to side in a rocking motion.

Getting in or out of a Chair

• To sit down, approach slowly with your back to the chair. When you reach the chair, bend forward and sit down slowly.

• To get up, put your feet under the chair, if possible. Rock forward once or twice in preparation; then bend forward and push up vigorously with your arms.

• If your favorite chair is too soft and too low to the floor, raise the back legs with blocks.

• If you need assistance in getting up, ask someone to help by pushing you from the back, not pulling you up by the arms. Sometimes, a slight touch is all that is necessary.

Getting out of Bed

• Rock into a sitting position by placing your arms over your head and swinging them forward and moving your legs toward the side of the bed. If you need further assistance, tie a knotted rope to the foot of the bed for use in pulling yourself up. You may want to raise the head of the bed by placing blocks under the legs.

Getting Dressed

• Avoid clothes that fasten up the back or have very small buttons.

• Practice buttoning and unbuttoning garments while watching television or listening to the radio. Another exercise to help straighten stiff fingers is to bounce a large ball with your open hand. Toss the ball against a wall or to another person.

• For help in putting on shoes, use a shoehorn. If your shoes have laces, try elastic or extra-long laces, or avoid laces entirely by wearing loafers or sneakers that have a Velcro closing.

TREATMENT

Although Parkinson's disease cannot be cured, medication can dramatically relieve the symptoms, often for years. The most important drug used to treat parkinsonism is levodopa (see chart on pages 300–304), which improves the supply of dopamine in the brain. Sometimes doctors also prescribe other drugs to boost the effectiveness of levodopa or as alternatives if levodopa's effectiveness seems to be wearing off (see charts on pages 304–321 for more details on these drugs).

OUTLOOK

Exercising, continuing your normal daily activities, and thinking positively are especially important for people with parkinsonism. Although you'll probably have to make some changes in your life to cope with the symptoms, most likely you'll be able to continue your usual activities. Hobbies that involve the use of the fingers (such as sewing or playing cards) are particularly useful to keep the hands

and fingers from stiffening. Your doctor can help you make other decisions about adapting to parkinsonism, such as whether you should continue driving a car. Good sources of information and support include the following:
• The American Parkinson's Disease Association, 116 John Street, New York, NY 10038, (212) 732-9550
• The Parkinson's Disease Foundation, Columbia-Presbyterian Medical Center, 640 West 168th Street, New York, NY 10032, (212) 923-4700

• The National Parkinson's Foundation, 111 Park Place, New York, NY 10007, (212) 374-1741 and 1501 Northwest Ninth Avenue, Miami, FL 33136, (800) 327-4545

• The United Parkinson's Foundation, 220 South State Street, Chicago, IL 60604, (312) 922-9734

• PEP-USA (Parkinson's Educational Program), 1800 Park Newport, #302, Newport Beach, CA 92660, (714) 640-0218

CONDITION: **PARKINSON'S DISEASE**

CATEGORY: **ANTIPARKINSON AGENTS**

GENERIC (CHEMICAL) NAME	BRAND (TRADE) NAME	DOSAGE FORMS AND STRENGTHS
Levodopa	DOPAR	Capsules: 100, 250, 500 mg
	LARODOPA	Capsules: 100, 250, 500 mg
		Tablets: 100, 250, 500 mg
Levodopa and carbidopa	SINEMET	Tablets: 10 mg carbidopa and 100 mg levodopa; 25 mg carbidopa and 100 mg levodopa; 25 mg carbidopa and 250 mg levodopa
	SINEMET CR	Tablets: 50 mg carbidopa and 200 mg levodopa

DRUG PROFILE

Levodopa or the combination of levodopa and carbidopa helps to improve muscle control in Parkinson's disease. Many experts think that the rigidity, shaking, and difficulty initiating movement characteristic of Parkinson's disease result from a deficiency of a chemical called dopamine in the brain. Levodopa is converted to dopamine in the brain, thereby helping restore the chemical balance that regulates the nervous system. Carbidopa helps more levodopa reach the brain.

BEFORE USING THIS DRUG

Let your doctor know *IF*

You have ever had allergic reactions or other problems with levodopa ■ the combination of levodopa and carbidopa ■ aspirin.

With Dopar only: ■ tartrazine (FD&C Yellow Dye No. 5).

You have ever had any of the following medical problems: ■ epilepsy or other seizure disorders ■ diabetes ■ asthma or other lung disease ■ glaucoma ■ heart or blood vessel disease ■ abnormal heart rhythms ■ hormone disturbances ■ kidney disease ■ liver disease ■ mental illness ■ skin cancer ■ stomach ulcer.

You are taking any of the following medicines: ■ other medicine for Parkinson's disease ■ amantadine ■ antacids ■ amphetamines ■ phenytoin (medicine for seizures) ■ medicine for high blood pressure ■ medicine for stomach pain or cramps ■ medicine for spasmodic conditions of the digestive or urinary tract ■ appetite suppressants ■ medicine for asthma or bronchitis ■ vitamin B_6 ■ tranquilizers ■ sinus medicines ■ antihistamines ■ medicine for nausea ■ medicine for depression (within the last two weeks) ■ muscle relaxants ■ sleep medicines ■ furazolidone (antibiotic) ■ papaverine (medicine for poor blood circulation) ■ methyldopa or clonidine (medicine for high blood pressure).

SPECIAL RESTRICTIONS WHILE TAKDING THIS DRUG

FOOD AND DRUG INTERACTIONS

Other Drugs	Vitamin B reduces the effects of levodopa (this does not occur with the combination of levodopa and carbidopa). If you are taking levodopa alone, do not take any vitamin supplement containing B_6 unless prescribed by your doctor.
Foods and Beverages	If you are taking levodopa alone, see the above warning regarding vitamin B_6. Foods with a high vitamin B_6 content, such as bacon, beef liver, pork, beans, peas, tuna, oatmeal, and avocados, should be eaten only in limited quantities. A diet too rich in protein may reduce the effectiveness of this medicine. You should limit your intake of meat, milk, cheese, and other high protein foods during the day. The recommended daily allowance of protein should be eaten at dinner or at an evening snack to decrease the interaction between protein and this medicine.

No special restrictions on alcohol use or smoking.

DAILY LIVING

Driving	This drug may cause drowsiness or loss of alertness. Be careful when driving, operating household appliances, or doing any other tasks that require alertness until you know how this drug affects you.
Exertion and Exercise	As your symptoms improve, be sure not to overdo physical activity. Let yourself gradually get used to your improving balance and coordination.
Examinations or Tests	It is important for you to keep all appointments with your doctor, even if your symptoms improve, so that your progress can be checked. Periodic blood and urine tests may be required.
Other Precautions	If you have diabetes, you may find that this medicine affects the results of urine tests for ketones or sugar; ask your doctor what kind of tests you should use.
	Tell any doctor or dentist you consult that you are taking this medicine, especially if you will be undergoing any type of surgery.
Helpful Hints	If this drug upsets your stomach, taking it with food should help.
	Dizziness or light-headedness may occur, especially when getting up from a reclining or sitting position. Getting up slowly may help prevent this.

No special restrictions on sun exposure or exposure to excessive heat or cold.

POSSIBLE SIDE EFFECTS

Although this list of adverse effects may seem somewhat intimidating, keep in mind that some are quite rare. Of course, should these or any other problems arise while you are on medication, it is always a good idea to consult your doctor.

IF YOU DEVELOP

breathing changes ■ hoarseness ■ blurred or double vision ■ changes in pupil size ■ spasm or closing of eyelids or any other eye problems ■ tiredness or weakness ■ unusual, uncontrollable movements of the body ■ clumsiness ■ disturbances in walking ■ slowing of movement ■ increased hand tremors ■ irregular heartbeat ■ dizziness or lightheadedness, especially when getting up from a reclining or sitting position ■ difficulty in urination ■ nausea or vomiting ■ stomach pain ■ hallucinations ■ delusions ■ agitation ■ paranoia (unreasonable fears) ■ depression

WHAT TO DO

May be serious Check with your doctor as soon as possible.

runny nose ■ anxiety, confusion, or nervousness ■ inability to concentrate ■ memory problems ■ restlessness ■ drowsiness ■ general ill feeling ■ headache ■ sleeplessness ■ nightmares ■ increased sweating ■ urinary frequency or incontinence ■ numbness ■ rash ■ hot flashes ■ vaginal bleeding ■ weight gain or loss ■ painful or persistent male erection ■ pain or swelling of hands or feet ■ hair loss ■ grinding of teeth ■ constipation ■ diarrhea ■ dark urine or sweat ■ dry mouth ■ loss of appetite ■ flushing ■ muscle twitching ■ gas ■ hiccups ■ bitter taste or taste changes ■ difficulty in swallowing ■ burning feeling in tongue ■ difficulty in opening mouth

If symptoms are disturbing or persist, let your doctor know.

STORAGE INSTRUCTIONS

Store in a cool, dark place (not in a bathroom medicine cabinet).

STOPPING OR INTERRUPTING THERAPY

Take this medicine exactly as directed by your doctor; do not stop taking it, even if your symptoms have not improved. In some people, it takes several weeks or even months before effects of this medicine are seen. If you miss a dose, take it as soon as possible. If it is within two hours of your next dose, skip the missed dose and resume your regular schedule. Do not take two doses at the same time.

When this medicine is suddenly stopped or the dose reduced there is the possibility of a serious reaction. If you abruptly stop taking this medicine or if your dose is reduced, notify your doctor if you develop any unusual symptoms such as muscle rigidity, fever, or mental changes.

SPECIAL CONSIDERATIONS FOR THOSE OVER SIXTY-FIVE

Older people may be especially sensitive to the side effects of this medicine. For those who have osteoporosis, it is particularly important not to overdo physical activity and to take special care to avoid falling.

CONDITION: **PARKINSON'S DISEASE**

CATEGORY: **ANTIPARKINSON AGENTS**

GENERIC (CHEMICAL) NAME	BRAND (TRADE) NAME	DOSAGE FORMS AND STRENGTHS
Selegiline hydrochloride	ELDEPRYL	Tablets: 5 mg

DRUG PROFILE

Selegiline, a drug which belongs to the MAO inhibitor group, is usually given in combination with levodopa/carbidopa to help improve the symptoms of Parkinson's disease. The rigidity, tremor, and difficulty initiating movement characteristic of Parkinson's disease results from a deficiency of a chemical called dopamine in the brain. Levodopa converts to dopamine in the brain, and selegiline is thought to prevent the natural breakdown process of the dopamine, thereby ensuring adequate levels and restoring the chemical balance that regulates the nervous system. (See levodopa, levodopa and carbidopa.)

BEFORE USING THIS DRUG

Let your doctor know *IF*

You have ever had allergic reactions or other problems with ■ selegiline, tranylcypromine, isocarboxazid, phenelzine sulfate, or any other MAO inhibitor drug ■ pargyline hydrochloride (medicine for high blood pressure).

You have ever had any of the following medical problems: ■ drug abuse, including alcohol and cocaine ■ heart disease, including angina (chest pain), coronary artery disease, and heart attack ■ diabetes ■ seizures ■ severe or frequent headaches ■ high blood pressure ■ kidney disease ■ liver disease ■ mental illness ■ overactive thyroid ■ stroke ■ glaucoma ■ pheochromocytoma (adrenal gland tumor) ■ asthma or other lung disease ■ anemia ■ angioneurotic edema (accumulation of excess fluid under the skin, often associated with hives, redness, or purplish or brownish-red spots).

You are taking any of the following medicines: ■ medicine for depression (within the past two weeks) ■ medicine for diabetes ■ medicine for high blood pressure ■ medicine for asthma ■ diuretics (water pills) ■ other medicine for Parkinson's disease ■ medicine for seizures ■ barbiturates ■ muscle relaxants ■ antihistamines ■ medicine for hay fever, coughs, or colds ■ appetite suppressants ■ narcotics or other prescription pain-killers ■ sleep medicines ■ any medicine containing alcohol ■ any medicine containing caffeine ■ amphetamines ■ methylphenidate (medicine for narcolepsy) ■ Antabuse (used in treatment of alcoholism) ■ tranquilizers.

SPECIAL RESTRICTIONS WHILE TAKING THIS DRUG

FOOD AND DRUG INTERACTIONS

Other Drugs	Your doctor may need to change your dosage of levodopa/carbidopa while you are taking selegiline; it is important to take each drug in the exact amount prescribed.
	Do not take any other drugs, including over-the-counter (OTC) drugs, before checking with your doctor. OTC drugs that may interact adversely with this drug include those used for colds, coughs, hay fever, and appetite suppression, as well as drugs containing caffeine.

Foods and Beverages	The combination of MAO inhibitors and foods or beverages that contain caffeine or the chemicals tyramine or tryptophan can result in serious problems. Foods to avoid include cheese (Cheddar, Camembert, Stilton, or processed cheese), sour cream, yogurt, liver (especially chicken liver), pickled herring, canned figs, raisins, bananas, avocados, soy sauce, meat tenderizers, fava beans, cured meats (eg, bologna, sausage, and salami) and yeast or meat extracts. Also, avoid large quantities of cocoa, coffee, tea, and cola beverages. Ask your doctor to provide you with a full list of foods to avoid; also, let your doctor know if you are on any special kind of diet. Continue to avoid the above foods and beverages for two weeks after stopping therapy with selegiline.
Alcohol	Avoid alcohol while taking this drug; the combination can cause serious reactions. Beer and Chianti wine are especially dangerous.

No special restrictions on smoking.

DAILY LIVING

Driving	This drug may cause drowsiness or loss of alertness. Be careful when driving, operating household appliances, or doing any other tasks that require alertness until you know how this drug affects you.
Examinations or Tests	It is important for you to keep all appointments with your doctor so that your progress can be checked.

Other Precautions	Tell any doctor or dentist you consult that you are taking this medicine, especially if you will be undergoing any type of surgery.

Helpful Hints	Dizziness or light-headedness may occur, especially when getting up from a reclining or sitting position. Getting up slowly may help prevent this.
	Also, take this drug with meals to prevent any gastrointestinal distress.
	Keep taking your medicine even if you do not at first notice any improvements.

No special restrictions on sun exposure, exertion and exercise, or exposure to excessive heat or cold.

POSSIBLE SIDE EFFECTS

Although this list of adverse effects may seem somewhat intimidating, keep in mind that some are quite rare. Of course, should these or any other problems arise while you are on medication, it is always a good idea to consult your doctor.

IF YOU DEVELOP

severe headache ■ stiff neck ■ chest pain ■ irregular, slow, or fast heartbeat ■ nausea or vomiting ■ abdominal pain ■ chills or fever ■ difficulty in breathing ■ confusion ■ hallucinations ■ body spasms ■ excessive sweating with clammy skin ■ increased sensitivity to light ■ enlarged pupils ■ severe dizziness, light-headedness, or fainting ■ seizures ■ severe anxiety ■ hyperactivity ■ agitation ■ jaw spasms or difficulty in opening mouth ■ muscle stiffness ■ slow reflexes ■ arching of torso ■ drowsiness

WHAT TO DO

Urgent Get in touch with your doctor immediately.

pounding heartbeat ■ swelling of hands, feet, or lower legs ■ rash ■ diarrhea ■ blurred or double vision ■ spasm or closing of eyelid or any other eye problems ■ tiredness ■ weakness ■ unusual, uncontrollable movements of the body ■ disturbances in walking ■ slowing of movement ■ increased hand tremor ■ delusions ■ anxiety ■ depression ■ nightmares ■ vivid dreams ■ severe insomnia ■ personality changes ■ unusual irritability

May be serious Check with your doctor as soon as possible.

constipation ■ difficulty in urinating ■ frequent urination ■ urinating at night ■ dizziness or light-headedness especially when getting up from a reclining or sitting position ■ dry mouth ■ restlessness ■ sleep disturbance ■ sexual problems ■ loss of appetite ■ weight loss ■ difficulty swallowing ■ heartburn ■ grinding of teeth ■ memory problems ■ general ill feeling ■ purplish or brownish-red spots

If symptoms are disturbing or persist, let your doctor know.

STORAGE INSTRUCTIONS

Store in a cool, dark place (not in a bathroom medicine cabinet).

STOPPING OR INTERRUPTING THERAPY

Take this medicine exactly as directed by your doctor. If you miss a dose wait until your next scheduled dose and then resume your regular dosage schedule.

SPECIAL CONSIDERATIONS FOR THOSE OVER SIXTY-FIVE

None.

CONDITION: **PARKINSON'S DISEASE**

CATEGORY: **ANTIPARKINSON AGENTS**

GENERIC (CHEMICAL) NAME	BRAND (TRADE) NAME	DOSAGE FORMS AND STRENGTHS
Amantadine hydrochloride	SYMMETREL	Capsules: 100 mg Syrup: 50 mg per tsp

DRUG PROFILE

Amantadine is used to treat Parkinson's disease and other movement disorders. Many experts think that the rigidity, shaking, and walking disturbances associated with these conditions result from a deficiency of a chemical called dopamine in the brain. Amantadine makes more dopamine available to the brain, thereby helping restore the chemical balance that regulates the nervous system. This drug is sometimes used along with levodopa or other medicine for Parkinson's disease.

BEFORE USING THIS DRUG

Let your doctor know *IF*

You have ever had allergic reactions or other problems with ■ amantadine.

You have ever had any of the following medical problems: ■ heart disease, including congestive heart failure ■ circulation problems ■ blood vessel disease of the brain ■ low blood pressure ■ swelling of feet or ankles ■ epilepsy or other seizure disorders ■ mental illness ■ kidney disease ■ liver disease ■ stomach or intestinal ulcers ■ recurring eczema.

You are taking any of the following medicines: ■ carbidopa and/or levodopa (other medicine for Parkinson's disease) ■ amphetamines ■ diet pills ■ medicine for depression ■ tranquilizers ■ medicine for nausea ■ sleep medicines ■ antihistamines ■ medicine for asthma, hay fever, allergies, or breathing problems ■ cough medicine ■ sinus medicine ■ medicine for diarrhea ■ medicine for stomach spasms or cramps ■ medicine for narcolepsy.

SPECIAL RESTRICTIONS WHILE TAKING THIS DRUG

FOOD AND DRUG INTERACTIONS

Other Drugs	Do not take any other drugs, including over-the-counter (OTC) drugs, before checking with your doctor. OTC drugs for appetite suppression, asthma, colds, cough, hay fever, or sinus problems should be avoided since these products can aggravate the stimulant effects of amantadine.
Alcohol	Drinking alcohol while taking this medicine may increase the risk of such side effects as dizziness, light-headedness, fainting, confusion, and circulation problems. Avoid alcohol unless your doctor has approved its use.

No special restrictions on foods and beverages or smoking.

DAILY LIVING

Driving	This drug may cause dizziness, light-headedness, or fainting. Be careful when driving, operating household appliances, or doing any other tasks that require alertness until you know how this drug affects you.
Exertion and Exercise	As your symptoms improve, be sure not to overdo physical activity. Let yourself gradually get used to your improving balance and coordination.
Examinations or Tests	It is important for you to keep all appointments with your doctor, even if your symptoms improve, so that your progress and reactions to this medicine can be checked.

Helpful Hints	If you have been taking this medicine for a while and feel that it is not working as well as it has in the past, let your doctor know.
	If your mouth or throat feels dry, chewing sugarless gum or sucking ice chips or sugarless hard candy will help.
	Dizziness or light-headedness may occur, especially when you get up from a reclining or sitting position. Getting up slowly may help prevent this.

No special restrictions on sun exposure or exposure to excessive heat or cold.

POSSIBLE SIDE EFFECTS

Although this list of adverse effects may seem somewhat intimidating, keep in mind that some are quite rare. Of course, should these or any other problems arise while you are on medication, it is always a good idea to consult your doctor.

IF YOU DEVELOP

confusion ■ hallucinations ■ slurred speech ■ fainting ■ difficulty in urination ■ sore throat or fever ■ depression ■ shakiness ■ clumsiness ■ uncontrollable facial movements ■ eye rolling ■ swelling of feet or lower legs ■ shortness of breath ■ difficulty in breathing ■ rapid weight gain ■ convulsions ■ sleeplessness or other sleep disturbances ■ feeling of drunkenness or detachment

WHAT TO DO

May be serious Check with your doctor as soon as possible.

dizziness or light-headedness, especially when getting up from a reclining or sitting position ■ nervousness ■ drowsiness ■ anxiety ■ inability to concentrate ■ memory problems ■ irritability ■ headache ■ tiredness or weakness ■ loss of appetite ■ nausea or vomiting ■ constipation ■ dry mouth, nose, or throat ■ purplish red, netlike, blotchy spots on skin ■ other rash ■ blurred vision or other visual disturbances ■ increased skin sensitivity to sunlight

If symptoms are disturbing or persist, let your doctor know.

STORAGE INSTRUCTIONS

Store in a cool, dark place (not in a bathroom medicine cabinet). If your medicine is in a liquid form, make sure that it does not freeze.

STOPPING OR INTERRUPTING THERAPY

It may take up to two weeks before you feel the helpful effects of this medicine. Do not stop taking it without consulting your doctor. Stopping this medicine suddenly may seriously worsen your medical condition. If you miss a dose, take it as soon as possible. If it is within four hours of your next scheduled dose, skip the missed dose and resume your regular schedule. Do not take two doses at the same time.

SPECIAL CONSIDERATIONS FOR THOSE OVER SIXTY-FIVE

Older people are more likely to experience such side effects as dizziness, confusion, and difficulty in urination. For those who have osteoporosis, it is particularly important not to overdo physical activity and to take special care to avoid falling.

CONDITION: **PARKINSON'S DISEASE**
CATEGORY: **ANTIPARKINSON AGENTS**

GENERIC (CHEMICAL) NAME	BRAND (TRADE) NAME	DOSAGE FORMS AND STRENGTHS
Benztropine mesylate	COGENTIN	Tablets: 0.5, 1, 2 mg
Biperiden	AKINETON	Tablets: 2 mg
Procyclidine	KEMADRIN	Tablets: 5 mg
Trihexyphenidyl hydrochloride	ARTANE	Controlled-release capsules: 5 mg Elixir: 2 mg per tsp Tablets: 2, 5 mg

DRUG PROFILE

These medicines are used to treat Parkinson's disease, as well as other movement disorders. They reduce rigidity, shakiness, and disturbances in walking. These drugs are often used along with levodopa or other medicine for Parkinson's disease.

BEFORE USING THIS DRUG

Let your doctor know *IF*

You have ever had allergic reactions or other problems with ■ benztropine ■ procyclidine ■ biperiden ■ trihexyphenidyl ■ other medicine for Parkinson's disease or movement disorders ■ any other medicine.

You have ever had any of the following medical problems: ■ heart or blood vessel disease, including congestive heart failure, abnormal heart rhythms, hardening of the arteries, or high blood pressure ■ stomach ulcer ■ hiatal hernia ■ esophageal reflux ■ intestinal blockage ■ diarrhea ■ ulcerative colitis or other digestive disorders ■ kidney disease ■ liver disease ■ myasthenia gravis

■ uncontrolled movements of hands, mouth, or tongue ■ difficulty in urination ■ enlarged prostate ■ glaucoma ■ overactive thyroid ■ recent fever ■ bleeding problems ■ mental illness.

You are taking any of the following medicines: ■ other medicine for Parkinson's disease ■ medicine for depression (within the last two weeks) ■ medicine for seizures ■ antihistamines ■ medicine for hay fever, allergies, or colds ■ barbiturates ■ narcotics or other prescription pain-killers ■ sedatives ■ tranquilizers ■ sleep medicines ■ muscle relaxants ■ medicine for stomach spasms or cramps ■ medicine for diarrhea ■ antacids ■ medicine for nausea ■ medicine for abnormal heart rhythms ■ medicine for high blood pressure ■ medicine or vaccine for flu.

SPECIAL RESTRICTIONS WHILE TAKING THIS DRUG

FOOD AND DRUG INTERACTIONS

Other Drugs	Do not take any other drugs, including over-the-counter (OTC) drugs, before checking with your doctor. This medicine increases the effect of drugs that depress the central nervous system—such as antihistamines; medicine for hay fever, allergies, or colds; sleep medicines; tranquilizers; narcotics or other prescription pain-killers; muscle relaxants; medicine for seizures—and worsens such side effects as dizziness, light-headedness, or drowsiness. Do not take antacids or medicine for diarrhea within one hour of taking benztropine, biperiden, procyclidine, or trihexyphenidyl.
Alcohol	Drinking alcohol while taking this medicine may increase the risk of such side effects as dizziness, light-headedness, or drowsiness. Avoid alcohol unless your doctor has approved its use.

No special restrictions on foods and beverages or smoking.

DAILY LIVING

Driving	This drug may cause dizziness, light-headedness, or blurred vision. Be careful when driving, operating household appliances, or doing any other tasks that require alertness until you know how this drug affects you.
Exertion and Exercise	This drug may cause you to sweat less than normally. Sweating is your body's natural way of cooling down, and not sweating enough can be dangerous. Use caution not to become overheated when you exert yourself.
Sun Exposure	Your eyes may become more sensitive to sunlight or other bright light while you are on this medicine. It is a good idea to avoid too much sun exposure. If your eyes become more sensitive to bright light, wearing dark glasses should lessen discomfort.
Excessive Heat	See "Exertion and Exercise"; use caution during hot weather, since overexertion may result in heat stroke. Avoid extremely hot baths or saunas. Also, check with your doctor if you develop a fever for any reason.
Examinations or Tests	It is important for you to keep all appointments with your doctor so that your progress and reactions to this drug can be checked. You may have to have your eyes checked before and during therapy with this medicine.
Other Precautions	Tell any doctor or dentist you consult that you are taking this medicine, especially if you will be undergoing any type of surgery.

Helpful Hints	If your mouth or throat feels dry, chewing sugarless gum or sucking ice chips or sugarless hard candy will help.
	Swallow the controlled-release capsules whole—do not break, crush, or chew them.

No special restrictions on exposure to excessive cold.

POSSIBLE SIDE EFFECTS

Although this list of adverse effects may seem somewhat intimidating, keep in mind that some are quite rare. Of course, should these or any other problems arise while you are on medication, it is always a good idea to consult your doctor.

IF YOU DEVELOP	WHAT TO DO
seizures ■ clumsiness or unsteadiness ■ severe drowsiness ■ severe dryness of mouth, nose, or throat ■ hallucinations ■ delirium ■ mood or mental changes ■ shortness of breath ■ difficulty in breathing ■ sleeplessness ■ irregular or fast heartbeat ■ warm skin or flushing ■ dry skin ■ fever	**Urgent** Get in touch with your doctor immediately.
confusion ■ disorientation ■ agitation ■ personality changes ■ rash ■ blood in urine ■ depression ■ constipation ■ diarrhea ■ nausea or vomiting ■ bloating ■ stomach pain	**May be serious** Check with your doctor as soon as possible.

weakness or inability to move certain muscles ■ blurred vision ■ increased skin sensitivity to sunlight ■ increased eye sensitivity to light ■ pupil changes ■ restlessness ■ dry or sore mouth, nose, or throat ■ decreased sweating ■ pain or difficulty in urination ■ headache ■ dizziness or lightheadedness, especially when getting up from a reclining or sitting position ■ nervousness or excitement ■ muscle cramps ■ numbness or weakness in hands or feet

If symptoms are disturbing or persist, let your doctor know.

STORAGE INSTRUCTIONS

Store in a cool, dark place (not in a bathroom medicine cabinet). If your medicine is in a liquid form, make sure that it does not freeze.

STOPPING OR INTERRUPTING THERAPY

Follow your doctor's instructions carefully on how to take this medicine. Stopping this medicine suddenly may worsen your medical condition. Your doctor will advise you on how to reduce your dosage gradually before stopping completely. If you miss a dose of this medicine, take it as soon as possible. If it is within two hours of your next dose, skip the missed dose and resume your regular schedule. Do not take two doses at the same time.

SPECIAL CONSIDERATIONS FOR THOSE OVER SIXTY-FIVE

Older people may be more susceptible to such side effects as mental changes and confusion, disorientation, agitation, excitement, hallucinations, and difficulty in urination. Thus, doctors may require regular checkups.

CONDITION: **PARKINSON'S DISEASE**

CATEGORY: **ANTIPARKINSON AGENTS**

GENERIC (CHEMICAL) NAME	BRAND (TRADE) NAME	DOSAGE FORMS AND STRENGTHS
Bromocriptine mesylate	PARLODEL	Capsules: 5 mg Tablets: 2.5 mg

DRUG PROFILE

Bromocriptine belongs to a family of drugs called ergot alkaloids. It is used to treat Parkinson's disease and is often given along with levodopa. Many experts think that the rigidity, shakiness, and disturbances in walking associated with Parkinson's disease result from a deficiency of a chemical called dopamine in the brain. Bromocriptine acts like dopamine, thereby helping to restore the regular activity of the nervous system. Bromocriptine may also be used to treat a variety of other medical problems, including tumors of the pituitary gland or pituitary hormone disturbances.

BEFORE USING THIS DRUG

Let your doctor know *IF*

You have ever had allergic reactions or other problems with ■ bromocriptine ■ any other ergot medicines (ergoloid mesylates, ergotamine, or methysergide).

You have ever had any of the following medical problems: ■ heart attack ■ abnormal heart rhythms ■ uncontrolled high blood pressure ■ liver disease ■ kidney disease ■ mental illness ■ low blood pressure ■ migraine headaches.

You are taking any of the following medicines: other medicine for Parkinson's disease ■ diuretics or other medicines for high blood pressure ■ hormones ■ medicine for nausea ■ medicine for depression or other mental illness ■ tranquilizers.

SPECIAL RESTRICTIONS WHILE TAKING THIS DRUG

FOOD AND DRUG INTERACTIONS

Other Drugs	Diuretics and medicine for high blood pressure may increase the risk of such side effects as dizziness and fainting while you are taking this medicine.
Alcohol	This medicine increases the effect of alcohol, a central nervous system depressant. Avoid alcohol unless your doctor has approved its use.

No special restrictions on foods and beverages or smoking.

DAILY LIVING

Driving	This drug may cause dizziness, drowsiness, light-headedness, confusion, faintness, or fainting. Be careful when driving, operating household appliances, or doing any other tasks that require alertness until you know how this drug affects you.
Examinations or Tests	It is important for you to keep all appointments with your doctor so that your progress and reactions to therapy can be checked. Periodic blood and urine tests may be required.
Helpful Hints	If this drug upsets your stomach, taking it with milk, meals, or snacks should help.

No special restrictions on exertion and exercise, sun exposure, or exposure to excessive heat or cold.

POSSIBLE SIDE EFFECTS

Although this list of adverse effects may seem somewhat intimidating, keep in mind that some are quite rare. Of course, should these or any other problems arise while you are on medication, it is always a good idea to consult your doctor.

IF YOU DEVELOP	WHAT TO DO
black, tarry stools ■ vomiting, with blood ■ seizures ■ weakness ■ irregular or fast heartbeat ■ chest pain	**Urgent** Get in touch with your doctor immediately.
dizziness or light-headedness, especially when getting up from a reclining or sitting position ■ fainting ■ confusion ■ behavior changes ■ hallucinations ■ uncontrollable movements of the face, tongue, arms, hands, head, or upper body ■ shortness of breath ■ swollen feet or ankles ■ clumsiness ■ pain, heat, or redness in feet or hands	**May be serious** Check with your doctor as soon as possible.
drowsiness or tiredness ■ headache (including migraine) ■ constipation ■ diarrhea ■ urinary frequency ■ urinary retention or incontinence ■ loss of appetite ■ stomach pain or cramps ■ indigestion ■ nausea or vomiting ■ dry mouth ■ metallic taste ■ difficulty in swallowing ■ stuffy nose ■ leg cramps ■ tingling or pain in fingers or toes, especially when exposed to cold ■ depression ■ sleeplessness ■ nightmares ■ nervousness ■ burning eyes or other eye problems ■ double vision or other visual disturbances ■ rash or hives ■ mottled skin	If symptoms are disturbing or persist, let your doctor know.

STORAGE INSTRUCTIONS

Store in a cool, dark place (not in a bathroom medicine cabinet).

STOPPING OR INTERRUPTING THERAPY

It may take several weeks before you feel the helpful effects of this medicine. Do not stop taking it without consulting your doctor. Stopping this medicine suddenly may worsen your medical condition. If you miss a dose, take it as soon as possible. If it is within four hours of your next scheduled dose, skip the missed dose and resume your regular schedule. Do not take two doses at the same time.

SPECIAL CONSIDERATIONS FOR THOSE OVER SIXTY-FIVE

Older people may be more susceptible to such side effects as confusion, hallucinations, and uncontrollable movements.

EPILEPSY

When we think about epilepsy, most of us see the image of a person losing consciousness, falling down, and jerking all over. That *is* what happens during a grand mal seizure. But in some people with epilepsy—a condition in which episodes of abnormal activity in some brain cells cause uncontrolled activity in the body—the seizure is just a twitching of one hand or foot. In others, the seizure consists of a feeling that one side of the body is numb or prickling. Or it is expressed as repeated behavior that has no purpose, like lip-smacking or hand-clapping. Sometimes epilepsy appears as just a few seconds of blinking or a vacant stare.

CAUSES

Brain cells, known as neurons, produce tiny electric charges that can be monitored through electrodes placed on the head. In epilepsy, the neurons periodically misfire. If the misfiring occurs in the part of the brain that controls vision, the seizure will consist of a hallucination. If it occurs in the part that directs the fingers, the fingers will twitch. Sometimes the abnormal electricity in one part of the brain sets off abnormal discharges elsewhere in the brain, sending several parts of the body into abnormal motion.

In most cases, the reason for the epilepsy is unknown. In others, it can be traced to an injury to the brain caused by oxygen deprivation, a blow to the head, a tumor, or a stroke. Most new cases of epilepsy show up in babies and young children, but brain injury can occur at any age. People who have never had a seizure before can suddenly develop the disorder when they are past fifty, sixty, or even eighty.

DIAGNOSIS

Your doctor will begin by taking a medical history and doing a physical exam. You will also be questioned about the circumstances in which the seizure occurred and whether it was preceded by an aura—a strange sensation that comes right before some types of seizures (and also before some migraine headaches). An aura may be just an ill-defined feeling, or something more specific such as visual disturbances or the impression of hearing peculiar sounds. If anyone was with you when the aura occurred, you should bring that person along to talk to the doctor, since you might not be able to recall much about the event.

Because epilepsy is marked by abnormal electrical activity in the brain, electroencephalogram (EEG) examinations are an important part of the diagnostic procedure. In addition to helping identify the cause of the seizure, they aid in selecting appropriate drug treatments. However, as valuable as the EEG is, it has certain limitations. Some people with epilepsy have abnormal brain waves only during the actual seizure; the rest of the time, their EEG record shows a regular pattern. Other people, who do not have epilepsy at all, sometimes produce abnormal tracings. Your doctor might, therefore, want you to have several EEGs to see whether the pattern is the same at different times of the day or after different kinds of stimulation.

Your doctor might also want you to have a computed axial tomography (CAT) scan, which provides a detailed image of your brain, or a positron emission tomography (PET) scan, which is an even newer method of detecting and mapping your brain's activity. Like the EEG, these tests are painless and noninvasive; there is no radiation to be concerned about, nor any physical probing inside your brain.

TREATMENT

If it's found that you do have epilepsy, these diagnostic tests should give your doctor a fairly good idea of the type it is and the location of the neurons that set it off. He or she can therefore prescribe the medicine that has the best chance of bringing your disorder entirely under control. If the first-choice drug does not work for you, or if it causes severe adverse reactions, the doctor can juggle drugs and doses until you get the relief you need. For information on anticonvulsant medicines, see the charts on pages 324–338. In those few cases in which medicine does not help, doctors and patients can explore the possibility of surgical removal of the part of the brain that is causing the problem. If the seizures always arise in a single area in the brain, surgery may provide a permanent cure.

OUTLOOK

Most people with epilepsy have to cope with it for the rest of their lives, though it can usually be controlled with drugs. There is no evidence that it gets either better or worse as a person gets older. But diagnostic and treatment techniques are getting better, giving hope of a more normal life, without the constant fear of seizures.

Caution: Some drugs in this section may affect pregnancy or fetal development. Check with your doctor if this concerns you.

CONDITION: **EPILEPSY AND SEIZURES**

CATEGORY: **ANTICONVULSANTS**

GENERIC (CHEMICAL) NAME	BRAND (TRADE) NAME	DOSAGE FORMS AND STRENGTHS
Carbamazepine	TEGRETOL	Chewable tablets: 100 mg Tablets: 200 mg Suspension: 100 mg per tsp

DRUG PROFILE

This drug is used to treat certain types of epilepsy. It prevents seizures or makes them occur less often by dampening the overactive nerve impulses in the brain. Carbamazepine is also used to treat trigeminal neuralgia (tic douloureux), which is a type of facial pain.

BEFORE USING THIS DRUG

Let your doctor know *IF*

You have ever had any allergic reactions or other problems with ■ carbamazepine ■ tricyclic antidepressants (medicine for depression).

You have ever had any of the following medical problems: ■ heart or blood vessel disease, including thrombophlebitis, congestive heart failure, high or low blood pressure, or heart attack ■ kidney disease ■ liver disease ■ blood disease ■ bone marrow depression ■ anemia ■ alcoholism ■ mental illness ■ diabetes ■ urinary problems ■ systemic lupus erythematosus ■ glaucoma.

You are taking any of the following medicines: ■ other medicines for seizures ■ medicine for depression (within the last two weeks) ■ anticoagulants (blood thinners) ■ barbiturates ■ tranquilizers ■ sleep medicines ■ muscle relaxants ■ narcotics and other prescription pain-killers ■ antibiotics ■ cimetidine (medicine for ulcers) ■ medicine for abnormal heart rhythms ■ tetracycline.

Any drug you have taken has ever affected your blood.

SPECIAL RESTRICTIONS WHILE TAKING THIS DRUG

FOOD AND DRUG INTERACTIONS

Other Drugs	Do not take any other drugs, including over-the-counter (OTC) drugs, before checking with your doctor. This drug affects the way many other drugs work, and your doctor may want to adjust the dose of carbamazepine or of the other drugs you may be taking.
Alcohol	Avoid alcohol unless your doctor has approved its use.

No special restrictions on foods and beverages or smoking.

DAILY LIVING

Driving	This drug may cause dizziness, light-headedness, or blurred vision. Be careful when driving, operating household appliances, or doing any other tasks that require alertness until you know how this drug affects you.
Sun Exposure	Your skin may become more sensitive to sunlight and more likely to develop a sunburn while taking this medicine. It is a good idea to apply a sunscreen to exposed skin surfaces before going outdoors.
Excessive Heat	Use caution during hot weather since overexertion may result in heat stroke. Avoid extremely hot baths and saunas.

Examinations or Tests	It is important for you to keep all appointments with your doctor so that your progress can be checked. Your dosage may have to be adjusted from time to time. Periodic blood and urine tests, as well as eye examinations, are usually required before and during therapy.
Other Precautions	Tell any doctor or dentist you consult that you are taking this medicine, especially if you will be undergoing any type of surgery or any kind of tests.

If you have diabetes, be aware that this drug may cause false urine-sugar tests. Discuss with your doctor what kind of home tests you should use. |
| Helpful Hints | If this medicine upsets your stomach, taking it with meals, snacks, or water should help.

If your mouth or throat feels dry, chewing sugarless gum or sucking ice chips or sugarless hard candy will help. |

No special restrictions on exertion and exercise or exposure to excessive cold.

POSSIBLE SIDE EFFECTS

Although this list of adverse effects may seem somewhat intimidating, keep in mind that some are quite rare. Of course, should these or any other problems arise while you are on medication, it is always a good idea to consult your doctor.

IF YOU DEVELOP

mouth sores ■ sore throat or fever ■ bleeding or bruising ■ chills ■ extreme tiredness or weakness

WHAT TO DO

Extremely Urgent: Stop taking this drug and get in touch with your doctor immediately.

fainting ■ collapse ■ stuffy nose ■ red, irritated eyes ■ swelling of the tip of the penis ■ swelling of lower legs or feet ■ pain, tenderness, or bluish color in legs or feet ■ dark urine ■ pale stools ■ yellowing of eyes or skin ■ seizures ■ irregular or fast heartbeat ■ severe dizziness or drowsiness ■ shortness of breath ■ irregular or shallow breathing ■ tremors ■ pain or difficulty in urination ■ rash, hives, or itching	**Urgent** Get in touch with your doctor immediately.
blurred or double vision ■ confusion ■ chest pain ■ slow or pounding heartbeat ■ back and forth eye movements or other eye problems ■ uncontrollable body movements ■ spasms ■ numbness, tingling, pain, or weakness in hands or feet ■ speech difficulties ■ swollen glands ■ restlessness and nervousness ■ depression ■ hallucinations ■ ringing in ears ■ increased sensitivity to sound ■ flushing ■ dilated pupils ■ urinary frequency ■ decreased urination ■ nausea or vomiting ■ stomach pain or discomfort ■ loss of appetite ■ diarrhea ■ constipation	**May be serious** Check with your doctor as soon as possible.
clumsiness or unsteadiness ■ light-headedness or dizziness ■ drowsiness ■ dry mouth or throat ■ tongue irritation ■ joint or muscle aches ■ leg cramps ■ headache ■ increased skin sensitivity to sunlight ■ changes in skin color ■ hair loss ■ male impotence ■ increased sweating ■ difficulty in swallowing	If symptoms are disturbing or persist, let your doctor know.

STORAGE INSTRUCTIONS

Store in a cool, dark place (not in a bathroom medicine cabinet).

STOPPING OR INTERRUPTING THERAPY

Do not stop taking this drug unless instructed to do so by your doctor. If you miss a dose, take it as soon as possible. If it is almost time for your next dose, skip the missed dose and resume your regular schedule. Do not take two doses at the same time. If you miss two or more doses in the same day, consult your doctor.

SPECIAL CONSIDERATIONS FOR THOSE OVER SIXTY-FIVE

Older people may be more susceptible to such side effects as confusion, nervousness, and restlessness.

CONDITION: **EPILEPSY AND SEIZURES**

CATEGORY: **ANTICONVULSANTS**

GENERIC (CHEMICAL) NAME	BRAND (TRADE) NAME	DOSAGE FORMS AND STRENGTHS
Phenytoin	DILANTIN	Capsules: 30,100 mg Suspension: 125 mg per tsp 30 mg per tsp Tablets: 50 mg
Phenytoin and phenobarbital	DILANTIN with phenobarbital	Kapseals: 100 mg phenytoin and ¼ grain phenobarbital, 100 mg phenytoin and ½ grain phenobarbital

DRUG PROFILE

Phenytoin is used to treat epilepsy and other types of seizure disorders. It prevents seizures or makes them occur less often by dampening the overactive nerve impulses in the brain.

BEFORE USING THIS DRUG

Let your doctor know *IF*

You have ever had any allergic reactions or other problems with ■ phenytoin ■ other medicine for seizures.

You have ever had any of the following medical problems: ■ diabetes ■ high blood sugar ■ liver disease ■ kidney disease ■ alcoholism ■ blood disease ■ bone disease.

You are taking any of the following medicines: ■ any other medicine for seizures ■ Antabuse (used in treatment of alcoholism) ■ barbiturates ■ tranquilizers ■ sleep medicines ■ muscle relaxants ■ medicine for depression ■ phenylbutazone (medicine for arthritis) ■ folic acid ■ vitamin D (calciferol) ■ antibiotics ■ cimetidine (medicine for ulcers) ■ anticoagulants (blood thinners) ■ corticosteroids ■ medicine for diabetes ■ medicine for tuberculosis ■ digoxin or digitalis (heart medicines) ■ hormones ■ propoxyphene (prescription pain-killer) ■ medicine for nausea ■ disopyramide/quinidine (medicine for abnormal heart rhythms) ■ any medicine containing alcohol ■ aminophylline, theophylline (medicine for asthma).

SPECIAL RESTRICTIONS WHILE TAKING THIS DRUG

FOOD AND DRUG INTERACTIONS

Other Drugs	Do not take any other drugs, including over-the-counter (OTC) drugs, before checking with your doctor. A number of drugs affect the way phenytoin works, and your doctor may want to adjust the dose of phenytoin or of the other drugs you may be taking. Also, do not switch to another brand or dosage form (eg, tablets to capsules) without consulting your doctor, since different forms of this medicine are absorbed by the body in different ways, and your dosage may have to be adjusted.
Foods and Beverages	Because this drug may cause folic acid deficiency, be sure to eat a well-balanced diet containing plenty of B vitamins. Your doctor may recommend that you take a multivitamin.
Alcohol	Drinking alcohol while taking this medicine may increase the risk of drowsiness and reduce the effects of the drug. Avoid alcohol unless your doctor has approved its use.

No special restrictions on smoking.

DAILY LIVING

Driving	This drug may cause drowsiness or loss of alertness. Be careful when driving, operating household appliances, or doing any other tasks that require alertness until you know how this drug affects you.
Examinations or Tests	It is important for you to keep all appointments for blood tests so that your progress and side effects can be checked.
Other Precautions	If you have diabetes, be aware that this medicine may affect blood-sugar levels. If you notice any change when testing sugar levels in your blood or urine, let your doctor know. Tell any doctor or dentist you consult that you are taking this medicine, especially if you will be undergoing any type of surgery.
Helpful Hints	If this medicine upsets your stomach, taking it with meals, snacks, or water should help. This medicine may cause your gums to become red and swollen. Practicing good oral hygiene (flossing and brushing carefully) can minimize this effect.

No special restrictions on exertion and exercise, sun exposure, or exposure to excessive heat or cold.

POSSIBLE SIDE EFFECTS

Although this list of adverse effects may seem somewhat intimidating, keep in mind that some are quite rare. Of course, should these or any other problems arise while you are on medication, it is always a good idea to consult your doctor.

IF YOU DEVELOP	WHAT TO DO
uncontrollable eye movements ■ crossed eyes or any other eye problems ■ blurred or double vision ■ rash ■ sore throat or fever ■ dark urine or gray stools ■ yellowing of eyes or skin ■ severe headache ■ swelling of the tip of the penis ■ enlarged lymph glands ■ stomach pain ■ bleeding or bruising ■ hallucinations ■ confusion ■ memory loss ■ severe dizziness or drowsiness ■ slurred speech ■ clumsiness ■ staggering walk ■ sleeplessness ■ behavior or personality changes ■ depression ■ pain in urination ■ urinary frequency ■ swelling of feet or hands ■ uncontrollable muscle movements	**Urgent** Get in touch with your doctor immediately.
irritability ■ restlessness ■ red, swollen gums ■ constipation ■ upset stomach ■ nausea or vomiting ■ diarrhea ■ loss of taste ■ difficulty in swallowing ■ loss of appetite ■ weight loss ■ acne ■ dizziness ■ drowsiness ■ hair growth ■ headache ■ muscle twitching ■ red eyes ■ stuffy nose	If symptoms are disturbing or persist, let your doctor know.

STORAGE INSTRUCTIONS

Store in a cool, dark place (not in a bathroom medicine cabinet). If your medicine is in a liquid form, make sure that it does not freeze.

STOPPING OR INTERRUPTING THERAPY

Since this drug does not cure your condition but only controls it, you may have to take this medicine for the rest of your life. Do not stop taking this medicine unless instructed to do so by your doctor. Suddenly stopping this medicine could trigger seizures; your doctor will advise you on how to reduce your dosage gradually before stopping completely. If you take phenytoin once a day and you miss a dose, take it as soon as possible and resume your regular schedule. If you do not remember until the following day, skip the missed dose and resume your regular schedule. If you take phenytoin several times a day and you miss a dose, take the missed dose as soon as possible. If your next dose is within four hours, skip the missed dose and resume your regular schedule. If you miss your dose for two or more days, check with your doctor.

SPECIAL CONSIDERATIONS FOR THOSE OVER SIXTY-FIVE

Older people may be more prone to such side effects as clumsiness and red, swollen gums. Also, the body's absorption of calcium may be lowered, leading to osteomalacia (softening of the bones), a condition to which this age group may be susceptible.

CONDITION: **EPILEPSY AND SEIZURES**

CATEGORY: **ANTICONVULSANTS**

GENERIC (CHEMICAL) NAME	BRAND (TRADE) NAME	DOSAGE FORMS AND STRENGTHS
Primidone	MYSOLINE	Suspension: 250 mg per tsp Tablets: 50, 250 mg

DRUG PROFILE

Primidone is used to treat epilepsy. It prevents seizures or makes them occur less often by dampening the overactive nerve impulses in the brain. Primidone can be used alone or with other medicine for more effective seizure control.

BEFORE USING THIS DRUG

Let your doctor know *IF*

You have ever had allergic reactions or other problems with ■ primidone
■ barbiturates.

You have ever had any of the following medical problems: ■ asthma or other lung disease ■ kidney disease ■ liver disease ■ porphyria.

You are taking any of the following medicines: ■ other medicine for seizures
■ corticosteroids ■ anticoagulants (blood thinners) ■ antihistamines ■ medicine for hay fever, allergies, or colds ■ barbiturates ■ narcotics or other prescription painkillers ■ tranquilizers ■ sleep medicines ■ medicine for fungal infection
■ doxycycline ■ muscle relaxants ■ quinidine (medicine for abnormal heart rhythms) ■ any medicine containing alcohol.

SPECIAL RESTRICTIONS WHILE TAKING THIS DRUG

FOOD AND DRUG INTERACTIONS

Other Drugs	This medicine increases the effects of drugs that depress the central nervous system—such as antihistamines; medicine for hay fever, allergies, or colds; sleep medicines; tranquilizers; narcotics or other prescription pain-killers; muscle relaxants; and other medicine for seizures.
Alcohol	Drinking alcohol may increase the effects of this medicine or cause dangerously high levels of this medicine in your body. Avoid alcohol unless your doctor has approved its use.

No special restrictions on foods and beverages or smoking.

DAILY LIVING

Driving	This drug may cause dizziness, light-headedness, or drowsiness. Be careful when driving, operating household appliances, or doing any other tasks that require alertness until you know how this drug affects you.
Examinations or Tests	It is important for you to keep all appointments with your doctor so that your progress and any side effects can be checked. Periodic blood tests may be required.
Other Precautions	Tell any doctor or dentist you consult that you are taking this drug, especially if you will be undergoing any type of surgery.

No special restrictions on exertion and exercise, sun exposure, or exposure to excessive heat or cold.

POSSIBLE SIDE EFFECTS

Although this list of adverse effects may seem somewhat intimidating, keep in mind that some are quite rare. Of course, should these or any other problems arise while you are on medication, it is always a good idea to consult your doctor.

IF YOU DEVELOP	WHAT TO DO
yellowing of eyes or skin ■ dark urine ■ pale stools ■ discoloration of skin	**Urgent** Get in touch with your doctor immediately.
wheezing or tightness in chest ■ extreme excitement ■ tiredness or weakness ■ rash or hives ■ swelling or twitching of eyelids ■ double vision ■ confusion ■ difficulty in breathing ■ emotional disturbances ■ mental changes, including depression ■ difficulty in swallowing ■ sore throat or fever ■ bleeding (including nosebleed) or bruising ■ swelling of the legs ■ speech difficulties ■ swelling of the tip of the penis ■ urinary problems	**May be serious** Check with your doctor as soon as possible.
clumsiness or unsteadiness ■ drowsiness ■ dizziness or light-headedness ■ male impotence ■ headache ■ loss of appetite ■ nausea or vomiting ■ upset stomach ■ constipation ■ diarrhea ■ loss of taste ■ hair loss ■ stuffy nose ■ red, itching eyes	If symptoms are disturbing or persist, let your doctor know.

STORAGE INSTRUCTIONS

Store in a cool, dark place (not in a bathroom medicine cabinet). If your medicine is in a liquid form, make sure that it does not freeze.

STOPPING OR INTERRUPTING THERAPY

It may be several weeks before you feel the beneficial effects of this drug. Do not suddenly stop taking this medicine, as this may trigger seizures. Your doctor will advise you on how to stop gradually and safely when you no longer need this medicine.

If you miss a dose, take it as soon as possible. If it is within an hour of your next dose, skip the missed dose and resume your regular schedule. Do not take two doses at the same time.

SPECIAL CONSIDERATIONS FOR THOSE OVER SIXTY-FIVE

Older people may be more prone to such side effects as dizziness, drowsiness, excitement, confusion, and depression.

CONDITION: **EPILEPSY AND SEIZURES**

CATEGORY: **ANTICONVULSANTS**

GENERIC (CHEMICAL) NAME	BRAND (TRADE) NAME	DOSAGE FORMS AND STRENGTHS
Divalproex sodium	DEPAKOTE	Delayed-release tablets: divalproex sodium equivalent to 125, 250, and 500 mg valproic acid Capsules, Sprinkle: 125 mg
Valproic acid	DEPAKENE	Capsules: 250 mg Syrup: 250 mg per tsp

DRUG PROFILE

Valproic acid and divalproex (which forms valproic acid in the body) are used to treat epilepsy and other types of seizure disorders. How they work is not exactly known. These drugs may be used in combination with other seizure medications.

BEFORE USING THIS DRUG

Let your doctor know *IF*

You have ever had allergic reactions or other problems with ■ divalproex ■ valproic acid.

You have ever had any of the following medical problems: ■ liver disease ■ kidney disease ■ gastrointestinal disease ■ blood disease ■ brain disease.

You are taking any of the following medicines: ■ other medicine for seizures ■ antihistamines ■ medicine for hay fever, coughs, or colds ■ barbiturates ■ narcotics or other prescription pain-killers ■ sleep medicine ■ muscle relaxants ■ tranquilizers ■ aspirin or other medicine for pain and swelling ■ acetaminophen ■ sulfinpyrazone (medicine for gout) ■ corticosteroids or corticotropin (ACTH) ■ amiodarone (medicine for abnormal heart rhythms) ■ medicine for cancer ■ Antabuse (used in the treatment of alcoholism) ■ Naltrexone (used in the treatment of narcotic addiction) ■ aminoquinolones (chloroquine, hydroxychloroquine) ■ medicine for tuberculosis ■ medicine for Parkinson's disease ■ anticoagulants (blood thinners) ■ pentoxifylline (medicine to improve blood flow) ■ thyroid medicine ■ antibiotics (medicine for infections) ■ etretinate (medicine for psoriasis) ■ insulin.

SPECIAL RESTRICTIONS WHILE TAKING THIS DRUG

FOOD AND DRUG INTERACTIONS

Other Drugs	This medicine increases the effects of drugs that depress the central nervous system—such as antihistamines; medicine for hay fever, allergies, or colds; sleep medicines; tranquilizers; narcotics or other prescription pain-killers; muscle relaxants; and other medicine for seizures.
Alcohol	Drinking alcohol may increase the effects of this medicine or cause dangerously high levels of this medicine in your body. Avoid alcohol unless your doctor has approved its use.

No special restrictions on foods and beverages or smoking.

DAILY LIVING

Driving	This drug may cause dizziness or drowsiness. Be careful when driving, operating household appliances, or doing any other tasks that require alertness until you know how this drug affects you.
Examinations or Tests	It is important for you to keep all appointments with your doctor so that your progress and any side effects can be checked. Periodic blood tests may be required.
Other Precautions	Tell any doctor or dentist you consult that you are taking this drug, especially if you will be undergoing any type of surgery.
	If you have diabetes, be aware that this medicine may affect blood-sugar levels. If you notice any change when testing sugar levels in your blood or urine, let your doctor know.
Helpful Hints	Take the capsule or tablet form of this medicine with a full glass of water. The capsule or delayed-release tablets should be swallowed whole, without crushing, breaking, or chewing. The sprinkle capsules may be taken whole or opened and added to a small amount of food. If this medicine upsets your stomach, taking it with meals or snacks should help. The syrup may be mixed with soft foods or liquids.

No special restrictions on exertion and exercise, sun exposure, or exposure to excessive heat or cold.

POSSIBLE SIDE EFFECTS

Although this list of adverse effects may seem somewhat intimidating, keep in mind that some are quite rare. Of course, should these or any other problems arise while you are on medication, it is always a good idea to consult your doctor.

IF YOU DEVELOP	WHAT TO DO
increase in seizures ■ clumsiness ■ loss of appetite ■ weight loss ■ nausea or vomiting ■ severe abdominal or stomach cramps ■ rash ■ itching ■ swelling of face, hands, or feet ■ bleeding or bruising ■ tiredness or weakness ■ yellowing of eyes or skin ■ trembling of hands or arms ■ dizziness ■ confusion ■ excitement	**May be serious** Check with your doctor as soon as possible.
diarrhea ■ constipation ■ abdominal or stomach cramps ■ indigestion ■ increased appetite ■ weight gain ■ hair loss ■ drowsiness ■ headache ■ depression ■ restlessness ■ irritability ■ mood changes ■ difficulty in speech ■ enlarged breasts ■ vision or eye problems	If symptoms are disturbing or persist, let your doctor know.

STORAGE INSTRUCTIONS

Store in a cool, dark place (not in a bathroom medicine cabinet). If your medicine is in a liquid form, make sure that it does not freeze.

STOPPING OR INTERRUPTING THERAPY

Since this drug does not cure your condition but only controls it, you may have to take this medicine for the rest of your life. Do not stop taking this medicine unless instructed to do so by your doctor. If you are taking this medicine once a day and you miss a dose, take it as soon as possible and resume your regular schedule. If you take this medicine more than once a day and you miss a dose, take the missed dose as soon as possible and take the rest of your doses for that day at regularly spaced intervals. Do not take two doses at the same time. Also, abruptly stopping this medicine may cause a seizure. Do not stop taking this medicine without talking to your doctor first.

SPECIAL CONSIDERATIONS FOR THOSE OVER SIXTY-FIVE

Because older people may be especially prone to the side effects of divalproex and valproic acid, doctors may start people over sixty-five on a lower dosage.

CONDITION: **EPILEPSY AND SEIZURES**

CATEGORY: **BARBITURATES**

GENERIC (CHEMICAL) NAME	BRAND (TRADE) NAME	DOSAGE FORMS AND STRENGTHS
Phenobarbital		Elixir: 20 mg per tsp Tablets: 8, 15, 30, 60, 100 mg

DRUG PROFILE

Phenobarbital is a barbiturate that is very effective in treating certain types of epilepsy. Barbiturates also have been used to treat insomnia and to relieve anxiety or nervousness. It is not known how barbiturates work, but some experts believe that these drugs act on the part of the brain responsible for wakefulness. Barbiturates are associated with daytime drowsiness and morning "hangover." Doctors usually prefer not to prescribe these drugs for older people since other drugs may be safer and more effective.

For complete information on this drug, see pages 586–590.

CONDITION: **EPILEPSY AND SEIZURES**

CATEGORY: **BENZODIAZEPINES**

GENERIC (CHEMICAL) NAME	BRAND (TRADE) NAME	DOSAGE FORMS AND STRENGTHS
Clonazepam	KLONOPIN	Tablets: 0.5, 1, 2 mg

DRUG PROFILE

Benzodiazepines are used to treat a number of conditions, including anxiety, insomnia, muscle spasm, and seizures. Exactly how these drugs work is a matter of some debate. However, what they all seem to have in common is that they reduce nerve cell activity in those areas of the central nervous system (CNS) and peripheral nervous system (PNS) thought to be responsible for the experience of anxiety and muscular tension. Low doses are usually prescribed for older people.

For complete information on this drug, see pages 580–585.

MYASTHENIA GRAVIS

Myasthenia gravis, a disease marked by muscle weakness, is most common among women in their twenties and thirties. In men, however, most cases of the disease occur after the age of forty.

CAUSES

Every voluntary movement, from scratching to swallowing to blinking your eyes, originates in the brain, which sends electrical signals along a complex network of nerve pathways leading to the muscles. In myasthenia gravis, the nerve-to-muscle transmission of these electrical impulses does not work properly because of a flaw in the muscles—specifically, in the structures known as receptors that are located on the muscle-cell surfaces. These receptors fail to bind a chemical messenger called acetylcholine (ACh), which is a vital link in the nerve-to-muscle pathway.

Myasthenia gravis is termed an autoimmune disease because the immune system produces antibodies that block off most of the ACh receptors. The result is mild to extreme muscle weakness. In many people with myasthenia gravis, the thymus gland appears to be involved. The thymus gland, which is located inside the chest, is part of the immune system. Seventy percent of people with myasthenia gravis have an enlarged thymus gland, and another 10 to 15 percent have tumors of the thymus gland.

DIAGNOSIS

Early symptoms of myasthenia gravis may be so subtle that they go unnoticed. In 50 percent of cases, double vision (which may be accompanied by drooping eyelids) first alerts the person that something is wrong. Within about a year, the symptoms generally progress to include weakness in the limbs, the facial muscles, and, in the most severe cases, the muscles involved in swallowing and breathing. Another feature of the disease is a feeling of tiredness after only slight use of the affected muscles. Most of the time, the symptoms are least severe in the morning, after a long period of rest. Weakness tends to become more pronounced with exercise and with emotional stress.

The course of myasthenia gravis varies widely. One of the hallmarks of the disease is the fluctuating nature of weakness: it varies considerably in a single day, from day to day, and from month to month. Remissions and exacerbations are common. Some people with the disease suffer a life-threatening near-paralysis of the respiratory muscles, while others have symptoms limited to the facial muscles. Early in the disease, about 25 percent of patients have spontaneous remissions, during which time symptoms improve markedly or disappear altogether. Such remissions, however, are never permanent in the absence of therapy.

If a pattern of symptoms leads the doctor to suspect that myasthenia gravis may be the problem, the diagnosis can be confirmed by injecting a small amount of a drug (neostigmine or edrophonium) that temporarily increases the activity of ACh. In a person who has myasthenia gravis, the injection will cause the symptoms to improve greatly for a short time. Further tests—including electromyography, which charts a muscle's response to electrical stimulation, and blood tests for certain antibodies—may also be performed.

TREATMENT

The treatment used most often for myasthenia gravis is aimed at reducing the disease's symptoms. Other therapies (thymectomy; corticosteroids or other drugs that suppress the immune system) may alter the course of the disease. Many people with myasthenia gravis are on long-term therapy with anticholinesterase drugs; these work the same way as the drug used in diagnosing the condition. One of the most common of these drugs is pyridostigmine bromide (see drug chart on pages 343–345). These medicines work best for people who understand their disease and know what activities and times of day are associated with the worst symptoms. Such people can gauge the amount of medicine they'll need, much as a person who has diabetes can calculate the amount of insulin required in different circumstances.

Other drugs sometimes used to treat myasthenia gravis are corticosteroids (see drug chart on pages 530–535) and adrenocorticotropic hormone (ACTH). These drugs suppress the immune system, thus reducing the level of circulating antibodies that block off ACh receptors. Another treatment that removes antibodies from the blood is plasma exchange, a process in which the plasma, which contains antibodies, is separated from other components of the blood.

Finally, thymectomy, or surgical removal of the thymus gland, is an option for many people with myasthenia gravis. After a thymectomy, medicine must be continued for some time—months to years, in some cases—but improvement eventually occurs in 80 percent of people who undergo the procedure. About one-third of those people experience total remission.

OUTLOOK

Myasthenia gravis varies greatly from person to person. Some individuals with the condition are severely disabled, while others are able to lead near-normal lives. The outlook for most people with myasthenia gravis has improved greatly in the past several years as treatments effective against even its worst symptoms have been developed. Current research efforts, directed at understanding and correcting the immune disorder that underlies myasthenia gravis, hold promise for even better therapeutic approaches to this chronic disease.

CONDITION: **MYASTHENIA GRAVIS**

CATEGORY: **MUSCLE STIMULANTS**

GENERIC (CHEMICAL) NAME	BRAND (TRADE) NAME	DOSAGE FORMS AND STRENGTHS
Pyridostigmine bromide	MESTINON	Controlled-release tablets: 180 mg Syrup: 60 mg per tsp Tablets: 60 mg

DRUG PROFILE

Pyridostigmine is used to treat the muscular weakness and fatigue associated with myasthenia gravis. This drug acts both directly and through the nervous system to increase muscle tone.

BEFORE USING THIS DRUG

Let your doctor know *IF*

You have ever had allergic reactions or other problems with ■ pyridostigmine.

You have ever had any of the following medical problems: ■ asthma ■ intestinal or urinary tract blockage ■ seizures ■ slow heartbeat ■ blood vessel disease ■ spastic disorder ■ overactive thyroid ■ abnormal heart rhythms ■ stomach ulcers.

You are taking any of the following medicines: ■ corticosteroids ■ antibiotics ■ medicine for abnormal heart rhythms ■ quinine (medicine for malaria).

SPECIAL RESTRICTIONS WHILE TAKING THIS DRUG

FOOD AND DRUG INTERACTIONS

No special restrictions on other drugs, foods and beverages, alcohol use, or smoking.

DAILY LIVING

Driving	This drug may cause double vision or other visual disturbances. Be careful when driving, operating household appliances, or doing any other tasks that require alertness until you know how this drug affects you.
Examinations or Tests	It is important for you to keep all appointments with your doctor so that your progress can be checked.
Other Precautions	Tell any doctor or dentist you consult that you are taking this drug, especially if you will be undergoing any type of surgery. The controlled-release tablet should be swallowed whole, without crushing, breaking, or chewing.

No special restrictions on exertion and exercise, sun exposure, or exposure to excessive heat or cold.

POSSIBLE SIDE EFFECTS

Although this list of adverse effects may seem somewhat intimidating, keep in mind that some are quite rare. Of course, should these or any other problems arise while you are on medication, it is always a good idea to consult your doctor.

IF YOU DEVELOP

seizures

difficulty in breathing ■ slow or fast heartbeat ■ muscle cramps or pain ■ weakness ■ muscle weakness, especially in the neck ■ nausea or vomiting ■ diarrhea ■ stomach cramps ■ dilated pupils ■ increased salivation ■ increased sweating ■ fainting ■ dizziness ■ double vision or other visual disturbances ■ increased urination ■ difficulty in chewing or in swallowing ■ agitation ■ restlessness ■ tearing eyes ■ increased phlegm production ■ clumsiness

WHAT TO DO

Urgent Get in touch with your doctor immediately.

May be serious Check with your doctor as soon as possible.

STORAGE INSTRUCTIONS

Store in a cool, dark place (not in a bathroom medicine cabinet). If your medicine is in a liquid form, make sure that it does not freeze.

STOPPING OR INTERRUPTING THERAPY

If you miss a dose, take it as soon as possible. If it is almost time for your next dose, skip the missed dose (unless you are experiencing muscular weakness) and resume your regular schedule. Do not take two doses at the same time.

SPECIAL CONSIDERATIONS FOR THOSE OVER SIXTY-FIVE

None.

HEADACHES

Headaches strike people of any age and either sex and occur at least once a month in 90 percent of the U.S. population. For most of these people, headaches are a fleeting discomfort caused by fatigue, hunger, or stress and are quickly relieved by aspirin or acetaminophen, fresh air, rest, or perhaps a gentle massage. But for others, headaches are a relentless fact of life that cannot be easily banished or easily borne.

The majority of headaches can be classified into three categories: organic headaches, muscle contraction (or tension) headaches, and vascular headaches.

ORGANIC HEADACHES

Although organic headaches are the least common type, they may indicate a serious disorder, such as high blood pressure or, rarely, a brain tumor. They should be considered a warning sign, and merit immediate medical attention. See a doctor if your headaches are sudden, severe, or progressive; are accompanied by confusion or loss of consciousness; recur in one area, such as an eye or temple; are accompanied by fever and stiff neck; or frequently awaken you from a sound sleep.

One variety of organic headache (actually a facial pain) that occurs more commonly in women than in men is caused by trigeminal neuralgia, often referred to as *tic douloureux*. This condition, a painful inflammation of the nerves in the cheek, most often begins between the ages of thirty and sixty. An attack of this disorder consists of repetitive painful jabs; this lasts one or more hours, and commonly occurs at night. Attacks may go on for several months and then ease up for a year or more. This condition is generally treated with medication. See pages 324–328 for a description of the drug most commonly used to relieve the distress of tic douloureux. In some cases, medical therapy eventually loses its effectiveness, and surgical techniques are used quite successfully to treat this condition.

TENSION HEADACHES

Muscle contraction, or tension, headaches are the most common type of headache. They often result from physical or emotional stress, which causes head and neck muscles to contract and feel tender. Poor posture or prolonged sitting may also lead to this type of headache. The steady, dull pain of a tension headache localizes in the forehead, back of the neck, or temples; sometimes the pain seems to wrap itself around the head like a steel band. Sufferers can often find quick relief from the tension through massage, heat, or a hot shower. Practicing relaxation techniques—such as meditation, yoga, or biofeedback—can often work magically. Also, aspirin or acetaminophen may effectively relieve the pain. For severe muscle tension headaches, slightly more potent drugs may be prescribed.

VASCULAR HEADACHES

Vascular headaches occur when blood vessels in the brain either constrict or dilate, causing the throbbing sensation characteristic of these headaches. Hangovers, hunger, and certain substances in food (such as monosodium glutamate, often used in Chinese cooking, and tyramine, found in red wine, certain shellfish and cheeses, and other foods), account for many of these headaches.

Migraine Headaches   Migraine headaches, a frightening form of vascular headache caused by blood vessel dilation, are excruciating and may incapacitate their victims for days at a time. Migraines usually start on one side of the head and remain there during the length of the attack. The intense throbbing is often accompanied by nausea, loss of appetite, and even vomiting. Two types of migraine headaches exist. The common variety has few or no warning symptoms and can occur two or three times a week if the patient is unduly stressed. The classic migraine headache, on the other hand, gives an unmistakable ten- to thirty-minute warning of its onset, with sensations known as auras—the victim may see flashing lights, zigzagging lines, or areas of total darkness. When the aura fades, the pain begins and can last from an hour or two to twenty-four or seventy-two hours.

Migraine headaches appear to run in families and to be associated with hard-driving, perfectionist personalities. Migraine therapy begins with pinpointing the headache's triggering factor—whether stress, fatigue, certain foods, flickering lights, or cigarette smoke, for example—and then attacking the condition with pharmacological, environmental, or psychological treatments. Biofeedback training has been effective in treating some cases of chronic migraine. Drug treatments are available that can either prevent a migraine from developing or stop it in its earliest stages. See the drug charts on pages 353–356 for a description of these agents.

Cluster Headaches   Cluster headaches, also caused by vascular irregularities, strike suddenly; recur repeatedly for a certain period (usually two to twelve weeks); and then disappear—only to return for another period of "clustered" pain. More common in men than in women, these headaches are associated with intense pain and have been known to cause some sufferers to bang their heads against a wall. Because it's important for therapy to begin early in an attack, drugs are often administered by injection or suppository to enable them to enter the bloodstream rapidly.

OUTLOOK

Although certain types of headaches merit prompt attention from a doctor, the vast majority are not symptoms of serious medical problems. Usually they can be controlled by the use of simple drugs and by changes in everyday habits.

Caution: Some drugs in this section may affect pregnancy or fetal development. Check with your doctor if this concerns you.

CONDITION: **HEADACHE**

CATEGORY: **ANALGESIC-BARBITURATE COMBINATIONS**

GENERIC (CHEMICAL) NAME	BRAND (TRADE) NAME	DOSAGE FORMS AND STRENGTHS
Butalbital, aspirin, and caffeine	FIORINAL	Capsules: 50 mg butalbital, 325 mg aspirin, and 40 mg caffeine Tablets: 50 mg butalbital, 325 mg aspirin, and 40 mg caffeine

DRUG PROFILE

The combination of butalbital (a barbiturate), aspirin, and caffeine is used to treat tension (muscle contraction) headaches. Aspirin blocks the production of naturally occurring triggers of pain and inflammation called prostaglandins. Butalbital produces a calming effect, and caffeine strengthens the action of aspirin.

BEFORE USING THIS DRUG

Let your doctor know *IF*

You have ever had allergic reactions or other problems with ■ any barbiturates ■ aspirin or any other salicylates ■ indomethacin ■ ibuprofen ■ caffeine ■ mefanic acid ■ phenylbutazone ■ sodium benzoate ■ tartrazine (FD&C Yellow Dye No. 5).

You have ever had any of the following medical problems: ■ hay fever ■ asthma or other lung disease ■ ulcers, gastritis, or any other digestive disorders ■ liver disease ■ kidney disease ■ systemic lupus erythematosus ■ glucose-6-phosphate dehydrogenase (G-6-PD) deficiency ■ vitamin K deficiency ■ pyruvate kinase deficiency ■ nasal polyps ■ chronic hives ■ chronic stuffy nose ■ rheumatic fever ■ heart or blood vessel disease ■ any bleeding disorder ■ recent oral surgery ■ diabetes ■ porphyria ■ mental illness ■ glaucoma ■ anemia ■ overactive thyroid ■ high or low blood pressure ■ drug abuse, including alcoholism.

You are taking any of the following medicines: ■ aspirin or aspirinlike medicine
■ medicine for arthritis or gout ■ anticoagulants (blood thinners) ■ corticosteroids
■ antacids ■ any medicine containing alcohol ■ beta-blockers (eg, propranolol,
atenolol, metoprolol) ■ medicine for high blood pressure ■ medicine for seizures
■ medicine for diabetes ■ methotrexate (medicine for cancer or severe psoriasis)
■ procarbazine (medicine for cancer) ■ other medicine for cancer ■ nitrates (medicine for chest pain) ■ medicine to make the urine more alkaline or more acidic
■ isoniazid (medicine for tuberculosis) ■ medicine for colds, cough, or hay fever
■ antihistamines ■ tranquilizers ■ sleep medicines ■ appetite suppressants
■ muscle relaxants ■ narcotics or other prescription pain-killers ■ barbiturates
■ medicine for depression ■ male hormones ■ thyroid hormones ■ digoxin or digitalis (heart medicines) ■ phenytoin (medicine for seizures) ■ quinidine (medicine
for abnormal heart rhythms) ■ theophylline (medicine for asthma) ■ penicillin, chloramphenicol, doxycycline, griseofulvin, or metronidazole (antibiotics) ■ vitamin D or K.

SPECIAL RESTRICTIONS WHILE TAKING THIS DRUG

FOOD AND DRUG INTERACTIONS

Other Drugs	Do not take any other drugs, including over-the-counter (OTC) drugs, before checking with your doctor. This medicine increases the effects of drugs that depress the central nervous system—such as antihistamines; medicine for hay fever, allergies, or colds; sleep medicines; tranquilizers; narcotics or other prescription pain-killers; muscle relaxants; and medicine for seizures.
	It is a good idea not to take other medicines that contain salicylates (even medicines that are applied to the skin). Check the labels of OTC products, such as special shampoos, lotions, and creams, to see if they contain aspirin, salicylic acid, or other salicylate drugs.
Foods and Beverages	Because this drug contains caffeine, you should probably limit your intake of caffeine-containing foods and beverages.

Alcohol	Avoid alcohol while taking this medicine; this combination can be dangerous, as well as irritating to the stomach.

No special restrictions on smoking.

DAILY LIVING

Driving	This drug may cause dizziness or loss of alertness. Be careful when driving, operating household appliances, or doing any other tasks that require alertness until you know how this drug affects you.
Examinations or Tests	It is important for you to keep all appointments with your doctor so that your progress can be checked. Ask your doctor every couple of months if you need to keep taking this medicine.
Other Precautions	Take this medicine exactly as prescribed by your doctor; taking it more often or for a longer period of time than prescribed may make it habit-forming. If you suspect that this medicine is not working, do not increase the dose without first checking with your doctor.
	If you accidentally take an overdose of this medicine, go to an emergency room immediately.
	Also, let your doctor know if you notice a buzzing or ringing sound in your ears, since this may be a sign that you are taking too much of this medicine.
	Tell any doctor or dentist you consult that you are taking this drug, especially if you will be undergoing any type of surgery.

If you have diabetes, be aware that false urine-sugar tests may occur while you are taking this drug. Check with your doctor before increasing the dose of any diabetes medicine you may be taking.

Helpful Hints	If this drug upsets your stomach, taking it with meals, milk, or water should help.

No special restrictions on exertion and exercise, sun exposure, or exposure to excessive heat or cold.

POSSIBLE SIDE EFFECTS

Although this list of adverse effects may seem somewhat intimidating, keep in mind that some are quite rare. Of course, should these or any other problems arise while you are on medication, it is always a good idea to consult your doctor.

IF YOU DEVELOP

cold, clammy skin ■ very slow or fast heartbeat ■ dizziness ■ drowsiness ■ light-headedness ■ confusion ■ slurred speech ■ chest pain ■ wheezing or other difficulty in breathing ■ loss of balance ■ fever ■ severe or continuing headache ■ swelling of the tip of the penis ■ pain in urination ■ blood in urine ■ decreased urination ■ seizures ■ diarrhea ■ extreme excitement or nervousness ■ hallucinations ■ talkativeness or incoherence ■ personality changes ■ tremors ■ severe or continuing nausea or vomiting ■ continuing stomach pain ■ increased sweating ■ increased thirst ■ visual disturbances ■ uncontrollable flapping movements of the hands ■ watery eyes ■ fainting

WHAT TO DO

Urgent Get in touch with your doctor immediately.

bleeding lip sores or other mouth sores ■ bleeding (including nosebleed) or bruising ■ muscle or joint pain, or any other pain ■ scaly, red skin ■ rash or hives ■ swollen eyes, face, or lips ■ red, itching eyes ■ stuffy nose ■ depression ■ agitation ■ extreme tiredness ■ yellowing of eyes or skin	**May be serious** Check with your doctor as soon as possible.
clumsiness ■ "hangover" feeling ■ anxiety ■ constipation ■ nausea or vomiting ■ nightmares ■ sleeplessness ■ irritability	If symptoms are disturbing or persist, let your doctor know.

STORAGE INSTRUCTIONS

Store in a cool, dark place (not in a bathroom medicine cabinet). If you notice a vinegarlike odor coming from the bottle, this means that the drug is breaking down and should be discarded.

STOPPING OR INTERRUPTING THERAPY

Take this medicine exactly as prescribed by your doctor. If you are taking this medicine on a regular schedule and you miss a dose, take it as soon as possible. If it is almost time for your next dose, skip the missed dose and resume your regular schedule.

SPECIAL CONSIDERATIONS FOR THOSE OVER SIXTY-FIVE

Older people may be especially prone to such side effects as difficulty in breathing, digestive upset, urinary problems, excitement, depression, and confusion.

CONDITION: **MIGRAINE HEADACHE**

CATEGORY: **ERGOT ALKALOIDS**

GENERIC (CHEMICAL) NAME	BRAND (TRADE) NAME	DOSAGE FORMS AND STRENGTHS
Ergotamine tartrate	ERGOSTAT	Sublingual tablets: 2 mg
	MEDIHALER ERGOTAMINE	Aerosol spray: 9 mg per ml
Ergotamine tartrate and caffeine	CAFERGOT	Capsules: 1 mg ergotamine tartrate and 100 mg caffeine
		Rectal suppositories: 2 mg ergotamine and 100 mg caffeine
	WIGRAINE	Tablets: 1 mg ergotamine tartrate and 100 mg caffeine
		Rectal suppositories: 2 mg ergotamine and 100 mg caffeine

DRUG PROFILE

Ergotamine is used to treat migraine headaches. By narrowing the blood vessels in the head, this drug relieves the pain of migraine (which results from an expansion of the blood vessels in the head). Some ergotamine preparations also contain caffeine, which, in addition to narrowing the blood vessels in the head, speeds up the absorption of ergotamine.

BEFORE USING THIS DRUG

Let your doctor know *IF*

You have ever had allergic reactions or other problems with ■ ergot alkaloids ■ caffeine.

You have ever had any of the following medical problems: ■ angina (chest pain) ■ phlebitis, hardening of the arteries, or Raynaud's syndrome (poor circulation in the fingers and toes) ■ high blood pressure ■ liver disease ■ kidney disease ■ sepsis or other infections ■ peptic ulcer ■ malnutrition.

With aerosol form of drug only: ■ asthma.

You are taking any of the following medicines: ■ methysergide ■ beta-blockers (eg, propranolol, atenolol, metoprolol).

SPECIAL RESTRICTIONS WHILE TAKING THIS DRUG

FOOD AND DRUG INTERACTIONS

Alcohol	Avoid alcohol, which can aggravate headache.
Smoking	Nicotine aggravates the narrowing of the blood vessels of the arms and legs that may occur with this drug. If you smoke, try to stop or at least cut down.

No special restrictions on other drugs or foods and beverages.

DAILY LIVING

Excessive Cold	Avoid exposure to excessive cold, which aggravates the narrowing of the blood vessels in the arms and legs that may occur with this drug.
Examinations or Tests	If you need to take this drug frequently, your doctor may wish to examine you regularly to make sure that the drug is not causing harmful narrowing of the blood vessels in your arms and legs.
Other Precautions	Be careful not to exceed the dose your doctor recommends. Taking too much of this medicine can cause serious side effects.

Let your doctor know if you develop an infection while taking this medicine.

Helpful Hints

This medicine works best if you take it at the first sign of a headache. Once you have taken your medicine, lie down and relax in a quiet, darkened room.

If you have been storing the suppository form of this medicine in a warm place, it may be too soft to use. Put it in the refrigerator for half an hour or run cold water over the wrapped suppository before use.

No special restrictions on driving, exertion and exercise, sun exposure, or exposure to excessive heat.

POSSIBLE SIDE EFFECTS

Although this list of adverse effects may seem somewhat intimidating, keep in mind that some are quite rare. Of course, should these or any other problems arise while you are on medication, it is always a good idea to consult your doctor.

IF YOU DEVELOP

seizures ■ coma ■ severe loss of alertness ■ fainting ■ chest pain ■ stomach pain or bloating ■ extreme thirst ■ red or purple blisters on the hands or feet

WHAT TO DO

Urgent Get in touch with your doctor immediately.

weak pulse ■ slow or fast heartbeat ■ weakness ■ muscle pain ■ numbness, coldness, or paleness of the arms or legs ■ swelling of the feet or legs ■ itching ■ arm, leg, or back pain ■ confusion ■ blurred vision

May be serious Check with your doctor as soon as possible.

After you STOP taking this medicine: headache

nausea or vomiting ■ drowsiness ■ sleep disturbances ■ diarrhea ■ dizziness	If symptoms are disturbing or persist, let your doctor know.

STORAGE INSTRUCTIONS

Store in a cool, dark place (not in a bathroom medicine cabinet). Suppositories should be stored in the refrigerator.

STOPPING OR INTERRUPTING THERAPY

If you have been taking this medicine frequently for a prolonged period, you should not suddenly stop taking it. Discuss with your doctor how to stop gradually to avoid unpleasant aftereffects.

SPECIAL CONSIDERATIONS FOR THOSE OVER SIXTY-FIVE

Older people may be more sensitive to the tendency of this drug to narrow the blood vessels of the arms and legs. Older people who have narrowed coronary arteries may also be more vulnerable to chest pain while taking this medicine.

CONDITION: **MIGRAINE HEADACHE**

CATEGORY: **ERGOT ALKALOIDS**

GENERIC (CHEMICAL) NAME	BRAND (TRADE) NAME	DOSAGE FORMS AND STRENGTHS
Methysergide	SANSERT	Tablets: 2 mg

DRUG PROFILE

Methysergide is used to prevent frequent or severe vascular headaches including migraine and cluster headaches. This drug cannot stop a vascular headache attack once it has started. Methysergide acts by narrowing the blood vessels in the head. (The head pain of migraine results from an expansion of those blood vessels.)

BEFORE USING THIS DRUG

Let your doctor know *IF*

You have ever had allergic reactions or other problems with ■ methysergide ■ ergot alkaloids ■ tartrazine (FD&C Yellow Dye No. 5).

You have ever had any of the following medical problems: ■ angina (chest pain) ■ hardening of the arteries ■ valvular or other heart or blood vessel disease ■ high blood pressure ■ asthma or other lung disease ■ liver disease ■ kidney disease ■ serious infection ■ rheumatoid arthritis ■ systemic lupus erythematosus ■ scleroderma ■ fibrotic diseases, including heart murmurs ■ peripheral vascular disease, including phlebitis and cellulitis.

You are taking any of the following medicines: ■ ergotamine or medicines containing ergotamine ■ beta-blockers (eg, propranolol, atenolol, metoprolol).

SPECIAL RESTRICTIONS WHILE TAKING THIS DRUG

FOOD AND DRUG INTERACTIONS

Alcohol	Avoid alcohol, which can aggravate headache.

No special restrictions on other drugs, foods and beverages, or smoking.

DAILY LIVING

Driving	This drug may cause drowsiness, light-headedness, and dizziness, and may also affect mental alertness and physical coordination. Be careful when driving, operating household appliances, or doing any other tasks that require alertness until you know how this drug affects you.
Excessive Cold	Try to avoid exposure to very cold temperatures while taking this medicine, since cold may increase the chance of negative side effects.

Examinations or Tests	It is important for you to keep all appointments with your doctor so that your progress can be checked.

Other Precautions	Do not take more than three tablets a day to prevent a migraine or four tablets a day to prevent cluster headaches. If the amount of medicine prescribed does not seem to be working, do not increase your intake without first checking with your doctor. Taking this medicine more often or for a longer period of time than prescribed by your doctor makes you more prone to developing side effects.
	If you develop edema (swelling due to water retention), consult your doctor, who may reduce your dosage of this drug or prescribe a diuretic. Limiting your salt intake may also help correct this problem.

Helpful Hints	This medicine may cause weight gain. Your doctor may suggest that you reduce your caloric intake.
	This medicine may upset your stomach; your doctor may advise you to take it with meals.

No special restrictions on exertion and exercise, sun exposure, or exposure to excessive heat.

POSSIBLE SIDE EFFECTS

Although this list of adverse effects may seem somewhat intimidating, keep in mind that some are quite rare. Of course, should these or any other problems arise while you are on medication, it is always a good idea to consult your doctor.

IF YOU DEVELOP	WHAT TO DO
chest pain ■ shortness of breath ■ swelling of hands, legs, or ankles ■ pale or cold hands or feet ■ loss of weight or appetite ■ fever ■ pain or cramps in flank, groin, leg, or lower back ■ numbness or coldness in fingers, toes, or face ■ weakness in legs ■ pain or difficulty in urination ■ decreased urination ■ severe dizziness ■ general ill feeling ■ fatigue	**Urgent** Get in touch with your doctor immediately.
itching ■ weak pulse ■ visual disturbances ■ changes in heart rate ■ feelings of excitement or unreality ■ cloudy thinking ■ hallucinations ■ nightmares ■ "high" feeling ■ restlessness ■ nervousness ■ confusion ■ hypersensitivity ■ muscle or joint pain ■ clumsiness	**May be serious** Check with your doctor as soon as possible.
dizziness or light-headedness, especially when getting up from a reclining or sitting position ■ drowsiness ■ sleeplessness ■ diarrhea ■ nausea, vomiting, or stomach pain ■ heartburn ■ constipation ■ depression ■ sleep disturbances ■ hair loss ■ flushing ■ weight gain ■ spots on the skin	If symptoms are disturbing or persist, let your doctor know.

STORAGE INSTRUCTIONS

Store in a cool, dark place (not in a bathroom medicine cabinet).

STOPPING OR INTERRUPTING THERAPY

If you miss a dose of this medicine, skip the missed dose, and resume your regular schedule. Do not take two doses at the same time. If you have been taking this medicine for several weeks, do not suddenly stop taking it without consulting your doctor. You may be advised to stop taking it gradually to avoid unpleasant side effects. Your doctor will probably not want you to take this medicine for more than six months at a time; if the doctor does suggest a rest from this medicine (usually about three to four weeks), follow instructions carefully. Let your doctor know if your headaches return after you have stopped taking this medicine.

SPECIAL CONSIDERATIONS FOR THOSE OVER SIXTY-FIVE

Older people, especially those with blood vessel problems, are more likely to experience side effects with this medicine.

CONDITION: **MIGRAINE HEADACHE**

CATEGORY: **BETABLOCKERS**

GENERIC (CHEMICAL) NAME	BRAND (TRADE) NAME	DOSAGE FORMS AND STRENGTHS
Propranolol hydrochloride	INDERAL	Tablets: 10, 20, 40, 60, 80, 90 mg
	INDERAL LA	Capsules: 60, 80, 120, 160 mg

DRUG PROFILE

Beta-adrenergic blocking drugs (beta-blockers) are used to control high blood pressure. Some are used for other conditions such as angina, heart arrhythmias, migraine headaches, and hypertrophic subaortic stenosis (a disease of the heart muscle). Some have also been found to improve a person's chance of survival for several years following a heart attack. By blocking certain nerve impulses, these medicines reduce the workload of the heart and help the heart to beat more regularly.

For complete information on this drug, see pages 59–64.

Chapter 3
Disorders of the Digestive System

PEPTIC ULCERS

Ulcers are small, craterlike sores that develop in the lining of the stomach (gastric ulcers) or the duodenum (duodenal ulcers), the first section of the small intestine. The term *peptic ulcer* is sometimes used to describe both types of ulcer. Learning how your ulcer may have developed and understanding what irritates it will help you work with your doctor to establish an effective treatment plan.

CAUSES

Peptic ulcers occur only in those regions of the digestive system that come in contact with digestive juices secreted by the stomach. These juices include stomach acid (hydrochloric acid) and a protein-digesting enzyme called pepsin. Many people with duodenal ulcers manufacture an excess of digestive juices. In contrast, many people with gastric ulcers have less stomach acid than would be expected. Scientists believe, therefore, that poor resistance of the protective mucous lining of the stomach and duodenum may be an important factor leading to the development of a peptic ulcer.

Duodenal ulcers are more common than gastric ulcers. It is estimated that the duodenal variety affects 10 percent of the male population at any one time (men are affected three times more frequently than women). People in their forties and fifties are the most likely to be affected. Gastric ulcers are about equally common in men and women, and they generally strike an older population. Peak incidence is in the fifties and sixties. Also, extensive use of aspirin or nonsteroidal anti-inflammatory drugs (NSAIDs) is known to increase the risk of peptic ulcers. This risk is particularly important in older people.

Helicobacter pylori is a recently discovered type of bacteria that is commonly found in the lining of the stomach. In some patients, infection with *Helicobacter pylori* seems to play a role in the development of ulcer disease.

DIAGNOSIS

The symptoms of ulcer disease are less specific in people over fifty, and the beginnings of the ulcer may be harder to pinpoint. The most common symptom of duodenal ulcer is pain. The pain, which is usually felt in the middle of the upper abdomen, between the breastbone and the navel, varies from a hunger pang to a continuous gnawing or burning sensation. It usually occurs two or three hours after eating, when the stomach is empty, and is usually relieved by antacids or eating. Other common symptoms include a bloated feeling after you eat.

Symptoms of a gastric ulcer are similar to those of a duodenal ulcer but tend to be less predictable. Again, there is pain, which may be felt in the same place as that of a duodenal ulcer or slightly higher. The pain sometimes occurs when the stomach is full, leading to a loss of appetite and weight loss. Other signs of a gastric ulcer include indigestion and occasionally even heartburn. Both duodenal and gastric ulcers can cause such serious complications as gastrointestinal bleeding, perforation (erosion of the ulcer all the way through the wall of the stomach or the duodenum), or obstruction of the digestive tract.

If you develop suspicious symptoms, your doctor will order some diagnostic tests. An X-ray film called an upper gastrointestinal series (or UGI) may be done. In this test, the person swallows a barium suspension, a thick, chalky liquid, which allows the radiologist to see the shape of the stomach and small intestine and to identify the ulcer. Another diagnostic procedure that may be done is known as endoscopy. Using a gastroscope—a flexible fiberoptic tube with a light at one end inserted through the mouth—the doctor can see the ulcer crater, photograph it for further study, and take tissue samples (biopsy) for study under the microscope.

TREATMENT

Several different types of drugs are available today for treating ulcers. A common treatment plan includes liquid antacids, which neutralize stomach acid, in addition to one of the following medicines called histamine H-2 blockers: cimetidine, ranitidine, famotidine, nizatidine, or a local protective agent like sucralfate. These drugs are effective in healing and controlling symptoms of peptic ulcer disease. Also, another drug, misoprostol, is used to block acid secretion and protect the stomach lining in patients who have to take large quantities of antiarthritis drugs. New drug therapies are being developed to treat ulcer disease related to infection with *Helicobacter pylori*. These therapies usually include antibiotics, bismuth subsalicylate (Pepto-Bismol), and an H-2 blocker. For more detailed information, see the charts on pages 365–385.

Your doctor may prescribe other medicines according to your specific needs. Rarely, drugs that prevent or relieve spasm—most often used for treating irritable bowel syndrome (see page 412)—may also be used in the treatment of peptic ulcers. However, most doctors do not recommend antispasmodics for older people because they can cause such potentially serious side effects as difficulty in swallowing and urinating, as well as constipation.

Antacids (available under many brand names) reduce the amount of acid in the upper digestive tract by neutralizing (buffering) it. Liquid antacids are generally more effective than tablets. Many doctors prescribe antacids to be taken one to three hours after meals and at bedtime (food acts as a buffer in the hour following a meal).

In most people, medicine will heal ulcers. But surgery is sometimes necessary, particularly if an ulcer complication occurs. Most people get along well following surgery—but it is only performed if medicine does not work or if a sudden serious complication develops.

There are things you can do—or not do—to help your ulcer heal. Smoking cigarettes has consistently been found to slow the healing of an ulcer, so you'd be wise to stop. Avoidance of aspirin and other antiarthritis drugs and alcohol is also advisable and important. As for your diet, consuming a lot of milk and cream is no longer considered an ulcer cure-all. Instead, the main dietary rule is to eat regular, nutritious meals. Avoid any foods that seem to bother you. Although the role of stress and anxiety in ulcer disease is not clear, it's a good idea to try to relax, avoid irritating situations, and work off tensions by exercising (at a level recommended by your doctor).

OUTLOOK

If you follow your doctor's recommendations, the chances are excellent that your ulcer will heal within a month or two. You may experience flare-ups from time to time, or you may go for years without feeling even a twinge of pain.

If your peptic ulcer recurs periodically, your doctor may put you on a low-dose maintenance therapy with one of the following antiulcer drugs: cimetidine, famotidine, nizatidine, or ranitidine. This may help reduce the recurrence of the ulcer and help control the disease.

CONDITION: **PEPTIC ULCERS**

CATEGORY: **ANTIULCER AGENTS**

GENERIC (CHEMICAL) NAME	BRAND (TRADE) NAME	DOSAGE FORMS AND STRENGTHS
Cimetidine	TAGAMET	Liquid: 300 mg per tsp Tablets: 200, 300, 400, 800 mg

DRUG PROFILE

Cimetidine, which blocks the release of stomach acid, is used to heal duodenal (intestinal) and gastric (stomach) ulcers. It is also used to prevent the recurrence of ulcers. This drug may also be prescribed for other conditions in which the stomach produces excess acid.

BEFORE USING THIS DRUG

Let your doctor know *IF*

You have ever had allergic reactions or other problems with ■ cimetidine, ranitidine, nizatidine, or famotidine.

You have ever had any of the following medical problems: ■ kidney disease ■ liver disease.

You are taking any of the following medicines: ■ other ulcer medicine ■ aspirin or other medicine for arthritis ■ anticoagulants (blood thinners) ■ theophylline (medicine for asthma) ■ diazepam or chlordiazepoxide (tranquilizers) ■ medicine for seizures (phenytoin) ■ medicine for high blood pressure ■ antacids ■ medicines with enteric coating ■ beta-blockers (propranolol, metoprolol, atenolol) ■ calcium channel blockers (eg, diltiazem, nifedipine, verapamil) ■ medicine for abnormal heart rhythm (procainamide, quinidine).

SPECIAL RESTRICTIONS WHILE TAKING THIS DRUG

FOOD AND DRUG INTERACTIONS

Other Drugs	Check with your doctor before taking any other drugs. A number of drugs can be affected by cimetidine. Your doctor may want to adjust the dose of cimetidine or the other medicines.
	Your doctor may advise you to avoid certain drugs, such as aspirin and any other medicine for arthritis and pain, that may aggravate your symptoms. However, if it is critical that you take this medicine, your doctor may instruct you to take cimetidine along with it.
	Allow at least one hour between the time you take this drug and the time you take an antacid.
Foods and Beverages	Your doctor may advise you to avoid certain foods and beverages (coffee, cola drinks, cocoa, chocolate) known to irritate the ulcer.
	If you are taking several doses of this medicine a day, you will probably be instructed to take them at meals and at bedtime.
Alcohol	Avoid alcohol, which can irritate an ulcer.
Smoking	Cigarette smoking irritates the stomach lining and can decrease the benefits of this drug. If you smoke, try to stop or at least cut down.

DAILY LIVING

Examinations or Tests	Your doctor may want to perform an endoscopy after a period of treatment in order to monitor the healing process, particularly if you have a gastric ulcer.

| Other Precautions | If the pain continues or worsens after several days of treatment, contact your doctor immediately. |

No special restrictions on driving, exertion and exercise, sun exposure, or exposure to excessive heat or cold.

POSSIBLE SIDE EFFECTS

Although this list of adverse effects may seem somewhat intimidating, keep in mind that some are quite rare. Of course, should these or any other problems arise while you are on medication, it is always a good idea to consult your doctor.

IF YOU DEVELOP	WHAT TO DO
confusion ■ depression ■ agitation ■ tiredness or weakness ■ drowsiness ■ bleeding or bruising ■ sore throat or fever ■ joint or muscle pain ■ rash or hives ■ difficulty in breathing ■ rapid or irregular heartbeat ■ severe stomach pain	**May be serious** Check with your doctor as soon as possible.
diarrhea ■ dizziness ■ headache ■ sore or enlarged breasts in men ■ male impotence ■ hair loss ■ nausea ■ vomiting ■ constipation	If symptoms are disturbing or persist, let your doctor know.

STORAGE INSTRUCTIONS

Store in a cool, dark place (not in a bathroom medicine cabinet). If your medicine is in a liquid form, make sure that it does not freeze.

STOPPING OR INTERRUPTING THERAPY

Take this drug for the full length of time prescribed (usually six to eight weeks), even if you feel better, unless otherwise directed by your doctor. If you miss a dose, take it as soon as possible. If it is almost time for your next dose, skip the missed dose and resume your regular schedule. Do not take two doses at the same time.

SPECIAL CONSIDERATIONS FOR THOSE OVER SIXTY-FIVE

Those older people who have reduced kidney function may require a reduction in dosage.

CONDITION: **PEPTIC ULCERS**

CATEGORY: **ANTIULCER AGENTS**

GENERIC (CHEMICAL) NAME	BRAND (TRADE) NAME	DOSAGE FORMS AND STRENGTHS
Nizatidine	AXID	Capsules: 150, 300 mg

DRUG PROFILE

Nizatidine, which blocks the release of stomach acid, is used to heal duodenal (intestinal) ulcers. It is also used to prevent ulcers from recurring.

BEFORE USING THIS DRUG

Let your doctor know *IF*

You have ever had allergic reactions or other problems with ■ cimetidine, famotidine, nizatidine, or ranitidine.

You have ever had any of the following medical problems: ■ kidney disease ■ liver disease.

You are taking any of the following medicines: ■ antacids ■ aspirin or other medicine for arthritis ■ ketoconazole (medicine for fungal infections).

SPECIAL RESTRICTIONS WHILE TAKING THIS DRUG

FOOD AND DRUG INTERACTIONS

Other Drugs	Your doctor may advise you to avoid certain drugs, such as aspirin and any other medicine for arthritis and pain, that may aggravate your symptoms. However, if it is crucial that you take this medicine, your

doctor may instruct you to take nizatidine along with it.

Allow at least one hour between the time you take this drug and the time you take an antacid.

Foods and Beverages	Your doctor may advise you to avoid certain foods and beverages (coffee, cola drinks, cocoa, chocolate) known to irritate the ulcers.
	If you are taking several doses of this medicine a day, you will probably be instructed to take them at meals and at bedtime.
Alcohol	Avoid alcohol, which can irritate an ulcer.
Smoking	Cigarette smoking irritates the stomach lining and can decrease the benefits of this drug. If you smoke, try to stop or at least cut down.
Driving	This drug may cause drowsiness. Be careful when driving, operating household appliances, or doing any other tasks that require alertness until you know how this drug affects you.
Examinations or Tests	Your doctor may want to perform an endoscopy after a period of treatment in order to monitor the healing process. Blood or urine tests may also be required.
Other Precautions	Tell any doctor you consult that you are taking this medicine, especially if skin tests for allergies or tests for stomach acid will be performed.
	If the pain continues or worsens after several days of treatment, contact your doctor immediately.

No special restrictions on exertion and exercise, sun exposure, or exposure to excessive heat or cold.

POSSIBLE SIDE EFFECTS

Although this list of adverse effects may seem somewhat intimidating, keep in mind that some are quite rare. Of course, should these or any other problems arise while you are on medication, it is always a good idea to consult your doctor.

IF YOU DEVELOP	WHAT TO DO
fast heartbeat ■ sore throat and fever ■ bleeding or bruising ■ tiredness or weakness	**May be serious** Check with your doctor as soon as possible.
drowsiness ■ swelling of breasts or breast tenderness (in both men and women) ■ rash, hives, or other skin problems ■ increased sweating ■ joint or muscle pain	If symptoms are disturbing or persist, let your doctor know.

STORAGE INSTRUCTIONS

Store in a cool, dark place (not in a bathroom medicine cabinet).

STOPPING OR INTERRUPTING THERAPY

Take this drug for the full length of time prescribed (usually four weeks), even if you feel better, unless otherwise directed by your doctor. If you miss a dose, take it as soon as possible. If it is almost time for your next dose, skip the missed dose and resume your regular schedule. Do not take two doses at the same time.

SPECIAL CONSIDERATIONS FOR THOSE OVER SIXTY-FIVE

None.

CONDITION: **PEPTIC ULCERS**

CATEGORY: **ANTIULCER AGENTS**

GENERIC (CHEMICAL) NAME	BRAND (TRADE) NAME	DOSAGE FORMS AND STRENGTHS
Ranitidine	ZANTAC	Syrup: 15 mg per ml Tablets: 150, 300 mg

DRUG PROFILE

Ranitidine, which blocks the release of stomach acid, is used to treat active duodenal (intestinal) and gastric (stomach) ulcers. It may also be prescribed for gastrointestinal reflux and for other conditions in which the stomach produces excess acid.

BEFORE USING THIS DRUG

Let your doctor know *IF*

You have ever had allergic reactions or other problems with ■ ranitidine, cimetidine, nizatidine, or famotidine.

You have ever had any of the following medical problems: ■ kidney disease ■ liver disease.

You are taking any of the following medicines: ■ antacids ■ medicine for asthma ■ medicine for high blood pressure ■ heart medicine ■ anticoagulants (blood thinners) ■ tranquilizers ■ muscle relaxants ■ acetaminophen ■ aspirin or other medicine for arthritis ■ medicines with enteric coating.

SPECIAL RESTRICTIONS WHILE TAKING THIS DRUG

FOOD AND DRUG INTERACTIONS

Other Drugs	Your doctor may advise you to avoid certain drugs, such as aspirin and any other medicine for arthritis and pain, that may aggravate your symptoms. However, if it is critical that you take this medicine, your doctor may instruct you to take ranitidine along with it. Allow at least an hour between the time you take this drug and the time you take an antacid.
Foods and Beverages	Your doctor may advise you to avoid certain foods and beverages (coffee, cola drinks, cocoa, chocolate) known to irritate an ulcer.
Alcohol	Avoid alcohol, which can irritate an ulcer.
Smoking	Cigarette smoking irritates the stomach lining and can decrease the benefits of this drug. If you smoke, try to stop or at least cut down.

DAILY LIVING

Examinations or Tests	Your doctor may want to perform an endoscopy after a period of treatment in order to monitor the healing process, especially if you have a gastric ulcer.
Other Precautions	If the pain continues or worsens after several days of treatment, contact your doctor immediately.

No special restrictions on driving, exertion and exercise, sun exposure, or exposure to excessive heat or cold.

POSSIBLE SIDE EFFECTS

Although this list of adverse effects may seem somewhat intimidating, keep in mind that some are quite rare. Of course, should these or any other problems arise while you are on medication, it is always a good idea to consult your doctor.

IF YOU DEVELOP	**WHAT TO DO**
confusion ■ depression ■ agitation ■ irregular or fast heartbeat ■ male impotence ■ general ill feeling ■ breast swelling in men ■ difficulty in breathing ■ yellowing of eyes or skin ■ pallor ■ weakness ■ fatigue ■ stomach pain ■ back pain ■ fever ■ dizziness ■ nausea ■ vomiting	**May be serious** Check with your doctor as soon as possible.
constipation ■ headache ■ rash ■ drowsiness	If symptoms are disturbing or persist, let your doctor know.

STORAGE INSTRUCTIONS

Store in a cool, dark place (not in a bathroom medicine cabinet).

STOPPING OR INTERRUPTING THERAPY

This drug should be taken without interruption for the full length of time prescribed by your doctor (usually about four weeks), even once you begin to feel better. If you miss a dose, take it as soon as possible. If it is almost time for your next dose, skip the missed dose and resume your regular schedule. Do not take two doses at the same time.

SPECIAL CONSIDERATIONS FOR THOSE OVER SIXTY-FIVE

Those older people who have reduced kidney function may require a reduction in dosage.

CONDITION: **PEPTIC ULCERS**

CATEGORY: **ANTIULCER AGENTS**

GENERIC (CHEMICAL) NAME	BRAND (TRADE) NAME	DOSAGE FORMS AND STRENGTHS
Famotidine	PEPCID	Suspension: 40 mg per tsp Tablets: 20, 40 mg

DRUG PROFILE

Famotidine, which blocks the release of stomach acid, is used to treat active duodenal (intestinal) and gastric (stomach) ulcers. It may also be prescribed for other conditions in which the stomach produces excess acid.

BEFORE USING THIS DRUG

Let your doctor know *IF*

You have ever had allergic reactions or other problems with ■ famotidine, cimetidine, nizatidine, or ranitidine.

You have ever had any of the following medical problems: ■ kidney disease ■ liver disease.

You are taking any of the following medicines: ■ medicines with enteric coating.

SPECIAL RESTRICTIONS WHILE TAKING THIS DRUG

FOOD AND DRUG INTERACTIONS

Other Drugs	Your doctor may advise you to avoid certain drugs, such as aspirin and any other medicine for arthritis and pain, that may aggravate your symptoms. However, if it is critical that you take this medicine, your

doctor may instruct you to take famotidine along
with it.

Allow at least an hour between the time you take this
drug and the time you take an antacid.

Foods and Beverages	Your doctor may advise you to avoid certain foods and beverages (coffee, cola drinks, cocoa, chocolate) known to irritate an ulcer.
Alcohol	Alcohol should be avoided because it irritates an ulcer.
Smoking	Cigarette smoking irritates the stomach lining and can decrease the benefits of this drug. If you smoke, try to stop or at least cut down.

DAILY LIVING

Examinations or Tests	Your doctor may want to perform an endoscopy after a period of treatment in order to monitor the healing process.
Other Precautions	If the pain continues or worsens after several days of treatment, contact your doctor immediately.

No special restrictions on driving, exertion and exercise, sun exposure, or exposure
to excessive heat or cold.

POSSIBLE SIDE EFFECTS

Although this list of adverse effects may seem somewhat intimidating, keep in mind that some are quite rare. Of course, should these or any other problems arise while you are on medication, it is always a good idea to consult your doctor.

IF YOU DEVELOP	WHAT TO DO
confusion ■ irregular or fast heartbeat ■ difficulty in breathing	**May be serious** Check with your doctor as soon as possible.
diarrhea ■ constipation ■ dizziness ■ headache ■ nausea or vomiting ■ rash or other skin problems ■ stomach discomfort	If symptoms are disturbing or persist, let your doctor know.

STORAGE INSTRUCTIONS

Store in a cool, dark place (not in a bathroom medicine cabinet).

STOPPING OR INTERRUPTING THERAPY

Famotidine should be taken without interruption for the full length of time prescribed by your doctor (usually about four weeks for an active ulcer), even after you begin to feel better. If you miss a dose, take it as soon as possible. If it is almost time for your next dose, skip the missed dose and resume your regular schedule. Do not take two doses at the same time.

SPECIAL CONSIDERATIONS FOR THOSE OVER SIXTY-FIVE

Those older people who have reduced kidney function may require a reduction in dosage.

CONDITION: **PEPTIC ULCERS**

CATEGORY: **ANTIULCER AGENTS**

GENERIC (CHEMICAL) NAME	BRAND (TRADE) NAME	DOSAGE FORMS AND STRENGTHS
Misoprostol	CYTOTEC	Tablets: 100 mcg, 200 mcg

DRUG PROFILE

This drug is used to prevent gastric (stomach) ulcers in people who are taking aspirin or other nonsteroidal anti-inflammatory drugs (NSAIDs) for arthritis and are therefore at risk of developing gastric ulcers. It works by blocking the release of stomach acid and also by protecting the lining of the stomach from the irritating effects of antiarthritis medications.

BEFORE USING THIS DRUG

Let your doctor know *IF*

You have ever had allergic reactions or other problems with ■ misoprostol.

You have ever had any of the following medical problems: ■ kidney disease.

You are taking any of the following medicines: ■ antacids.

SPECIAL RESTRICTIONS WHILE TAKING THIS DRUG

FOOD AND DRUG INTERACTIONS

Other Drugs	Antacids that contain magnesium increase the chance of diarrhea as a side effect while you are taking misoprostol. Do not take magnesium-containing antacids.

Foods and Beverages	This medicine should be taken with meals and at bedtime.
Alcohol	Avoid alcohol, which can weaken the protective lining of the stomach.
Smoking	Cigarette smoking irritates the lining of the stomach and can decrease the benefits of this drug. If you smoke, try to stop or at least cut down.
Other Precautions	Read the patient information leaflet that accompanies the medication. Misoprostol should not be taken by women who can become pregnant because it can cause a miscarriage and possibly dangerous bleeding. Women who have the potential of getting pregnant should have a negative pregnancy test and be on an effective contraceptive before receiving misoprostol. Do not give this drug to anyone else, and especially not to a friend or relative who may be or want to get pregnant.

No special restrictions on driving, exertion and exercise, sun exposure, or exposure to excessive heat or cold.

POSSIBLE SIDE EFFECTS

Although this list of adverse effects may seem somewhat intimidating, keep in mind that some are quite rare. Of course, should these or any other problems arise while you are on medication, it is always a good idea to consult your doctor.

IF YOU DEVELOP

severe drowsiness, dizziness, or light-headedness shakiness ■ seizures ■ shortness of breath ■ abdominal pain ■ diarrhea ■ fever ■ slow or pounding heartbeat

WHAT TO DO

Urgent Get in touch with your doctor immediately.

vaginal bleeding ■ nausea or vomiting ■ gas ■ headache ■ constipation ■ indigestion

May be serious Check with your doctor as soon as possible.

STORAGE INSTRUCTIONS

Store in a cool, dark place (not in a bathroom medicine cabinet).

STOPPING OR INTERRUPTING THERAPY

Misoprostol should be taken for as long as you are taking your aspirin or other medicine for arthritis. If you miss a dose, take it as soon as possible. If it is almost time for your next dose, skip the missed dose and resume your regular schedule. Do not take two doses at the same time.

SPECIAL CONSIDERATIONS FOR THOSE OVER SIXTY-FIVE

None.

CONDITION: **PEPTIC ULCERS**

CATEGORY: **ANTIULCER AGENTS**

GENERIC (CHEMICAL) NAME	BRAND (TRADE) NAME	DOSAGE FORMS AND STRENGTHS
Sucralfate	CARAFATE	Tablets: 1 g

DRUG PROFILE

Sucralfate is used to treat duodenal (intestinal) and occasionally gastric (stomach) ulcers. This drug forms a protective coating over the ulcer, which gives the duodenal lining time to heal. It is also used to prevent the recurrence of ulcers.

BEFORE USING THIS DRUG

Let your doctor know *IF*

You have ever had allergic reactions or other problems with ■ sucralfate.

You have ever had the following medical problem: ■ constipation.

You are taking any of the following medicines: ■ other medicine for ulcers ■ antacids ■ tetracycline ■ phenytoin (medicine for seizures) ■ digoxin or digitalis (heart medicines) ■ ciprofloxacin (Cipro) ■ norfloxacin (Noroxin) ■ theophylline.

SPECIAL RESTRICTIONS WHILE TAKING THIS DRUG

FOOD AND DRUG INTERACTIONS

Other Drugs	Antacids should be taken at least thirty minutes before or after taking your dose of sucralfate. If these medicines are taken close together, sucralfate will not be as effective.
Foods and Beverages	Your doctor may advise you to avoid certain foods and beverages (coffee, cola drinks, cocoa, chocolate) known to irritate an ulcer.
Alcohol	Avoid alcohol, which can irritate an ulcer.
Smoking	Ulcers generally heal faster if you do not smoke. Cigarette smoking irritates the stomach lining and can decrease the benefits of this drug. If you are being treated for an ulcer and you smoke, try to stop or at least cut down.

DAILY LIVING

Helpful Hints	Take this medicine on an empty stomach, one hour before meals and at bedtime, unless instructed otherwise by your doctor.

Do not chew tablets; instead, swallow them with water for best results. If you have difficulty swallowing the tablets, you may crush them in warm water and drink the mixture.

No special restrictions on driving, exertion and exercise, sun exposure, or exposure to excessive heat or cold.

POSSIBLE SIDE EFFECTS

Although this list of adverse effects may seem somewhat intimidating, keep in mind that some are quite rare. Of course, should these or any other problems arise while you are on medication, it is always a good idea to consult your doctor.

IF YOU DEVELOP

dizziness ■ drowsiness ■ dry mouth ■ constipation ■ nausea ■ stomach discomfort ■ back pain ■ rash or itching ■ diarrhea ■ vomiting ■ gas ■ headache

WHAT TO DO

If symptoms are disturbing or persist, let your doctor know.

STORAGE INSTRUCTIONS

Store in a cool, dark place (not in a bathroom medicine cabinet).

STOPPING OR INTERRUPTING THERAPY

This drug should be taken without interruption for the full length of time prescribed by your doctor (usually four to eight weeks), even if your symptoms disappear. If you miss a dose, take it as soon as possible. If it is less than one hour before a meal, skip the missed dose and resume your regular schedule. Do not take two doses at the same time.

SPECIAL CONSIDERATIONS FOR THOSE OVER SIXTY-FIVE

Older people may be more prone to constipation with this drug.

CONDITION: **PEPTIC ULCERS**

CATEGORY: **ANTIULCER AGENTS**

GENERIC (CHEMICAL) NAME	BRAND (TRADE) NAME	DOSAGE FORMS AND STRENGTHS
Propantheline bromide	PRO-BANTHINE	Tablets: 7.5, 15 mg

DRUG PROFILE

Propantheline is used along with other drugs to treat peptic ulcers. This drug works by reducing the amount of acid produced by the stomach.

BEFORE USING THIS DRUG

Let your doctor know *IF*

You have ever had allergic reactions or other problems with ■ propantheline.

You have ever had any of the following medical problems: ■ digestive problems, including colitis or severe diarrhea ■ asthma or other lung disease ■ difficulty in urination or other urinary problems ■ enlarged prostate ■ glaucoma ■ heart or circulatory problems ■ abnormal heart rhythms ■ hiatal hernia ■ high blood pressure ■ kidney disease ■ liver disease ■ myasthenia gravis ■ overactive thyroid.

You are taking any of the following medicines: ■ other medicine for ulcers ■ antacids or medicine for stomach spasms and cramps ■ medicine for diarrhea ■ medicine for Parkinson's disease ■ tranquilizers ■ medicine for nausea ■ medicine for seizures ■ antihistamines ■ medicine for hay fever, coughs, or colds ■ narcotics or other prescription pain-killers ■ sleep medicines ■ medicine for depression ■ digoxin or digitalis (heart medicines) ■ medicine for abnormal heart rhythms ■ potassium-containing medicines or supplements ■ acetaminophen ■ medicine for fungal infections ■ beta-blockers (eg, propranolol, atenolol, metoprolol) ■ thiazide diuretics ■ nitrofurantoin (medicine for urinary tract infections) ■ corticosteroids.

SPECIAL RESTRICTIONS WHILE TAKING THIS DRUG

FOOD AND DRUG INTERACTIONS

Other Drugs	Do not take any other drugs, including over-the-counter (OTC) drugs, before checking with your doctor. This drug may affect how fast your body absorbs other drugs; it also increases the effect of drugs that depress the central nervous system, such as antihistamines; medicine for hay fever, allergies, or colds; sleep medicines; tranquilizers; narcotics or other prescription pain-killers; muscle relaxants; and medicine for seizures. Allow one to two hours between the time you take this drug and the time you take an antacid.
Alcohol	This medicine increases the effect of alcohol, a central nervous system depressant. Avoid alcohol unless your doctor has approved its use.

No special restrictions on foods and beverages or smoking.

DAILY LIVING

Driving	This drug may cause dizziness, drowsiness, or blurred vision. Be careful when driving, operating household appliances, or doing any other tasks that require alertness until you know how this drug affects you.
Exertion and Exercise	This drug may cause you to sweat less. Sweating is your body's natural way of cooling down, and not sweating enough can be dangerous. Use caution not to become overheated when you exercise or exert yourself.

Excessive Heat	See above; use caution during hot weather, since overexertion may result in heat stroke. Avoid extremely hot baths or saunas. Also, check with your doctor if you develop a fever for any reason.
Other Precautions	Tell any doctor or dentist you consult that you are taking this drug, especially if you will be undergoing any type of surgery.
	Take this medicine exactly as prescribed by your doctor; taking it more often or for a longer period of time than prescribed makes you more prone to developing side effects.
Helpful Hints	If your mouth or throat feels dry, chewing sugarless gum or sucking ice chips or sugarless hard candy should help.
	This medicine is generally taken one half to one hour before meals.

No special restrictions on sun exposure or exposure to excessive cold.

POSSIBLE SIDE EFFECTS

Although this list of adverse effects may seem somewhat intimidating, keep in mind that some are quite rare. Of course, should these or any other problems arise while you are on medication, it is always a good idea to consult your doctor.

IF YOU DEVELOP	WHAT TO DO
fever ■ delirium ■ confusion ■ nervousness ■ rash or hives ■ irregular or fast heartbeat	**Urgent** Get in touch with your doctor immediately.
constipation ■ difficulty in urination ■ eye pain ■ flushing ■ restlessness ■ excitement ■ behavior changes	**May be serious** Check with your doctor as soon as possible.

bloating ■ nausea or vomiting ■ dry mouth ■ dizziness ■ headache ■ blurred vision ■ changes in pupil size ■ increased eye sensitivity to light ■ drowsiness ■ weakness ■ decreased sweating ■ loss of taste ■ male impotence ■ sleeplessness

If symptoms are disturbing or persist, let your doctor know.

STORAGE INSTRUCTIONS

Store in a cool, dark place (not in a bathroom medicine cabinet).

STOPPING OR INTERRUPTING THERAPY

If you miss a dose, take it as soon as possible. If it is almost time for your next dose, skip the missed dose and resume your regular schedule. Do not take two doses at the same time.

SPECIAL CONSIDERATIONS FOR THOSE OVER SIXTY-FIVE

Older people may be more prone to such side effects as confusion, excitement, difficulty in urination, blurred vision, and constipation. For this reason, a doctor may want to start treatment with a lower dosage and check the person frequently.

INDIGESTION

You may have noticed that you're just not enjoying mealtimes as much as you used to. This may have nothing to do with the quality of the cuisine but everything to do with the digestive ailments you've been experiencing during or soon after eating. Some people can't get through a meal without feeling gnawing pains in the abdomen. Others get that gassy feeling, even if baked beans weren't on the menu. Still others make it through the meal all right, only to experience a burning chest pain and a sour taste in the mouth. Indigestion is the culprit that can turn mealtime into a medley of digestive complaints. Indigestion is not a precise medical term; it is used to refer to a whole spectrum of abdominal aches, pains, twinges, and discomforts that can detract from your dining pleasure.

Most conditions that cause indigestion are harmless, and you can ease your distress through some self-help measures outlined here. If these measures don't work, consult your doctor for advice. Less frequently, there may be something more serious behind your mealtime miseries, and you should be alert to those symptoms that signal a more urgent need for a medical consultation.

HEARTBURN

Perhaps one of the most universal symptoms of indigestion is heartburn, which occurs when food, stomach acid, and digestive enzymes back up from the stomach into the esophagus. In addition to a temporary burning pain behind the breastbone, there is often an acidic aftertaste and sometimes belching, bloating, nausea, and vomiting. Known medically as gastroesophageal reflux, heartburn is usually caused by a weakness in the lower esophagus; this allows stomach acid and other irritating substances to flow up into the esophagus. Normally, the refluxed material is quickly returned to the stomach. If the irritating substances remain in the lower esophagus too long, they may damage and further weaken this portion of the esophagus.

In other instances, heartburn occurs because digested food is not emptied efficiently from the stomach into the intestines. The longer the food stays in the stomach, the more opportunity there is for it to back up into the esophagus. (It used to be thought that hiatal hernias cause heartburn, but it is now known that the majority of normal people past the age of fifty have a hiatal hernia—a condition in which part of the stomach slides up through the diaphragm into the chest cavity. This condition by itself does not cause heartburn.)

Useful self-help measures to combat heartburn include the shedding of some extra pounds if you're overweight; the avoidance of lifting, bending, and lying down after eating; and wearing clothes that do not bind the waist and abdomen. You may find that not eating for two to three hours before bedtime and elevating the head of your bed six inches or so will prevent your discomfort. (The head of the bed itself should be raised. It is not advised to simply prop up your head with an extra, fluffy pillow.) You may also find that altering your diet by staying away from foods that weaken the lower esophagus (such as fatty foods, chocolate, alcohol, and peppermint) and avoiding foods that irritate the lining of the esophagus (such as acidic fruit juice and spicy tomato drinks) might help relieve the symptoms of heartburn.

Over-the-counter (OTC) antacids can provide quick, short-term relief, curbing the pain within ten minutes or so. If the pain persists past that time, it's a clue that the burning sensation is not heartburn at all but a more severe condition. In either case, it is prudent to check with your doctor.

Another common remedy to relieve heartburn is a combination of antacids and an ingredient called alginic acid (Gaviscon). This compound acts to form a foam barrier that floats on top of the stomach contents and prevents reflux from occurring. Your doctor may be able to prescribe a medicine for heartburn, such as metoclopramide to improve emptying of the stomach (see page 390) or possibly an H-2 blocker such as cimetidine, famotidine, nizatidine, or ranitidine (see pages 368–376) if simpler remedies are not successful. In cases where reflux of stomach contents causes damage to the esophagus and cannot be controlled with other therapies (eg, antacids, alginic acid, and H-2

blockers) a therapy is available. The agent is called omeprazole (Prilosec) and is very effective in reducing acid production by the stomach.

Not every symptom that occurs under the rib cage signals gastroesophageal reflux. If food seems to stick in your throat when you try to swallow, or if your symptoms of heartburn don't go away with the treatment outlined here, your doctor may order some diagnostic tests to rule out other diagnoses (such as peptic ulcer) or complications of the heartburn (such as esophageal scarring or ulcer). During the early phase of evaluation, an upper gastrointestinal series may be performed, which is a special X-ray test that shows the esophagus, stomach, and duodenum. In many cases, additional tests such as endoscopy are needed.

INTESTINAL GAS

It can be painful. Even worse, it can be embarrassing. However, unless it occurs at a socially inappropriate moment, it is usually harmless. And perhaps the best news about gas—a problem familiar to all of us—is that it is often preventable.

Technically known as flatus, gas is shapeless and usually odorless matter that is produced in the digestive system. Gas may cause distress in the upper or lower digestive tract. Upper gas, which lodges in the stomach, is usually caused by swallowing too much air while talking, eating, drinking, or simply chewing. The faster these actions are performed, the more air is swallowed, and the more gas results.

The other type, lower gas, is formed in the large intestine by the action of bacteria on undigested food particles.

Upper gas—with its accompanying belching—can be combated by changing some everyday habits. You'll swallow less air if you don't chew gum, don't use a straw to drink, and don't talk a lot while you eat. If you're in the habit of taking effervescent OTC medicines, you may be making matters worse, not better. The added carbonation in these products increases the amount of swallowed air—and the amount of belching.

What you consume also affects the amount of gas passed rectally, and beans are not the only culprit. Cabbage, broccoli, brussels sprouts, and onions are also gassy, as are carbonated drinks and coffee. Ingestion of milk and milk products, which contain a sugar called lactose, may produce gas in persons who lack the intestinal enzyme that digests lactose. This condition, known as lactose-intolerance, is common in older people because in many people as they get older the intestine no longer produces this enzyme. Also, after any illness with diarrhea, there is a temporary decrease in the function of this enzyme and you may experience gas when ingesting milk and milk products.

You may also find that you've been particularly gassy while dieting. This is because many artificial sweeteners are nondigestible carbohydrates; the bacteria in the lower bowel act upon these sugars, resulting in the production of rectal gas.

What you *should* do, in the way of diet, is eat slowly and moderately and include whole grains, root vegetables, and raw fruits on your daily menu. These foods will help you move your bowels freely and will prevent the entrapment of gas. Exercise is also important. The abdominal muscles overlying the intestines help reduce feelings of distention and bloating, but with increasing age, decreasing physical activity, or both, these muscles become lax. Doing such exercises as sit-ups will tighten these muscles and reduce your bloated feeling after meals.

You may find that some OTC medicines, such as those containing simethicone, will relieve your discomfort. Activated charcoal has also been marketed as an antiflatulent. Most people, however, find that diet modification is the most effective way to relieve the pain, and embarrassment, of too much gas.

If your gas pain continues despite your best efforts, you should check with your doctor. Gas pains can be quite sharp and usually occur in the left or right upper abdomen under the ribs or in the back. Persistent abdominal pains may mean that an obstruction is blocking the normal passage of gas out of the rectum or that something other than gas is causing your symptoms.

PANCREATITIS

Indigestion can also be caused by other conditions, such as irritable bowel syndrome (see page 412), gallbladder disease (see pages 462–463), or peptic ulcer (see pages 362–364). Still another possible cause is pancreatitis, which is an inflammation of the pancreas gland. This disorder usually results either from the lodging of a gallstone in the pancreatic ducts or excessive intake of alcohol over a long period of time. The major symptom of pancreatitis is severe pain above and around the navel; there may also be nausea, vomiting, fever, and chills. Pancreatitis can be a serious disease, but most people who have it recover completely. It is important to get medical help at once if you develop the above symptoms. Some people develop chronic pancreatitis and may suffer from indigestion between their attacks of pain. The damaged pancreas can no longer manufacture certain enzymes required for digestion or produce insulin to control the blood sugar levels. In these cases, doctors may prescribe pancrelipase (see pages 409–411), or other agents with pancreatic enzymes (see pages 405–408). These medicines—combinations of enzymes that are naturally produced by the pancreas—help the body digest food properly.

Occasionally, some people with chronic pancreatitis undergo surgery to remove the damaged pancreatic tissue or sever the nerves that carry the pain. If a significant portion of the pancreas is removed, insulin injections and medicines containing pancreatic enzymes may be necessary.

OUTLOOK

Indigestion is a common digestive disorder that has many causes. Dietary modification and some simple self-help measures are generally sufficient to relieve the pain and other symptoms. Over-the-counter medications may also play a role in easing your distress. But sometimes this is not enough. If your symptoms persist, if an unexplained new symptom develops, or if you have any of these additional symptoms (loss of appetite, weight loss, back pain along with abdominal distress, change in bowel habits, or bleeding from the digestive tract), consult your doctor. Indigestion can be more than it seems.

CONDITION: **HEARTBURN**

CATEGORY: **PROMOTILITY DRUGS**

GENERIC (CHEMICAL) NAME	BRAND (TRADE) NAME	DOSAGE FORMS AND STRENGTHS
Metoclopramide	REGLAN	Syrup: 5 mg per tsp Tablets: 5, 10 mg

DRUG PROFILE

Metoclopramide is used to relieve symptoms such as nausea, vomiting, loss of appetite, and continued feeling of fullness after eating that is due to failure of the stomach to empty properly. The drug, called a promotility agent, acts by increasing the contractions of the stomach and intestines, thus quickening the pace at which food empties from the stomach and moves through the intestines. It is also prescribed for gastroesophageal reflux (heartburn), diabetic gastroparesis (a condition in which the stomach loses its ability to contract), and prevention of nausea associated with chemotherapy.

For complete information on this drug, see pages 458–461.

CONDITION: **HEARTBURN**

CATEGORY: **ANTISECRETORY**

GENERIC (CHEMICAL) NAME	BRAND (TRADE) NAME	DOSAGE FORMS AND STRENGTHS
Omeprazole	PRILOSEC	Delayed-release capsules: 20 mg

DRUG PROFILE

Omeprazole, which blocks the release of stomach acid, is used to treat severe gastroesophageal reflux (heartburn) and Zollinger-Ellison syndrome, a rare condition in which the stomach produces excess acid.

BEFORE USING THIS DRUG

Let your doctor know *IF*

You have ever had allergic reactions or other problems with ■ omeprazole.

You are taking any of the following medicines: ■ diazepam (tranquilizer) ■ phenytoin (medicine for seizures) ■ warfarin (blood thinner).

SPECIAL RESTRICTIONS WHILE TAKING THIS DRUG

FOOD AND DRUG INTERACTIONS

Other Drugs	Check with your doctor or pharmacist if you are taking other medicines. Because this medicine affects stomach acidity it may interfere with the absorption of other medicines.
	Avoid drugs like ibuprofen and aspirin because they may aggravate your condition.
Foods and Beverages	Take this medicine before eating unless otherwise instructed by your doctor.
	Your doctor may advise you to avoid certain foods and beverages (coffee, cola drinks, cocoa, chocolate) that can aggravate your condition.
Alcohol	Avoid alcohol, which can further irritate the stomach lining.

Smoking	Cigarette smoking irritates the stomach lining and can worsen your condition. If you smoke, try to stop or at least cut down.

DAILY LIVING

Helpful Hints	These timed-release capsules should be swallowed whole; do not open, crush, or chew them.

No special restrictions on driving, exertion and exercise, sun exposure, or exposure to excessive heat or cold.

POSSIBLE SIDE EFFECTS

Although this list of adverse effects may seem somewhat intimidating, keep in mind that some are quite rare. Of course, should these or any other problems arise while you are on medication, it is always a good idea to consult your doctor.

IF YOU DEVELOP

headache ■ dizziness ■ diarrhea ■ abdominal pain ■ nausea or vomiting ■ constipation ■ rash ■ cough ■ back pain ■ fever ■ tiredness ■ weakness

WHAT TO DO

If symptoms are disturbing or persist, let your doctor know.

STORAGE INSTRUCTIONS

Store in a cool, dark place (not in a bathroom medicine cabinet).

STOPPING OR INTERRUPTING THERAPY

This drug should be taken for exactly the length of time directed by your doctor, generally for four to eight weeks. Do not take it for a longer period than that prescribed. This medicine should not be used for maintenance therapy in the treatment of gastroesophageal reflux. If you miss a dose, take it as soon as possible. If it almost time for your next dose, skip the missed dose and resume your regular schedule. Do not take two doses at the same time.

SPECIAL CONSIDERATIONS FOR THOSE OVER SIXTY-FIVE

None.

CONDITION: **INDIGESTION**

CATEGORY: **ANTISPASMODICS**

GENERIC (CHEMICAL) NAME	BRAND (TRADE) NAME	DOSAGE FORMS AND STRENGTHS
Chlordiazepoxide hydrochloride and clidinium bromide	LIBRAX	Capsules: 5 mg chlordiazepoxide and 2.5 mg clidinium

DRUG PROFILE

Chlordiazepoxide/clidinium is a combination drug used to treat peptic ulcers and irritable bowel syndrome (spastic colon). It relaxes the digestive system, reduces stomach acid, and provides a sedative effect.

BEFORE USING THIS DRUG

Let your doctor know *IF*

You have ever had allergic reactions or other problems with ■ chlordiazepoxide or any other benzodiazepines ■ clidinium.

You have ever had any of the following medical problems: ■ difficulty in urination ■ asthma or other lung disease ■ glaucoma ■ enlarged prostate ■ kidney disease ■ liver disease ■ depression or severe mental illness ■ intestinal blockage ■ myasthenia gravis ■ drug or alcohol addiction ■ constipation ■ high blood pressure ■ heart disease including abnormal heart rhythms ■ overactive thyroid.

You are taking any of the following medicines: ■ medicine for spasmodic conditions of the intestinal or urinary tract ■ tranquilizers ■ medicine for diarrhea ■ medicine for Parkinson's disease ■ medicine for seizures ■ antihistamines ■ barbiturates ■ muscle relaxants ■ narcotics or other prescription pain-killers ■ sleep medicines ■ medicine for depression.

SPECIAL RESTRICTIONS WHILE TAKING THIS DRUG

FOOD AND DRUG INTERACTIONS

Other Drugs	Do not take any other drugs, including over-the-counter (OTC) drugs, before checking with your doctor. This medicine increases the effect of drugs that depress the central nervous system, such as antihistamines; medicine for hay fever, allergies, or colds; sleep medicines; tranquilizers; narcotics or other prescription pain-killers; muscle relaxants; and medicine for seizures. If you are taking any medicine for diarrhea, allow at least one hour between the time you take that medicine and the time you take chlordiazepoxide/clidinium.
Foods and Beverages	If you are being treated for an ulcer, your doctor may advise you to avoid certain foods and beverages (coffee, cola drinks, cocoa, chocolate) known to irritate an ulcer.
Alcohol	This medicine increases the effect of alcohol, a central nervous system depressant. Avoid alcohol unless your doctor has approved its use.
Smoking	Ulcers generally heal faster if you do not smoke. If you are being treated for an ulcer and you smoke, try to stop or at least cut down.

DAILY LIVING

Driving	This medicine may cause dizziness or drowsiness. Be careful when driving, operating household appliances, or doing any other tasks that require alertness until you know how this drug affects you.

Exertion and Exercise	This drug may cause you to sweat less than normally. Sweating is your body's natural way of cooling down, and not sweating enough can be dangerous. Use caution not to become overheated when you exercise or exert yourself.
Excessive Heat	See above; use caution during hot weather, since overexertion may result in heat stroke. Avoid extremely hot baths or saunas. Also, check with your doctor if you develop a fever for any reason.
Other Precautions	Take this medicine exactly as prescribed by your doctor; taking it more often or for a longer period of time than prescribed may make it habit forming.
Helpful Hints	If your mouth or throat feels dry, chewing sugarless gum or sucking ice chips or sugarless hard candy will help.
	Take this medicine before meals and at bedtime unless instructed otherwise by your doctor.

No special restrictions on sun exposure or exposure to excessive cold.

POSSIBLE SIDE EFFECTS

Although this list of adverse effects may seem somewhat intimidating, keep in mind that some are quite rare. Of course, should these or any other problems arise while you are on medication, it is always a good idea to consult your doctor.

IF YOU DEVELOP

confusion ■ difficulty in urination ■ severe drowsiness ■ fast heartbeat ■ flushing ■ skin dryness ■ fainting ■ rash ■ shortness of breath ■ yellowing of eyes or skin

WHAT TO DO

Urgent Get in touch with your doctor immediately.

constipation ■ severely dry mouth, nose, or throat ■ blurred vision ■ depression ■ excitement ■ agitation ■ nervousness ■ irritability ■ clumsiness ■ tiredness or weakness ■ sleep disturbances ■ mood changes	**May be serious** Check with your doctor as soon as possible.
dizziness ■ drowsiness ■ nausea ■ dry mouth ■ headache ■ vivid dreams ■ decreased or increased sweating ■ increased or diminished sex drive	If symptoms are disturbing or persist, let your doctor know.

STORAGE INSTRUCTIONS

Store in a cool, dark place (not in a bathroom medicine cabinet).

STOPPING OR INTERRUPTING THERAPY

Do not stop taking this medicine abruptly without consulting your doctor. If you miss a dose take it as soon as possible. If it is almost time for your next dose, skip the missed dose and resume your regular schedule. Do not take two doses at the same time. If you have been taking this medicine for a long period of time, or in large doses, your doctor will probably want you to gradually reduce the amount rather than stop abruptly.

SPECIAL CONSIDERATIONS FOR THOSE OVER SIXTY-FIVE

Older people may be more sensitive to this medicine and may be particularly prone to confusion, agitation, drowsiness, excitement, difficulty in urination, or blurred vision.

CONDITION: **INDIGESTION**

CATEGORY: **ANTISPASMODICS**

GENERIC (CHEMICAL) NAME	BRAND (TRADE) NAME	DOSAGE FORMS AND STRENGTHS
Dicyclomine	BENTYL	Capsules: 10 mg Syrup: 10 mg per tsp Tablets: 20 mg

This drug is available under many other brand names as well.

DRUG PROFILE

Dicyclomine is used to treat irritable bowel syndrome (spastic colon). It reduces the production of stomach acid and relieves intestinal spasms. It is not known exactly how this drug works.

BEFORE USING THIS DRUG

Let your doctor know *IF*

You have ever had allergic reactions or other problems with ■ dicyclomine.

You have ever had any of the following medical problems: ■ digestive problems, including severe diarrhea ■ difficulty in urination or other urinary problems ■ enlarged prostate ■ glaucoma ■ heart disease, including abnormal heart rhythms or fast heartbeat ■ kidney disease ■ liver disease ■ overactive thyroid ■ myasthenia gravis ■ asthma or other lung disease.

You are taking any of the following medicines: ■ medicine for stomach spasms or cramps ■ medicine for Parkinson's disease ■ medicine for diarrhea ■ tranquilizers ■ medicine for nausea ■ narcotics or other prescription pain-killers ■ sleep medicines ■ medicine for depression ■ medicine for abnormal heart rhythms.

SPECIAL RESTRICTIONS WHILE TAKING THIS DRUG

FOOD AND DRUG INTERACTIONS

Other Drugs	Do not take any other drugs, including over-the-counter (OTC) drugs, before checking with your doctor. This drug may increase the effect of drugs that depress the central nervous system, such as antihistamines; medicine for hay fever, allergies, or colds; sleep medicines; tranquilizers; narcotics or other prescription pain-killers; muscle relaxants; and medicine for seizures. Allow at least one hour between the time you take this drug and the time you take an antacid.
Foods and Beverages	If you are being treated for an ulcer, your doctor may advise you to avoid certain foods and beverages (coffee, cola drinks, cocoa, chocolate) known to irritate an ulcer.
Alcohol	This medicine increases the effect of alcohol, a central nervous system depressant. Avoid alcohol unless your doctor has approved its use.
Smoking	Ulcers generally heal faster if you do not smoke. If you are being treated for an ulcer and you smoke, try to stop or at least cut down.

DAILY LIVING

Driving	This medicine may cause dizziness or drowsiness. Be careful when driving, operating household appliances, or doing any other tasks that require alertness until you know how this drug affects you.

Exertion and Exercise	This medicine may cause you to sweat less than normally. Sweating is your body's natural way of cooling down, and not sweating enough can be dangerous. Use caution when you exercise or exert yourself.
Excessive Heat	See above; use caution during hot weather, as over-exertion may result in heat stroke. Avoid extremely hot baths and saunas. Also, check with your doctor if you develop a fever for any reason.
Other Precautions	Take this medicine exactly as prescribed by your doctor; taking it more often or for a longer period of time than prescribed makes you more prone to developing side effects. Be sure to let your doctor know if you develop constipation. Tell any doctor or dentist you consult that you are taking this medicine, especially if you will be undergoing any type of surgery.
Helpful Hints	Take this medicine before meals and at bedtime, unless otherwise instructed by your doctor.

No special restrictions on exposure to excessive cold.

POSSIBLE SIDE EFFECTS

Although this list of adverse effects may seem somewhat intimidating, keep in mind that some are quite rare. Of course, should these or any other problems arise while you are on medication, it is always a good idea to consult your doctor.

IF YOU DEVELOP	WHAT TO DO
constipation ■ difficulty in urination ■ rash ■ irregular or fast heartbeat ■ flushing ■ eye pain ■ hallucinations	**May be serious** Check with your doctor as soon as possible.
bloating ■ nausea or vomiting ■ stomach pain ■ dry mouth ■ dizziness ■ headache ■ blurred vision ■ changes in pupil size ■ increased sensitivity to light ■ confusion ■ male impotence ■ drowsiness ■ light-headedness ■ weakness ■ nervousness ■ excitement ■ decreased sweating ■ loss of taste	If symptoms are disturbing or persist, let your doctor know.

STORAGE INSTRUCTIONS

Store in a cool, dark place (not in a bathroom medicine cabinet). If your medicine is in a liquid form, make sure that it does not freeze.

STOPPING OR INTERRUPTING THERAPY

This medicine should be taken exactly as prescribed by your doctor. If you miss a dose, take it as soon as possible. If it is almost time for your next dose, skip the missed dose and resume your regular schedule. Do not take two doses at the same time.

SPECIAL CONSIDERATIONS FOR THOSE OVER SIXTY-FIVE

Older people may be more prone to the side effects of constipation, confusion, and excitement. For this reason, doctors may wish to check their progress frequently.

CONDITION: **INDIGESTION**

CATEGORY: **ANTISPASMODICS**

GENERIC (CHEMICAL) NAME	BRAND (TRADE) NAME	DOSAGE FORMS AND STRENGTHS
Belladonna alkaloids (atropine, hyoscyamine, and hyoscine [scopolamine]) and barbiturates (phenobarbital)	DONNATAL	Capsules: 16.2 mg phenobarbital, 0.1037 mg hyoscyamine, 0.0194 mg atropine, and 0.0065 mg hyoscine Controlled-release tablets: 48.6 mg phenobarbital, 0.3111 mg hyoscyamine, 0.0582 mg atropine, and 0.0195 mg hyoscine Elixir: 16.2 mg phenobarbital, 0.1037 mg hyoscyamine, 0.0194 mg atropine, and 0.0065 mg hyoscine per tsp No. 2 Tablets: 32.4 mg phenobarbital, 0.1037 mg hyoscyamine, 0.0194 mg atropine, and 0.0065 mg hyoscine Tablets: 16.2 mg phenobarbital, 0.1037 mg hyoscyamine, 0.0194 mg atropine, and 0.0065 mg hyoscine

KINESED	Chewable tablets: 16 mg phenobarbital, 0.12 mg hyoscyamine, 0.12 mg atropine, and 0.007 mg scopolamine

This combination drug is available under a variety of other brand names as well.

DRUG PROFILE

The combination of belladonna alkaloids and a barbiturate is used to relieve stomach and intestinal cramping and spasms. It is used along with other drugs to treat irritable bowel syndrome and intestinal inflammation (enterocolitis). Belladonna prevents muscular contraction and excessive acid secretion in the stomach and intestines, while phenobarbital acts on the brain to provide a calming effect.

BEFORE USING THIS DRUG

Let your doctor know *IF*

You have ever had allergic reactions or other problems with ■ belladonna alkaloids, such as atropine, hyoscyamine, or scopolamine ■ barbiturates.

You have ever had any of the following medical problems: ■ digestive problems, including colitis or severe diarrhea ■ asthma or other lung disease ■ difficulty in urination or other urinary problems ■ enlarged prostate ■ glaucoma ■ heart disease, including abnormal heart rhythms or fast heartbeat ■ kidney disease ■ liver disease ■ overactive thyroid ■ myasthenia gravis ■ porphyria.

You are taking any of the following medicines: ■ medicine for stomach spasm or cramps ■ medicine for Parkinson's disease ■ medicine for diarrhea ■ tranquilizers ■ medicine for nausea ■ medicine for seizures ■ antihistamines ■ narcotics or other prescription pain-killers ■ sleep medicines ■ medicine for depression ■ medicine for abnormal heart rhythms ■ digoxin or digitalis (heart medicines).

SPECIAL RESTRICTIONS WHILE TAKING THIS DRUG

FOOD AND DRUG INTERACTIONS

Other Drugs	Do not take any other drugs, including over-the-counter (OTC) drugs, before checking with your doctor. This medicine increases the effect of drugs that depress the central nervous system, such as antihistamines; medicine for hay fever, allergies, or colds; sleep medicines; tranquilizers; narcotics or other prescription pain-killers; muscle relaxants; and medicine for seizures. Allow at least one hour between the time you take this drug and the time you take an antacid or medicine for diarrhea.
Alcohol	This medicine increases the effect of alcohol, a central nervous system depressant. Avoid alcohol unless your doctor has approved its use.

No special restrictions on foods and beverages or smoking.

DAILY LIVING

Driving	This medicine may cause dizziness, drowsiness, or blurred vision. Be careful when driving, operating household appliances, or doing any other tasks that require alertness until you know how this drug affects you.
Exertion and Exercise	This drug may cause you to sweat less than normally. Sweating is your body's natural way of cooling down, and not sweating enough can be dangerous. Use caution not to become overheated when you exercise or exert yourself.

Excessive Heat	See above; use caution during hot weather, since overexertion may result in heat stroke. Avoid extremely hot baths or saunas.
	Check with your doctor if you develop any kind of fever.
Other Precautions	Be sure to let your doctor know if you develop constipation.
	Getting up from a reclining or sitting position may cause you to become dizzy.
Helpful Hints	If your mouth or throat feels dry, chewing sugarless gum or sucking ice chips or sugarless hard candy will help.

No special restrictions on sun exposure or exposure to excessive cold.

POSSIBLE SIDE EFFECTS

Although this list of adverse effects may seem somewhat intimidating, keep in mind that some are quite rare. Of course, should these or any other problems arise while you are on medication, it is always a good idea to consult your doctor.

IF YOU DEVELOP

continual blurred vision ■ seizures ■ confusion ■ severe drowsiness ■ hallucinations ■ difficulty in breathing ■ slurred speech ■ fast heartbeat ■ palpitations ■ flushing ■ fever ■ rash or hives ■ difficulty in urination

After you STOP taking this medicine: delirium ■ seizures

eye pain ■ changes in pupil size ■ sore throat ■ nervousness ■ excitement ■ sleeplessness ■ restlessness ■ irritability

WHAT TO DO

Urgent Get in touch with your doctor immediately.

May be serious Check with your doctor as soon as possible.

constipation ■ decreased sweating ■ dizziness ■ drowsiness ■ dry mouth, nose, throat, or skin ■ increased eye sensitivity to light ■ loss of taste ■ bloating ■ nausea or vomiting ■ headache ■ male impotence

If symptoms are disturbing or persist, let your doctor know.

STORAGE INSTRUCTIONS

Store in a cool, dark place (not in a bathroom medicine cabinet). If your medicine is in a liquid form, make sure that it does not freeze.

STOPPING OR INTERRUPTING THERAPY

This medicine should be taken without interruption for the length of time prescribed by your doctor. If you miss a dose, take it as soon as possible. If it is almost time for your next dose, skip the missed dose and resume your regular schedule. Do not take two doses at the same time.

SPECIAL CONSIDERATIONS FOR THOSE OVER SIXTY-FIVE

Older people may be more sensitive to this drug combination and more likely to experience such side effects as confusion, constipation, difficulty in urination, drowsiness, nervousness, irritability, and restlessness, even with small doses.

CONDITION: **INDIGESTION**

CATEGORY: **DIGESTANTS**

GENERIC (CHEMICAL) NAME	BRAND (TRADE) NAME	DOSAGE FORMS AND STRENGTHS
Pancreatic enzyme and digestant combinations	DONNAZYME	Tablets: 300 mg pancreatin, 150 mg pepsin, 150 mg bile salts, 0.0518 mg hyoscyamine, 0.0097 mg atropine, 0.0033 mg scopolamine, 8.1 mg phenobarbital

DRUG PROFILE

These preparations of enzymes normally produced by the pancreas are used to treat miscellaneous digestive disorders. Some of these preparations also contain drugs that relax the digestive system.

BEFORE USING THIS DRUG

Let your doctor know *IF*

You have ever had allergic reactions or other problems with ■ belladonna alkaloids such as atropine, hyoscyamine, or scopolamine ■ barbiturates ■ pancrelipase or pancreatin ■ pork products ■ beef products.

You have ever had any of the following medical problems: ■ asthma or other lung disease ■ digestive problems, including severe diarrhea ■ difficulty in urination or other urinary problems ■ enlarged prostate ■ glaucoma ■ heart disease, including abnormal heart rhythms or fast heartbeat ■ kidney disease ■ liver disease ■ overactive thyroid ■ myasthenia gravis.

You are taking any of the following medicines: ■ medicine for stomach spasm or cramps ■ medicine for Parkinson's disease ■ medicine for diarrhea ■ tranquilizers ■ medicine for nausea ■ medicine for seizures ■ antihistamines ■ narcotics or other prescription pain-killers ■ sleep medicines ■ medicine for depression ■ medicine for abnormal heart rhythms ■ digoxin or digitalis (heart medicines).

SPECIAL RESTRICTIONS WHILE TAKING THIS DRUG

FOOD AND DRUG INTERACTIONS

Other Drugs	Do not take any other drugs, including over-the-counter (OTC) drugs, before checking with your doctor. This medicine increases the effect of drugs that depress the central nervous system, such as antihistamines; medicine for hay fever, allergies, or colds; sleep medicines; tranquilizers; narcotics or other prescription pain-killers; muscle relaxants; and medicine for seizures.

Allow at least one hour between the time you take this drug and the time you take an antacid or medicine for diarrhea.

Alcohol	This medicine increases the effect of alcohol, a central nervous system depressant. Avoid alcohol unless your doctor has approved its use.

No special restrictions on foods and beverages, smoking, driving, exertion and exercise, sun exposure, or exposure to excessive heat or cold.

POSSIBLE SIDE EFFECTS

Although this list of adverse effects may seem somewhat intimidating, keep in mind that some are quite rare. Of course, should these or any other problems arise while you are on medication, it is always a good idea to consult your doctor.

IF YOU DEVELOP

blood in urine ■ joint pain ■ difficulty in breathing ■ stuffy nose ■ continual blurred vision ■ convulsions ■ confusion ■ severe drowsiness ■ hallucinations ■ slurred speech ■ fast heartbeat ■ palpitations ■ flushing ■ fever ■ voice changes ■ restlessness ■ clumsiness ■ staggering

WHAT TO DO

Urgent Get in touch with your doctor immediately.

rash or hives ■ diarrhea ■ nausea or vomiting ■ stomach cramps or pain ■ sore throat ■ eye pain ■ changes in pupil size ■ bleeding or bruising ■ yellowing of eyes or skin ■ difficulty in urination ■ nervousness ■ excitement ■ agitation ■ irritability ■ sleeplessness

May be serious Check with your doctor as soon as possible.

constipation ■ decreased sweating ■ dizziness ■ drowsiness ■ dry mouth, nose, throat, or skin ■ increased eye sensitivity to light ■ loss of taste ■ bloating ■ headache ■ male impotence ■ aching muscles or bones

If symptoms are disturbing or persist, let your doctor know.

STORAGE INSTRUCTIONS

Store in a cool, dark place (not in a bathroom medicine cabinet).

STOPPING OR INTERRUPTING THERAPY

This medicine should be taken without interruption for the full length of time prescribed by your doctor. If you miss a dose, take it as soon as possible. If it is almost time for your next dose, skip the missed dose and resume your regular schedule. Do not take two doses at the same time.

SPECIAL CONSIDERATIONS FOR THOSE OVER SIXTY-FIVE

Older people may be more sensitive to this medicine and more likely to experience such side effects as confusion, difficulty in urination, drowsiness, nervousness, agitation, irritability, and restlessness.

CONDITION: **INDIGESTION**

CATEGORY: **DIGESTANTS**

GENERIC (CHEMICAL) NAME	BRAND (TRADE) NAME	DOSAGE FORMS AND STRENGTHS
Pancrelipase	COTAZYM	Capsules: 8,000 units lipase, 30,000 units protease, and 30,000 units amylase
	COTAZYM-S	Capsules: 5,000 units lipase, 20,000 units protease, and 20,000 units amylase
	ILOZYME	Tablets: 11,000 units lipase, 30,000 units protease, and 30,000 units amylase
	PANCREASE	Capsules: 4,000 units lipase, 20,000 units amylase, and 25,000 units protease
	PANCREASE MT 4	Capsules: 4,000 units lipase, 12,000 units amylase, 12,000 units protease
	PANCREASE MT 10	Capsules: 10,000 units lipase, 30,000 units amylase, 30,000 units protease
	PANCREASE MT 16	Capsules: 16,000 units lipase, 48,000 units amylase, 48,000 units protease
	VIOKASE	Powder: 16,800 units lipase, 70,000 units protease, and 70,000 units amylase per 1/4 tsp Tablets: 8,000 units lipase, 30,000 units protease, and 30,000 units amylase

DRUG PROFILE

Pancrelipase, a combination of enzymes that are naturally produced by the pancreas, helps the body digest food properly. It is prescribed for people who have insufficient amounts of these enzymes as a result of inflammation of the pancreas (pancreatitis) or have had their pancreas surgically removed (pancreatectomy).

BEFORE USING THIS DRUG

Let your doctor know *IF*

You have ever had allergic reactions or other problems with ■ pancrelipase ■ pancreatin ■ pork products.

SPECIAL RESTRICTIONS WHILE TAKING THIS DRUG

FOOD AND DRUG INTERACTIONS

Foods and Beverages	Your doctor will probably prescribe a special diet to follow while taking this medicine.

No special restrictions on other drugs, alcohol use, or smoking.

DAILY LIVING

Helpful Hints	Avoid touching or inhaling the powder form of this drug, because it can be quite irritating.

No special restrictions on driving, exertion and exercise, sun exposure, or exposure to excessive heat or cold.

POSSIBLE SIDE EFFECTS

Although this list of adverse effects may seem somewhat intimidating, keep in mind that some are quite rare. Of course, should these or any other problems arise while you are on medication, it is always a good idea to consult your doctor.

IF YOU DEVELOP	WHAT TO DO
blood in urine ■ joint pain ■ swollen feet or legs ■ difficulty in breathing ■ stuffy nose	**Urgent** Get in touch with your doctor immediately.
rash ■ diarrhea ■ nausea ■ stomach cramps or pain	**May be serious** Check with your doctor as soon as possible.

STORAGE INSTRUCTIONS

Store in a cool, dark place (not in a bathroom medicine cabinet).

STOPPING OR INTERRUPTING THERAPY

This medicine should be taken without interruption for the full length of time prescribed by your doctor. If you miss a dose, take it as soon as possible. If it is almost time for your next dose, skip the missed dose and resume your regular schedule. Do not take two doses at the same time.

SPECIAL CONSIDERATIONS FOR THOSE OVER SIXTY-FIVE

None.

DIARRHEA

You may have found yourself, of late, making more trips to the bathroom than you would like. Your friends may be constantly complaining of constipation, but you sometimes experience the opposite—frequent and loose bowel movements. This is a problem that can be treated in different ways, depending on its cause. Sometimes it's just a matter of drinking fluids to avoid dehydration until the disorder resolves itself. In other cases there's more that you—and your doctor—can do to alleviate your distress.

IRRITABLE BOWEL SYNDROME

Diarrhea may be a symptom of a disorder known as irritable bowel syndrome, or IBS. This syndrome is one of the most common digestive disorders seen in medical practice. Also referred to as spastic colon, mucous colitis, and irritable colon, it occurs twice as frequently in women as in men and can strike any age group.

IBS occurs when the contractions of the colon—which are usually gentle and rhythmic—become irregular and poorly coordinated. When this happens, the fecal material does not proceed normally along the five-foot length of the colon toward the rectum. Instead, it is either expelled too soon from the colon or retained too long.

The most common symptom of IBS is pain, which usually worsens soon after eating. It typically occurs in the lower left side of the abdomen but may occur on the right side or higher up. Other common symptoms of irritable bowel syndrome include bloating, heartburn, belching, gas, and loss of appetite. And, of course, there is the disturbance in bowel function that may produce diarrhea, constipation, or alternating bouts of each.

It's important that you inform your doctor of any change in your normal bowel habits or the appearance of blood in your stools. If your doctor diagnoses IBS, there's a lot you can do to keep the condition under control. By adding fiber to your diet, avoiding fats, and exercising, you will go a long way toward freeing yourself of the disabling symptoms of this digestive disorder. Milk, milk products, or caffeine may worsen this condition, so reducing these components in your diet may be helpful. It's also a good idea to avoid emotionally charged situations that produce anxiety; anxiety and tension seem to trigger the diarrhea and constipation of IBS. Your doctor may suggest you take medicine to treat the problem. The medicines available for people with IBS are discussed on pages 393–405.

INFECTIOUS GASTROENTERITIS

This is the term for poisoning or invasion of the intestines by bacteria or viruses that produce the symptoms of an upset stomach. You may experience a mild attack of nausea followed by diarrhea, or you may feel severely ill, with recurrent attacks of watery diarrhea, abdominal cramps, fever, and extreme weakness.

Severe cases of gastroenteritis can be particularly dangerous to older people with chronic illnesses because diarrhea can cause dehydration—the loss of body fluid without adequate replacement. It is important that an older person continually replace these lost fluids and take in some sugar along with liquids (drinking juice or sweetened tea will help the intestine to absorb water and salt). Other things you should do during an attack are stay at home, rest, and eat only when you are hungry.

Some over-the-counter medicines may help relieve the diarrhea once the nausea and vomiting have subsided. But don't take aspirin or other painkillers because they may worsen the condition. If you don't feel better after two or three days or if there's any blood, mucus, or pus in your stool, consult your doctor. He or she will question you about your symptoms and may send a sample of your bowel movements to a laboratory for analysis to establish or confirm a diagnosis. Depending on the findings, you may receive a prescription for an antispasmodic drug, a drug that slows down bowel activity, or an antibiotic. Those prescription medicines are discussed on pages 393–405.

TRAVELER'S DIARRHEA

Traveler's diarrhea is a type of gastroenteritis that usually lasts about three to five days—just long enough to have ruined many a vacation. Known also as "turista" and "Montezuma's revenge," it is noted mainly for the watery diarrhea it produces. The high-risk areas for contracting this ailment are developing countries in Latin America, Africa, the Mediterranean areas, and the Middle and Far East.

It used to be thought that traveler's diarrhea is caused by a general change in the bacteria inhabiting the intestines or by eating spicy, unfamiliar foods. But its most frequent cause is actually a bacterium called *Escherichia coli*, or *E. coli*. If you consume food or water (or ice) contaminated by this organism, your small intestine may become infected. A likely result is not only diarrhea but also abdominal cramps, nausea, vomiting, and a low fever.

Wise dietary precautions to take while traveling include the avoidance of raw meats, raw seafood, raw vegetables, and unpeeled raw fruits. Stick to such drinks as bottled carbonated beverages without ice, beer, wine, hot coffee, and hot tea. Only drink water that's been bottled or treated with chlorine or iodine.

If you're careful, you'll lower your chances of developing traveler's diarrhea, but you can't eliminate them altogether. If you do find yourself laid low by this condition, try to avoid dehydration and stay out of the sun as much as possible. You may find that resting in bed lessens the abdominal cramping. Generally, if you experience one to three loose stools a day and feel well otherwise, no treatment is required. If you have three to five loose stools a day and feel well otherwise, two tablespoons of bismuth subsalicylate (Pepto-Bismol) every half hour for up to eight doses in 24 hours should help clear up your symptoms. If you are experiencing sixor more loose stools a day, and if you have a fever or there is blood in the stools, you should check with a doctor.

Antidiarrheal medicine should be used sparingly, if at all. In some cases, a doctor may prescribe one of the drugs discussed on pages 415–422.

TREATMENT

Although the conditions described in this section are often managed without medicine, your doctor may find it appropriate to put you on medicine to relieve your discomfort. A variety of medicines are available to help your gastrointestinal system function more normally.

OUTLOOK

An attack of infectious gastroenteritis or traveler's diarrhea is generally a passing phenomenon. If you take effective measures to prevent dehydration, you should be none the worse for it. If the diarrhea is prolonged, however, or if there is fever or severe and persistent pain in the abdomen, check with a doctor; a more serious abdominal disorder may be the cause of your symptoms.

Irritable bowel syndrome, in contrast, may be a recurrent problem. Doctors are now able to control many of its unpleasant symptoms, enabling you to lead a normal life. As you pay more attention to your diet and your need for exercise and try to avoid stressful situations, you may even feel healthier than ever.

CONDITION: **DIARRHEA**

CATEGORY: **ANTIDIARRHEAL AGENTS**

GENERIC (CHEMICAL) NAME	BRAND (TRADE) NAME	DOSAGE FORMS AND STRENGTHS
Diphenoxylate and atropine sulfate	LOMOTIL	Liquid: 2.5 mg diphenoxylate and 0.025 mg atropine per tsp Tablets: 2.5 mg diphenoxylate and 0.025 mg atropine

DRUG PROFILE

This drug is used along with other therapy to treat severe diarrhea and intestinal cramping. Diphenoxylate is thought to reduce the movements of the stomach and intestines.

BEFORE USING THIS DRUG

Let your doctor know *IF*

You have ever had allergic reactions or other problems with ■ diphenoxylate ■ atropine.

You have ever had any of the following medical problems: ■ severe colitis ■ severe bleeding ■ kidney disease ■ liver disease ■ drug addiction ■ fever (at present) ■ rectal bleeding.

You are taking any of the following medicines: ■ other medicine for diarrhea ■ antacids ■ medicine for stomach spasms or cramps ■ medicine for Parkinson's disease ■ medicine for nausea ■ tranquilizers ■ medicine for seizures ■ antihistamines ■ narcotics or other prescription pain-killers ■ sleep medicines ■ medicine for depression ■ medicine for abnormal heart rhythms ■ digoxin or digitalis (heart medicines) ■ acetaminophen ■ antibiotics.

You have recently traveled to a foreign country.

SPECIAL RESTRICTIONS WHILE TAKING THIS DRUG

FOOD AND DRUG INTERACTIONS

Other Drugs	Do not take any other drugs, including over-the-counter (OTC) drugs, before checking with your doctor. This medicine increases the effect of drugs that depress the central nervous system, such as antihistamines; medicine for hay fever, allergies, or colds; sleep medicines; tranquilizers; narcotics or other prescription pain-killers; muscle relaxants; and medicine for seizures.
Alcohol	This medicine increases the effect of alcohol, a central nervous system depressant. Avoid alcohol unless your doctor has approved its use.

No special restrictions on foods and beverages or smoking.

DAILY LIVING

Driving	This medicine may cause dizziness, drowsiness, or blurred vision. Be careful when driving, operating household appliances, or doing any other tasks that require alertness until you know how this drug affects you.
Other Precautions	Take this medicine exactly as prescribed by your doctor; taking it more often or for a longer period of time than prescribed may make it habit-forming.

Let your doctor know if your diarrhea does not stop within a few days, or if you develop a fever or rectal bleeding.

Tell any doctor or dentist you consult that you are taking this drug, especially if you will be undergoing any type of surgery. |

No special restrictions on exertion and exercise, sun exposure, or exposure to excessive heat or cold.

POSSIBLE SIDE EFFECTS

Although this list of adverse effects may seem somewhat intimidating, keep in mind that some are quite rare. Of course, should these or any other problems arise while you are on medication, it is always a good idea to consult your doctor.

IF YOU DEVELOP

blurred vision ■ severe drowsiness ■ severely dry mouth ■ difficulty in breathing ■ fast heartbeat ■ flushing ■ severe bloating ■ constipation ■ severe nausea or vomiting ■ stomach pain ■ fever ■ changes in pupil size ■ rectal bleeding ■ difficulty in urination ■ swelling of face, hands, or feet ■ rash, hives, or itching

WHAT TO DO

Urgent Get in touch with your doctor immediately.

---

dizziness ■ drowsiness ■ headache ■ depression ■ feeling of euphoria ■ weakness ■ general ill feeling ■ numbness in hands or feet ■ dry mouth, throat, nose, or skin ■ increased thirst ■ swollen gums ■ nausea or vomiting ■ stomach discomfort or bloating ■ loss of appetite ■ restlessness ■ sleeplessness

May be serious Check with your doctor as soon as possible.

STORAGE INSTRUCTIONS

Store in a cool, dark place (not in a bathroom medicine cabinet). If your medicine is in a liquid form, make sure that it does not freeze.

STOPPING OR INTERRUPTING THERAPY

If you miss a dose, take it as soon as possible. If it is almost time for your next dose, skip the missed dose and resume your regular schedule. Do not take two doses at the same time.

SPECIAL CONSIDERATIONS FOR THOSE OVER SIXTY-FIVE

Older people may be more prone to constipation with this drug.

CONDITION: **DIARRHEA**

CATEGORY: **ANTIDIARRHEAL AGENTS**

GENERIC (CHEMICAL) NAME	BRAND (TRADE) NAME	DOSAGE FORMS AND STRENGTHS
Loperamide hydrochloride	IMODIUM	Capsules: 2 mg
	IMODIUM A-D	Liquid: 1 mg per tsp Caplets: 2 mg

DRUG PROFILE

Loperamide is used to treat mild acute (short-term) diarrhea as well as chronic (long-term) diarrhea resulting from intestinal resection or irritable bowel syndrome. Imodium A-D is available as an over-the-counter preparation.

BEFORE USING THIS DRUG

Let your doctor know *IF*

You have ever had allergic reactions or other problems with ■ loperamide.

You have ever had any of the following medical problems: ■ colitis ■ liver disease ■ fever (at present) ■ rectal bleeding.

You are taking any of the following medicines: ■ antibiotics ■ diphenoxylate and atropine sulfate (Lomotil).

SPECIAL RESTRICTIONS WHILE TAKING THIS DRUG

FOOD AND DRUG INTERACTIONS

Foods and Beverages	Your doctor may suggest changes in your diet. Tell your doctor if you find that certain foods or beverages cause a diarrheal attack.

No special restrictions on other drugs, alcohol use, or smoking.

DAILY LIVING

Driving	May cause drowsiness, dizziness or blurred vision. Be careful when driving, operating household appliances, or doing other tasks that require alertness until you know how this drug affects you.
Examinations or Tests	If you are taking this drug on a long-term basis, your doctor may want to check your progress periodically.
Other Precautions	Let your doctor know if your diarrhea does not stop within a few days or if you develop a fever or rectal bleeding.

No special restrictions on exertion and exercise, sun exposure, or exposure to excessive heat or cold.

POSSIBLE SIDE EFFECTS

Although this list of adverse side effects may seem somewhat intimidating, keep in mind that some are quite rare. Of course, should these or any other problems arise while you are on medication, it is always a good idea to consult your doctor.

IF YOU DEVELOP	WHAT TO DO
rectal bleeding	**Urgent** Get in touch with your doctor immediately.

bloating ■ constipation ■ dizziness ■ drowsiness ■ tiredness ■ dry mouth ■ fever ■ nausea or vomiting ■ rash ■ stomach pain or discomfort

May be serious Check with your doctor as soon as possible.

STORAGE INSTRUCTIONS

Store in a cool, dark place (not in a bathroom medicine cabinet). If your medicine is in a liquid form, make sure that it does not freeze.

STOPPING OR INTERRUPTING THERAPY

Take this drug exactly as prescribed by your doctor. If you miss a dose, take it as soon as possible. If it is almost time for your next dose, skip the missed dose and resume your regular schedule. Do not take two doses at the same time.

SPECIAL CONSIDERATIONS FOR THOSE OVER SIXTY-FIVE

Older people may be more prone to constipation with this drug.

CONDITION: **DIARRHEA**

CATEGORY: **ANTIBIOTICS**

GENERIC (CHEMICAL) NAME	BRAND (TRADE) NAME	DOSAGE FORMS AND STRENGTHS
Vancomycin hydrochloride	VANCOCIN HCl	Capsules: 125, 250 mg Solution: 1, 10 g

DRUG PROFILE

Vancomycin is an antibiotic that is used to treat special types of colitis caused by certain types of bacteria. This drug works by suppressing the growth of the bacteria that are responsible for the inflammation of the bowel.

BEFORE USING THIS DRUG

Let your doctor know *IF*

You have ever had allergic reactions or other problems with ■ vancomycin.

You have ever had any of the following medical problems: ■ kidney disease ■ deafness or hearing problems ■ intestinal blockage ■ other inflammatory bowel disease.

You are taking any of the following medicines: ■ cholestyramine or colestipol ■ aminoglycosides (gentamicin, tobramycin) ■ amphotericin B (medicine for fungal infections) ■ bacitracin, colistin, polymyxin B (medicine for fungal infections) ■ cyclosporine ■ bumetanide ■ ethacrynic acid or furosemide (diuretics).

SPECIAL RESTRICTIONS WHILE TAKING THIS DRUG

FOOD AND DRUG INTERACTIONS

Other Drugs	If you are also taking cholestyramine or colestipol, allow three to four hours between taking either of these drugs and a dose of vancomycin.
	If you are taking vancomycin for diarrhea associated with antibiotic therapy, do not take any other diarrhea medicine without checking with your doctor. Some antidiarrhea medicines may make your condition worse while you are taking vancomycin.

No special restrictions on foods and beverages, smoking, or alcohol use.

DAILY LIVING

Examination or Tests	It is important for you to keep all appointments with your doctor so that your progress can be checked. Blood, urine, and/or hearing tests may be required.
Other Precautions	If your symptoms persist or worsen after a few days of treatment, contact your doctor immediately.

No special restrictions on driving, exertion and exercise, sun exposure, or exposure to excessive heat or cold.

POSSIBLE SIDE EFFECTS

Although this list of adverse effects may seem somewhat intimidating, keep in mind that some are quite rare. Of course, should these or any other problems arise while you are on medication, it is always a good idea to consult your doctor.

IF YOU DEVELOP	WHAT TO DO
hearing loss ■ ringing, buzzing, or "full" feeling in ears ■ chills ■ fever ■ rash, hives, or other skin problems ■ dizziness ■ nausea or vomiting	**Urgent** Get in touch with your doctor immediately.
unpleasant taste	If symptoms are disturbing or persist, let your doctor know.

STORAGE INSTRUCTIONS

Store in a cool, dark place (not in a bathroom medicine cabinet). If your medicine is in a liquid form, make sure that it does not freeze.

STOPPING OR INTERRUPTING THERAPY

If you miss a dose, take it as soon as possible. If it is almost time for your next dose, skip the missed dose and resume your regular schedule. Do not take two doses at the same time. Make sure you take your full supply of medicine, even if your symptoms improve before all your medicine is used.

SPECIAL CONSIDERATIONS FOR THOSE OVER SIXTY-FIVE

Older people may be more sensitive to the side effects of this medicine. If side effects are troublesome, contact your doctor, who can adjust your dosage accordingly. Because kidney function sometimes decreases with age, doctors may want to start people over sixty-five on a lower dosage.

CONSTIPATION

The seemingly endless supply of laxative commercials that appear in the media give eloquent testimony to the importance people place on regular bowel movements. Real constipation is not as widespread as the ads would lead you to believe. A daily bowel movement is not a requirement for good health, and bowel movements that are reasonably regular are considered normal (even two or three times a week is adequate).

If, however, bowel movements are very infrequent, are difficult, the resulting stool is hard and dry, or your abdomen still feels full after defecating, then you are constipated. The condition may be a short-term problem caused by temporary disruption in your diet or schedule, or it may be chronic, brought on by poor eating habits, lack of exercise, or certain medications. In some extreme cases, overuse of laxatives can cause a type of chronic constipation that is particularly hard to remedy.

Many people are more prone to developing constipation as they grow older because they become less physically active, and eat less, both of which may contribute to constipation. In addition, lifelong overuse of laxatives begins to take its toll in the middle years, by which time the muscle tone of the colon (a tubelike organ in the lower abdomen through which stool passes before being eliminated) may have become almost completely lax.

How Constipation Develops

After food has been digested, the remaining waste products pass from the small intestine into the colon, where fluids and salts are absorbed. The resulting semi-soft fecal matter then passes into the rectum, initiating the urge to defecate.

A number of problems along the way can slow the process, thus contributing to constipation. If, for example, you don't drink enough fluids, the stool may be particularly dry. Or, if your diet is low in fiber (the nondigestible portion of whole grains, vegetables, and fruits) and high in fat and sugar, the stool produced will have considerably less bulk and take longer to pass through the colon.

Ignoring the urge to defecate can also lead to constipation. When not acted upon, the urge passes, and the stool remains in the rectum, becoming harder and drier—and dry stool can itself cause constipation.

Certain drugs can also promote constipation. Antidepressants, blood pressure medications, certain pain medications, aluminum-containing antacids, and mineral supplements such as calcium and iron are among the most common constipation-inducing medications. Repeated use of irritating laxatives over a number of years can cause the colon to lose its ability to contract and propel stool into the rectum naturally. The colon becomes, in effect, dependent on the artificial stimulation the laxative provides—but in time, even a laxative will not do the trick.

The Natural Approach

Constipation can often be remedied by simple changes in diet—specifically, by increasing the intake of fiber and fluids. About 15-30 grams of fiber per day are necessary for bowel regularity. If you've been in the habit of eating mostly refined foods, it may take a concerted effort to consume that much fiber.

Fresh fruits and vegetables are a good source of fiber. Contrary to popular belief, however, they are not the best source. To get enough fiber, you need to eat bran and whole grain cereals, breads, and pasta. A serving of bran cereal every morning will provide much of the needed fiber, but your diet should also include whole grain breads. In addition to eating fresh fruits and vegetables, dried fruits such as prunes and raisins are also helpful. It is important to drink at least four glasses of juice or water every day. Coffee and tea shouldn't be counted as part of this amount, since these beverages have a diuretic effect that can actually worsen constipation by speeding up elimination of fluids.

These changes will help only if you let them. That means allowing time for bowel movements and responding to the urge to defecate when it occurs. Some doctors recommend a breakfast of bran cereal and a warm beverage to stimulate the bowel first thing in the morning.

Other Treatments

When constipation occurs because of travel, bed rest from illness or injury, or emotional upset, dietary modification may not be enough to restore regularity and you may need a laxative or suppository.

The safest type of laxative is a bulk former. It is usually sold as a powder to be mixed in water. Bulk-forming laxatives may be taken several times a day with no ill effects. However, they do not work immediately. Because many of these preparations contain sugar, diabetics should either avoid using them or make allowances in other areas of their diets.

Other types of laxatives are stool lubricants and softeners. Mineral oil is a stool lubricant, while a stool softener may contain a mild detergent. These are rarely more effective than a high-fiber diet. Stool softeners are available in suppository and oral forms.

Avoid laxatives that contain irritants or stimulants. Many over-the-counter laxatives contain these agents; active ingredients include cascara sagrada, senna, magnesium hydroxide, and castor oil. These products lead, over time, to laxative dependence and can, in the short run, worsen conditions such as appendicitis.

Osmotic laxatives, which are available by prescription, work by means of substances such as lactulose that increase the water content of the stool. These drugs are discussed more fully on pages 426–428.

Enemas are generally not recommended unless a person is undergoing treatment for some medical procedure such as a barium enema or a colonoscopy. If you must use an enema, use plain water or a mild commercial formula.

When To See Your Doctor

Any sudden change in bowel habits, including constipation, may indicate presence of a serious illness and should be reported to your doctor immediately. If constipation is a chronic problem, your doctor may also be able to help you manage it effectively.

CONDITION: **CONSTIPATION**

CATEGORY: **LAXATIVES**

GENERIC (CHEMICAL) NAME	BRAND (TRADE) NAME	DOSAGE FORMS AND STRENGTHS
Lactulose	CHRONULAC	Syrup: 10 g lactulose per tbsp (15 ml)

DRUG PROFILE

This drug is used for treatment of chronic constipation that is not treatable by other therapies. By drawing water into the bowel from surrounding tissues, it softens the stool, making its passage easier. Lactulose is also used in the treatment of a form of liver disease.

BEFORE USING THIS DRUG

Let your doctor know *IF*

You have ever had allergic reactions or other problems with ■ galactose ■ lactose.

You have ever had any of the following medical problems: ■ diabetes ■ kidney disease ■ high or low blood levels of potassium, chloride, or carbon dioxide ■ heart disease ■ high blood pressure ■ colostomy or ileostomy ■ intestinal blockage ■ rectal bleeding.

You are taking any of the following medicines: ■ other laxatives ■ antibiotics ■ antacids ■ anticoagulants (blood thinners) ■ heart medicine ■ any other drugs.

You are on a low-sugar diet.

SPECIAL RESTRICTIONS WHILE TAKING THIS DRUG

FOOD AND DRUG INTERACTIONS

Other Drugs	If you are taking any other medicines, allow two hours between taking them and your dose of lactulose. Do not take any other laxatives while taking lactulose without first checking with your doctor.
Foods and Beverages	If you are taking this drug for constipation, your doctor may recommend a diet that includes plenty of liquid and roughage (bran, whole-grain cereals and breads, and leafy green vegetables). You may be instructed to avoid foods that worsen constipation such as cakes, pastries, cheese, and candy.

No special restrictions on smoking or alcohol use.

DAILY LIVING

Exertion and Exercise	Regular exercise will help maintain a healthy bowel. Be sure to check with your doctor before starting out on any new exercise program.
Examinations or Tests	Periodic blood tests may be required.
Other Precautions	Tell any doctor you consult that you are taking this medicine, especially if you will be undergoing any diagnostic procedures involving the bowel such as protoscopy or colonoscopy.
Helpful Hints	If you find the taste of this medicine unpleasant, you can mix it with fruit juice, water, or milk.

No special restrictions on driving, sun exposure, or exposure to excessive heat or cold.

POSSIBLE SIDE EFFECTS

Although this list of adverse effects may seem somewhat intimidating, keep in mind that some are quite rare. Of course, should these or any other problems arise while you are on medication, it is always a good idea to consult your doctor.

IF YOU DEVELOP	WHAT TO DO
confusion ■ extreme tiredness or weakness ■ rash ■ irregular heartbeat ■ muscle cramps	**Urgent** Get in touch with your doctor immediately.
diarrhea ■ intestinal cramps ■ gas ■ belching ■ nausea or vomiting ■ increased thirst	If symptoms are disturbing or persist, let your doctor know.

STORAGE INSTRUCTIONS

Store in a cool, dark place (not in a bathroom medicine cabinet) and make sure that it does not freeze. It is particularly important to avoid exposing this medicine to hot temperatures, as heat may change its pharmacological properties.

STOPPING OR INTERRUPTING THERAPY

If you miss a dose, take it as soon as possible. If it is almost time for your next dose, skip the missed dose and resume your regular schedule. Do not take two doses at the same time.

SPECIAL CONSIDERATIONS FOR THOSE OVER SIXTY-FIVE

Older people may be more prone to develop low potassium levels while taking this medication. Your doctor may want to order periodic blood tests.

INFLAMMATORY BOWEL DISEASE

Among the most serious and least understood of all the problems of the digestive tract, inflammatory bowel disease is really two diseases—ulcerative colitis and Crohn's disease. More than two million Americans suffer from the disabling effects of these diseases, and each year one hundred thousand new cases are diagnosed.

You may have heard that these disorders are "young people's" diseases, but about 10 to 20 percent of cases occur in individuals over the age of fifty. So, if you've just been told you have ulcerative colitis or Crohn's disease, you are certainly not alone in your age group.

CAUSES

Just what *are* ulcerative colitis and Crohn's disease? Ulcerative colitis is a chronic disorder characterized by inflammation and sores on the inner lining of the large intestine, or colon. It does not involve the small intestine. Crohn's disease typically affects the ileum, the lower portion of the small intestine, and/or the colon. This disorder causes the intestinal wall to become inflamed and deeply scarred. In severe cases, small openings (fistulas) develop in the intestinal wall, and infected contents may leak out.

Ulcerative colitis and Crohn's disease are grouped together under the same name (inflammatory bowel disease) because of their similarities and because the causes of both disorders are unknown. But there are several telling differences between the two conditions. For example, the presence of fistulas occurs only in Crohn's disease. In Crohn's disease, the rectum frequently is normal, and there are often "skip areas" in the colon—patches of normal-appearing intestine interspersed with the areas of disease. In chronic ulcerative colitis, by contrast, the rectum is always affected, and inflammation in the colon is continuous.

Crohn's disease expresses itself somewhat differently in older people than in their younger counterparts, as it is more likely to affect the colon in this older population. Crohn's disease of the colon alone may have a better outlook than the form of the disease that affects the small intestine.

DIAGNOSIS

Ulcerative colitis usually begins gradually. However, an initial attack or a flare-up may occur suddenly, giving no preliminary warning. The most common symptom is bloody diarrhea. Severe cases may involve painful abdominal cramps, fever, loss of appetite, anemia, and frequent loose stools containing blood and pus. Some people with ulcerative colitis experience such serious complications as hemorrhage or distention and rupture of the bowel. In most people, the pattern of the disease is a cyclical one of alternating flare-ups and periods of improvement.

The typical symptoms of Crohn's disease are also diarrhea, abdominal pain, low-grade fever, poor appetite, and gradual weight loss. Sometimes this disease is confused with ulcerative colitis because of the similarity of symptoms. People with Crohn's disease are less likely to have blood in their stool. Many people with Crohn's disease develop a noncancerous mass in their right lower abdomen that may be painful to the touch. In advanced Crohn's disease, the drainage of nutrients from the damaged intestinal wall may lead to malnutrition.

Many doctors are unaware of the occurrence of inflammatory bowel disease in older people and may attribute bowel symptoms to other conditions, such as diverticular disease of the colon or cancer. This will lead to a delay in diagnosis. But inflammatory bowel disease can be distinguished from other problems that affect the intestines through a careful history of your symptoms, a thorough physical examination, and appropriate diagnostic tests.

The initial diagnostic test done is often a sigmoidoscopy. This is a simple procedure performed in the doctor's office in which a fiberoptic tube with a light at one end is passed through the anus to inspect the rectum and lower part of the colon. Looking through the viewing end, the doctor can see the lining of the rectum and lower colon quite clearly. A specimen of tissue may also be obtained (biopsy) that can be studied under the microscope to help the doctor make a diagnosis.

If the symptoms seem to point to Crohn's disease and the disease appears to be higher up in your bowel, the doctor may decide to perform a similar procedure known as a colonoscopy. Your doctor may also request that you have an upper gastrointestinal or small bowel series and a barium-enema X-ray examination to find out the extent of the disease. For these tests, a radiopaque dye is swallowed or introduced into the rectum through a short enema tube. The dye passes through the entire small or large intestine, and the features of the bowels can be seen on the developed X rays.

TREATMENT

As yet, there is no drug known to cure inflammatory bowel disease, but various medicines can effectively relieve symptoms and keep them in check. Drug treatment consists of steroids, antibiotics and certain anti-inflammatory agents. Sulfasalazine has been shown to be moderately successful in treatment of patients with ulcerative colitis. Unfortunately, it contains sulfapyridine, a sulfalike drug that has been shown to be a cause of the major side effects associated with sulfasalazine. Recently, new drugs have been developed that do not contain sulfapyridine, but only the active component of sulfasalazine, a chemical substance called 5-aminosalicylic acid (5-ASA). Two of these new drugs are mesalamine (Rowasa) and olsalazine (Dipentum). These new drugs may be useful in patients who are sensitive to sulfa-medications or sulfasalazine. For more information on the available medicines for this disorder, see the drug charts on pages 432–439.

Your doctor may decide that surgery is necessary if medicine can no longer control the symptoms of your illness, if your intestines become blocked, or if your ulcerative colitis is considered likely to progress to cancer. (People who have had colitis involving the entire colon for ten years or more are at an increased risk of developing colon cancer.) Surgery for ulcerative colitis entails removing all or most of the colon. Surgery for Crohn's disease is usually less extensive; only the most severely affected portions of the intestine are removed.

OUTLOOK

Inflammatory bowel disease is a potentially serious intestinal disorder that can affect young and old alike. Fortunately, the great majority of cases can be kept under control with medicine and, sometimes, surgery.

While this can be an emotionally trying illness, the support of family and friends can be enormously helpful to you in coping with this disease and in dealing with recovery from any necessary surgery. In the case of ulcerative colitis, a complete cure through surgery is possible. Otherwise, inflammatory bowel disease is a remittent illness. During the months or even years that it stays dormant, you can lead a normal life in every way.

FOR MORE INFORMATION

A good source for further information on inflammatory bowel disease is the National Foundation for Ileitis and Colitis, Inc., which has chapters located in many states. For the location of the chapter nearest you, contact the national office at 295 Madison Avenue, New York, NY 10017; (212) 685-3440. You can also obtain a free pamphlet, *Inflammatory Bowel Disease*, by writing to the Gastrointestinal Research Foundation, University of Chicago Medical Center, 5841 S. Maryland Avenue, Chicago, IL 60637.

CONDITION: **INFLAMMATORY BOWEL DISEASE**

CATEGORY: **SULFONAMIDES**

GENERIC (CHEMICAL) NAME	BRAND (TRADE) NAME	DOSAGE FORMS AND STRENGTHS
Sulfasalazine	AZULFIDINE	Coated tablets: 500 mg Suspension: 250 mg per tsp Tablets: 500 mg
Mesalamine	ROWASA	Enema: 4 g per 60 ml Rectal suppositories: 500 mg
Olsalazine	DIPENTUM	Capsules: 250 mg

DRUG PROFILE

Sulfasalazine is used to treat inflammatory bowel disease—ulcerative colitis and Crohn's disease. In the body, sulfasalazine is converted to mesalamine. Mesalamine is used to treat mild cases of ulcerative colitis in the lower colon. These drugs relieve inflammation within the colon. Olsalazine is used for maintenance treatment in patients who cannot tolerate sulfasalazine.

BEFORE USING THIS DRUG

Let your doctor know *IF*

You have ever had allergic reactions or other problems with ■ sulfasalazine ■ mesalamine ■ sulfonamides (sulfa drugs) ■ thiazide diuretics ■ medicine for diabetes ■ aspirin or other salicylate drugs ■ sulfites ■ olsalazine.

You have ever had any of the following medical problems: ■ glucose-6-phosphate dehydrogenase (G-6-PD) deficiency ■ porphyria ■ kidney disease ■ liver disease ■ blood disease ■ asthma or severe allergies ■ intestinal blockage ■ urinary tract blockage.

You are taking any of the following medicines: ■ other sulfa drugs ■ any drugs you take by mouth containing para-aminobenzoic acid (PABA) ■ phenytoin (medicine for seizures) ■ digoxin or digitalis (heart medicines) ■ sulfinpyrazone or probenicid (medicines for gout) ■ aspirin, aspirinlike medicine, or other medicine for pain and inflammation ■ methotrexate (medicine for cancer and severe psoriasis) ■ anticoagulants (blood thinners) ■ folic acid ■ medicine for diabetes ■ medicine for depression ■ antibiotics for urinary tract infections.

SPECIAL RESTRICTIONS WHILE TAKING THIS DRUG

FOOD AND DRUG INTERACTIONS

No special restrictions on other drugs, foods and beverages, alcohol use, or smoking.

DAILY LIVING

Sun Exposure	Your skin may become more sensitive to sunlight and more likely to sunburn while taking this medicine. It is a good idea to apply a sunscreen to exposed skin surfaces before going outdoors.
Examinations or Tests	It is important for you to keep all appointments with your doctor so that your progress can be checked. Blood or urine tests may be required.
Other Precautions	Tell any doctor or dentist you consult that you are taking this medicine, especially if you will be undergoing any type of surgery or diagnostic testing.
	If you have diabetes, be aware that this drug may affect urine-sugar and ketone tests. Check with your doctor to see if you should use a different type of test.
	Let your doctor know if you are taking the coated tablets and you notice whole tablets in your stool; you may be unable to digest this dosage form.

Helpful Hints

If this medicine upsets your stomach, taking it with meals should help. If this does not help, then contact your doctor. The doctor may feel that a slight adjustment in dosage may be helpful.

For maximum benefit, take this drug on an empty stomach (one hour before or two hours after meals). Be sure to drink four to six glasses of water a day while taking this drug.

No special restrictions on driving, exertion and exercise, or exposure to excessive heat or cold.

POSSIBLE SIDE EFFECTS

Although this list of adverse effects may seem somewhat intimidating, keep in mind that some are quite rare. Of course, should these or any other problems arise while you are on medication, it is always a good idea to consult your doctor.

IF YOU DEVELOP

seizures ■ bluish tinge to skin ■ rash ■ hives, itching or other skin conditions ■ difficulty in breathing ■ sore throat or fever ■ swollen tongue or vocal cords ■ chest pain ■ blood in urine

numbness, tingling, or pain in hands or feet ■ paleness ■ chills ■ bleeding or bruising ■ severe headache ■ mouth sores ■ red, itching eyes with runny nose ■ swelling around eyes, neck, or ears ■ swelling of the tip of the penis ■ joint pain ■ yellowing of eyes or skin ■ stomach pain ■ blood in urine ■ decreased or increased urination ■ amber color to urine or skin ■ pain or burning in urination ■ low-back pain ■ clumsiness ■ depression ■ confusion ■ hallucinations ■ behavior changes ■ tiredness or weakness ■ ringing or buzzing sound in ears or other hearing problems

WHAT TO DO

Urgent Get in touch with your doctor immediately.

May be serious Check with your doctor as soon as possible.

upset stomach ■ nausea or vomiting ■ increased skin sensitivity to sunlight ■ headache ■ dizziness ■ drowsiness ■ restlessness ■ sleeplessness ■ loss of appetite ■ diarrhea ■ diarrhea, with blood ■ anxiety

If symptoms are disturbing or persist, let your doctor know.

STORAGE INSTRUCTIONS

Store in a cool, dark place (not in a bathroom medicine cabinet). If your medicine is in a liquid form, make sure that it does not freeze.

STOPPING OR INTERRUPTING THERAPY

If you miss a dose, take it as soon as possible. If it is almost time for your next dose, skip the missed dose and resume your regular schedule. Do not take two doses at the same time.

SPECIAL CONSIDERATIONS FOR THOSE OVER SIXTY-FIVE

None.

CONDITION: **INFLAMMATORY BOWEL DISEASE**

CATEGORY: **CORTICOSTEROIDS**

GENERIC (CHEMICAL) NAME	BRAND (TRADE) NAME	DOSAGE FORMS AND STRENGTHS
Hydrocortisone	CORTENEMA	Suspension: 100 mg per 60 ml unit

This drug is available under other brand names as well.

DRUG PROFILE

Hydrocortisone enema is used to treat ulcerative colitis. It reduces swelling and provides relief for the inflamed colon.

BEFORE USING THIS DRUG

Let your doctor know *IF*

You have ever had allergic reactions or other problems with ■ corticosteroids ■ any other drugs.

You have ever had any of the following medical problems: ■ rectal infection or bleeding ■ pain, burning, itching, or blisters in the rectal area ■ colitis or diverticulitis ■ diabetes ■ bone disease, such as osteoporosis ■ fungal infection ■ herpes eye infection ■ high blood pressure ■ kidney disease ■ liver disease ■ myasthenia gravis ■ peptic ulcer ■ stomach cramps ■ tuberculosis ■ underactive thyroid ■ mental illness ■ seizures.

You are taking any of the following medicines: ■ antibiotics ■ diuretics or medicine for high blood pressure ■ medicine for inflammation, such as arthritis (including aspirin) ■ insulin or other medicine for diabetes ■ anticoagulants (blood thinners) ■ medicine for seizures ■ estrogens.

You have recently had a vaccination.

SPECIAL RESTRICTIONS WHILE TAKING THIS DRUG

FOOD AND DRUG INTERACTIONS

Other Drugs	Corticosteroids interact with many other drugs. Tell your doctor if you are taking any of the drugs listed above.
Foods and Beverages	Your doctor will probably suggest some changes in your diet to avoid aggravating your inflammatory bowel condition. A low-salt, high-potassium diet may also be recommended to counterbalance some corticosteroid side effects, such as fluid retention.

No special restrictions on alcohol use or smoking.

DAILY LIVING

Examinations or Tests	Your doctor may perform a sigmoidoscopy (examination of the colon with a lighted instrument) to check whether your condition is responding to treatment.
Other Precautions	Tell your doctor if you develop burning, itching, or pain in the rectum during treatment with this medicine.
	Tell any doctor or dentist you consult that you are taking this medicine, especially if you are going to have a vaccination or immunization or if you will be undergoing any type of surgery or allergy skin tests.
	If you have diabetes, be aware that this medicine may raise blood-sugar levels. If you notice any change when testing sugar levels in your blood or urine, let your doctor know.
Helpful Hints	When using a hydrocortisone enema, it is best to retain the fluid for at least one hour (preferably overnight) for maximum benefit. The medicine comes with complete instructions for use.

No special restrictions on driving, exertion and exercise, sun exposure, or exposure to excessive heat or cold.

POSSIBLE SIDE EFFECTS

Although this list of adverse effects may seem somewhat intimidating, keep in mind that some are quite rare. Of course, should these or any other problems arise while you are on medication, it is always a good idea to consult your doctor.

IF YOU DEVELOP	WHAT TO DO
severe abdominal pain ■ seizures	**Urgent** Get in touch with your doctor immediately.
rash, hives, or other skin changes ■ blood in stools ■ bloating ■ diarrhea ■ constipation ■ stomach pain ■ rectal pain or burning ■ rectal bleeding ■ depression ■ personality changes ■ "high" feeling ■ mood changes ■ sleeplessness ■ swelling of hands, feet, or ankles ■ palpitations ■ difficulty breathing ■ poor wound healing ■ unusual roundness of the face	**May be serious** Check with your doctor as soon as possible.
dizziness ■ headache	If symptoms are disturbing or persist, let your doctor know.

STORAGE INSTRUCTIONS

Store in a cool, dark place (not in a bathroom medicine cabinet). Make sure that your medicine does not freeze.

STOPPING OR INTERRUPTING THERAPY

Do not stop using this medicine without consulting your doctor. If you miss a dose, take it as soon as possible. If it is almost time for your next dose, skip the missed dose and resume your regular schedule.

SPECIAL CONSIDERATIONS FOR THOSE OVER SIXTY-FIVE

Long-term use of corticosteroids by mouth may cause gradual bone loss, which can be serious in older people, particularly women, who are vulnerable to osteoporosis. However, corticosteroid enemas are usually used only for a limited time.

CONDITION: **INFLAMMATORY BOWEL DISEASE**

CATEGORY: **CORTICOSTEROIDS**

GENERIC (CHEMICAL) NAME	BRAND (TRADE) NAME	DOSAGE FORMS AND STRENGTHS
Prednisone	DELTASONE	Tablets: 2.5, 5, 10, 20, 50 mg

DRUG PROFILE

Oral corticosteroids (also known as steroids) are used to treat a wide variety of inflammatory diseases, such as arthritis, and other rheumatic disorders, such as lupus. They are also used in conjunction with immunosuppressive agents to prevent reactions from kidney and heart transplants. Although these multifaceted drugs do not cure the underlying disease, they suppress the redness, swelling, and heat that signal inflammation.

For complete information on this drug, see pages 530–535.

NAUSEA AND VOMITING

When your body tries to get rid of irritating or disease-causing substances in the digestive tract, nausea and vomiting may occur. These substances can be viruses or bacteria that have lodged in your intestine or things you've eaten that for one reason or another don't agree with you.

Or you might become nauseated during an attack of vertigo, or dizziness, which can result from a disturbance in the balance-maintaining structures of the inner ear or from a distortion of vision. Nausea and vomiting are also symptoms of motion sickness, which makes some people miserable when they take a cruise or even just ride in a car; for unknown reasons, some people are more prone to motion sickness than others. And sometimes emotional stress can make you feel that you want to throw up.

Persistent nausea can be a sign of liver inflammation or gallbladder disease. Also, if you suffer nausea after starting on a new medicine, it may be an adverse effect of that medicine.

As unpleasant as they are, nausea and vomiting are usually mild and self-limiting; that is, you feel bad and throw up a few times, but then you feel better in a day or two. However, nausea and vomiting can also be symptoms of serious disease, or they can lead to a dangerous loss of fluids or an imbalance of vital body chemicals. This is a special problem for older people who are chronically ill or who rely on daily medicines to preserve their well-being. If you are in either of these categories, an attack of vomiting should be a signal for you to call your doctor right away.

CAUSES

Infectious gastroenteritis is the general term for infections in the stomach and intestine. Cramps, diarrhea, and loss of appetite may accompany the nausea and vomiting. You can get gastroenteritis if you eat improperly cooked or refrigerated food in which bacteria have been multiplying; it can happen when the normal bacteria in your own body are upset or unbalanced by another illness; and it can also be the result of a contagious viral infection that we generally refer to as stomach or intestinal flu.

Similar symptoms occur with *gastritis*, an inflammation of the stomach lining, which can be caused by a viral infection but is more often the result of smoking, drinking, using too much aspirin or other anti-inflammatory drugs, overeating, or eating something that you're allergic to or that's too spicy or acidic for you.

In addition, a number of other conditions can cause the symptoms of nausea and vomiting, including pancreatitis (inflammation of the pancreas), gallstones, cholecystitis (inflammation of the gallbladder), gastritis, gastric obstruction, ulcers, certain types of cancer, and some diseases of the central nervous system.

TREATMENT AND OUTLOOK

Most cases of gastroenteritis and gastritis clear up if you just take it easy for a day or two, staying in bed if you can. You will probably not want to eat anything, but you should make an effort to take in fluids like water, weak tea, or fruit juice. If you have recognized a particular food or behavior that has caused your problem, you should abstain from it even after you feel better; if you think one of your medicines is causing the difficulty, talk to your doctor before discontinuing its use.

You should also ask your doctor for help if your symptoms seem unusually severe, if they persist for more than a couple of days, or if they recur several times in a week. And you should get immediate medical attention if your nausea and vomiting are accompanied by any of the following:

• Severe pain in your abdomen that does not go away when you throw up; this might be a sign of appendicitis, inflammation of the pancreas, or gallbladder disease.

• Pain in one eye and blurred vision; these are symptoms of acute glaucoma.

• The appearance of blood or black particles ("coffee grounds") in your vomit; this is a sign of internal bleeding.

• A feeling that you are parched or dried out, along with infrequent urination, or if you feel dizzy; these are signs of dehydration.

Also, if you had received a blow to the head within twenty-four hours of the time you started feeling nauseated, see a doctor to find out if any brain injury has occurred.

Drugs are available that will relieve nausea and stop the vomiting, but your doctor may want to examine you before prescribing to be sure you do not have something that requires some other kind of treatment. Medicines that will prevent motion sickness and its accompanying symptoms are also available, so if you suspect or know that you are subject to that disorder, check with your doctor before you set out on your next trip. For more information on the available medicines for nausea and vomiting, see the drug charts on pages 442–461.

CONDITION: **NAUSEA AND VOMITING**

CATEGORY: **ANTIHISTAMINES**

GENERIC (CHEMICAL) NAME	BRAND (TRADE) NAME	DOSAGE FORMS AND STRENGTHS
Meclizine hydrochloride	ANTIVERT	Chewable tablets: 25 mg Tablets: 12.5, 25, 50 mg

DRUG PROFILE

Meclizine, which belongs to the category of drugs called antihistamines, is used to prevent the nausea, vomiting, and dizziness that are associated with motion sickness. This medicine also is used to treat dizziness resulting from inner-ear disturbances. Meclizine works by reducing the sensitivity of the nerves in the inner ear that control balance; it also blocks the nerve pathways to the part of the brain that controls vomiting.

For complete information on this drug, see pages 294-296.

CONDITION: **NAUSEA AND VOMITING**

CATEGORY: **ANTINAUSEANTS**

GENERIC (CHEMICAL) NAME	BRAND (TRADE) NAME	DOSAGE FORMS AND STRENGTHS
Dimenhydrinate	DRAMAMINE	Liquid: 12.5 mg per 4 ml Tablets: 50 mg Chewable Tablets: 50 mg

This drug is available by prescription and over the counter under many other brand names as well.

DRUG PROFILE

Dimenhydrinate, which belongs to the category of drugs called antihistamines, is used to prevent nausea, vomiting, and dizziness associated with motion sickness. This drug works by reducing the sensitivity of the nerves in the inner ear that control balance. It also blocks the nerve pathways to the part of the brain that controls vomiting.

BEFORE USING THIS DRUG

Let your doctor know *IF*

You have ever had allergic reactions or other problems with ■ dimenhydrinate ■ other antihistamines.

You have ever had any of the following medical problems: ■ asthma or other lung disease ■ enlarged prostate ■ difficulty in urination or other urinary problems ■ glaucoma ■ irregular or fast heartbeat.

You are taking any of the following medicines: ■ medicine for Parkinson's disease ■ medicine for seizures ■ aspirin or aspirinlike medicine ■ medicine for cancer ■ antibiotics ■ digoxin or digitalis (heart medicines) ■ medicine for abnormal heart rhythms ■ barbiturates ■ muscle relaxants ■ antihistamines ■ narcotics or other prescription pain-killers ■ sleep medicines ■ tranquilizers ■ medicine for depression ■ medicine for high blood pressure ■ appetite suppressants.

SPECIAL RESTRICTIONS WHILE TAKING THIS DRUG

FOOD AND DRUG INTERACTIONS

Other Drugs	Do not take any other drugs, including over-the-counter (OTC) drugs, before checking with your doctor. This medicine increases the effect of drugs that depress the central nervous system such as antihistamines; medicine for hay fever, allergies, or colds; sleep medicines; tranquilizers; narcotics or other prescription pain-killers; muscle relaxants; and medicine for seizures. This drug may mask ringing in the ears caused by aspirin. Let your doctor know if you are taking aspirin or aspirinlike medicine.

Alcohol	This medicine increases the effect of alcohol, a central nervous system depressant. Avoid alcohol unless your doctor has approved its use.

No special restrictions on foods and beverages or smoking.

DAILY LIVING

Driving	This medicine may cause dizziness, drowsiness, weakness, or blurred vision. Be careful when driving, operating household appliances, or doing any other tasks that require alertness until you know how this drug affects you.
Other Precautions	This drug, because it controls nausea and vomiting, can mask some of the symptoms of appendicitis. If you have sharp stomach or lower abdominal pain, be sure to let your doctor know at once. If you are going to be tested for allergies, tell the doctor in charge that you are taking this drug, since it affects the results of allergy tests.
Helpful Hints	Taking this drug with food, milk, or water will lessen the chance of upset stomach. For maximum benefit, take it one to two hours before traveling. If your mouth or throat feels dry, chewing sugarless gum or sucking ice chips or sugarless hard candy will help.

No special restrictions on exertion and exercise, sun exposure, or exposure to excessive heat or cold.

POSSIBLE SIDE EFFECTS

Although this list of adverse effects may seem somewhat intimidating, keep in mind that some are quite rare. Of course, should these or any other problems arise while you are on medication, it is always a good idea to consult your doctor.

IF YOU DEVELOP	WHAT TO DO
seizures ■ unsteadiness or clumsiness ■ severe drowsiness ■ fainting ■ flushing ■ hallucinations ■ difficulty in breathing ■ dilation of pupils ■ insomnia ■ confusion ■ difficulty in speaking or swallowing ■ nervousness ■ irritability ■ restlessness ■ excitement or other mood changes ■ weakness ■ tremors ■ tightness of chest	**Urgent** Get in touch with your doctor immediately.
tiredness ■ palpitations	**May be serious** Check with your doctor as soon as possible.
drowsiness ■ dizziness ■ thickened phlegm ■ blurred vision or other visual disturbances ■ pain or difficulty in urination ■ urinary frequency ■ dry mouth, throat, or nose ■ increased skin sensitivity to sunlight ■ nightmares ■ rash ■ fast heartbeat ■ loss of appetite ■ upset stomach ■ constipation ■ diarrhea ■ nausea or vomiting ■ male sexual problems ■ chills ■ increased sweating ■ ringing in the ears or other hearing problems	If symptoms are disturbing or persist, let your doctor know.

STORAGE INSTRUCTIONS

Store in a cool, dark place (not in a bathroom medicine cabinet). If your medicine is in a liquid form, make sure that it does not freeze.

STOPPING OR INTERRUPTING THERAPY

This medicine should be taken without interruption for the full length of time prescribed by your doctor. If you miss a dose, take it as soon as possible. If it is almost time for your next dose, skip the missed dose and resume your regular schedule. Do not take two doses at the same time.

SPECIAL CONSIDERATIONS FOR THOSE OVER SIXTY-FIVE

Older people taking this medicine may be more prone to develop confusion, pain or difficulty in urination, dizziness, drowsiness, fainting, or dry mouth. Nightmares, restlessness, and irritability are also more apt to occur in those over sixty-five.

CONDITION: **NAUSEA AND VOMITING (MOTION SICKNESS)**

CATEGORY: **ANTINAUSEANTS**

GENERIC (CHEMICAL) NAME	BRAND (TRADE) NAME	DOSAGE FORMS AND STRENGTHS
Scopolamine	TRANSDERM-SCŌP	Patch: 1.5 mg

DRUG PROFILE

Scopolamine is used to prevent the dizziness, nausea, and vomiting associated with motion sickness. The medicine is contained in a disclike patch, which is placed behind the ear and worn for up to three days. The active ingredient is slowly released from the patch and absorbed through the skin.

BEFORE USING THIS DRUG

Let your doctor know *IF*

You have ever had allergic reactions or other problems with ■ scopolamine ■ atropine ■ belladonna ■ hyoscyamine.

You have ever had any of the following medical problems: ■ severe bleeding problems ■ colitis ■ severe dry mouth ■ enlarged prostate ■ glaucoma ■ heart disease ■ high blood pressure ■ hiatal hernia ■ intestinal blockage or other intestinal problems ■ kidney disease ■ liver disease ■ asthma or other lung disease ■ myasthenia gravis ■ urinary blockage or other urinary problems.

You are taking any of the following medicines: ■ medicine for depression ■ antihistamines ■ medicine for hay fever, allergies, or colds ■ muscle relaxants ■ narcotics or other prescription pain-killers ■ tranquilizers ■ sleep medicines ■ medicine for seizures.

SPECIAL RESTRICTIONS WHILE TAKING THIS DRUG

FOOD AND DRUG INTERACTIONS

Other Drugs	Do not take any other drugs, including over-the-counter (OTC) drugs, before checking with your doctor. This medicine increases the effect of drugs that depress the central nervous system, such as antihistamines; medicine for hay fever, allergies, or colds; sleep medicines; tranquilizers; narcotics or other prescription pain-killers; muscle relaxants; and medicine for seizures.
Alcohol	This medicine increases the effect of alcohol, a central nervous system depressant. Avoid alcohol unless your doctor has approved its use.

No special restrictions on foods and beverages or smoking.

DAILY LIVING

Driving	This drug may cause blurred vision or drowsiness. Be careful when driving, operating household appliances, or doing any other tasks that require alertness until you know how this drug affects you.
Exertion and Exercise	This drug may cause you to sweat less than normally. Sweating is your body's natural way of cooling down, and not sweating enough can be dangerous. Use caution not to become overheated when you exercise or exert yourself.
Sun Exposure	This medicine may make your eyes unusually sensitive to sunlight; sunglasses may help relieve this problem.

Excessive Heat	See "Exertion and Exercise"; use caution during hot weather, since overexertion may result in heat stroke. Avoid extremely hot baths or saunas.
Other Precautions	Tell any doctor or dentist you consult that you are taking this medicine, especially if you will be undergoing any type of surgery.
	Before using this medicine, read the directions for use carefully. Wash and dry your hands thoroughly before and after handling a patch to avoid accidentally getting some of the medicine in your eye. Apply the patch to the hairless area of the skin behind the ear; be sure you do not place it over any skin that has been irritated or cut.
Helpful Hints	Plan to wear a patch for at least four hours before you will need it. Although you can swim or bathe with a patch on, try to keep the patch as dry as possible so it will not fall off. If the patch does loosen, remove it and replace it with a new one.
	If your mouth or throat feels dry, chewing sugarless gum or sucking ice chips or sugarless hard candy will help.

No special restrictions on exposure to excessive cold.

POSSIBLE SIDE EFFECTS

Although this list of adverse effects may seem somewhat intimidating, keep in mind that some are quite rare. Of course, should these or any other problems arise while you are on medication, it is always a good idea to consult your doctor.

IF YOU DEVELOP	WHAT TO DO
clumsiness ■ confusion ■ dizziness ■ severe drowsiness ■ seizures ■ slurred speech ■ extremely dry mouth, nose, or throat ■ fever ■ hallucinations ■ shortness of breath ■ difficulty in breathing ■ extreme excitement, nervousness, restlessness, or anxiety ■ fast heartbeat ■ extremely dry or warm skin ■ flushing	**Urgent** Get in touch with your doctor immediately.
eye pain ■ rash or hives	**May be serious** Get in touch with your doctor as soon as possible.
constipation ■ dry mouth, nose, throat, or skin ■ difficulty in swallowing ■ decreased sweating ■ increased eye sensitivity to sunlight ■ blurred vision ■ drowsiness ■ weakness ■ headache ■ problems with urination ■ bloating ■ nausea or vomiting ■ unusual euphoria ■ memory problems ■ sleep disturbances *After you STOP taking this medicine*: increased eye sensitivity to sunlight ■ anxiety ■ irritability ■ sleep disturbances or nightmares	If symptoms are disturbing or persist, let your doctor know.

STORAGE INSTRUCTIONS

Store in a cool, dark place (not in a bathroom medicine cabinet).

STOPPING OR INTERRUPTING THERAPY

A patch can be worn for up to three days. If you still need this medicine, remove the old patch before putting on a new one. Never wear two patches at the same time.

SPECIAL CONSIDERATIONS FOR THOSE OVER SIXTY-FIVE

Older people may be more prone to such side effects as confusion, drowsiness, nervousness, constipation, problems with urination, and dry mouth, nose, throat, or skin.

CONDITION: **NAUSEA AND VOMITING**

CATEGORY: **ANTINAUSEANTS**

GENERIC (CHEMICAL) NAME	BRAND (TRADE) NAME	DOSAGE FORMS AND STRENGTHS
Dronabinol	MARINOL	Capsules: 2.5, 5, 10 mg

DRUG PROFILE

Dronabinol is used to prevent the side effects of nausea and vomiting in patients who are receiving chemotherapy. This drug is thought to work by suppressing the mechanism in the brain that controls vomiting. It is used only when all other drugs for nausea or vomiting are not effective or not tolerated.

BEFORE USING THIS DRUG

Let your doctor know *IF*

You have ever had allergic reactions or other problems with ■ dronabinol ■ marijuana or products containing marijuana ■ sesame oil.

You have ever had any of the following medical problems: ■ heart disease ■ drug abuse, including alcoholism ■ high blood pressure ■ schizophrenia ■ manic depression.

You are taking any of the following medicines: ■ medicine for seizures ■ barbiturates ■ muscle relaxants ■ antihistamines ■ narcotics or other prescription pain-killers ■ sleep medicines ■ tranquilizers ■ medicine for depression ■ alcohol-containing medicines, such as some cough preparations.

SPECIAL RESTRICTIONS WHILE TAKING THIS DRUG

FOOD AND DRUG INTERACTIONS

Other Drugs	Do not take any other drugs, including over-the-counter (OTC) drugs, before checking with your doctor. This medicine increases the effect of drugs that depress the central nervous system such as antihistamines; medicine for hay fever, allergies, or colds; sleep medicines; tranquilizers; narcotics or other prescription pain-killers; muscle relaxants; and medicine for seizures.
Alcohol	This medicine increases the effect of alcohol, a central nervous system depressant. It is a good idea to avoid alcohol completely while you are taking this medicine.

No special restrictions on foods and beverages or smoking.

DAILY LIVING

Driving	This medicine may cause dizziness, drowsiness, light-headedness, mood changes, weakness, or blurred vision. Be careful when driving, operating household appliances, or doing any other tasks that require alertness until you know how this drug affects you.
Examinations or Tests	Your doctor will probably want to supervise you closely while you are taking this medicine. Electrocardiograms and blood pressure tests may be required.
Other Precautions	Tell any doctor or dentist you consult that you are taking this medicine, especially if you will be undergoing any type of surgery.

This medicine, because it controls nausea and vomiting, can mask some of the symptoms of appendicitis. If you have sharp stomach or lower abdominal pain, be sure to let your doctor know at once.

If dizziness or light-headedness is a problem, use caution when getting up from a sitting or lying-down position.

Overdose with this drug can be extremely dangerous. If you suspect that you may have taken an overdose, get in touch with your doctor immediately.

Helpful Hints

If your mouth or throat feels dry, chewing sugarless gum or sucking ice chips or sugarless hard candy will help.

No special restrictions on exertion and exercise, sun exposure, or exposure to excessive heat or cold.

POSSIBLE SIDE EFFECTS

Although this list of adverse effects may seem somewhat intimidating, keep in mind that some are quite rare. Of course, should these or any other problems arise while you are on medication, it is always a good idea to consult your doctor.

IF YOU DEVELOP	**WHAT TO DO**
mood changes ■ confusion ■ hallucinations ■ depression ■ anxiety ■ nervousness ■ fast or pounding heartbeat ■ severe dizziness or fainting ■ irrational fears ■ irritability ■ behavior or personality changes	**May be serious** Check with your doctor as soon as possible.
clumsiness ■ unsteadiness ■ dizziness ■ drowsiness ■ trouble concentrating ■ dry mouth ■ blurred vision or other vision changes ■ dizziness or light-headedness when getting up from a sitting or reclining position ■ tiredness or weakness ■ muscle pain ■ false sense of well-being ■ ringing in ears ■ headache ■ trouble speaking ■ increased sweating ■ flushing ■ sleep problems ■ restlessness ■ memory problems ■ "weird" feeling ■ fecal incontinence ■ tingling or burning sensations	If symptoms are disturbing or persist, let your doctor know.

STORAGE INSTRUCTIONS

Dronabinol capsules should be stored in the refrigerator, but be careful not to let them freeze. It is especially important to keep these medicines out of the reach of children.

STOPPING OR INTERRUPTING THERAPY

This medicine should be taken exactly as your doctor instructs you. If you miss a dose, take it as soon as possible. If it is almost time for your next dose, skip the missed dose and resume your regular schedule. Do not take two doses at the same time.

SPECIAL CONSIDERATIONS FOR THOSE OVER SIXTY-FIVE

Older people taking this medicine may be more prone to experience dizziness or light-headedness, especially when getting up from a sitting or reclining position.

CONDITION: **NAUSEA AND VOMITING**
CATEGORY: **PHENOTHIAZINES**

GENERIC (CHEMICAL) NAME	BRAND (TRADE) NAME	DOSAGE FORMS AND STRENGTHS
Prochlorperazine	COMPAZINE	Controlled-release capsules: 10, 15, 30 mg Rectal suppositories: 2.5, 5, 25 mg Syrup: 5 mg per tsp Tablets: 5, 10, 25 mg Ampule: 5 mg per ml Vial: 5 mg per ml
Thiethylperazine maleate	TORECAN	Rectal suppositories: 10 mg Tablets: 10 mg Ampule: 5 mg per ml

DRUG PROFILE

Phenothiazines are used to treat a variety of emotional disorders, including very severe anxiety, agitation, depression, and sleep disturbances. Some phenothiazines (prochlorperazine, thiethylperazine, and chlorpromazine) are also used to treat nausea and vomiting. These drugs are thought to work by inhibiting the action of dopamine, a chemical messenger, in the part of the brain that is the seat of the emotions as well as in the zone of the brain that controls nausea and vomiting.

For complete information on these drugs, see pages 606–612.

CONDITION: **NAUSEA AND VOMITING**

CATEGORY: **ANTICHOLINERGIC DRUGS**

GENERIC (CHEMICAL) NAME	BRAND (TRADE) NAME	DOSAGE FORMS AND STRENGTHS
Trimethobenzamide hydrochloride	TIGAN	Capsules: 100, 250 mg Rectal suppositories: 100, 200 mg Ampule: 100 mg per ml Vial: 100 mg per ml

DRUG PROFILE

Trimethobenzamide is used to treat nausea and vomiting. Although it is not known exactly how this drug works, it is thought to affect the nerve pathways in the part of the brain that controls vomiting.

BEFORE USING THIS DRUG

Let your doctor know *IF*

You have ever had allergic reactions or other problems with ■ trimethobenzamide ■ benzocaine or other local anesthetics.

You have ever had any of the following medical problems: ■ intestinal problems ■ encephalitis or any other brain disease.

You are taking any of the following medicines: ■ other medicine for nausea ■ aspirin ■ medicine for convulsions ■ antihistamines ■ barbiturates ■ narcotics or other prescription pain-killers ■ tranquilizers ■ sleep medicines ■ medicine for depression ■ medicine for stomach pain or cramps.

You currently have a fever.

SPECIAL RESTRICTIONS WHILE TAKING THIS DRUG

FOOD AND DRUG INTERACTIONS

Other Drugs	Do not take any other drugs, including over-the-counter (OTC) drugs, before checking with your doctor. This medicine increases the effect of drugs that depress the central nervous system, such as antihistamines; medicine for hay fever, allergies, or colds; sleep medicines; tranquilizers; narcotics and other prescription pain-killers; muscle relaxants; and medicine for seizures.
	Because this drug prevents nausea and vomiting, it may mask the overdosage symptoms of other drugs you may be taking. This drug may also mask ringing in the ears caused by aspirin.
Alcohol	This medicine increases the effect of alcohol, a central nervous system depressant. Avoid alcohol unless your doctor has approved its use.

No special restrictions on foods and beverages or smoking.

DAILY LIVING

Driving	This medicine may cause dizziness, drowsiness, or blurred vision. Use caution when driving, operating household appliances, or doing any other tasks that require alertness until you know how this drug affects you.
Other Precautions	This medicine, because it controls nausea and vomiting, can mask some of the symptoms of appendicitis. If you have sharp stomach or lower abdominal pain, be sure to let your doctor know at once.

Helpful Hints

If you have been storing the suppository form of this medicine in a warm place, it may be too soft to use. Put it in the refrigerator for half an hour or run cold water over the wrapped suppository before use.

No special restrictions on exertion and exercise, sun exposure, or exposure to excessive heat or cold.

POSSIBLE SIDE EFFECTS

Although this list of adverse effects may seem somewhat intimidating, keep in mind that some are quite rare. Of course, should these or any other problems arise while you are on medication, it is always a good idea to consult your doctor.

IF YOU DEVELOP	WHAT TO DO
seizures	**Urgent** Get in touch with your doctor immediately.
depression ■ confusion shakiness or tremors ■ sore throat or fever ■ tiredness ■ increased nausea or severe vomiting ■ yellowing of eyes or skin	**May be serious** Check with your doctor as soon as possible.
drowsiness ■ blurred vision ■ diarrhea ■ dizziness ■ headache ■ muscle cramps	If symptoms are disturbing or persist, let your doctor know.

STORAGE INSTRUCTIONS

Store in a cool, dark place (not in a bathroom medicine cabinet). Suppositories should be stored in the refrigerator.

STOPPING OR INTERRUPTING THERAPY

Trimethobenzamide should be taken without interruption for the full length of time prescribed by your doctor. If you miss a dose, take it as soon as possible. If it is almost time for your next dose, skip the missed dose and resume your regular schedule. Do not take two doses at the same time.

SPECIAL CONSIDERATIONS FOR THOSE OVER SIXTY-FIVE

Older people with fever and/or dehydration may be more susceptible to the adverse effects of this drug.

CONDITION: **NAUSEA AND VOMITING**

CATEGORY: **PROMOTILITY DRUGS**

GENERIC (CHEMICAL) NAME	BRAND (TRADE) NAME	DOSAGE FORMS AND STRENGTHS
Metoclopramide	REGLAN	Syrup: 5 mg per tsp Tablets: 5, 10 mg

DRUG PROFILE

Metoclopramide is used to relieve symptoms such as nausea, vomiting, loss of appetite, and continued feeling of fullness after eating that is due to failure of the stomach to empty properly. The drug acts by increasing the contractions of the stomach and intestines, thus quickening the pace at which food empties from the stomach and moves through the intestines. It is also prescribed for gastroesophageal reflux (heartburn), diabetic gastroparesis (a condition in which the stomach loses its ability to contract), and prevention of nausea associated with chemotherapy.

BEFORE USING THIS DRUG

Let your doctor know *IF*

You have ever had allergic reactions or other problems with ■ metoclopramide ■ procaine ■ procainamide (medicine for abnormal heart rhythms).

You have ever had any of the following medical problems: ■ stomach surgery ■ intestinal or stomach bleeding ■ epilepsy or other seizure disorders ■ intestinal blockage or adhesions ■ kidney disease ■ liver disease ■ Parkinson's disease ■ pheochromocytoma (adrenal gland tumor).

You are taking any of the following medicines: ■ other medicine for nausea and vomiting ■ medicine for Parkinson's disease ■ tranquilizers ■ medicine for seizures ■ antihistamines ■ barbiturates ■ narcotics or other prescription pain-killers ■ sleep medicines ■ medicine for depression ■ insulin (medicine for diabetes) ■ sodium bicarbonate (baking soda) ■ medicine for intestinal spasms ■ medicine for severe emotional and behavior disorders (haloperidol, chlorpromazine) ■ heart medicine (digoxin).

SPECIAL RESTRICTIONS WHILE TAKING THIS DRUG

FOOD AND DRUG INTERACTIONS

Other Drugs	Do not take any other drugs, including over-the-counter (OTC) drugs, before checking with your doctor. This medicine increases the effect of drugs that depress the central nervous system, such as antihistamines; medicine for hay fever, allergies, or colds; sleep medicines; tranquilizers; narcotics or other prescription pain-killers; muscle relaxants; and medicine for seizures.
Alcohol	This medicine increases the effect of alcohol, a central nervous system depressant. Avoid alcohol unless your doctor has approved its use.

No special restrictions on foods and beverages or smoking.

DAILY LIVING

Driving	This medicine may cause dizziness, drowsiness, or blurred vision. Be careful when driving, operating household appliances, or doing any other tasks that require alertness until you know how this drug affects you.

Other Precautions

Tell any doctor or dentist you consult that you are taking this drug, especially if you will be undergoing any type of surgery.

If you have diabetes, you may need to adjust the timing or amount of insulin dosages, since this medicine hastens the body's passage of food through the intestine and the rise of sugar levels in the bloodstream.

Helpful Hints

If this medicine upsets your stomach, ask your doctor if you can take it with food.

No special restrictions on exertion and exercise, sun exposure, or exposure to excessive heat or cold.

POSSIBLE SIDE EFFECTS

Although this list of adverse effects may seem somewhat intimidating, keep in mind that some are quite rare. Of course, should these or any other problems arise while you are on medication, it is always a good idea to consult your doctor.

IF YOU DEVELOP

confusion ■ severe drowsiness ■ muscle spasms ■ shuffling walk ■ uncontrollable movements of hands, face, tongue, jaw, or mouth ■ other uncontrollable muscle changes ■ change in facial expression ■ slurred speech ■ trembling or shaking of hands ■ tongue inflammation ■ swelling of eye area ■ seizures ■ hallucinations ■ difficulty in breathing ■ mood changes ■ fever ■ rash ■ yellowing of the eyes or skin

WHAT TO DO

May be serious Check with your doctor as soon as possible.

drowsiness ■ restlessness ■ tiredness ■ dizziness ■ constipation ■ diarrhea ■ headache ■ nausea or vomiting ■ upset stomach ■ sleeplessness ■ anxiety or agitation ■ depression ■ visual disturbances ■ urinary frequency or incontinence ■ dry mouth ■ breast swelling in men

If symptoms are disturbing or persist, let your doctor know.

STORAGE INSTRUCTIONS

This drug should be kept in a cool, dark place (not in a bathroom medicine cabinet). If your medicine is in a liquid form, make sure that it does not freeze.

STOPPING OR INTERRUPTING THERAPY

Take this drug exactly as directed by your doctor. Do not increase the dose or take it for longer than prescribed. If you miss a dose, take it as soon as possible. If it is almost time for your next dose, skip the missed dose and resume your regular schedule. Do not take two doses at the same time.

SPECIAL CONSIDERATIONS FOR THOSE OVER SIXTY-FIVE

Older individuals are more sensitive to metoclopramide and more likely to experience some of the side effects. Your doctor, therefore, may decide to begin treatment with a lower dosage.

GALLSTONES

Gallstone disease is nothing new. Its symptoms and possible causes were discussed extensively in the medical literature of the last century. But many older people experience it for the first time because the incidence of the disease increases with advancing years. This condition is about two to four times more likely to develop in women than in men, is especially prevalent in obese individuals, and is most common in persons of both sexes over forty years of age. It is estimated that 30 percent of women and 15 percent of men over the age of seventy have gallstones.

Many people who have gallstone disease are not even aware they have this problem because they don't have any symptoms. Others do experience symptoms severe enough to require medical attention. The center of all this attention—the gallbladder—is a small, pear-shaped organ that is located in the upper right abdomen, tucked partway underneath the liver. Its purpose is to concentrate the bile, and then store it until it is needed for digestive work.

CAUSES

Researchers have found that the main culprit in gallstone disease is abnormal bile. There are three basic components of bile: cholesterol, bile acids, and phospholipids. In healthy people, these components are in proper balance, and the bile is in a freely moving, fluid state. But for reasons not yet understood, this chemical balance is disturbed in some people. The ratio of cholesterol to bile acids increases, causing the bile to become supersaturated with cholesterol. This can lead to the formation of stones. (Although there are other types of gallstones, cholesterol stones are the most common.)

Incidentally, the development of these stones is not caused by a high cholesterol level in the blood. Nor does it appear to be related to the amount of fat in the diet.

DIAGNOSIS

Depending on their number, size, and location, gallstones may cause either no problems at all, only mild discomfort, or the typical symptoms of a gallbladder attack—severe pain in the right upper or middle portion of the abdomen, sometimes accompanied by nausea, vomiting, and fever. Most often, this happens when one or more gallstones become lodged in the duct that carries bile to the duodenum. When this duct is blocked, the normal flow of bile is interrupted. As a result, the gallbladder may become severely inflamed or even infected.

If your doctor suspects that you might have gallstones, he or she will order some specific tests to confirm the diagnosis. A highly accurate test for this purpose, known as ultrasonography, involves transmitting high-pitched sound waves through the body over the area of the gallbladder.

A transducer, which is a sound-producing device, is placed over the skin and moved around from location to location. If you have a stone in the gallbladder or duct an echo will be generated in that area. The echo is then transmitted through a computer onto a video screen, and a visual record is made from that image. Ultrasonography does not involve X rays.

TREATMENT

How your doctor manages your gallstone problem depends on various factors, including how severe your symptoms are, how long you have had gallbladder trouble, your overall health, and your age. The risks of surgically removing the gallbladder are higher in an older person, so more consideration might be given to a nonsurgical approach to the problem. If the gallstones have caused no symptoms, medical or surgical treatment may not be necessary.

Drugs   Chenodiol and ursodiol are currently the only drugs on the market in the United States that are able to dissolve cholesterol gallstones in humans. For more detailed information on these drugs, refer to the chart on pages 464–466.

Surgery   Because of the current limitations of drug therapy and because people can function quite well without a gallbladder, gallstones are still most often treated by surgically removing the entire organ. This operation, called a cholecystectomy, is one of the safest and most frequently performed of all abdominal procedures. At the same time that the gallbladder is removed, any stones found in the bile duct are also extracted. Gallbladder surgery generally cures the gallstone problem but, like any form of major emergency surgery, there is a risk of complications, especially in older people.

OUTLOOK

Therapy with gallstone-dissolving drugs can, over time, eliminate the stones that are causing the difficulty; with long-term treatment, recurrence of the problem can be prevented. While this does not constitute a cure, it does mean relief from the severe pain and other symptoms of a gallbladder attack.

Caution: Some drugs in this section may affect pregnancy or fetal development. Check with your doctor if this concerns you.

CONDITION: **GALLSTONES**

CATEGORY: **DISSOLVING AGENTS**

GENERIC (CHEMICAL) NAME	BRAND (TRADE) NAME	DOSAGE FORMS AND STRENGTHS
Chenodiol	CHENIX	Tablets: 250 mg
Ursodiol	ACTIGALL	Capsules: 300 mg

DRUG PROFILE

Chenodiol and ursodiol are used to dissolve gallstones in patients in whom surgery is not necessary or should be avoided. These drugs are part of the body's naturally occurring bile acids. When taken as directed, they create an environment that dissolves gallstones and prevents new ones from forming.

BEFORE USING THIS DRUG

Let your doctor know *IF*

You have ever had allergic reactions or other problems with ■ chenodiol ■ ursodiol.

You have ever had any of the following medical problems: ■ any other disease of the gallbladder or bile ducts ■ inflammatory bowel disease ■ liver disease ■ pancreas disease.

You are taking any of the following medicines: ■ antacids ■ estrogens (female hormones) ■ medicine for high cholesterol.

SPECIAL RESTRICTIONS WHILE TAKING THIS DRUG

FOOD AND DRUG INTERACTIONS

Foods and Beverages	Your doctor may prescribe a high-fiber diet to help stones dissolve faster and prevent new stones from forming. A weight-reduction diet may also be advised.

No special restrictions on other drugs, alcohol use, or smoking.

DAILY LIVING

Examinations or Tests	Your doctor will order regular blood tests and X rays or ultrasound tests to check whether the gallstones are dissolving and the liver is functioning properly.
Other Precautions	If you have severe pain in your upper right side, or if you have fever, severe nausea and vomiting, yellowing of eyes or skin, or change in urine or stool color, contact your doctor immediately. These symptoms may reflect a worsening of your gallbladder condition.
Helpful Hints	Take this medicine with food or milk unless your doctor instructs you otherwise. This medicine often causes mild diarrhea; this will probably not last very long. If it bothers you, your doctor can reduce your dosage.

No special restrictions on driving, exertion and exercise, sun exposure, or exposure to excessive heat or cold.

POSSIBLE SIDE EFFECTS

Although this list of adverse effects may seem somewhat intimidating, keep in mind that some are quite rare. Of course, should these or any other problems arise while you are on medication, it is always a good idea to consult your doctor.

IF YOU DEVELOP	WHAT TO DO
severe diarrhea	**May be serious** Check with your doctor as soon as possible.
mild diarrhea ■ frequent urge for bowel movements ■ constipation ■ gas ■ loss of appetite ■ nausea or vomiting ■ stomach pain or cramps ■ heartburn	If symptoms are disturbing or persist, let your doctor know.

STORAGE INSTRUCTIONS

Store in a cool, dark place (not in a bathroom medicine cabinet).

STOPPING OR INTERRUPTING THERAPY

Chenodiol and ursodiol should be taken without interruption for the full length of time prescribed by your doctor, even once you begin to feel better. If stopped too soon, gallstones may not dissolve completely. If you miss a dose, take it as soon as possible. If it is almost time for your next dose, skip the missed dose and resume your regular schedule. Do not take two doses at the same time.

SPECIAL CONSIDERATIONS FOR THOSE OVER SIXTY-FIVE

None.

Chapter 4
Pain and Discomfort

PAIN

Pain is nature's distress signal, alerting us that something may be seriously awry and should be tended to. It's easy to forget, however, that pain is a symptom, not a disease. While it's important to relieve pain, it's even more important to discover what's causing it. As one grows older, one becomes more susceptible to certain conditions that cause pain. While medicine can sometimes help, relief is not always just a pill away.

THE MECHANISM OF PAIN

There are two types of pain—acute and chronic. Acute pain, which comes on suddenly and may last from a few hours to a few weeks, may be caused by such circumstances as an infection, accident, or surgery. Chronic pain, which may last for several months or persist throughout one's life, can be caused by a variety of conditions. In some cases, the underlying problem may defy detection.

Although there is a great deal still to be learned about the mechanism of pain, the basic way in which the "distress signal" is communicated to the brain is relatively clear. Apparently, a two-part process is involved. First, to trigger the body's protective reflexes, specialized nerve endings, known as pain receptors, pick up the sensation of injury and relay it via the spinal cord to the brain. Next, there is a more diffused and prolonged ache, perhaps a reminder of the damage that has been done. Chemicals are the actual communicators in the alarm system. Tissue damage—caused by burning a finger, for example—releases tiny bursts of powerful substances that activate pain in nerve endings.

The alarm system is accompanied by another system—one that censors the messages of pain. When the body has been injured, the brain triggers the release of pain-killing chemicals known as endorphins. These natural pain-killers inhibit pain messages on their way up the spine.

THE PSYCHOLOGY OF PAIN

The way in which you experience pain is completely subjective. What is very painful to someone else may cause you only minor discomfort. Our experience of pain is modified by a number of factors. Some people have a higher or lower pain tolerance than others. For example, when stuck by a needle, some people will perceive the pain more strongly than others will—that is, they have a lower threshold.

Tolerance to pain depends, in part, on a general attitude toward pain; a high threshold may have been developed during childhood by such admonitions as "keep a stiff upper lip." Also, pain tolerance can be diminished by negative factors such as stress, fatigue, fear, anxiety, and depression.

Pain tolerance can be increased by positive factors, chief among which is distraction. Other positive factors that can modify pain include hypnosis and meditation. A study on the chemistry of pain indicates that men are less sensitive to pain than are women—and, interestingly, older people less sensitive than the young.

TREATMENT

Treatment for acute or chronic pain can range from relaxation techniques to acupuncture or biofeedback training to such drugs as aspirin, codeine, or stronger pain-killers. With chronic pain in particular, your doctor may design a regimen that incorporates both drug and nondrug therapies. By learning to minimize pain through distraction and relaxation, it is possible to keep doses of pain-killers at low levels, so side effects can be avoided or minimized.

Pain relief medicines fall into two categories—narcotics and others. *Nonnarcotic analgesics* are the most frequent drugs taken by older people, with aspirin the most popular choice. Aspirin is capable of reducing both fever and inflammation, as are other derivatives of salicylic acid (see chart on pages 471–475). You may prefer, however, using either acetaminophen or ibuprofen, which are also nonnarcotic drugs available over the counter. Acetaminophen (see chart on pages 476–478) has little anti-inflammatory effect, but you may use it to reduce a fever or relieve pain if you find that aspirin upsets your stomach. Note, however, that, like many drugs, it tends to remain in an older person's system for a relatively long time, so any adverse reaction to the drug may be prolonged. Ibuprofen (see chart on pages 486–488), like aspirin, reduces pain, fever, and inflammation. Trial and error will help you determine which product works best for you.

Ibuprofen belongs to the group of pain-killers known as nonsteroidal anti-inflammatory agents. They are frequently used for arthritis, as well as other types of painful inflammatory conditions.

Keep in mind that no drug—including aspirin—is completely without potential side effects. Nevertheless, nonnarcotics are generally safe if the instructions given on the package are followed.

Narcotic analgesics are available *only* with a doctor's prescription. These are potent drugs that should be used only in specific circumstances, such as to relieve acute pain after an injury or surgery or to ease the pain of the terminally ill (see pages 479–485). Narcotic analgesics include codeine (and the similar drugs hydrocodone and oxycodone), meperidine, and hydromorphone. In older people, lower dosages are used. Common side effects of these drugs are drowsiness and constipation. In general, older people are more sensitive to the side effects of these medicines.

One hallmark of a narcotic is that the body builds up a tolerance to it, meaning that more drug is needed to produce the same effect over time. The danger of addiction after prolonged use is possible.

When all else fails, people who continue to suffer from chronic pain can seek help from a clinic specializing in pain disorders. At a multidisciplinary pain clinic, a team of specialists can prescribe or adjust medicines to achieve greater effectiveness without the dangers of abuse. Psychotherapy and behavioral modification may also be used. They may also offer such unconventional pain-reduction methods as acupuncture; nerve blocks, in which nerve paths are interrupted by injections; cryoanalgesia, the freezing of nerve fibers; and TENS (transcutaneous electrical nerve stimulation). Medicines may be prescribed or adjusted to achieve greater effectiveness with less danger of abuse. There are now estimated to be several hundred of these clinics around the country, some of which offer more comprehensive programs than others.

OUTLOOK

The search continues for a more complete understanding of the complexities of pain, as well as for potent pain-killers that don't have the drawbacks of narcotics. With all the innovative research being done in this area—and the increasing attention it is receiving from medical scientists—the next decade will likely produce more effective solutions to the challenges of pain management.

Caution: Some drugs in this section may affect pregnancy or fetal development. Check with your doctor if this concerns you.

CONDITION: **PAIN**

CATEGORY: **ANALGESICS**

GENERIC (CHEMICAL) NAME	BRAND (TRADE) NAME	DOSAGE FORMS AND STRENGTHS
Aspirin and other salicylate drugs		

Aspirin and aspirin-containing drugs are available over the counter under a variety of brand names, dosage forms, and strengths. Some of these preparations have a special coating to help protect the lining of the stomach against possible irritation. Because of the importance of aspirin in the treatment of chronic pain, even though they are most often nonprescription drugs, they are included in this book for reader reference.

DRUG PROFILE

Aspirin and other drugs in the salicylate family are used to relieve pain, inflammation, and fever. Large doses are used to treat symptoms of arthritis and rheumatism such as swelling, stiffness, and joint pain. Aspirin is thought to control pain and swelling by blocking the production of naturally occurring triggers of pain and inflammation, called prostaglandins. These drugs also relieve fever by changing the way the body regulates its temperature.

BEFORE USING THIS DRUG

Let your doctor know *IF*

You have ever had allergic reactions or other problems with ■ aspirin or aspirin-containing medicine ■ indomethacin ■ ibuprofen or any other nonsteroidal anti-inflammatory drugs ■ any other substance to which you are hypersensitive.

You have ever had any of the following medical problems: ■ hay fever ■ asthma ■ ulcers, gastritis, or any other stomach or intestinal problems ■ liver disease ■ kidney disease ■ systemic lupus erythematosus ■ glucose-6-phosphate dehydrogenase (G-6-PD) deficiency ■ vitamin K deficiency ■ anemia ■ nasal polyps ■ pyruvate kinase deficiency ■ chronic hives ■ chronic stuffy nose ■ rheumatic fever ■ disease of the blood vessels ■ any bleeding disorder ■ recent oral surgery ■ diabetes ■ tinnitus (ringing in ears).

You are taking any of the following medicines: ■ acetaminophen ■ medicine for gout ■ medicine for arthritis ■ anticoagulants (blood thinners) ■ corticosteroids ■ antacids ■ any medicine containing magnesium ■ any medicine containing alcohol ■ beta-blockers ■ medicine for high blood pressure ■ diuretics ■ captopril (medicine for high blood pressure and congestive heart failure) ■ medicine for glaucoma ■ medicine for seizures ■ medicine for diabetes ■ methotrexate (medicine for severe psoriasis and cancer) ■ nitrates (medicine for chest pain) ■ medicine to make the urine more alkaline or more acidic ■ medicine for tuberculosis ■ medicine for nausea or vomiting ■ medicine for diabetes.

With a buffered aspirin or salicylate: ■ tetracycline.

SPECIAL RESTRICTIONS WHILE TAKING THIS DRUG

FOOD AND DRUG INTERACTIONS

Other Drugs	Be especially careful about using other medicines that contain aspirin. Check the labels of all other drugs you are taking, including over-the-counter (OTC) products. If you use any laxative containing cellulose, take it at least two hours before or after your dose of aspirin.
Foods and Beverages	If you are on a low-salt diet, check with your doctor before taking buffered effervescent aspirin tablets or sodium salicylate because these preparations contain sodium. Caffeine can worsen the irritant effects of aspirin. Reduce your intake of caffeine-containing products (eg, coffee, tea, cola drinks).
Alcohol	It is a good idea to cut down on alcohol while taking aspirin-containing medicine. Alcohol may add to the irritant effects of salicylates on your stomach.

Smoking	Smoking also creates excess stomach acid, which may worsen the stomach irritation caused by aspirin.

DAILY LIVING

Examinations or Tests	It is important for you to keep all appointments with your doctor so that your progress can be checked. If you are on long-term therapy with a salicylate drug, periodic blood or urine tests may be required.
Other Precautions	If you have diabetes, be aware that false urine-sugar tests may occur while you are taking aspirin. Check with your doctor before increasing the dose of any diabetes medicine you may be taking.

Tell any doctor or dentist you consult that you are taking aspirin, especially if you will be undergoing any type of surgery.

Let your doctor know if you notice a buzzing or ringing sound in your ears, since this may be a sign of aspirin overdose. If you should accidentally take an overdose of this drug, go to a hospital emergency room immediately.

If you are taking aspirin or another salicylate for a fever that does not subside after three days, check with your doctor.

Do not take aspirin during the last trimester of pregnancy unless prescribed by your doctor.

Aspirin or other salicylates should not be given to children or teenagers with chickenpox or the flu because of the possibility of developing a serious life-threatening condition called Reye's Syndrome.

Helpful Hints	Take this medicine with a snack, after meals, or with milk or an antacid to reduce its irritant effects on your stomach. Also, do not skip meals while you are on aspirin therapy.
	The coated tablets should be swallowed whole without crushing, chewing, or breaking.
	The liquid may be mixed with fruit juice; drink a full glass of water afterwards.

No special restrictions on driving, exertion and exercise, sun exposure, or exposure to excessive heat or cold.

POSSIBLE SIDE EFFECTS

Although this list of adverse effects may seem somewhat intimidating, keep in mind that some are quite rare. Of course, should these or any other problems arise while you are on medication, it is always a good idea to consult your doctor.

IF YOU DEVELOP

seizures ■ confusion ■ severe or continuing headache ■ blood in urine or decreased urination ■ fast heartbeat ■ dizziness or light-headedness ■ severe drowsiness ■ personality changes ■ severe or continuing nausea or vomiting ■ difficulty in breathing or breathing changes ■ continuing stomach pain ■ fever ■ increased sweating ■ tearing eyes ■ fainting ■ rectal bleeding ■ shock (sweating, faintness, rapid pulse, nausea, panting, and pale, cold, moist skin) ■ bloody or black, tarry stools ■ vomiting, with blood or vomit that looks like coffee grounds ■ wheezing ■ rash, hives, or itching

WHAT TO DO

Urgent Get in touch with your doctor immediately.

stomach pain or tenderness ■ nausea or vomiting ■ ringing or buzzing in ears ■ tightness in chest ■ tiredness or weakness ■ bleeding or bruising ■ loss of taste for cigarettes

May be serious Check with your doctor as soon as possible.

heartburn ■ loss of appetite

With preparations that contain caffeine: sleeplessness or nervousness

With salicylamide only: drowsiness

If symptoms are disturbing or persist, let your doctor know.

STORAGE INSTRUCTIONS

Store in a cool, dark place (not in a bathroom medicine cabinet). If your medicine is in a liquid form, make sure that it does not freeze. If you notice a vinegarlike odor from a bottle of pills, this means that the drug is breaking down and should be discarded.

STOPPING OR INTERRUPTING THERAPY

If you are taking aspirin for arthritis, you may have to take it for the rest of your life, since this medicine controls but does not cure arthritis. If you miss a dose, take it as soon as possible. If it is almost time for your next dose, skip the missed dose and resume your regular schedule. Do not take two doses at the same time.

SPECIAL CONSIDERATIONS FOR THOSE OVER SIXTY-FIVE

Those older people who have reduced kidney function tend not to eliminate the salicylates as readily as people with normal kidney function. In this case, a doctor may schedule regular checkups to make sure the person is receiving the proper dosage and that too much drug is not accumulating in the body.

CONDITION: **PAIN**

CATEGORY: **ANALGESICS**

GENERIC (CHEMICAL) NAME	BRAND (TRADE) NAME	DOSAGE FORMS AND STRENGTHS
Acetaminophen	Regular Strength ANACIN-3	Tablets: 325 mg
	Maximum Strength ANACIN-3	Caplets: 500 mg Tablets: 500 mg
	Aspirin-free ARTHRITIS PAIN FORMULA	Tablets: 500 mg
	Extra Strength DATRIL	Caplets: 500 mg Tablets: 500 mg
	PANADOL	Caplets: 500 mg Tablets: 500 mg
	Maximum Strength ST. JOSEPH Aspirin-Free	Tablets: 500 mg
	Regular Strength TYLENOL	Caplets: 325 mg Tablets: 325 mg
	Extra-Strength TYLENOL	Caplets: 500 mg Gelcaps: 500 mg Liquid: 500 mg per tbsp Tablets: 500 mg

DRUG PROFILE

Acetaminophen is used to relieve fever and pain. It is thought to work by blocking pain centers in the central nervous system and by resetting the body's thermostat to its normal temperature.

BEFORE USING THIS DRUG

Let your doctor know *IF*

You have ever had severe allergic reactions or other problems with
  ■ acetaminophen.

You have ever had any of the following medical problems: ■ anemia ■ asthma or other lung disease ■ kidney disease ■ liver disease.

You are taking any of the following medicines: ■ anticoagulants (blood thinners) ■ barbiturates ■ medicine for seizures ■ charcoal ■ antibiotics ■ sulfinpyrazone ■ medicine for Parkinson's disease ■ medicine for stomach cramps, ulcers, or irritable bowel syndrome ■ medicine for urinary tract spasms ■ medicine for asthma ■ scopolamine (medicine for motion sickness).

SPECIAL RESTRICTIONS WHILE TAKING THIS DRUG

FOOD AND DRUG INTERACTIONS

Other Drugs	Be especially careful about using other medicines that contain acetaminophen. Check the labels of all other drugs you are taking, including over-the-counter (OTC) medicines.
Alcohol	Drinking large amounts of alcohol during long-term therapy with acetaminophen may lead to liver problems and should be avoided.

No special restrictions on foods and beverages or smoking.

DAILY LIVING

Examinations or Tests	It is important for you to keep all appointments with your doctor so that your progress can be checked.
Other Precautions	Take this medicine exactly as instructed on the package labeling. If you are taking acetaminophen for a fever that does not subside after three days, check with your doctor.

No special restrictions on driving, exertion and exercise, sun exposure, or exposure to excessive heat or cold.

POSSIBLE SIDE EFFECTS

Although this list of adverse effects may seem somewhat intimidating, keep in mind that some are quite rare. Of course, should these or any other problems arise while you are on medication, it is always a good idea to consult your doctor.

IF YOU DEVELOP	WHAT TO DO
hoarseness ■ nausea or vomiting ■ stomach cramps or pain ■ excitement ■ delirium ■ severe dizziness or drowsiness ■ clammy skin ■ fast, shallow breathing ■ fast, weak, irregular pulse ■ yellowing of eyes or skin ■ diarrhea ■ loss of appetite ■ fever or sore throat ■ stomach swelling and tenderness ■ bloody or cloudy urine ■ decreased urination ■ pain or difficulty in urination	**Urgent** Get in touch with your doctor immediately.
bleeding or bruising ■ rash, hives, or itching ■ tiredness or weakness	**May be serious** Check with your doctor as soon as possible.

STORAGE INSTRUCTIONS

Store in a cool, dark place (not in a bathroom medicine cabinet). If your medicine is in a liquid form, make sure that it does not freeze.

STOPPING OR INTERRUPTING THERAPY

Take this medicine exactly as directed on the package label unless otherwise instructed by your doctor.

SPECIAL CONSIDERATIONS FOR THOSE OVER SIXTY-FIVE

Exceeding recommended doses is dangerous because liver damage can occur more easily in this age group if too much acetaminophen is taken.

CONDITION: **PAIN**

CATEGORY: **ANALGESICS**

GENERIC (CHEMICAL) NAME	BRAND (TRADE) NAME	DOSAGE FORMS AND STRENGTHS
Codeine sulfate		Tablets: 15, 30, 60 mg
Codeine phosphate and acetaminophen	PHENAPHEN with Codeine	Capsules: 325 mg acetaminophen and 15, 30, or 60 mg codeine phosphate
	PHENAPHEN-650 with Codeine	Tablets: 650 mg acetaminophen and 30 mg codeine phosphate
	TYLENOL with Codeine	Elixir: 120 mg acetaminophen and 12 mg codeine phosphate
		Tablets: 300 mg acetaminophen and 7.5, 15, 30, or 60 mg codeine phosphate
Codeine phosphate and aspirin	EMPIRIN with Codeine	Tablets: 325 mg aspirin and 15, 30, or 60 mg codeine phosphate
Fentanyl	DURAGESIC	Transdermal patch: 25 μg per hr., 50 μg per hr., 75 μg per hr., 100 μg per hr.
Hydrocodone bitartrate and acetaminophen	VICODIN	Tablets: 5 mg hydrocodone bitartrate and 500 mg acetaminophen
	VICODIN ES	Tablets: 7.5 mg hydrocodone bitartrate and 750 mg acetaminophen

	LORTAB	Tablets: 2.5 mg hydrocodone bitartrate and 500 mg acetaminophen, 5 mg hydrocodone bitartrate and 500 mg acetaminophen, 7.5 mg hydrocodone bitartrate and 500 mg acetaminophen
		Liquid: 2.5 mg hydrocodone bitartrate and 120 mg acetaminophen
	LORCET Plus	Tablets: 7.5 mg hydrocodone bitartrate and 650 mg acetaminophen
	ANEXSIA	Tablets: 5 mg hydrocodone bitartrate and 500 mg acetaminophen, 7.5 mg hydrocodone bitartrate and 650 mg acetaminophen
	HYDROCET	Capsules: 5 mg hydrocodone bitartrate and 500 mg acetaminophen
Hydromorphone hydrochloride	DILAUDID	Rectal suppositories: 3 mg Tablets: 1, 2, 3, 4 mg
Meperidine hydrochloride	DEMEROL	Syrup: 50 mg per tsp Tablets: 50, 100 mg
Meperidine hydrochloride and promethazine hydrochloride	MEPERGAN Fortis	Capsules: 50 mg meperidine hydrochloride and 25 mg promethazine hydrochloride
Methadone hydrochloride	DOLOPHINE Hydrochloride	Tablets: 5, 10 mg
Oxycodone hydrochloride and acetaminophen	PERCOCET	Tablets: 5 mg oxycodone hydrochloride and 325 mg acetaminophen

Oxycodone hydrochloride and acetaminophen	TYLOX	Capsules: 5 mg oxycodone hydrochloride and 500 mg acetaminophen
Oxycodone hydrochloride, oxycodone terephthalate, and aspirin	PERCODAN	Tablets: 4.5 mg oxycodone hydrochloride, 0.38 mg oxycodone terephthalate, and 325 mg aspirin
	PERCODAN-Demi	Tablets: 2.25 mg oxycodone hydrochloride, 0.19 mg oxycodone terephthalate, and 325 mg aspirin
Propoxyphene hydrochloride	DARVON	Capsules: 65 mg
Propoxyphene hydrochloride and acetaminophen	WYGESIC	Tablets: 65 mg propoxyphene hydrochloride and 650 mg acetaminophen
Butalbital, aspirin, caffeine, and codeine phosphate	FIORINAL with Codeine	Capsules: 50 mg butalbital; 325 mg aspirin; 40 mg caffeine; and 30 mg (No. 3) codeine phosphate
Propoxyphene hydrochloride, aspirin, and caffeine	DARVON COMPOUND–65	Capsules: 65 mg propoxyphene hydrochloride, 389 mg aspirin, and 32.4 mg caffeine
Propoxyphene napsylate	DARVON-N	Suspension: 50 mg per tsp Tablets: 100 mg

Propoxyphene napsylate and acetaminophen DARVOCET-N	Tablets: 100 mg propoxyphene napsylate and 650 mg acetaminophen

DRUG PROFILE

This class of drugs is used to relieve pain. These medicines alter the perception of pain; although it is not known exactly how they work, they are thought to act on nerves located in the brain and spinal cord that transmit the sensation of pain.

BEFORE USING THIS DRUG

Let your doctor know *IF*

You have ever had allergic reactions or other problems with ■ any prescription pain-killers.

You have ever had any of the following medical problems: ■ drug dependence ■ head injury ■ seizures ■ asthma or other lung disease ■ enlarged prostate ■ urinary problems ■ glaucoma ■ kidney disease ■ liver disease ■ abnormal heart rhythms ■ stomach or intestinal disorders ■ underactive thyroid ■ Addison's disease ■ alcoholism ■ heart attack.

You are taking any of the following medicines: ■ other pain-killers ■ medicine for glaucoma ■ antihistamines ■ medicine for coughs, colds, or hay fever ■ medicine for seizures ■ barbiturates ■ muscle relaxants ■ tranquilizers ■ sleep medicines ■ medicine for depression (within the last two weeks) ■ cimetidine (medicine for ulcers) ■ anticoagulants (blood thinners) ■ amphetamines.

SPECIAL RESTRICTIONS WHILE TAKING THIS DRUG

FOOD AND DRUG INTERACTIONS

Other Drugs	These medicines increase the effect of drugs that affect the central nervous system, such as antihistamines; medicine for hay fever, allergies, or colds;

sleep medicines; tranquilizers; other narcotics or pre-scription pain-killers; muscle relaxants, or medicines for seizures. Do not take any other drugs, including over-the-counter (OTC) drugs, before checking with your doctor.

You may need to take stool softeners while on these drugs to help with constipation.

Alcohol	These medicines increase the effect of alcohol, which is a central nervous system depressant. Avoid alcohol unless your doctor has approved its use.

No special restrictions on foods and beverages or smoking.

DAILY LIVING

Driving	These drugs may cause drowsiness, light-headedness, and dizziness and also affect mental alertness and physical coordination. Be careful when driving, operating household appliances, or doing any other tasks that require alertness until you know how this drug affects you.
Examinations or Tests	It is important for you to keep all appointments with your doctor so that your progress can be checked.
Other Precautions	Tell any doctor or dentist you consult that you are taking this medicine, especially if you will be undergoing any type of surgery.
	Take this medicine exactly as prescribed by your doctor; taking it more often or for a longer period of time than prescribed may make it habit-forming.
	If you accidentally take an overdose of this medicine, call your doctor or go to an emergency room immediately.

Helpful Hints

These drugs may cause constipation. To help avoid this condition, you should eat a diet rich in fiber, drink plenty of water, and exercise regularly.

You may vomit or feel nauseated when you first start taking this medicine. If this happens, lie down until you feel better. You also may experience dizziness and light-headedness, especially when getting up from a reclining or sitting position. Getting up slowly may help prevent this problem.

If you have been storing the suppository form of this medicine in a warm place, it may be too soft to use. Put it in the refrigerator for half an hour or run cold water over the wrapped suppository before use.

No special restrictions on exertion and exercise, sun exposure, or exposure to excessive heat or cold.

POSSIBLE SIDE EFFECTS

Although this list of adverse effects may seem somewhat intimidating, keep in mind that some are quite rare. Of course, should these or any other problems arise while you are on medication, it is always a good idea to consult your doctor.

IF YOU DEVELOP

difficulty in breathing ■ severe dizziness or drowsiness ■ seizures ■ blurred vision or other visual disturbances ■ extreme restlessness or nervousness ■ severe weakness ■ irregular, slow, or fast heartbeat ■ shakiness, tremors, or other unusual body movements

WHAT TO DO

Urgent Get in touch with your doctor immediately.

inability to concentrate ■ confusion ■ depression ■ "high" feeling or other mood changes ■ weakness ■ faintness ■ agitation or nervousness ■ sleeplessness ■ delirium ■ eye pain ■ rash, hives, or itching ■ dry mouth ■ hallucinations

May be serious Check with your doctor as soon as possible.

nausea or vomiting ■ constipation ■ dizziness or light-headedness, especially when getting up from a reclining or sitting position ■ drowsiness ■ flushing ■ sexual problems ■ difficulty in urination or decreased urination ■ increased sweating

With oxycodone only: headache

If symptoms are disturbing or persist, let your doctor know.

STORAGE INSTRUCTIONS

Store in a cool, dark place (not in a bathroom medicine cabinet). If your medicine is in a liquid form, make sure that it does not freeze. Suppositories should be stored in the refrigerator.

STOPPING OR INTERRUPTING THERAPY

If you have been taking this medicine regularly for several weeks, do not abruptly stop taking it; your doctor will advise you on how to decrease your dosage gradually.

SPECIAL CONSIDERATIONS FOR THOSE OVER SIXTY-FIVE

Older people may be more susceptible to such side effects of this medicine as difficulty in breathing, confusion or difficulty in thinking, agitation, drowsiness, weakness, nausea, difficulty in urination, and constipation.

CONDITION: **PAIN**

CATEGORY: **NONSTEROIDAL ANTI-INFLAMMATORY DRUGS (NSAIDs)**

GENERIC (CHEMICAL) NAME	BRAND (TRADE) NAME	DOSAGE FORMS AND STRENGTHS
Diclofenac	VOLTAREN	Tablets: 25, 50, 75 mg
Diflunisal	DOLOBID	Tablets: 250, 500 mg
Etodolac	LODINE	Capsules: 200, 300 mg
Fenoprofen calcium	NALFON	Capsules: 200, 300 mg Tablets: 600 mg
Flurbiprofen	ANSAID	Tablets: 50, 100 mg
Ibuprofen	ADVIL (OTC)	Caplets: 200 mg Tablets: 200 mg
	MEDIPREN	Tablets: 200 mg
	MOTRIN	Tablets: 300, 400, 600, 800 mg
	NUPRIN (OTC)	Caplets: 200 mg Tablets: 200 mg
	RUFEN	Tablets: 400, 600, 800 mg
Ketoprofen	ORUDIS	Capsules: 25, 50, 75 mg
Indomethacin	INDOCIN	Capsules: 25, 50 mg Rectal suppositories: 50 mg Suspension: 25 mg per tsp

	INDOCIN SR	Controlled-release capsules: 75 mg
Meclofenamate sodium	MECLOMEN	Capsules: meclofenamate sodium equivalent to 50 or 100 mg meclofenamic acid
Mefenamic acid	PONSTEL	Kapseals: 250 mg
Naproxen	NAPROSYN	Tablets: 250, 375, 500 mg
Naproxen sodium	ANAPROX	Tablets: 275 mg Suspension: 125 mg per tsp.
	ANAPROX DS	Tablets: 550 mg
Phenylbutazone	BUTAZOLIDIN	Capsules: 100 mg Tablets: 100 mg
Piroxicam	FELDENE	Capsules: 10, 20 mg
Sulindac	CLINORIL	Tablets: 150, 200 mg
Tolmetin sodium	TOLECTIN	Tablets: tolmetin sodium equivalent to 200 mg tolmetin
	TOLECTIN DS	Capsules: tolmetin sodium equivalent to 400 mg tolmetin
	TOLECTIN 600	Tablets: tolmetin sodium equivalent to 600 mg tolmetin

DRUG PROFILE

Nonsteroidal anti-inflammatory drugs, or NSAIDs, help relieve swelling, stiffness, joint pain, and inflammation in the long-term treatment of arthritis. These drugs are thought to act by blocking the production of naturally occurring pain and inflammation triggers called prostaglandins.

For complete information on these drugs, see pages 524–530.

Chapter 5
Disorders of the Muscles, Bones, and Joints

BACKACHE

Just about everyone has a backache at some time in life. For most people, back trouble is annoying but temporary and not disabling. For others, however, back pain is so chronic and intense that normal living is impossible.

CAUSES

The cause of a backache is often not clear, but an understanding of the structure of the back can suggest some possible reasons for discomfort or pain. The bones of the back, or vertebrae, are like hollow spools with the spinal cord threaded through the holes. Nerves sprout off the spinal cord, emerging from smaller holes at the back of the vertebrae, to carry messages back and forth between the body parts and the cord. Between the vertebrae are little pads called discs, which are composed of a cushiony, elastic material inside a membrane.

Strong bands of tissue (ligaments) and the muscles of the back support this vertebral stack, holding it in a double curve that swoops gently outward at the mid-back area and arches inward at the neck and at the waistline.

Back problems can start in any part of the back and then expand to involve other structures. Discs don't really "slip," but they can bulge out of alignment, or their membranes can tear so that the material inside begins to ooze. In either case, nearby nerves can be squeezed, causing a painful "pinching." If the sciatic nerve, which extends from the lower back and runs down the leg to the foot, is the one that's being pinched, pain may be felt along the entire leg. This is sometimes called sciatica.

In other cases of back trouble, muscles of the back tighten in spasm as the body tries to realign the vertebrae surrounding the disc. Pain then occurs in the lower back, a condition that used to be referred to as "lumbago."

Back pain can also be associated with poor posture or excess weight, which causes the abdomen to sag forward, pulling on the muscles of the lower back. Or, muscles grown weak from lack of exercise can be strained if you lift a heavy parcel or simply turn or bend. Osteoporosis, arthritis, tumors, infections, and injuries can also lead to vertebral degeneration and pain in the back.

DIAGNOSIS AND TREATMENT

If you complain of back pain and your doctor suspects that you may have a spinal tumor, an infection, or an injury that requires specific kinds of therapy, he or she may order special tests, including X rays. Most backaches can be relieved. First, you and your doctor should agree on a nondrug approach that might include heat or cold application, weight loss (if necessary), supervised exercise, environmental adjustments, the use of a bed-board and, perhaps, physical therapy. You may be advised to sleep on your back with a pillow under your knees or on your side with your knees drawn up; this relieves pressure on the nerves in your back.

If your pain is severe your doctor may prescribe pain medications or medications that have a pain-relieving (analgesic) and an anti-inflammatory action (NSAIDs). If you experience muscle spasms, your doctor may prescribe muscle relaxants. These medications are discussed in detail in the drug charts on pages 492–519.

If the pain is severe or has persisted for a long time, you might have to spend a short time at bed rest. Prolonged bed rest produces complications in older people, including deconditioning and muscle wasting, which only aggravate the problem. An older person needs non-weight-bearing exercise during bed rest. If possible, early mobilization with the aid of a back brace or corset may be cautiously attempted.

If none of these relatively mild measures provides you much relief, the next step might be traction. This means that you must lie in bed on your back while a system of weights and pulleys straightens your back. This can be done on a continuous basis in the hospital or on an outpatient basis for about a half hour a day. If that doesn't help, you and your doctor might want to consider an operation.

OUTLOOK

When your pain is gone, ask your doctor whether you should consult a physical therapist who can show you some back-strengthening exercises and can instruct you in back-sparing ways of standing, moving, lifting, and doing your daily tasks. If you modify some of the habits that contributed to your back pain, it's likely you'll be able to maintain a healthy back.

Caution: Some drugs in this section may affect pregnancy or fetal development. Check with your doctor if this concerns you.

CONDITION: **MUSCLE INJURIES**

CATEGORY: **BENZODIAZEPINES**

GENERIC (CHEMICAL) NAME	BRAND (TRADE) NAME	DOSAGE FORMS AND STRENGTHS
Diazepam	VALIUM	Tablets: 2, 5, 10 mg
	VALRELEASE	Controlled-release capsules: 15 mg

DRUG PROFILE

Benzodiazepines may be used to treat anxiety, insomnia, muscle spasm, and seizures. Exactly how these drugs work is not known. However, what they all seem to have in common is that they reduce nerve cell activity in those areas of the central nervous system (CNS) and peripheral nervous system (PNS) thought to be responsible for the experience of anxiety and muscular tension. In the elderly person, benzodiazepines can cause profound side effects and should be avoided if possible. If prescribed, they should be for short-term use only.

For complete information on this drug, see pages 580–585.

CONDITION: **MUSCLE INJURIES**

CATEGORY: **MUSCLE RELAXANTS**

GENERIC (CHEMICAL) NAME	BRAND (TRADE) NAME	DOSAGE FORMS AND STRENGTHS
Carisoprodol	SOMA	Tablets: 350 mg
	RELA	Tablets: 350 mg
Methocarbamol	ROBAXIN	Tablets: 500, 750 mg

DRUG PROFILE

Carisoprodol and methocarbamol are used to relieve acute muscle pain and discomfort from strains, sprains, and other muscle injuries. They work by relaxing the muscles. These medicines are used as part of a treatment program that includes rest, physical therapy, and other drugs.

BEFORE USING THIS DRUG

Let your doctor know *IF*

You have ever had allergic reactions or other problems with ■ carisoprodol ■ methocarbamol ■ carbromal ■ mebutamate ■ meprobamate ■ tybamate.

You have ever had any of the following medical problems: ■ kidney disease ■ liver disease.

With carisoprodol only: ■ drug abuse, including alcoholism ■ porphyria.

With methocarbamol only: ■ myasthenia gravis.

You are taking any of the following medicines: ■ other muscle relaxants ■ barbiturates ■ medicine for depression (within the last two weeks) ■ medicine for seizures ■ antihistamines ■ medicine for hay fever, coughs, or colds ■ sleep medicines ■ narcotics or other prescription pain-killers ■ tranquilizers.

With methocarbamol only: ■ medicine for myasthenia gravis.

SPECIAL RESTRICTIONS WHILE TAKING THIS DRUG

FOOD AND DRUG INTERACTIONS

Other Drugs	Do not take any other drugs, including over-the-counter (OTC) drugs, before checking with your doctor. This medicine increases the effect of other drugs that depress the central nervous system, and therefore may cause drowsiness or confusion. Some medicines to be careful with are: other muscle relaxants;

antihistamines; medicine for hay fever, allergies, or colds; sleep medicines; tranquilizers; narcotics or other prescription pain-killers; and medicine for seizures.

Alcohol	This drug increases the effect of alcohol, a central nervous system depressant. Avoid alcohol unless your doctor has approved its use.

No special restrictions on foods and beverages or smoking.

DAILY LIVING

Driving	This drug may cause dizziness, light-headedness, or faintness. Be careful when driving, operating household appliances, or doing any other tasks that require alertness until you know how this drug affects you.
Exertion and Exercise	Discuss with your doctor which kinds of physical exercise are safe for you to undertake.
Examinations or Tests	It is important for you to keep all appointments with your doctor so that your progress can be checked.
Other Precautions	Tell any doctor or dentist you consult that you are taking either of these drugs, especially if you will be undergoing any type of surgery.
Helpful Hints	If you are taking methocarbamol, your urine may turn a black, brown, or green color. This is a harmless reaction and will subside once you have stopped taking this medicine. If you find methocarbamol tablets difficult to swallow, try crushing them and mixing the powder with a little food or liquid.

No special restrictions on sun exposure or exposure to excessive heat or cold.

POSSIBLE SIDE EFFECTS

Although this list of adverse effects may seem somewhat intimidating, keep in mind that some are quite rare. Of course, should these or any other problems arise while you are on medication, it is always a good idea to consult your doctor.

IF YOU DEVELOP

inability to walk ■ extreme weakness ■ double vision or other visual disturbances ■ speech difficulties ■ confusion ■ difficulty in breathing ■ fever

With carisoprodol only: "high" feeling

WHAT TO DO

Urgent Get in touch with your doctor immediately.

---

fast heartbeat ■ fainting ■ smarting eyes ■ rash, hives, or itching ■ other skin problems ■ depression ■ excitement ■ anxiety ■ muscle weakness ■ bleeding or bruising ■ sore throat ■ swelling of face, lips, or tongue ■ yellowing of skin ■ bloody or black, tarry stools ■ tiredness or weakness

With carisoprodol only: flushing

After you STOP taking carisoprodol: stomach cramps ■ sleeplessness ■ chills ■ headache ■ nausea

May be serious Check with your doctor as soon as possible.

---

dizziness or light-headedness, especially when getting up from a reclining or sitting position ■ drowsiness ■ clumsiness ■ nausea or vomiting ■ more frequent bowel movements ■ hiccups ■ stomach cramps and pain ■ heartburn ■ constipation ■ diarrhea ■ stuffy nose ■ headache ■ tremors ■ restlessness ■ irritability ■ sleeplessness ■ loss of appetite

If symptoms are disturbing or persist, let your doctor know.

STORAGE INSTRUCTIONS

Store in a cool, dark place (not in a bathroom medicine cabinet).

STOPPING OR INTERRUPTING THERAPY

Do not suddenly stop taking this medicine; your doctor will advise you on how to decrease your dosage gradually. If you miss a dose of this medicine, take it as soon as possible. If it is not within an hour of the scheduled time for the missed dose, skip it and resume your regular schedule. Do not take two doses at the same time.

SPECIAL CONSIDERATIONS FOR THOSE OVER SIXTY-FIVE

Since this drug is excreted by the liver, and liver function sometimes decreases with age, your doctor may begin treatment at a lower dosage.

CONDITION: **MUSCLE INJURIES**

CATEGORY: **MUSCLE RELAXANTS**

GENERIC (CHEMICAL) NAME	BRAND (TRADE) NAME	DOSAGE FORMS AND STRENGTHS
Cyclobenzaprine hydrochloride	FLEXERIL	Tablets: 10 mg

DRUG PROFILE

Cyclobenzaprine is used to relieve acute painful muscle spasms. It works by relaxing the muscles. Cyclobenzaprine is used as part of a treatment program that may include rest, physical therapy, and other drugs.

BEFORE USING THIS DRUG

Let your doctor know *IF*

You have ever had allergic reactions or other problems with ■ cyclobenzaprine.

You have ever had any of the following medical problems: ■ glaucoma ■ heart or blood vessel disease (especially recent heart attack, abnormal heart rhythms, or congestive heart failure) ■ overactive thyroid ■ difficulty in urination.

You are taking any of the following medicines: ■ other muscle relaxants ■ medicine for seizures ■ medicine for depression (within the last two weeks) ■ antihistamines ■ medicine for hay fever, coughs, or colds ■ appetite suppressants ■ barbiturates ■ sleep medicines ■ tranquilizers ■ medicine for narcolepsy ■ medicine for high blood pressure ■ medicine for asthma ■ thyroid hormones ■ anticoagulants (blood thinners) ■ narcotics or other prescription pain-killers.

SPECIAL RESTRICTIONS WHILE TAKING THIS DRUG

FOOD AND DRUG INTERACTIONS

Other Drugs	Do not take any other drugs, including over-the-counter (OTC) drugs, before checking with your doctor. This medicine increases the effect of other drugs that depress the central nervous system, such as other muscle relaxants; antihistamines; medicine for hay fever, allergies, or colds; sleep medicines; tranquilizers; narcotics or other prescription pain-killers; and medicine for seizures.
Alcohol	This drug increases the effects of alcohol, a central nervous system depressant. Avoid alcohol unless your doctor has approved its use.

No special restrictions on foods and beverages or smoking.

DAILY LIVING

Driving	This drug may cause dizziness, light-headedness, or faintness. Be careful when driving, operating household appliances, or doing any other tasks that require alertness until you know how this drug affects you.
Exertion and Exercise	Discuss with your doctor which kinds of physical exercise are safe for you to undertake.
Examinations or Tests	It is important for you to keep all appointments with your doctor so that your progress can be checked.
Other Precautions	Tell any doctor or dentist you consult that you are taking this drug, especially if you will be undergoing any type of surgery.
Helpful Hints	If your mouth or throat feels dry, chewing sugarless gum or sucking ice chips or sugarless hard candy will help.

No special restrictions on sun exposure or exposure to excessive heat or cold.

POSSIBLE SIDE EFFECTS

Although this list of adverse effects may seem somewhat intimidating, keep in mind that some are quite rare. Of course, should these or any other problems arise while you are on medication, it is always a good idea to consult your doctor.

IF YOU DEVELOP

swelling of face, lips, or tongue ■ irregular or fast heartbeat ■ severe drowsiness ■ fainting ■ hallucinations ■ muscle stiffness

WHAT TO DO

Urgent Get in touch with your doctor immediately.

clumsiness or unsteadiness ■ confusion
■ depression ■ difficulty in urination ■ urinary
frequency ■ ringing or buzzing in ears ■ rash, hives,
or itching ■ yellowing of eyes or skin ■ nervousness
■ agitation ■ anxiety ■ excitement ■ strange thoughts
or dreams

May be serious Check with
your doctor as soon as
possible.

fatigue or weakness ■ dizziness or light-headedness
■ drowsiness ■ dry mouth ■ muscle twitching or
weakness ■ increased thirst ■ increased sweating
■ numbness, tingling, or pain in hands or feet
■ tremors ■ sleeplessness ■ speech difficulties
■ headache ■ constipation ■ nausea ■ indigestion
■ bad taste in mouth or other taste changes
■ general feeling of unwellness ■ loss of appetite
■ diarrhea ■ stomach pain ■ gas ■ blurred vision

If symptoms are disturbing
or persist, let your doctor
know.

After you STOP taking this medicine: nausea
■ headache ■ general ill feeling

STORAGE INSTRUCTIONS

Store in a cool, dark place (not in a bathroom medicine cabinet).

STOPPING OR INTERRUPTING THERAPY

Do not suddenly stop taking this medicine; your doctor will advise you on how to
gradually decrease your dosage. If you miss a dose of this medicine, take it as soon
as possible. If it is not within an hour of the scheduled time for the missed dose, skip
it and resume your regular schedule. Do not take two doses at the same time.

SPECIAL CONSIDERATIONS FOR THOSE OVER SIXTY-FIVE

Older people may be more prone to such side effects as dry mouth, difficulty in urination (male patients), and constipation.

CONDITION: **MUSCLE INJURIES**

CATEGORY: **MUSCLE RELAXANT**

GENERIC (CHEMICAL) NAME	BRAND (TRADE) NAME	DOSAGE FORMS AND STRENGTHS
Chlorzoxazone	PARAFLEX PARAFON Forte DSC	Tablets: 250 mg Caplets: 500 mg

DRUG PROFILE

Chlorzoxazone is used to relieve pain and discomfort from acute strains, sprains, and other muscle injuries. Chlorzoxazone relaxes the muscles. It is used as part of a treatment program that includes rest, physical therapy, and other drugs.

BEFORE USING THIS DRUG

Let your doctor know *IF*

You have ever had allergic reactions or other problems with ■ chlorzoxazone ■ any other drug.

You have ever had any of the following medical problems: ■ eczema, hay fever, hives, or other allergic reactions ■ asthma or other lung disease ■ kidney disease ■ liver disease ■ heart disease ■ anemia.

You are taking any of the following medicines: ■ other muscle relaxants ■ antibiotics ■ charcoal ■ sleep medicines ■ tranquilizers ■ medicine for depression (within the last two weeks) ■ narcotics or other prescription pain-killers.

SPECIAL RESTRICTIONS WHILE TAKING THIS DRUG

FOOD AND DRUG INTERACTIONS

Other Drugs	Do not take any other drugs, including over-the-counter (OTC) drugs, particularly aspirin or a drug such as ibuprofen, before checking with your doctor.

This medicine increases the effect of other drugs that depress the central nervous system and therefore may cause drowsiness or confusion. Some drugs to be careful with are: other muscle relaxants; antihistamines; medicines for hay fever, allergies, or colds; sleep medicines; tranquilizers; narcotics or other prescription pain-killers; and medicine for seizures. Check the labels of all other drugs you are taking.

Alcohol	This drug increases the effect of alcohol, a central nervous system depressant. The risk of liver problems is also increased with alcohol. Avoid alcohol unless your doctor has approved its use.

No special restrictions on foods and beverages or smoking.

DAILY LIVING

Driving	This drug may cause dizziness, light-headedness, or faintness. Be careful when driving, operating household appliances, or doing any other tasks that require alertness until you know how this drug affects you.
Exertion and Exercise	Discuss with your doctor which kinds of physical exercise are safe for you to undertake.
Examinations or Tests	It is important for you to keep all appointments with your doctor so that your progress can be checked.
Other Precautions	If overdose of this medicine is suspected, call your doctor or go to a hospital emergency room immediately.
	Tell any doctor or dentist you consult that you are taking this drug, especially if you will be undergoing any type of surgery.

Helpful Hints	This drug may cause your urine to turn orange or reddish-purple. This effect will disappear once you stop taking this drug.
	Tablets may be crushed and mixed with soft foods, milk, or fruit juice.

No special restrictions on sun exposure or exposure to excessive heat or cold.

POSSIBLE SIDE EFFECTS

Although this list of adverse effects may seem somewhat intimidating, keep in mind that some are quite rare. Of course, should these or any other problems arise while you are on medication, it is always a good idea to consult your doctor.

IF YOU DEVELOP	WHAT TO DO
swelling of lips, face, or tongue ■ shallow or fast breathing ■ increased sweating ■ muscle weakness ■ stomach cramps or pain ■ nausea or vomiting ■ diarrhea ■ loss of appetite ■ hoarseness ■ delirium ■ severe dizziness or drowsiness ■ clammy skin ■ fast, weak, or irregular pulse ■ yellowing of the eyes or skin	**Urgent** Get in touch with your doctor immediately.
bloody or black, tarry stools ■ bloody or cloudy urine or other changes in urination ■ tiredness or weakness ■ skin redness, itching, rash, or hives	**May be serious** Check with your doctor as soon as possible.
drowsiness ■ dizziness or light-headedness ■ excitement ■ restlessness ■ anxiety ■ headache ■ constipation ■ upset stomach ■ general ill feeling	If symptoms are disturbing or persist, let your doctor know.

STORAGE INSTRUCTIONS

Store in a cool, dark place (not in a bathroom medicine cabinet).

STOPPING OR INTERRUPTING THERAPY

Take this medicine exactly as instructed by your doctor. Do not take more of it or for a longer period of time than prescribed. If you miss a dose, take it as soon as possible. If it is almost time for your next dose, skip the missed dose and resume your regular schedule. Do not take two doses at the same time.

SPECIAL CONSIDERATIONS FOR THOSE OVER SIXTY-FIVE

None.

CONDITION: **MUSCLE INJURIES**

CATEGORY: **MUSCLE RELAXANT—ANALGESIC COMBINATIONS**

GENERIC (CHEMICAL) NAME	BRAND (TRADE) NAME	DOSAGE FORMS AND STRENGTHS
Orphenadrine citrate, aspirin, and caffeine	NORGESIC	Tablets: 25 mg orphenadrine citrate, 385 mg aspirin, and 30 mg caffeine
	NORGESIC Forte	Tablets: 50 mg orphenadrine citrate, 770 mg aspirin, and 60 mg caffeine

DRUG PROFILE

The combination of orphenadrine, aspirin, and caffeine is used to relieve acute pain and discomfort from acute strains, sprains, or other muscle injuries. Orphenadrine reduces muscle spasm, while aspirin controls pain and swelling by blocking the production of naturally occurring triggers of pain and inflammation, called prostaglandins. Caffeine strengthens the action of the aspirin. This medicine is used as part of a treatment program that includes rest, physical therapy, and additional drugs.

BEFORE USING THIS DRUG

Let your doctor know *IF*

You have ever had allergic reactions or other problems with ■ orphenadrine ■ caffeine ■ aspirin or any other salicylate drug ■ medicine called NSAIDs (eg, indomethacin, ibuprofen, naproxen, etc.) ■ sodium benzoate.

You have ever had any of the following medical problems: ■ hay fever ■ asthma ■ ulcers or gastritis ■ lesions of the digestive tract ■ liver disease ■ kidney disease ■ systemic lupus erythematosus ■ glucose-6-phosphate dehydrogenase (G-6-PD) deficiency ■ vitamin K deficiency ■ nasal polyps ■ pyruvate kinase deficiency ■ chronic hives ■ chronic stuffy nose ■ rheumatic fever ■ disease of the blood vessels ■ any bleeding disorder ■ recent oral surgery ■ diabetes ■ overactive thyroid ■ heart disease, including abnormal heart rhythms ■ high blood pressure ■ enlarged prostate ■ difficulty in urination ■ congestive heart failure ■ glaucoma.

You are taking any of the following medicines: ■ any other pain-killers ■ medicine for gout ■ medicine for arthritis ■ anticoagulants (blood thinners) ■ corticosteroids ■ antacids ■ any medicine containing magnesium ■ any medicine containing alcohol ■ beta-blockers ■ medicine for high blood pressure ■ thiazide diuretics (water pills) ■ captopril (medicine for congestive heart failure and high blood pressure) ■ medicine for glaucoma ■ medicine for seizures ■ medicine for diabetes ■ methotrexate (medicine for severe psoriasis, severe rheumatoid arthritis, or cancer) ■ nitrates (medicine for chest pain) ■ medicine to make the urine more alkaline or more acidic ■ medicine for tuberculosis ■ phenothiazines (medicine for nausea or severe anxiety) ■ acetaminophen ■ tranquilizers ■ digoxin or digitalis (heart medicines) ■ antibiotics ■ medicine for Parkinson's disease ■ sleep medicines ■ quinidine or disopyramide (medicine for abnormal heart rhythms) ■ potassium-containing medicines or supplements ■ cimetidine (medicine for ulcers) ■ barbiturates ■ medicine for stomach cramps ■ medicine for hay fever, coughs, or colds ■ antihistamines ■ medicine for depression ■ nitrofurantoin (medicine for urinary tract infections).

SPECIAL RESTRICTIONS WHILE TAKING THIS DRUG

FOOD AND DRUG INTERACTIONS

Other Drugs	Do not take any other drugs, including over-the-counter (OTC) drugs, especially aspirin, acetaminophen, or ibuprofen, before checking with your

doctor. This medicine increases the effect of other drugs that depress the central nervous system, such as other muscle relaxants; antihistamines; medicines for hay fever, allergies, or colds; sleep medicines; tranquilizers; narcotics or other prescription pain-killers; and medicine for seizures. In addition, be especially careful about using other medicines that contain salicylates. Check the labels of all other drugs you are taking, as well as such products as special shampoos, lotions, and creams, to see if they contain aspirin, salicylic acid, or other salicylate drugs.

Alcohol	This drug increases the effect of alcohol, a central nervous system depressant. Alcohol may also add to the irritant effects of aspirin on your stomach. Avoid alcohol unless your doctor has approved its use.

No special restrictions on foods and beverages or smoking.

DAILY LIVING

Driving	This drug may cause dizziness, light-headedness, or faintness. Be careful when driving, operating household appliances, or doing any other tasks that require alertness until you know how this drug affects you.
Exertion and Exercise	Discuss with your doctor which kinds of physical exercise are safe for you to undertake.
Examinations or Tests	It is important for you to keep all appointments with your doctor so that your progress can be checked.
Other Precautions	If you have diabetes, be aware that false urine-sugar tests may occur while you are taking an aspirin-containing drug. Check with your doctor before increasing the dose of any diabetes medicine you may be taking.

Tell any doctor or dentist you consult that you are taking this drug, especially if you will be undergoing any type of surgery.

Let your doctor know if you notice a buzzing or ringing sound in your ears, since this may be a sign of aspirin overdose.

If you accidentally take an overdose of this drug, go to a hospital emergency room immediately.

Helpful Hints

To reduce risk of possible stomach upset, take this drug with meals, snacks, or a full glass of water.

If your mouth or throat feels dry, chewing sugarless gum or sucking ice chips or sugarless hard candy will help.

No special restrictions on sun exposure or exposure to excessive heat or cold.

POSSIBLE SIDE EFFECTS

Although this list of adverse effects may seem somewhat intimidating, keep in mind that some are quite rare. Of course, should these or any other problems arise while you are on medication, it is always a good idea to consult your doctor.

IF YOU DEVELOP

seizures ■ confusion ■ severe or continuing headache ■ blood in urine or decreased urination
■ irregular or fast heartbeat ■ diarrhea ■ severe dizziness, light-headedness, or drowsiness ■ extreme
excitement or nervousness ■ hallucinations
■ delirium ■ unusual talkativeness or incoherence
■ personality changes ■ tremors ■ severe or continuing nausea or vomiting ■ difficulty in breathing
■ rapid, deep breathing ■ continuing stomach pain
■ fever ■ increased sweating ■ increased thirst
■ blurred vision or other visual disturbances
■ uncontrollable flapping movements of the hands
■ tearing eyes ■ fainting

WHAT TO DO

Urgent Get in touch with
your doctor immediately.

---

stomach pain or tenderness ■ nausea or vomiting
■ bloody or black, tarry stools ■ vomiting, with blood
or vomit that looks like coffee grounds ■ ringing or
buzzing in ears ■ tightness in chest ■ wheezing
■ rash, hives, or itching ■ tiredness or weakness
■ bleeding or bruising ■ loss of taste for cigarettes
■ hoarseness ■ flushing ■ eye pain ■ hallucinations
■ excitement, nervousness, or restlessness
■ sleeplessness

May be serious Check with
your doctor as soon as
possible.

---

dry mouth ■ heartburn or indigestion ■ loss of appetite ■ anxiety ■ drowsiness, dizziness, or
light-headedness ■ constipation ■ difficulty in
urination ■ increased eye sensitivity to light
■ decreased sweating ■ loss of taste ■ bloating

If symptoms are disturbing
or persist, let your doctor
know.

STORAGE INSTRUCTIONS

Store in a cool, dark place (not in a bathroom medicine cabinet). If you notice a
vinegarlike odor from the bottle, this means that the drug is breaking down and
should be discarded.

STOPPING OR INTERRUPTING THERAPY

If you miss a dose of this medicine, take it as soon as possible. If it is not within an hour of the scheduled time for the missed dose, skip it and resume your regular schedule. Do not take two doses at the same time.

SPECIAL CONSIDERATIONS FOR THOSE OVER SIXTY-FIVE

Those older people who have reduced kidney function tend not to eliminate the salicylates as readily as people with normal kidney function. For this reason, doctors may check such people regularly to make sure they are receiving the proper dosage and that too much drug is not accumulating in the body.

CONDITION: **MUSCLE INJURIES**

CATEGORY: **MUSCLE RELAXANT—ANALGESIC COMBINATIONS**

GENERIC (CHEMICAL) NAME	BRAND (TRADE) NAME	DOSAGE FORMS AND STRENGTHS
Carisoprodol and aspirin	SOMA COMPOUND	Tablets: 200 mg carisoprodol and 325 mg aspirin
Methocarbamol and aspirin	ROBAXISAL	Tablets: 400 mg methocarbamol and 325 mg aspirin

DRUG PROFILE

These combination drugs are used to relieve pain and discomfort from strains, sprains, or other muscle injuries. Carisoprodol and methocarbamol relax the muscles, while aspirin controls pain by blocking the production of naturally occurring triggers of pain and inflammation, called prostaglandins. These medicines are used as part of a treatment program that may include rest, physical therapy, and other drugs.

BEFORE USING THIS DRUG

Let your doctor know *IF*

You have ever had allergic reactions or other problems with ■ carisoprodol ■ methocarbamol ■ carbromal ■ mebutamate ■ tybamate ■ aspirin or any other salicylate drug ■ medicine called NSAIDs (eg, indomethacin, ibuprofen, naproxen, etc.) ■ sodium benzoate ■ tartrazine (FD&C Yellow Dye No. 5).

You have ever had any of the following medical problems: ■ hay fever ■ asthma ■ ulcers or gastritis ■ lesions of the digestive tract ■ liver disease ■ kidney disease ■ systemic lupus erythematosus ■ glucose-6-phosphate dehydrogenase (G-6-PD) deficiency ■ vitamin K deficiency ■ pyruvate kinase deficiency ■ nasal polyps ■ chronic hives ■ chronic stuffy nose ■ rheumatic fever ■ disease of the blood vessels ■ any bleeding disorder ■ recent oral surgery ■ diabetes ■ hypoglycemia ■ hearing problems ■ anemia.

With carisoprodol only: ■ drug abuse, including alcoholism ■ porphyria.

With methocarbamol only: ■ myasthenia gravis.

If you are taking any of the following medicines: ■ other muscle relaxants ■ medicine for gout ■ medicine for arthritis ■ anticoagulants (blood thinners) ■ corticosteroids ■ antacids ■ any medicine containing magnesium ■ any medicine containing alcohol ■ beta-blockers ■ medicine for high blood pressure ■ diuretics ■ captopril (medicine for congestive heart failure) ■ medicine for glaucoma ■ medicine for seizures ■ medicine for diabetes ■ methotrexate (medicine for severe psoriasis, severe rheumatoid arthritis, or cancer) ■ nitrates (medicine for chest pain) ■ medicine to make the urine more alkaline or more acidic ■ medicine for tuberculosis ■ medicine for nausea or vomiting ■ acetaminophen ■ barbiturates ■ medicine for depression (within the last two weeks) ■ antihistamines ■ medicine for hay fever, coughs, or colds ■ sleep medicines ■ narcotics or other prescription pain-killers ■ tranquilizers.

With methocarbamol only: ■ medicine for myasthenia gravis.

SPECIAL RESTRICTIONS WHILE TAKING THIS DRUG

FOOD AND DRUG INTERACTIONS

Other Drugs	Do not take any other drugs, including over-the-counter (OTC) drugs such as aspirin, acetaminophen, or ibuprofen, before checking with your doctor. This medicine increases the effect of other drugs that depress the central nervous system, such as other muscle relaxants; antihistamines; medicine for hay fever, allergies, and colds; sleep medicines; tranquilizers; narcotics or other prescription pain-killers; and medicine for seizures. In addition, be especially careful about using other medicines that contain salicylates. Check the labels of all other drugs you are taking, as well as such products as special shampoos, lotions, and creams, to see if they contain aspirin, salicylic acid, or other salicylate drugs.
Alcohol	This drug increases the effect of alcohol, a central nervous system depressant. Alcohol may also add to the irritant effects of aspirin on your stomach. Avoid alcohol unless your doctor has approved its use.

No special restrictions on foods and beverages or smoking.

DAILY LIVING

Driving	This drug may cause dizziness, light-headedness, or faintness. Be careful when driving, operating household appliances, or doing any other tasks that require alertness until you know how this drug affects you.
Exertion and Exercise	Discuss with your doctor which kinds of physical exercise are safe for you to undertake.

Examinations or Tests	It is important for you to keep all appointments with your doctor so that your progress can be checked.

Other Precautions	If you have diabetes, be aware that false urine-sugar tests may occur while you are taking an aspirin-containing drug. Check with your doctor before increasing the dose of any diabetes medicine you may be taking.
	Tell any doctor or dentist you consult that you are taking either of these drugs, especially if you will be undergoing any type of surgery.
	Let your doctor know if you notice a buzzing or ringing sound in your ears, as this may be a sign of aspirin overdose. If you accidentally take an overdose of either of these drugs, go to a hospital emergency room immediately.

Helpful Hints	If you are taking methocarbamol, your urine may turn a black, brown, or green color. This is a harmless reaction and will subside once you have stopped taking this medicine.

No special restrictions on sun exposure or exposure to excessive heat or cold.

POSSIBLE SIDE EFFECTS

Although this list of adverse effects may seem somewhat intimidating, keep in mind that some are quite rare. Of course, should these or any other problems arise while you are on medication, it is always a good idea to consult your doctor.

IF YOU DEVELOP

seizures ■ confusion ■ severe or continuing head-ache ■ blood in urine or decreased urination ■ fast heartbeat ■ diarrhea ■ severe dizziness, light-headedness, or drowsiness ■ extreme excitement or nervousness ■ hallucinations ■ talkativeness, inco-herence, or speech difficulties ■ personality changes ■ tremors ■ severe or continuing nausea or vomiting ■ difficulty in breathing ■ rapid, deep breathing ■ continuing stomach pain ■ fever ■ increased sweating ■ increased thirst ■ uncontrollable flapping movements of the hands ■ tearing eyes ■ fainting ■ inability to walk ■ extreme weakness ■ blurred or double vision

With carisoprodol only: "high" feeling

WHAT TO DO

Urgent: Stop taking the drug and get in touch with your doctor immediately.

---

stomach pain or tenderness ■ nausea or vomiting ■ bloody or black, tarry stools ■ vomiting, with blood, or vomit that looks like coffee grounds ■ ringing or buzzing in ears ■ tightness in chest ■ wheezing ■ rash, hives, itching, or other skin problems ■ tiredness or weakness ■ bleeding or bruising ■ loss of taste for cigarettes ■ smarting eyes ■ depression ■ excitement ■ anxiety ■ muscle weak-ness ■ swelling of face, lips, or tongue ■ yellowing of eyes or skin

With carisoprodol only: flushing

After you STOP taking carisoprodol: stomach cramps ■ sleeplessness ■ chills ■ headache ■ nausea

May be serious Check with your doctor as soon as possible.

dizziness or light-headedness, especially when getting up from a reclining or sitting position ■ drowsiness ■ clumsiness ■ more frequent bowel movements ■ hiccups ■ headache ■ restlessness ■ irritability ■ sleeplessness ■ loss of appetite ■ heartburn or indigestion ■ diarrhea ■ constipation ■ stuffy nose ■ sore throat

If symptoms are disturbing or persist, let your doctor know.

STORAGE INSTRUCTIONS

Store in a cool, dark place (not in a bathroom medicine cabinet). If you notice a vinegarlike odor from the bottle, this means that the drug is breaking down and should be discarded.

STOPPING OR INTERRUPTING THERAPY

Do not suddenly stop taking this medicine; your doctor will advise you on how to gradually decrease your dosage. If you miss a dose of either of these medicines, take it as soon as possible. If it is not within an hour of the scheduled time for the missed dose, skip it and resume your regular schedule. Do not take two doses at the same time.

SPECIAL CONSIDERATIONS FOR THOSE OVER SIXTY-FIVE

Those older people who have decreased kidney or liver function tend not to eliminate the salicylates as readily as people with normal kidney or liver function. For this reason, doctors may check such people regularly to make sure they are receiving the proper dosage and that too much drug is not accumulating in the body.

CONDITION: **NIGHT CRAMPS**

CATEGORY: **MUSCLE RELAXANTS**

GENERIC (CHEMICAL) NAME	BRAND (TRADE) NAME	DOSAGE FORMS AND STRENGTHS
Quinine sulfate	QUINAMM	Tablets: 260 mg

DRUG PROFILE

Quinine is used to treat nighttime leg muscle cramps. This drug acts directly on the muscles to make them less excitable by nerve impulses.

BEFORE USING THIS DRUG

Let your doctor know *IF*

You have ever had allergic reactions or other problems with ■ quinine ■ quinidine.

You have ever had any of the following medical problems: ■ asthma ■ eye disease, including optic neuritis ■ glucose-6-phosphate dehydrogenase (G-6-PD) deficiency ■ blood disease ■ hearing problems (especially noises in the ear) ■ heart disease, including abnormal heart rhythms ■ blackwater fever.

You are taking any of the following medicines: ■ any medicine containing quinine (includes some cold products) ■ quinidine (medicine for abnormal heart rhythms) ■ digoxin or digitalis (heart medicines) ■ medicine to make the urine less acidic ■ antacids containing aluminum ■ anticoagulants (blood thinners) ■ medicine for myasthenia gravis ■ tranquilizers ■ calcium blockers ■ antihistamines ■ NSAIDs ■ aminoglycosides (amikacin, gentamicin, streptomicin) ■ furosemide ■ aspirin.

SPECIAL RESTRICTIONS WHILE TAKING THIS DRUG

FOOD AND DRUG INTERACTIONS

Other Drugs	If you are taking any heart drugs (digoxin or digitalis), consult your doctor, since the combination with quinine may result in dangerously high levels of these drugs.
	Avoid antacids that contain aluminum, since they may interfere with the body's absorption of quinine.

No special restrictions on foods and beverages, alcohol use, or smoking.

DAILY LIVING

Examinations or Tests	It is important for you to keep all appointments with your doctor so that your progress can be checked.
Other Precautions	Tell any doctor or dentist you consult that you are taking this drug, especially if you will be undergoing any type of surgery.
Helpful Hints	If this medicine upsets your stomach, taking it with milk, meals, or snacks should help.

No special restrictions on driving, exertion and exercise, or exposure to excessive heat or cold. To avoid a reaction to the sun, wear sunglasses and avoid prolonged exposure to bright sunlight.

POSSIBLE SIDE EFFECTS

Although this list of adverse effects may seem somewhat intimidating, keep in mind that some are quite rare. Of course, should these or any other problems arise while you are on medication, it is always a good idea to consult your doctor.

IF YOU DEVELOP

chest pain ■ irregular heartbeat ■ seizures ■ ringing or buzzing in the ears or other hearing disturbances ■ blurred vision or other visual disturbances ■ rash, hives, or itching ■ wheezing ■ shortness of breath ■ difficulty in breathing ■ fever ■ flushing ■ confusion ■ fainting

WHAT TO DO

Urgent Get in touch with your doctor immediately.

---

dizziness ■ severe headache ■ swelling of face ■ increased sweating ■ feeling of dread ■ restlessness ■ increased eye sensitivity to light

May be serious Check with your doctor as soon as possible.

diarrhea ■ nausea or vomiting ■ stomach cramps or pain	If symptoms are disturbing or persist, let your doctor know.

STORAGE INSTRUCTIONS

Store in a cool, dark place (not in a bathroom medicine cabinet).

STOPPING OR INTERRUPTING THERAPY

If you miss a dose of this medicine, take it as soon as possible. If it is not within an hour of the scheduled time for the missed dose, skip it and resume your regular schedule. Do not take two doses at the same time.

SPECIAL CONSIDERATIONS FOR THOSE OVER SIXTY-FIVE

Since this drug is excreted by the liver and liver function sometimes decreases with age, your doctor may begin treatment at a lower dosage.

CONDITION: **MUSCLE CRAMPING AND STIFFENING**
CATEGORY: **ANTISPASTICITY DRUGS**

GENERIC (CHEMICAL) NAME	BRAND (TRADE) NAME	DOSAGE FORMS AND STRENGTHS
Baclofen	LIORESAL	Tablets: 10, 20 mg

DRUG PROFILE

Baclofen is used to relieve the spasm, cramping, and stiffening of muscles caused by multiple sclerosis or spinal cord injuries. This drug is thought to act on the spinal cord, blocking certain nerve impulses. Baclofen is used as part of a treatment program that may include rest, physical therapy, and other drugs.

BEFORE USING THIS DRUG

Let your doctor know *IF*

You have ever had allergic reactions or other problems with ■ baclofen.

You have ever had any of the following medical problems: ■ seizures ■ kidney disease ■ mental or emotional problems ■ stroke ■ stomach ulcer ■ diabetes.

You are taking any of the following medicines: ■ other muscle relaxants ■ medicine for seizures ■ antihistamines ■ medicine for hay fever, coughs, or colds ■ barbiturates ■ medicine for depression (within the last two weeks) ■ narcotics or other prescription pain-killers ■ tranquilizers ■ sleep medicines ■ medicine for diabetes.

SPECIAL RESTRICTIONS WHILE TAKING THIS DRUG

FOOD AND DRUG INTERACTIONS

Other Drugs	Do not take any other drugs, including over-the-counter (OTC) drugs, before checking with your doctor. This medicine increases the effect of other drugs that depress the central nervous system, such as other muscle relaxants; antihistamines; medicine for hay fever, allergies, or colds; sleep medicines; tranquilizers; narcotics or other prescription pain-killers; and medicine for seizures.
Alcohol	This drug increases the effect of alcohol, a central nervous system depressant. Avoid alcohol unless your doctor has approved its use.

No special restrictions on foods and beverages or smoking.

DAILY LIVING

Driving	This drug may cause dizziness, light-headedness, or faintness. Be careful when driving, operating household appliances, or doing any other tasks that require alertness until you know how this drug affects you.
Exertion and Exercise	Discuss with your doctor which kinds of physical exercise are safe for you to undertake.
Examinations or Tests	It is important for you to keep all appointments with your doctor so that your progress can be checked.
Other Precautions	Tell any doctor or dentist you consult that you are taking this drug, especially if you will be undergoing any type of surgery.

If you have diabetes, be aware that this medicine may affect blood-sugar levels. If you notice any change when testing sugar levels in your blood or urine, let your doctor know. |

No special restrictions on sun exposure or exposure to excessive heat or cold.

POSSIBLE SIDE EFFECTS

Although this list of adverse effects may seem somewhat intimidating, keep in mind that some are quite rare. Of course, should these or any other problems arise while you are on medication, it is always a good idea to consult your doctor.

IF YOU DEVELOP

seizures ■ difficulty in breathing ■ irregular heartbeat ■ blurred or double vision or other visual disturbances

WHAT TO DO

Urgent Get in touch with your doctor immediately.

chest pain ■ bloody or dark urine ■ fainting ■ hallucinations ■ depression ■ anxiety ■ ringing or buzzing in ears ■ rash or itching ■ clumsiness ■ speech difficulties ■ tremors ■ rigid muscles ■ twitching ■ vomiting

May be serious Check with your doctor as soon as possible.

drowsiness, dizziness, or light-headedness ■ muscle weakness, pain, or stiffness ■ uncontrollable movements ■ nausea ■ confusion ■ weight gain ■ swelling of ankles ■ stomach pain ■ constipation ■ diarrhea ■ loss of appetite ■ numbness or tingling in hands or feet ■ slurred speech ■ male impotence ■ inability to ejaculate ■ excitement ■ "high" feeling ■ sleeplessness ■ stuffy nose ■ dry mouth ■ taste changes ■ positive test for occult blood in stool ■ pain or difficulty in urination ■ urinary frequency ■ increased sweating ■ tiredness

If symptoms are disturbing or persist, let your doctor know.

STORAGE INSTRUCTIONS

Store in a cool, dark place (not in a bathroom medicine cabinet).

STOPPING OR INTERRUPTING THERAPY

Do not suddenly stop taking this medicine; your doctor will advise you on how to decrease your dosage gradually. If you miss a dose of this medicine, take it as soon as possible. If it is not within an hour of the scheduled time for the missed dose, skip it and resume your regular schedule. Do not take two doses at the same time.

SPECIAL CONSIDERATIONS FOR THOSE OVER SIXTY-FIVE

Older people are more prone to such mental and emotional side effects as hallucinations, confusion, depression, anxiety, and excitement, as well as drowsiness. Extreme sleepiness or sedation may occur and affect your ability to function normally. Also, since this drug is excreted by the kidneys and kidney function decreases with age, your doctor may begin treatment at a lower dosage.

ARTHRITIS

Arthritis is a common ailment, affecting more than thirty-six million people in the United States. This single term actually refers to a host of different disorders.

Arthritis occurs when the delicate architecture of the joints—the meeting places of bones—is damaged. Just a few joints can be affected or many; within a joint, the destruction of key components (such as the tough, shock-absorbing cartilage between bones) can be partial or total. The condition is marked by pain and sometimes by inflammation (swelling, redness, heat) in the joints. Arthritis sometimes causes disfigurement, ranging from gnarled fingers to a curved spine. Fortunately, though, new treatments reduce these crippling effects.

CAUSES

By far the most common form of the disease is osteoarthritis (OA). This condition affects an estimated sixteen million people in the United States, mainly older people. Older patients often assume that their symptoms are due to growing old; however, much OA results from a combination of the biological changes of aging, traumatic injuries to the body, and metabolic, immunologic, or inherited structural changes. Many doctors think that the major cause of osteoarthritis is the gradual wear and tear our joints experience over the years.

The main symptoms of OA are pain and stiffness in one or more joints.

The joints most often affected include those of the fingers, the base of the thumb, the neck, the hips, the lower back, and the knees. The pain, which can range from dull aches to occasional sharp peaks, is often strongest first thing in the morning. Some people claim they can predict the weather by the severity of their pain. You may not want to plan a picnic by it, but arthritis pain sometimes is influenced by prevailing weather conditions.

Although the word *arthritis* literally means "joint inflammation," OA often occurs without significant inflammation. Swelling of the knee may occur, but there is no fever or other systemic symptom of inflammation.

The next most common type of arthritis is rheumatoid arthritis (RA), which affects about seven million people in the United States. This is the form of the disease most likely to be crippling. Although RA can strike at any age, it most often occurs in early to middle adulthood. However, it is not unusual for persons sixty to seventy years old to get it. About three-quarters of its victims are women. Researchers suspect that RA is an autoimmune disease, in which the body mistakenly perceives some of its own tissues as foreign and the immune system launches an attack against them. No one knows precisely what triggers this attack.

Unlike osteoarthritis, rheumatoid arthritis can sometimes develop quite rapidly, and it *always* involves inflammation of the joints. In some cases, tissues other than joints become inflamed as well. Joints in the hands and feet are most commonly affected, but any and all joints can fall prey. The symptoms of the disease may subside for unpredictable lengths of time, only to flare up again.

Of the many other forms of arthritis, the most common in older people is gout. Gout usually strikes men over forty and involves acute pain in a single joint, usually the big toe. (See pages 542–543 for more on gout.) Another form, polymyalgia rheumatica, affects mostly people over sixty. Common symptoms are fever; weight loss; and pain in the neck, back, shoulders, upper arms, or thighs. An accompanying condition, known as giant-cell arteritis, may cause blindness.

DIAGNOSIS AND TREATMENT

If you have persistent pain, stiffness, or inflammation in any of your joints, see your doctor. A careful medical examination, along with various blood tests and possibly X rays, can help him or her determine whether you are suffering from arthritis and, if so, what form of the disease you have. Depending on the situation, your doctor may refer you to an arthritis specialist (rheumatologist).

Your treatment plan should be tailored to your particular case. One key to living with arthritis is to neither overwork nor underwork the affected joints; therefore, appropriate doses of moderate exercise and rest are likely to be part of your therapy program. A more formal physical therapy program may be part of your treatment plan.

Electric blankets and other sources of heat may also be recommended to help ease your joint pain; at other times, your doctor may suggest you use cold compresses to relieve inflammation.

In some cases, joint-protection devices such as splints are useful both for relieving pain and preventing deformity. Your doctor will probably stress the importance of well-balanced meals and, if you are overweight, the need to cut calories.

The basic therapy for arthritis is rest, physical therapy, heat, patient education, and an anti-inflammatory drug, which is usually aspirin or an aspirinlike drug. If the aspirin causes stomach upset, then an enteric-coated aspirin may be prescribed. An interesting study recently reported that the use of acetaminophen can be just as effective as ibuprofen (a nonsteroidal anti-inflammatory drug or NSAID) in treating pain due to osteoarthritis. Since the NSAIDs have many potential side effects, you may wish to ask your doctor about this as an alternative.

In the management of rheumatoid arthritis, if the basic therapy described above is not effective, then additional medications can be incorporated into the treatment program. The NSAIDs can be very patient-specific and your doctor may have to try several different medications before finding one that is helpful to you. In very severe, unresponsive cases, antimalarials or gold compounds (eg, auranofin) might be used. If these latter agents are unsuccessful, then penicillamine, corticosteroids or methotrexate may be prescribed. As a treatment of last resort, surgery, such as hip replacement, can provide great relief for some types of arthritis. For detailed information on these drugs, see charts on pages 523–541.

Even if you have a mild case of arthritis, don't try to diagnose and treat the problem yourself. Some people make the mistake of simply taking aspirin or a nonprescription-strength, nonsteroidal anti-inflammatory drug like ibuprofen on their own. But the dosages they're using may be too low for effectiveness or too high for safety, and the medicine they choose may not be the ideal one for their condition. A doctor's judgment is crucial in designing the treatment plan and in monitoring its effectiveness.

OUTLOOK

There is currently no cure for any form of arthritis. But the treatments and therapies available for making life livable with arthritis—even when severe—have grown in number and effectiveness in recent years. Meanwhile, our understanding of the various processes that can cause joint-tissue deterioration is steadily advancing. There's every reason to expect that modern medicine will continue to brighten the outlook for people who have an arthritic condition.

Caution: Some drugs in this section may affect pregnancy or fetal development. Check with your doctor if this concerns you.

CONDITION: **ARTHRITIS**

CATEGORY: **SALICYLATE DRUGS**

GENERIC (CHEMICAL) NAME	BRAND (TRADE) NAME	DOSAGE FORMS AND STRENGTHS
Salsalate	DISALCID	Capsules: 500 mg Tablets: 500, 750 mg
	SALFLEX	Tablets: 500, 750 mg
Choline magnesium trisalicylate	TRILISATE	Liquid: 500 mg per tsp Tablets: 500, 750, 1000 mg

Aspirin and other
salicylate drugs

Aspirin and other salicylate drugs are available over the counter under a variety of brand names, dosage forms, and strengths. Some of these preparations have a special coating to help protect the lining of the stomach against possible irritation. Because of the importance of salicylate drugs in the treatment of chronic pain, even though they are most often nonprescription drugs, they are included in this book for reader reference.

Salsalate and trisalicylate are primarily used for treatment of arthritis and rheumatism and are not available as over-the-counter (OTC) drugs.

DRUG PROFILE

Aspirin and other drugs in the salicylate family are used to relieve pain, inflammation, and fever. Large doses are used to treat symptoms of arthritis and rheumatism such as swelling, stiffness, and joint pain. Aspirin and other salicylates are thought to control pain and swelling by blocking the production of naturally occurring triggers of pain and inflammation, called prostaglandins. These drugs relieve fever by changing the way the body regulates its temperature.

For complete information on these drugs, see pages 471–475.

CONDITION: **ARTHRITIS**

CATEGORY: **NONSTEROIDAL ANTI-INFLAMMATORY DRUGS**

GENERIC (CHEMICAL) NAME	BRAND (TRADE) NAME	DOSAGE FORMS AND STRENGTHS
Diclofenac	VOLTAREN	Tablets: 25, 50, 75 mg
Diflunisal	DOLOBID	Tablets: 250, 500 mg
Etodolac	LODINE	Capsules: 200, 300 mg
Fenoprofen calcium	NALFON	Capsules: 200, 300 mg Tablets: 600 mg
Flurbiprofen	ANSAID	Tablets: 50, 100 mg
Ibuprofen	ADVIL (OTC)	Caplets: 200 mg Tablets: 200 mgs
	MEDIPREN	Tablets: 200 mg
	MOTRIN	Tablets: 300, 400, 600, 800 mg
	NUPRIN (OTC)	Caplets: 200 mg Tablets: 200 mg
	RUFEN	Tablets: 400, 600, 800 mg
Ketoprofen	ORUDIS	Capsules: 25, 50, 75 mg
Indomethacin	INDOCIN	Capsules: 25, 50 mg Rectal suppositories: 50 mg

	INDOCIN SR	Suspension: 25 mg per tsp Controlled-release capsules: 75 mg
Meclofenamate sodium	MECLOMEN	Capsules: meclofenamate sodium equivalent to 50 or 100 mg meclofenamic acid
Mefenamic acid	PONSTEL	Kapseals: 250 mg
Naproxen sodium Naproxen	ANAPROX ANAPROX DS NAPROSYN NAPROSYN	Tablets: 275 mg Tablets: 550 mg Suspension: 125 mg per tsp Tablets: 250, 375, 500 mg
Phenylbutazone	BUTAZOLIDIN	Capsules: 100 mg Tablets: 100 mg
Piroxicam	FELDENE	Capsules: 10, 20 mg
Sulindac	CLINORIL	Tablets: 150, 200 mg
Tolmetin sodium	TOLECTIN TOLECTIN DS TOLECTIN 600	Tablets: tolmetin sodium equivalent to 200 mg tolmetin Capsules: tolmetin sodium equivalent to 400 mg tolmetin Tablets: tolectin sodium equivalent to 600 mg tolmetin

DRUG PROFILE

Nonsteroidal anti-inflammatory drugs, or NSAIDs, help relieve swelling, stiffness, joint pain, and inflammation in the long-term treatment of arthritis. These drugs are thought to act by blocking the production of naturally occurring triggers of pain and inflammation, called prostaglandins.

BEFORE USING THIS DRUG

Let your doctor know *IF*

You have ever had allergic reactions or other problems with ■ the medicine prescribed for you or any other nonsteroidal anti-inflammatory agent ■ other medicines for arthritis or gout including aspirin or other salicylates.

You have ever had any of the following medical problems: ■ asthma or broncho-spasm ■ bleeding disorders ■ dizziness ■ heart disease ■ high blood pressure ■ congestive heart failure ■ kidney disease ■ liver disease ■ nasal polyps ■ water retention ■ stomach ulcer, intestinal bleeding, colitis, or other digestive disorders ■ diabetes.

With indomethacin and phenylbutazone only: ■ seizures ■ mental illness ■ Parkinson's disease.

You are taking any of the following medicines: ■ acetaminophen ■ potassium supplements ■ anticoagulants (blood thinners) ■ medicine for diabetes ■ beta-blockers (medicine for high blood pressure) ■ aspirin or aspirinlike products ■ diuretics (water pills: furosemide, bumetanide) ■ lithium ■ methotrexate ■ ibuprofen ■ ciprofloxacin or norfloxacin.

With diclofenac only: ■ digoxin (heart medicine) ■ cyclosporine.

With diflunisal only: ■ medicine containing aluminum.

With fenoprofen only: ■ barbiturates.

With flurbiprofen only: ■ antacids ■ beta-blockers ■ cimetidine (medicine for peptic ulcer).

With ibuprofen only: ■ medicine for seizures.

With indomethacin only: triamterene, or thiazide diuretics (water pills) ■ medicine called ACE inhibitors (eg, captopril, enalapril, lisinopril, etc.) ■ cimetidine (medicine for ulcers) ■ digoxin or digitalis (heart medicines) ■ probenecid (medicine for gout) ■ medicine for asthma ■ decongestants.

With ketoprofen only: ■ probenecid (medicine for gout), methotrexate.

With naproxen only: ■ probenecid.

With phenylbutazone only: ■ male hormones ■ barbiturates ■ digoxin or digitalis (heart medicines) ■ medicine for seizures.

SPECIAL RESTRICTIONS WHILE TAKING THIS DRUG

FOOD AND DRUG INTERACTIONS

Other Drugs	It is important to let your doctor know if you are taking any other drug, especially blood thinners or lithium, since their effects may be increased when taken with some NSAIDs. Also, be sure to tell your doctor if you have ever experienced asthma or an allergic reaction to aspirin or any other type of arthritis medicine.
Alcohol	Drinking alcohol while taking this drug may cause stomach upset. Avoid alcohol unless your doctor has approved its use.

No special restrictions on foods and beverages or smoking.

DAILY LIVING

Driving	This type of drug may cause drowsiness or loss of alertness. Be careful when driving, operating household appliances, or doing any other tasks that require alertness until you know how this drug affects you.
Examinations or Tests	It is important for you to keep all appointments with your doctor so that your progress can be checked.

Other Precautions

If you have diabetes, be aware that these medicines may cause fluctuations in blood-sugar levels. Your doctor may want to monitor your blood-sugar levels carefully during the first few weeks of use.

Taking aspirin regularly with NSAIDs may cause stomach upset. If the drug you are taking upsets your stomach, ask your doctor if you can take it with an antacid.

If there are any signs of intestinal bleeding, such as black, tarry bowel movements or vomiting blood that looks either red, brown, or resembles coffee grounds, call your doctor immediately.

Helpful Hints

NSAIDs reach the bloodstream more quickly if your stomach is empty. However, to reduce stomach irritation they are usually taken with food or immediately after meals.

If you have been storing the suppository form of this medicine in a warm place, it may be too soft to use. Put it in the refrigerator for half an hour or run cold water over the wrapped suppository before use.

No special restrictions on exertion and exercise, sun exposure, or exposure to excessive heat or cold.

POSSIBLE SIDE EFFECTS

Although this list of adverse effects may seem somewhat intimidating, keep in mind that some are quite rare. Of course, should these or any other problems arise while you are on medication, it is always a good idea to consult your doctor.

IF YOU DEVELOP	WHAT TO DO
fever ■ rash, hives, or itching ■ difficulty in breathing ■ severe nausea or vomiting ■ vomiting, with blood ■ black, tarry stools ■ swelling of hands or feet ■ decreased urination	**Urgent** Get in touch with your doctor immediately.
stomach pain ■ blurred vision or other visual disturbances ■ ringing or buzzing in ears or other hearing problems ■ yellowing of eyes or skin ■ any change in color of urine or stool ■ increased sweating ■ confusion ■ nervousness ■ agitation	**May be serious** Check with your doctor as soon as possible.
indigestion ■ heartburn ■ nausea or vomiting ■ diarrhea ■ constipation ■ loss of appetite ■ gas or bloating ■ drowsiness ■ sleeplessness ■ headache ■ dizziness, light-headedness, or faintness	If symptoms are disturbing or persist, let your doctor know.

STORAGE INSTRUCTIONS

Store in a cool, dark place (not in a bathroom medicine cabinet). Suppositories should be stored in the refrigerator.

STOPPING OR INTERRUPTING THERAPY

Because these medicines control but do not cure arthritis, you may have to take them for a long period of time. Your symptoms could take from one to four weeks to abate. Do not take more of this medicine or take it for a longer period of time than recommended by your doctor or the package labeling. If you are supposed to take your medicine once a day and you miss a dose, take it as soon as possible. If it is not within six hours of the scheduled time for the missed dose, skip it and resume your regular schedule. If you are supposed to take your medicine two or more times a day and you miss a dose, take it as soon as possible. If it is not within two hours of the scheduled time for the missed dose, skip it and resume your regular schedule.

SPECIAL CONSIDERATIONS FOR THOSE OVER SIXTY-FIVE

Because kidney function sometimes decreases with age, older people may be susceptible to urinary problems with these drugs. Your doctor may therefore start your medication at a lower dosage. Indomethacin and meclofenamate should be used with great care by those over sixty-five, since side effects are more likely to occur.

CONDITION: **ARTHRITIS**
CATEGORY: **CORTICOSTEROIDS**

GENERIC (CHEMICAL) NAME	BRAND (TRADE) NAME	DOSAGE FORMS AND STRENGTHS
Betamethasone	CELESTONE	Syrup: 0.6 mg per tsp Tablets: 0.6 mg
Cortisone acetate		Tablets: 5, 10, 25 mg
Dexamethasone	DECADRON	Elixir: 0.5 mg per tsp Tablets: 0.25, 0.5, 0.75, 1.5, 4, 6 mg
Hydrocortisone Hydrocortisone cypionate	CORTEF CORTEF Oral Suspension	Tablets: 5, 10, 20 mg Suspension: hydrocortisone cypionate equivalent to 10 mg hydrocortisone per tsp
Methylprednisolone	MEDROL	Tablets: 2, 4, 8, 16, 24, 32 mg
Prednisolone	DELTA-CORTEF PRELONE	Tablets: 5 mg Syrup: 15 mg per tsp

Prednisone	DELTASONE	Tablets: 2.5, 5, 10, 20, 50 mg
Triamcinolone	ARISTOCORT	Tablets: 1, 2, 4, 8 mg
	KENACORT	Tablets: 4, 8 mg
Triamcinolone diacetate	ARISTOCORT	Syrup: 2 mg per tsp
	KENACORT	Syrup: 4 mg per tsp

DRUG PROFILE

Oral corticosteroids (also known as steroids) are used to treat a wide variety of inflammatory diseases, such as arthritis, and other rheumatic disorders, such as lupus. (These are not the drugs that are used first in the treatment of arthritis.) They are also used in conjunction with immunosuppressive agents to prevent reactions from kidney and heart transplants. Although these multifaceted drugs do not cure the underlying disease, they suppress the redness, swelling, and heat that signal inflammation.

BEFORE USING THIS DRUG

Let your doctor know *IF*

You have ever had allergic reactions or other problems with ■ any corticosteroids ■ corticotropin (ACTH).

You have ever had any of the following medical problems: ■ peptic ulcer or intestinal bleeding ■ diabetes ■ bone disease such as osteoporosis ■ slow healing of wounds ■ high blood pressure ■ mental illness ■ recent fungal infection ■ recent viral infection ■ herpes eye infection ■ colitis or diverticulitis ■ glaucoma ■ heart disease ■ disease of the blood vessels ■ kidney disease ■ liver disease ■ myasthenia gravis ■ congestive heart failure ■ tuberculosis ■ underactive thyroid ■ seizures ■ high cholesterol.

You are taking any of the following medicines: ■ other medicine for arthritis or other inflammatory conditions, including aspirin or aspirinlike medicine ■ antibiotics ■ digoxin or digitalis (heart medicines) ■ medicine for abnormal heart rhythms ■ diuretics ■ medicine for high blood pressure ■ medicine for asthma ■ insulin or other medicine for diabetes ■ anticoagulants (blood thinners) ■ medicine for Parkinson's disease ■ barbiturates ■ medicine for seizures ■ female hormones (estrogens) ■ medicine for myasthenia gravis ■ antacids

■ muscle relaxants ■ medicine for high cholesterol ■ medicine for tuberculosis
■ potassium-containing medicines or supplements.

You have recently had a vaccination.

You are subjected to unusual stress in your daily life.

SPECIAL RESTRICTIONS WHILE TAKING THIS DRUG

FOOD AND DRUG INTERACTIONS

Other Drugs	These drugs interact with many other drugs; do not take any other drug, including over-the-counter (OTC) drugs, before checking with your doctor.
	These drugs may affect how your body absorbs medicine for diabetes, and your dosage may need to be adjusted.
	Let your doctor know if you are planning to receive any kind of vaccine or immunization.
Foods and Beverages	Tell your doctor if you are on any kind of special diet. Your doctor may recommend a low-salt, high-potassium diet to counterbalance some of the side effects of this drug such as bloating.
	Long-term therapy with this drug makes you more prone to osteoporosis (thinning of the bones). Your doctor may recommend that you include more calcium in your diet or may prescribe a calcium supplement for you.
	You may also be advised to take vitamin A and/or C supplements while on this drug.
Alcohol	Drinking alcohol while taking this drug may cause stomach upset. Avoid alcohol unless your doctor has approved its use.

No special restrictions on smoking.

DAILY LIVING

Exertion and Exercise	Discuss with your doctor which kinds of physical exercises are safe for you to undertake.
Examinations or Tests	It is important for you to keep all appointments with your doctor so that your progress can be checked. Periodic blood, urine, and eye tests may be required.
Other Precautions	Tell any doctor or dentist you consult that you are presently taking or have taken any of these drugs in the past year, especially if you will be undergoing any type of surgery. If you are undergoing some sort of unusual stress, or if you develop any signs of infection (fever, sore throat, muscle aches, pain in urination), call your doctor.
Helpful Hints	If this medicine upsets your stomach, taking it with milk, meals, or snacks should help. If you continue to experience distress, let your doctor know.

No special restrictions on sun exposure or exposure to excessive heat or cold.

POSSIBLE SIDE EFFECTS

Although this list of adverse effects may seem somewhat intimidating, keep in mind that some are quite rare. Of course, should these or any other problems arise while you are on medication, it is always a good idea to consult your doctor.

IF YOU DEVELOP

seizures ■ stomach pain ■ dizziness or faintness
■ fever ■ loss of appetite with weight loss ■ muscle or
joint pain or weakness ■ nausea or vomiting
■ difficulty in breathing ■ tiredness ■ slow or fast
heartbeat ■ palpitations ■ swelling of mouth or
tongue ■ speech difficulties ■ pain in urination
■ urinary frequency

After you STOP taking this medicine: loss of appetite
and/or weight loss ■ nausea or vomiting
■ drowsiness ■ headache ■ fever ■ joint or muscle
pain ■ peeling of skin ■ dizziness ■ depression

back, hip, or rib pain ■ acne ■ increased sweating
■ hair growth ■ skin redness, rash, or hives ■ scaly
skin or other skin changes ■ bruising ■ depression
■ nervousness or restlessness ■ anxiety ■ "high"
feeling ■ other mood changes ■ blood in stools
■ bloating ■ halos around lights or other visual disturbances ■ sore throat or hoarseness ■ wounds that
take a long time to heal ■ swelling of hands, feet, or
ankles ■ diarrhea ■ constipation ■ reactivation of an
ulcer ■ any lung or throat infection ■ white patches in
mouth or throat

indigestion ■ increase in appetite with weight gain
■ eruptions on mouth or lips ■ sleeplessness
■ headache ■ unusual roundness of the face

WHAT TO DO

Urgent Get in touch with
your doctor immediately.

May be serious Check with
your doctor as soon as
possible.

If symptoms are disturbing
or persist, let your doctor
know.

STORAGE INSTRUCTIONS

Store in a cool, dark place (not in a bathroom medicine cabinet). If your medicine is
in a liquid form, make sure that it does not freeze.

STOPPING OR INTERRUPTING THERAPY

Corticosteroids affect many organs and tissues in the body. For this reason take this
medicine exactly as prescribed by your doctor. Do not suddenly stop taking this

medicine; your doctor will advise you on how to gradually reduce your dosage. Ask your doctor what to do if you miss a dose. You may experience side effects from corticosteroids for up to a year after stopping therapy; let your doctor know if this should happen.

SPECIAL CONSIDERATIONS FOR THOSE OVER SIXTY-FIVE

Long-term use of corticosteroids may cause gradual bone loss; this can be serious in older people, particularly women, who are vulnerable to osteoporosis. This age group is particularly susceptible to adverse effects on the muscles and nerves as well.

CONDITION: **ARTHRITIS**

CATEGORY: **OTHER ANTIARTHRITIC AGENTS**

GENERIC (CHEMICAL) NAME	BRAND (TRADE) NAME	DOSAGE FORMS AND STRENGTHS
Auranofin	RIDAURA	Capsules: 3 mg

DRUG PROFILE

Auranofin is a gold compound used to treat rheumatoid arthritis. It is not known exactly how this drug works to relieve joint pain and inflammation. Because of its relatively serious potential side effects, auranofin is reserved for people who do not respond to therapy with nonsteroidal anti-inflammatory drugs and should be prescribed only by doctors who are familiar with its use.

BEFORE USING THIS DRUG

Let your doctor know *IF*

You have ever had allergic reactions or other problems with ■ auranofin or other gold compounds ■ gold or other metals.

You have ever had any of the following medical problems: ■ blood diseases, including bone marrow depression ■ kidney disease ■ liver disease ■ systemic lupus erythematosus ■ skin disease, including rash, hives, or eczema ■ colitis bleeding disease ■ any reaction to a drug that affected your blood, lungs, or digestive tract ■ irritable bowel disease ■ blood vessel disease.

You are taking any of the following medicines: ■ other arthritis medicine, especially penicillamine or phenylbutazone ■ medicine for cancer ■ medicine for malaria ■ phenytoin (medicine for seizures).

You have recently received radiation therapy.

SPECIAL RESTRICTIONS WHILE TAKING THIS DRUG

FOOD AND DRUG INTERACTIONS

No special restrictions on other drugs, foods and beverages, alcohol use, or smoking.

DAILY LIVING

Exertion and Exercise	Discuss with your doctor which kinds of physical exercise are safe for you to undertake.
Sun Exposure	If you experience skin problems with auranofin, prolonged exposure to sunlight will aggravate the problem. It is a good idea to apply a sunscreen to exposed skin surfaces before going outdoors.
Examinations or Tests	It is important for you to keep all appointments with your doctor so that your progress can be checked. Periodic blood and urine tests are usually required before and during therapy.
Other Precautions	Take this medicine exactly as instructed by your doctor; taking more than your prescribed dose may increase your chances of developing side effects.
	Let your doctor know if any side effect becomes bothersome. If you experience diarrhea, a dose change or even a break from taking this drug may be

possible. Medicine for diarrhea or an oral iron preparation may be prescribed for you.

No special restrictions on driving or exposure to excessive heat or cold.

POSSIBLE SIDE EFFECTS

Although this list of adverse effects may seem somewhat intimidating, keep in mind that some are quite rare. Of course, should these or any other problems arise while you are on medication, it is always a good idea to consult your doctor.

IF YOU DEVELOP

red marks on skin ■ puffy face, hands, or feet ■ coughing, wheezing, or other difficulty in breathing

WHAT TO DO

Urgent Get in touch with your doctor immediately.

severe diarrhea or diarrhea lasting more than three days ■ rash, hives, or itching ■ sores or white spots in mouth or throat ■ bloody or cloudy urine ■ bleeding or bruising ■ vomiting, with blood or vomit that looks like coffee grounds ■ difficulty in swallowing ■ headache ■ dizziness ■ fever ■ irritation or soreness of tongue or gums ■ metallic taste ■ severe stomach pain ■ bloody or black, tarry stools ■ yellowing of eyes or skin ■ numbness, tingling, pain, or weakness in hands or feet ■ tiredness ■ sore throat

May be serious Check with your doctor as soon as possible.

nausea or vomiting ■ stomach cramps or pain ■ increased bowel movements, loose stools, or diarrhea ■ indigestion ■ gas or bloating ■ loss of appetite ■ constipation ■ taste changes ■ hair loss ■ positive test for occult blood in stool

If symptoms are disturbing or persist, let your doctor know.

STORAGE INSTRUCTIONS

Store in a cool, dark place (not in a bathroom medicine cabinet).

STOPPING OR INTERRUPTING THERAPY

It may be three to six months before you see any improvement in your symptoms. If you are supposed to take your medicine once a day and miss a dose, take it as soon as possible. If you do not remember until the following day, skip the missed dose and resume your regular schedule. If you are supposed to take your medicine twice or more a day and miss a dose, take it as soon as possible. If it is almost time for your next dose, skip it and resume your regular schedule. Do not take two doses at the same time.

SPECIAL CONSIDERATIONS FOR THOSE OVER SIXTY-FIVE

None.

CONDITION: **ARTHRITIS**

CATEGORY: **OTHER ANTIARTHRITIC AGENTS**

GENERIC (CHEMICAL) NAME	BRAND (TRADE) NAME	DOSAGE FORMS AND STRENGTHS
Penicillamine	CUPRIMINE DEPEN	Capsules: 125, 250 mg Tablets: 250 mg

DRUG PROFILE

Penicillamine (a chemical relative of penicillin) is used in the treatment of several medical problems, including rheumatoid arthritis. With long-term use, this drug can reduce the swelling, stiffness, and joint pain of arthritis. How it works is not known, and penicillamine does not cure arthritis. Because of its relatively serious potential side effects, penicillamine is reserved for people who have not responded to other treatments.

BEFORE USING THIS DRUG

Let your doctor know *IF*

You have ever had allergic reactions or other problems with ■ penicillamine ■ penicillin ■ chrysotherapy (gold salts).

You have ever had any of the following medical problems: ■ kidney disease ■ liver disease ■ stomach ulcer.

You are taking any of the following medicines ■ phenylbutazone or gold (other medicines for arthritis) ■ medicine for cancer ■ medicine or vitamins containing iron or magnesium ■ medicine for malaria ■ digoxin or digitalis (heart medicines) ■ antacids containing aluminum ■ probenecid (medicine for gout) ■ medicine to prevent reactions after organ transplants ■ aspirin or aspirinlike medicine ■ corticosteroids.

SPECIAL RESTRICTIONS WHILE TAKING THIS DRUG

FOOD AND DRUG INTERACTIONS

Other Drugs	Do not take any other drugs, including over-the-counter (OTC) drugs, before checking with your doctor. If you require any drug or vitamin that contains iron, do not take it within two hours of your penicillamine dose, since iron can interfere with the action of penicillamine. If you are taking any other drug, do not take it within an hour of taking penicillamine.

No special restrictions on foods and beverages, alcohol use, or smoking.

DAILY LIVING

Examinations or Tests	It is important for you to keep all appointments with your doctor so that your progress can be checked. You will probably require blood and urine tests every two weeks during the first six months on penicillamine and monthly thereafter.
Helpful Hints	Penicillamine should be taken on an empty stomach —at least an hour before or more than two hours after eating—to speed its absorption into the body. If this drug upsets your stomach, however, taking it with milk, meals, or snacks should help.

No restrictions on driving, exertion and exercise, sun exposure, or exposure to excessive heat or cold.

POSSIBLE SIDE EFFECTS

Although this list of adverse effects may seem somewhat intimidating, keep in mind that some are quite rare. Of course, should these or any other problems arise while you are on medication, it is always a good idea to consult your doctor.

IF YOU DEVELOP

WHAT TO DO

sore throat or fever ■ chills ■ bleeding ■ bruising, wounding, or dark spots on skin ■ spitting up blood ■ difficulty in breathing ■ wheezing ■ unexplained cough ■ difficulty in speech ■ difficulty in chewing or swallowing ■ yellowing of eyes or skin ■ sores or white spots in mouth or gums ■ any change in color of urine or stool

Urgent Get in touch with your doctor immediately.

joint pain ■ rash, hives, or itching ■ wrinkling or any other skin problems ■ swelling of lymph glands ■ swelling of feet or lower legs ■ weight gain ■ tiredness or weakness ■ ringing in the ears ■ blurred vision or other visual disturbances ■ muscle weakness ■ tongue inflammation

May be serious Check with your doctor as soon as possible.

nausea or vomiting ■ stomach pain ■ loss of appetite ■ diarrhea ■ decreased sense of taste ■ upset stomach ■ hair loss ■ dry and scaly corners of the mouth ■ soreness of the vagina or vulva

If symptoms are disturbing or persist, let your doctor know.

STORAGE INSTRUCTIONS

Store in a cool, dark place (not in a bathroom medicine cabinet).

STOPPING OR INTERRUPTING THERAPY

Take this medicine exactly as prescribed, since it has been especially tailored to you and your particular symptoms. It may be two to three months before you notice improvement in your symptoms. If you are supposed to take this medicine once a day and miss a dose, take it as soon as possible. If you do not remember until the next day, skip the missed dose and resume your regular schedule. If you are supposed to take your medicine twice a day and miss a dose, take it as soon as possible. If it is almost time for your next dose, skip the missed dose and resume your regular schedule. If you are supposed to take penicillamine more than twice a day and miss a dose, take the missed dose within two hours of the scheduled time for that dose. If a longer time has passed, skip the missed dose and resume your regular schedule.

SPECIAL CONSIDERATIONS FOR THOSE OVER SIXTY-FIVE

Older people may be more prone to the side effects of this medicine, especially rashes and taste changes. Doctors may start people over sixty-five on a lower dosage and build it up gradually.

CONDITION: **ARTHRITIS**

CATEGORY: **OTHER ANTIARTHRITIC AGENTS**

GENERIC (CHEMICAL) NAME	BRAND (TRADE) NAME	DOSAGE FORMS AND STRENGTHS
Methotrexate	RHEUMATREX	Tablets: 2.5 mg

DRUG PROFILE

Methotrexate is used to treat certain types of leukemia, cancer of the lymph nodes, cancer of the breast, and certain cancers of the head, neck, skin, and lung. This drug is also sometimes used to treat severe rheumatoid arthritis and severe cases of psoriasis—a skin disorder. Methotrexate slows and halts the growth and spread of cancer cells by interfering with one of the steps in cell growth.

For complete information on this drug, see pages 1072–1076.

GOUT

Gout ranks high among human biology's great sources of exquisite agony. And much of the old folklore surrounding this disease is at least partly true. For example, gout has often been regarded as a disease of rotund gentlemen who ingest food and alcohol with abandon. Indeed, the disease almost exclusively strikes men over forty; obesity and alcohol can contribute to its risks, though they are *not* prerequisites. And the traditional caricatures of gout sufferers as having tender, swollen big toes do indeed show one of the main targets of the disease.

For nearly two million people in the United States, gout is no source of amusement. Rather, it is the cause of flare-ups of extreme pain and inflammation in the joints of large toes as well as other weight-bearing joints. Its sufferers' main consolation is that a variety of medicines can effectively relieve symptoms as well as treat the underlying problem.

CAUSES

At the root of gout is an excess of uric acid in the blood. Uric acid is produced naturally in the body and is also derived from foods containing substances called purines. Usually there is a proper balance between the production of uric acid and its disposal in the urine. Levels can rise because of overproduction, impaired excretion, or both.

Under certain conditions, excess uric acid in the blood will form tiny needle-shaped crystals, which typically settle in the joints of the legs and feet. This then triggers the body to dispatch white blood cells to attack the crystals, causing the swelling, redness, and extreme sensitivity in the affected joint. A doctor's clearest evidence of gout comes from a combination of white blood cells and uric acid crystals in a sample of fluid taken from the joint.

For a lucky few, the first flare-up of gout is also the last. Generally, though, gout attacks tend to recur and can increase in severity. Left uncorrected, high uric acid levels can collect in the kidneys, and may damage the kidneys' delicate blood-filtering apparatus and possibly form painful kidney stones. Over the years, untreated gout may lead to a condition called tophaceous gout, in which small clumps of uric acid crystals can trigger inflammation, pain, and tissue damage throughout the body—notably in the big toe, elbow, and inner ear.

Pseudogout is a condition similar to gout, but in this case calcium-containing crystals, instead of uric acid crystals, settle in the joints of the legs, feet, and hands. These crystals can trigger the body to dispatch white blood cells and cause swelling, redness, and pain in much the same way as classic gout. Because of the similarities between this condition and classic gout this condition is often called pseudogout. Evidence of pseudogout comes from the identification of the calcium-containing crystals in fluid taken from the painful joint. Treatment of an attack of pseudogout generally includes use of a nonsteroidal anti-inflammatory drug.

TREATMENT

A number of treatments can relieve the pain of gout and the potential tissue damage caused by excess uric acid. Colchicine is one of the oldest medicines for quelling the inflammation and pain of an acute gout attack; also, small doses may be used to prevent acute gout attacks (see the chart on pages 544–546). As alternatives, a doctor may recommend one of the nonsteroidal anti-inflammatory drugs (NSAIDs) for use during attacks (see the charts on pages 524–530).

For long-term treatment of gout, several other medicines can help lower blood levels of uric acid in two ways—by helping the body get rid of uric acid through the urine and by inhibiting the production of uric acid in the first place (see the charts on pages 546–556).

Your doctor will advise you to avoid foods containing very high levels of purines—including organ meats such as liver, pancreas, or brain—and to use moderation in your eating habits. Losing weight, if you are obese, should also help. Other useful measures include controlling high blood pressure, high blood fat levels, and diabetes. Finally, alcohol helps block the excretion of uric acid, so you would be wise to cut back or abstain.

OUTLOOK

Managing gout and other uric acid-related disorders is a lifetime affair. If, after study, your doctor recommends drugs that help lower blood levels of uric acid, those agents should be taken indefinitely; uric acid levels can rise quickly when the drugs are discontinued. But the gains from sticking to antigout therapy, once begun, are great in preventing both the extreme pain of gout and the potential damage to various parts of the body.

Caution: Some drugs in this section may affect pregnancy or fetal development. Check with your doctor if this concerns you.

CONDITION: **GOUT**

CATEGORY: **ANTIGOUT AGENTS (DRUGS FOR ACUTE ATTACKS)**

GENERIC (CHEMICAL) NAME	BRAND (TRADE) NAME	DOSAGE FORMS AND STRENGTHS
Colchicine		Tablets: 0.5 mg ($\frac{1}{120}$ grain), 0.6 mg ($\frac{1}{100}$ grain)

DRUG PROFILE

Colchicine is used to treat acute attacks of gouty arthritis and to prevent attacks from recurring. It may also be used to treat chronic gouty arthritis. This drug works by reducing inflammation.

BEFORE USING THIS DRUG

Let your doctor know *IF*

You have ever had allergic reactions or other problems with ■ colchicine.

You have ever had any of the following medical problems: ■ heart disease ■ kidney disease ■ liver disease ■ blood disease ■ stomach ulcer or other digestive disorders.

You are taking any of the following medicines: ■ vitamin B_{12} ■ NSAIDs (especially phenylbutazone) ■ diuretics (water pills).

You are receiving: ■ radiation therapy.

SPECIAL RESTRICTIONS WHILE TAKING THIS DRUG

FOOD AND DRUG INTERACTIONS

Alcohol	Avoid alcohol while taking this drug; alcohol may increase the amount of uric acid in the blood, thus worsening your condition.

No special restrictions on other drugs, foods and beverages, or smoking.

DAILY LIVING

Examinations or Tests	It is important for you to keep all appointments with your doctor so that your progress can be checked. Periodic blood and urine tests may be required.
Helpful Hints	Be sure to drink plenty of fluids (at least ten to twelve full glasses of water a day) to prevent the formation of kidney stones.

No special restrictions on driving, exertion and exercise, sun exposure, or exposure to excessive heat or cold.

POSSIBLE SIDE EFFECTS

Although this list of adverse effects may seem somewhat intimidating, keep in mind that some are quite rare. Of course, should these or any other problems arise while you are on medication, it is always a good idea to consult your doctor.

IF YOU DEVELOP

numbness, tingling, pain, or weakness in hands or feet ■ rash or other skin problems ■ fever ■ bleeding or bruising ■ sore throat ■ severe muscle weakness ■ blood in urine ■ decreased urination

WHAT TO DO

Urgent Get in touch with your doctor immediately.

diarrhea ■ nausea or vomiting ■ stomach pain or discomfort	**May be serious** *Stop taking this medicine* and check with your doctor as soon as possible.
hair loss	If symptoms are disturbing or persist, let your doctor know.

STORAGE INSTRUCTIONS

Store in a cool, dark place (not in a bathroom medicine cabinet).

STOPPING OR INTERRUPTING THERAPY

Your doctor may tell you to stop taking this drug when pain is relieved, or at the first sign of diarrhea, vomiting, or stomach pain. If you are on long-term therapy with this drug and you miss a dose, take it as soon as possible. If it is almost time for your next dose, skip the missed dose and resume your regular schedule. Do not take two doses at the same time.

SPECIAL CONSIDERATIONS FOR THOSE OVER SIXTY-FIVE

Older people may be more prone to the side effects of colchicine.

CONDITION: **GOUT**

CATEGORY: **ANTIGOUT AGENTS (URIC ACID REDUCERS)**

GENERIC (CHEMICAL) NAME	BRAND (TRADE) NAME	DOSAGE FORMS AND STRENGTHS
Allopurinol	LOPURIN	Tablets: 100, 300 mg
	ZYLOPRIM	Tablets: 100, 300 mg

DRUG PROFILE

Allopurinol is used in such conditions as gout and kidney stones caused by an excess amount of uric acid in the body. This drug blocks xanthine oxidase, an enzyme necessary for the production of uric acid, and may be used in combination with other drugs. Although allopurinol can prevent gout attacks, it does not actually cure gout and cannot stop a gout attack in progress.

BEFORE USING THIS DRUG

Let your doctor know *IF*

You have ever had allergic reactions or other problems with ■ allopurinol ■ thiazide diuretics.

You have ever had any of the following medical problems: ■ kidney disease ■ liver disease ■ hemochromatosis (excess iron in the blood).

You are taking any of the following medicines: ■ other medicine for gout or gouty arthritis ■ penicillin or any drug in the penicillin family, including amoxicillin, ampicillin, bacampicillin, and hetacillin ■ medicine for asthma ■ anticoagulants (blood thinners) ■ azathioprine, dacarbazine, mercaptopurine (medicines for cancer) ■ chlorpropamide (medicine for diabetes) ■ medicine for high blood pressure ■ diuretics (water pills) ■ medicine to make the urine more acidic ■ pyrazinamide (medicine for tuberculosis) ■ co-trimoxazole (medicine for urinary tract infections) ■ medicine for seizures ■ captopril (medicine for congestive heart failure).

SPECIAL RESTRICTIONS WHILE TAKING THIS DRUG

FOOD AND DRUG INTERACTIONS

Alcohol	Avoid alcohol while taking this drug; alcohol may increase the amount of uric acid in the blood, thus worsening your condition.

No special restrictions on other drugs, foods and beverages, or smoking.

DAILY LIVING

Driving

This drug may cause drowsiness. Be careful when driving, operating household appliances, or doing any other tasks that require alertness until you know how this drug affects you.

Examinations or Tests

It is important for you to keep all appointments with your doctor so that your progress can be checked. Periodic blood and urine tests may be required.

Other Precautions

It may be several months before you notice the effects of this medicine, but continue to take it as instructed. Should you experience more frequent gout attacks during the first few months of treatment, your doctor may prescribe an additional medicine, such as colchicine.

Helpful Hints

If this drug upsets your stomach, taking it with milk, meals, or snacks should help. If you continue to experience distress, let your doctor know.

Be sure to drink plenty of fluids (at least ten to twelve full glasses) while taking this drug.

No special restrictions on exertion and exercise, sun exposure, or exposure to excessive heat or cold.

POSSIBLE SIDE EFFECTS

Although this list of adverse effects may seem somewhat intimidating, keep in mind that some are quite rare. Of course, should these or any other problems arise while you are on medication, it is always a good idea to consult your doctor.

IF YOU DEVELOP	WHAT TO DO
rash, hives, or itching ■ chills ■ fever ■ muscle aches and pains ■ nausea or vomiting occurring shortly after rash ■ general ill feeling ■ pain in urination ■ blood in urine ■ decreased urination ■ eye irritation ■ swelling of lips and mouth ■ red, thickened, or scaly skin ■ boils on nose ■ bleeding (including nosebleed) or bruising ■ yellowing of eyes or skin ■ loosening of fingernails ■ small red marks on skin	**Urgent** Get in touch with your doctor immediately.
numbness, tingling, pain, or weakness in hands or feet ■ increase in gout attacks ■ loss of appetite ■ weight loss ■ swelling of hands or feet ■ hearing problems	**May be serious** Check with your doctor as soon as possible.
drowsiness ■ diarrhea ■ stomach pain ■ nausea or vomiting (without rash) ■ taste changes ■ upset stomach	If symptoms are disturbing or persist, let your doctor know.

STORAGE INSTRUCTIONS

Store in a cool, dark place (not in a bathroom medicine cabinet).

STOPPING OR INTERRUPTING THERAPY

Take this medicine exactly as instructed by your doctor. If you are supposed to take this medicine once a day and miss a dose, take it as soon as possible. If you do not remember until the next day, skip the missed dose and resume your regular schedule. Do not take two doses at the same time. If you are supposed to take this drug twice or more a day and miss a dose, take it as soon as possible. If it is almost time for your next dose and your dose is one 100 mg tablet, double the next dose; if your dose is two 100 mg tablets, take three tablets for your next dose. Then go back to your regular schedule.

SPECIAL CONSIDERATIONS FOR THOSE OVER SIXTY-FIVE

Those older people who have reduced kidney function tend not to eliminate this drug as readily as people with normal kidney function. Doctors may check such people regularly to make sure they are receiving the proper dosage and that too much drug is not accumulating in the body.

CONDITION: **GOUT**

CATEGORY: **ANTIGOUT AGENTS (URIC ACID REDUCERS)**

GENERIC (CHEMICAL) NAME	BRAND (TRADE) NAME	DOSAGE FORMS AND STRENGTHS
Probenecid	BENEMID	Tablets: 0.5 g

DRUG PROFILE

Probenecid increases the elimination of uric acid from the body through urination in people susceptible to chronic gout and gouty arthritis. Probenecid does not actually cure gout and cannot stop a gout attack in progress. Probenecid is also sometimes prescribed along with penicillin for the treatment of infections because it helps achieve extra "mileage" from a penicillin dose.

BEFORE USING THIS DRUG

Let your doctor know *IF*

You have ever had allergic reactions or other problems with ■ probenecid.

You have ever had any of the following medical problems: ■ blood disease ■ kidney disease, including kidney stones ■ stomach ulcer ■ glucose-6-phosphate dehydrogenase (G-6-PD) deficiency.

You are taking any of the following medicines: ■ other medicine for gout or gouty arthritis ■ any medicine for pain and inflammation ■ aspirin or aspirinlike medicine ■ methotrexate (medicine for severe psoriasis, severe rheumatoid arthritis, or cancer) ■ captopril (medicine for congestive heart failure) ■ clofibrate (medicine for high cholesterol) ■ medicine for diabetes ■ water pills (diuretics) ■ medicine for asthma ■ antibiotics ■ medicine for high blood pressure ■ pyrazinamide (medicine for tuberculosis) ■ vitamin B preparations ■ medicine for herpes infections.

SPECIAL RESTRICTIONS WHILE TAKING THIS DRUG

FOOD AND DRUG INTERACTIONS

Other Drugs	Do not take aspirin or aspirinlike medicines, since they reduce the effectiveness of probenecid. If you have pain or a fever, take acetaminophen instead.
	If you have diabetes and are taking an oral diabetes medicine, you may develop low blood sugar while on this drug. If this happens, stop taking the oral diabetes medicine and inform your doctor immediately.
	If you are taking cholestyramine (medicine for high cholesterol), take your dose of probenecid one hour before or four to six hours following your dose of cholestyramine.
Alcohol	Avoid alcohol while taking this drug; alcohol may increase the amount of uric acid in the blood, thus worsening your condition.

No special restrictions on smoking.

DAILY LIVING

Examinations or Tests	It is important for you to keep all appointments with your doctor so that your progress can be checked. Periodic blood and urine tests may be required.
Other Precautions	Tell any doctor or dentist you consult that you are taking this drug, especially if you will be undergoing any type of surgery or any kind of diagnostic tests.
	It may be several weeks before you notice the effects of this medicine, but you should continue to

take it as instructed. If you do experience gout attacks, your doctor will prescribe appropriate medicine to stop an attack in progress.

If you have diabetes, be aware that this drug may interfere with certain urine-sugar tests. Ask your doctor what kind of test is best to use while taking this medicine.

Helpful Hints

Be sure to drink plenty of fluids (at least ten to twelve full glasses of water a day) while taking this drug to help prevent the formation of kidney stones.

If this drug upsets your stomach, taking it with milk, meals, or snacks should help. If you continue to experience distress, let your doctor know.

No special restrictions on driving, exertion and exercise, sun exposure, or exposure to excessive heat or cold.

POSSIBLE SIDE EFFECTS

Although this list of adverse effects may seem somewhat intimidating, keep in mind that some are quite rare. Of course, should these or any other problems arise while you are on medication, it is always a good idea to consult your doctor.

IF YOU DEVELOP	WHAT TO DO
blood in urine ■ pain in urination ■ lower back pain ■ fever ■ extreme dizziness ■ tiredness ■ difficulty in breathing ■ sore throat ■ decreased urination ■ bleeding or bruising ■ skin rash or itching	**May be serious** Check with your doctor as soon as possible.
nausea or vomiting ■ loss of appetite ■ headache ■ urinary frequency ■ sore gums ■ flushing ■ upset stomach	If symptoms are disturbing or persist, let your doctor know.

STORAGE INSTRUCTIONS

Store in a cool, dark place (not in a bathroom medicine cabinet).

STOPPING OR INTERRUPTING THERAPY

Take this medicine exactly as instructed by your doctor. If you miss a dose, take it as soon as possible. If it is almost time for your next dose, skip the missed dose and resume your regular schedule. Do not take two doses at the same time.

SPECIAL CONSIDERATIONS FOR THOSE OVER SIXTY-FIVE

None.

CONDITION: **GOUT**

CATEGORY: **ANTIGOUT AGENTS (URIC ACID REDUCERS)**

GENERIC (CHEMICAL) NAME	BRAND (TRADE) NAME	DOSAGE FORMS AND STRENGTHS
Sulfinpyrazone	ANTURANE	Capsules: 200 mg Tablets: 100 mg

DRUG PROFILE

Sulfinpyrazone increases the elimination of uric acid from the body through urination in people susceptible to gouty arthritis. It is used to treat chronic gouty arthritis. Sulfinpyrazone does not actually cure gouty arthritis and cannot stop an attack in progress.

BEFORE USING THIS DRUG

Let your doctor know *IF*

You have ever had allergic reactions or other problems with ■ sulfinpyrazone
■ phenylbutazone.

You have ever had any of the following medical problems: ■ blood disease ■ kidney disease, including kidney stones ■ stomach ulcer or other digestive disorders.

You are taking any of the following medicines: ■ other medicine for gout or gouty arthritis ■ any medicine for pain and inflammation ■ aspirin or aspirinlike medicine ■ medicine for cancer ■ medicine for high cholesterol ■ medicine for diabetes ■ water pills (diuretics) ■ medicine for asthma ■ antibiotics, especially sulfa drugs ■ medicine for high blood pressure ■ pyrazinamide (medicine for tuberculosis) ■ acetaminophen ■ niacin ■ verapamil (medicine for chest pain or high blood pressure) ■ cholestyramine ■ anticoagulants (blood thinners).

SPECIAL RESTRICTIONS WHILE TAKING THIS DRUG

FOOD AND DRUG INTERACTIONS

Other Drugs	Do not take aspirin or aspirinlike medicine, as they reduce the effectiveness of this drug. If you have pain or a fever, take acetaminophen instead.
	If you are taking cholestyramine for high cholesterol, take your dose of this drug at least one hour before or four to six hours after your dose of cholestyramine.
Alcohol	Avoid alcohol while taking this drug; alcohol may increase the amount of uric acid in the blood, thus worsening your condition.

No special restrictions on smoking.

DAILY LIVING

Examinations or Tests	It is important for you to keep all appointments with your doctor so that your progress can be checked. Periodic blood and urine tests may be required.

Other Precautions	It may be several weeks before you notice the effects of this medicine, but you should continue to take it as instructed. If you do experience gout attacks, your doctor will prescribe appropriate medicine to stop an attack in progress.
Helpful Hints	Take sulfinpyrazone with milk or meals to avoid stomach upset. Be sure to drink plenty of fluids (at least ten to twelve full glasses of water a day) to help prevent the formation of kidney stones.

No special restrictions on driving, exertion and exercise, sun exposure, or exposure to excessive heat or cold.

POSSIBLE SIDE EFFECTS

Although this list of adverse effects may seem somewhat intimidating, keep in mind that some are quite rare. Of course, should these or any other problems arise while you are on medication, it is always a good idea to consult your doctor.

IF YOU DEVELOP	WHAT TO DO
bleeding or bruising ■ clumsiness or unsteadiness ■ difficulty in breathing ■ seizures ■ diarrhea ■ severe or continuing nausea, vomiting, or stomach pain ■ sore throat ■ fever ■ tiredness or weakness	**Urgent** Get in touch with your doctor immediately.
rash ■ bloody or black, tarry stools ■ blood in urine ■ reactivation of stomach ulcer ■ dizziness ■ hearing problems ■ swelling of face, feet, or hands ■ yellowing of eyes or skin ■ lower back pain ■ pain or difficulty in urination	**May be serious** Check with your doctor as soon as possible.

nausea or vomiting ■ stomach pain ■ indigestion	If symptoms are disturbing or persist, let your doctor know.

STORAGE INSTRUCTIONS

Store in a cool, dark place (not in a bathroom medicine cabinet).

STOPPING OR INTERRUPTING THERAPY

Take this medicine exactly as instructed by your doctor. If you miss a dose, take it as soon as possible. If it is almost time for your next dose, skip the missed dose and resume your regular schedule. Do not take two doses at the same time.

SPECIAL CONSIDERATIONS FOR THOSE OVER SIXTY-FIVE

None.

OSTEOPOROSIS

One out of every four women over the age of sixty is affected by osteoporosis, which has been called a silent epidemic. Bones weakened by osteoporosis cannot withstand normal strains and break easily, often during such routine activities as bending or lifting. There are 1.3 million osteoporosis-related fractures each year in people over forty-five. Although all bones are affected, fractures of the spine, wrist, and hip are most common.

CAUSES

What happens as we age to make us prone to osteoporosis? To understand this, let's first look at the relationship between calcium and bone. Your body has between two and four pounds of calcium. Most of it—98 percent—is found in your bones. Contrary to popular opinion, bone is *not* lifeless but a constantly changing, living tissue. Calcium is its most important component, giving bones their strength and solidity. Each day, new bone is added as old bone is broken down and removed from the body through a process called remodeling. The amount of bone present in the body is the result of a balance between the formation of new bone and the breakdown of old bone.

When we reach our mid-thirties, the balance tips a bit, and more bone is lost than gained. Some bone loss is a normal part of aging and affects both men and women, but osteoporosis involves a more extreme loss that results in dangerous weakening of the bones.

Women are far more likely to develop osteoporosis than men, however, for reasons that include inadequate amounts of calcium-rich foods during childbearing years, smaller frames, and a decrease in the level of estrogen that occurs after menopause. (Although the connection between estrogen and bone loss is not completely understood, researchers think that estrogen is needed to maintain the balance between deposit and loss of calcium in the bones.) Inactivity may also contribute to the development of osteoporosis in both sexes. Other, less important, reasons that affect both sexes are inadequate amounts of vitamin D in the diet and inadequate exposure to sunlight. Sunlight helps the body manufacture vitamin D, which is necessary for calcium absorption.

Fair-skinned white women and Asian women are more likely to develop osteoporosis than are black women. Thin women with small frames are also likely candidates. In addition, women who have an early menopause and who smoke are more susceptible to this condition.

DIAGNOSIS

An early sign of osteoporosis is a gradual loss of height, which results from the compression of weakened bones of the spine. In its extreme form, this leads to the development of a curved spine. Often, the gradual loss of bone isn't recognized until a bone fractures. Your doctor may confirm the diagnosis of osteoporosis with X rays or with advanced techniques for measuring bone thickness and density.

TREATMENT

Because it is difficult, if not impossible, to replace lost bone, the goal of treatment is to stop further bone loss. A dietary approach may be one way to do this. Because your body cannot make calcium, you must supply it by eating calcium-rich foods. The current Recommended Dietary Allowance (RDA) for calcium is 1000 mg (milligrams). Most researchers believe that's less than what's needed, particularly for women past menopause, and probably for older men as well. They recommend increasing the amount to 1,500 mg a day. One cup of milk has about 300 mg, one ounce of cheese has about 200 mg, and eight sardines have about 350 mg of calcium.

Because many people don't eat enough calcium-rich food each day, doctors may recommend a calcium supplement to ensure an adequate daily supply. Keep in mind, however, that calcium supplements are not recommended for people who have ever had kidney stones and may not be advisable for people with a family history of this condition. If the calcium tablets are too large to swallow whole, you can crush them and mix them with something easy to swallow like applesauce or cottage cheese. Turn to the drug chart on pages 566–568 for more information on calcium supplements.

Recent research indicates that calcium supplementation is not, in itself, adequate for preventing bone loss during and after menopause. Estrogen replacement therapy has been found to be the most important preventive in postmenopausal women. The hormone estrogen is often prescribed for women in this category. Except in women who have undergone a hysterectomy, estrogen is given with intermittent doses of progesterone. Such hormonal treatment has been effective in limiting osteoporosis in some postmenopausal women.

There may be another important benefit of estrogen replacement therapy in addition to preventing bone loss. Estrogens seem to lower levels of cholesterol in the blood, in particular LDL (low-density lipoprotein—the so-called bad cholesterol). Estrogens also seem to raise levels of HDL (high-density lipoprotein—the "good" cholesterol). Over the long term, these improvements in cholesterol levels may help reduce the risk of developing heart disease. The drug chart on pages 560–565 will provide you with more information on estrogen.

The best regimen for preventing osteoporosis appears to be a combination of estrogen replacement therapy and calcium supplementation. The use of calcium supplements may permit a reduced dose of estrogen—and a lowered risk of unpleasant side effects connected with estrogen therapy, such as uterine bleeding and migraine headaches.

Make sure you get enough sunlight so that your body can manufacture vitamin D. If you can't get out into the sun for fifteen minutes to an hour a day or if you live in a climate where the sun doesn't shine every day, drink vitamin D–fortified milk, or ask your doctor about supplements. Although high dose vitamin D supplements (25,000 to 50,000 units) are often used to treat osteoporosis, they may not be beneficial and may actually worsen this condition. These doses can also lead to dangerous toxicity. Do not decide on your own to take a vitamin D supplement.

Exercise regularly. Inactivity leads to bone loss, no matter what your age. Any weight-bearing exercise such as walking, dancing, or tennis is beneficial because it places stress on the skeleton, stimulating the formation of bone. Of course, it's wise to check with your doctor if you're contemplating embarking on a new exercise program.

OUTLOOK

Although we don't yet know how to reverse calcium loss from bones, we do know that further loss can be halted by weight-bearing exercise. For women, estrogen replacement is another possibility.

Combinations of substances (such as the hormone calcitonin) that show promise in reversing the bone loss of osteoporosis are currently under investigation. If they prove safe and effective, they may one day soon help to end this silent epidemic.

CONDITION: **OSTEOPOROSIS**

CATEGORY: **ESTROGENS**

GENERIC (CHEMICAL) NAME	BRAND (TRADE) NAME	DOSAGE FORMS AND STRENGTHS
Conjugated estrogens	PREMARIN	Tablets: 0.3, 0.625, 0.9, 1.25, 2.5 mg
Chlorotrianisene	TACE	Capsules: 12, 25, 72 mg
Diethylstilbestrol (DES)		Tablets: 1, 5 mg
Estradiol	ESTRACE ESTRADERM	Tablets: 1, 2 mg Skin patch: 0.05, 0.1 mg per 24 hours
Estropipate	OGEN	Tablets: 0.625, 1.25, 2.5, 5 mg
Ethinyl estradiol	ESTINYL	Tablets: 0.02, 0.05, 0.5 mg
Quinestrol	ESTROVIS	Tablets: 100 mcg

DRUG PROFILE

Estrogens (female hormones) are used to help treat the bone loss that occurs in women after menopause or after surgical removal of the uterus and/or ovaries, when the body no longer produces natural estrogens. These drugs are also used in other medical conditions such as breast cancer or prostate cancer as well as for atrophic vaginitis (dryness of the vagina) and other symptoms of menopause. Estrogens help the bones to retain the calcium they need to stay healthy. Many studies have shown that estrogen deficiency contributes to bone loss after menopause. Estrogens are usually administered in low doses in a cycle: three weeks on therapy and one week off therapy. You may be given a low dose of progesterone along with estrogens, which will help counteract some of estrogen's side effects. Estrogens are used as part of a treatment program for osteoporosis that may include diet, calcium supplements, and exercise. Although estrogens can prevent further bone loss, they cannot rebuild bones or straighten bones that have already become thin. Exactly how these hormones work is not known, but they probably increase the absorption of calcium from the intestine and/or decrease the removal of calcium from the bone.

BEFORE USING THIS DRUG

Let your doctor know *IF*

You have ever had allergic reactions or other problems with ■ estrogens.

With Estinyl and Estrace only: ■ tartrazine (FD&C Yellow Dye No. 5) ■ aspirin.

You have ever had any of the following medical problems: ■ asthma or other lung disease ■ circulation disorders or blood clots ■ breast lumps or breast cancer or a family history of breast cancer ■ any other kind of cancer ■ endometriosis ■ diabetes ■ epilepsy or other seizure disorders ■ gallbladder disease or gallstones ■ heart disease, including heart attacks ■ high blood pressure or a family history of high blood pressure ■ high blood calcium levels ■ jaundice ■ kidney disease ■ liver disease ■ depression ■ migraine headaches ■ stroke ■ high cholesterol or a family history of high cholesterol ■ high blood pressure or toxemia during pregnancy ■ weight gain or fluid retention in combination with menstrual cycle ■ abnormal bleeding from the vagina ■ bleeding gums.

You are taking any of the following medicines: ■ corticosteroids or corticotropin (ACTH) ■ medicine for diabetes ■ medicine for seizures ■ barbiturates ■ rifampin (antibiotic) ■ antidepressants ■ vitamin C ■ anticoagulants (blood thinners) ■ aminocaproic acid (medicine for excessive bleeding) ■ chenodiol (medicine for gallstones) ■ dantrolene (muscle relaxant) ■ mineral oil ■ tamoxifen (medicine for cancer) ■ vitamin A ■ vitamin B ■ thyroid hormones ■ meprobamate (sedative and muscle relaxant) ■ cyclosporine (a drug used for organ transplantation).

SPECIAL RESTRICTIONS WHILE TAKING THIS DRUG

FOOD AND DRUG INTERACTIONS

Foods and Beverages	Your doctor may prescribe a diet to help maintain healthy bones, which you should follow carefully. Such a diet is usually high in calcium; if it is difficult for you to include enough calcium in your diet, your doctor may suggest that you take a calcium supplement.
Smoking	Smoking increases the chance of developing such serious side effects as blood clot, heart attack, and stroke with estrogen therapy. If you smoke, try to stop or at least cut down.

No special restrictions on other drugs or alcohol use.

DAILY LIVING

Exertion and Exercise	You should try to include some regular physical activity in your daily life to strengthen your bones. Discuss with your doctor which kinds of exercise are appropriate for you.
Sun Exposure	You may find that you sunburn more easily or that you develop brown, blotchy spots on your skin after exposure to the sun while taking estrogens. Try to minimize sun exposure. It is a good idea to apply a sunscreen to exposed skin surfaces before going outdoors.
Examinations or Tests	It is important for you to keep all appointments with your doctor so that your progress can be checked. You will need periodic gynecologic examinations, including Pap smears, breast examinations, and annual mammograms.

Periodic blood pressure or blood and urine tests may be required while you are on estrogen therapy.

Other Precautions

Tell any doctor or dentist you consult that you are on estrogen therapy, especially if you will be undergoing any type of surgery or any kind of diagnostic testing.

If you wear contact lenses, you may find your eyes becoming sensitive to them during estrogen therapy. If this happens, discuss with your eye doctor whether it may be necessary for you to wear eyeglasses while you are on estrogen.

Estrogen therapy has been associated with a number of serious side effects. Long-term use of estrogens in women after menopause increases the possibility of developing endometrial cancer (cancer of the uterus [womb]). If you develop any abnormal bleeding from the vagina, let your doctor know. (If your uterus has been surgically removed [hysterectomy], there is no chance of you developing endometrial cancer.) Your doctor may be able to tailor your dosage schedule to minimize such a risk.

Studies of women taking oral contraceptives (which contain higher doses of estrogen and progesterone than are prescribed for women after menopause) have shown an increased risk of noncancerous liver tumors, blood clots, heart attacks, and stroke. If you develop any warning sign of a blood clot (see "Possible Side Effects"), call your doctor or go to an emergency room immediately.

Helpful Hints

Tablets and capsules. You may feel nauseated during the first few weeks of estrogen therapy. If this is a problem, try taking your daily dose during or directly after meals or with snacks.

Skin patch. Immediately after opening the package, apply the patch to a clean, dry, hairless area of skin.

Avoid the breast area and waistline (wearing tight clothing may dislodge the patch). The skin at the site should not be open, irritated, or oily. If the patch becomes loose or falls off, reapply it or, if necessary, apply a new one. Apply patches to different areas of the body, allowing at least one week between applications to a particular site.

No special restrictions on driving or exposure to excessive heat or cold.

POSSIBLE SIDE EFFECTS

Although this list of adverse effects may seem somewhat intimidating, keep in mind that some are quite rare. Of course, should these or any other problems arise while you are on medication, it is always a good idea to consult your doctor.

IF YOU DEVELOP	WHAT TO DO
Possible signs of a blood clot: pain or heavy feeling in chest; pains in groin or legs (especially the calf); weakness or numbness in arms or legs; severe and sudden headache, sometimes with vomiting; visual disturbances; difficulty in speech; sudden dizziness or faintness; unexplained cough or shortness of breath	**Urgent** Get in touch with your doctor immediately.
pain, swelling, or tenderness in stomach or side ■ vaginal bleeding ■ vaginal discharge ■ vaginitis ■ breast lumps ■ discharge from nipples ■ depression ■ uncontrollable, jerky movements ■ yellowing of eyes or skin ■ bleeding ■ fever ■ joint pain ■ rash	**May be serious** Check with your doctor as soon as possible.

nausea or vomiting ■ increased or decreased appetite ■ weight gain or loss ■ swelling of arms or legs ■ tenderness and swelling of breasts ■ stomach cramps or bloating ■ diarrhea ■ headache, including migraine headaches ■ dizziness ■ change in sexual drive ■ hair growth or loss ■ intolerance to contact lenses or other eye problems ■ increased skin sensitivity to sunlight, including development of brown, blotchy spots

With patch only: redness and irritation at patch site ■ skin redness or other skin problems

If symptoms are disturbing or persist, let your doctor know.

STORAGE INSTRUCTIONS

Store in a cool, dark place (not in a bathroom medicine cabinet).

STOPPING OR INTERRUPTING THERAPY

If you miss a dose of the oral form of this medicine, take it as soon as possible. If you do not remember until the following day, skip the missed dose and resume your regular schedule. Do not take two doses at the same time.

SPECIAL CONSIDERATIONS FOR THOSE OVER SIXTY-FIVE

None.

CONDITION: **OSTEOPOROSIS**

CATEGORY: **CALCIUM SUPPLEMENTS**

GENERIC (CHEMICAL) NAME	BRAND (TRADE) NAME	DOSAGE FORMS AND STRENGTHS
Calcium carbonate	CALTRATE	Tablets: 600 mg
	OS-CAL	Chewable tablets: 500 mg
		Tablets: 250, 500 mg
	TUMS	Chewable tablets: 500, 750 mg
Calcium phosphate	POSTURE	Tablets: 300, 600 mg
Dibasic calcium phosphate		Capsules: 500 mg

DRUG PROFILE

Calcium supplements are used along with estrogen as part of a treatment program to prevent the bone loss from osteoporosis for people who find it difficult to include sufficient calcium in their diets. Calcium is a major component of bone; a deficiency of this mineral can lead to the weakening of bones that is the hallmark of osteoporosis. Although calcium supplements are not prescription drugs, they are included in this book because of their importance in helping decrease bone loss in older women after menopause.

BEFORE USING THIS DRUG

Let your doctor know *IF*

You have ever had any of the following medical problems: ■ heart disease ■ kidney disease, including kidney stones ■ severe constipation ■ sarcoidosis ■ hyperparathyroidism.

You are taking any of the following medicines: ■ aspirin, indomethacin, or other medicine for arthritis ■ sodium polystyrene sulfonate (medicine to lower the amount of potassium in the body) ■ tranquilizers ■ medicine for ulcers (eg, cimetidine, ranitidine) ■ digoxin or digitalis (heart medicines) ■ iron preparations ■ ketoconazole (medicine for fungal infections) ■ tetracyclines ■ levodopa (medicine for Parkinson's disease) ■ quinidine (medicine for abnormal heart rhythms) ■ beta-blockers ■ ACE inhibitors (eg, captopril, enalapril, etc.) ■ corticosteroids ■ medicine for seizures ■ verapamil (medicine for chest pain) ■ thiazide diuretics.

SPECIAL RESTRICTIONS WHILE TAKING THIS DRUG

FOOD AND DRUG INTERACTIONS

Other Drugs	Calcium preparations may interfere with the absorption of other drugs. If you are taking any other medicine by mouth, space your dose one to two hours before or after taking your calcium supplement.
Foods and Beverages	Avoid large amounts of foods that may interfere with the effectiveness of this medicine, such as spinach, rhubarb, bran, and whole-grain cereals.

No special restrictions on alcohol use or smoking.

DAILY LIVING

Examinations or Tests	It is important for you to keep all appointments with your doctor so that your progress can be checked.

No special restrictions on driving, exertion and exercise, sun exposure, or exposure to excessive heat or cold.

POSSIBLE SIDE EFFECTS

Although this list of adverse effects may seem somewhat intimidating, keep in mind that some are quite rare. Of course, should these or any other problems arise while you are on medication, it is always a good idea to consult your doctor.

IF YOU DEVELOP	WHAT TO DO
severe and continuing constipation ■ pain or difficulty in urination ■ tiredness ■ continuing headache ■ loss of appetite ■ anxiety ■ mood or mental changes ■ muscle pain or twitching	**May be serious** Check with your doctor as soon as possible.
mild constipation ■ gas or bloating ■ belching	If symptoms are disturbing or persist, let your doctor know.

STORAGE INSTRUCTIONS

Store in a cool, dark place (not in a bathroom medicine cabinet).

STOPPING OR INTERRUPTING THERAPY

If you miss a dose of this medicine, take it as soon as possible. If you do not remember until the following day, skip the missed dose and resume your regular schedule.

SPECIAL CONSIDERATIONS FOR THOSE OVER SIXTY-FIVE

Older people may be especially prone to constipation with calcium supplements.

PAGET'S DISEASE

Paget's disease is the second most common bone disease next to osteoporosis. It is a slowly progressive condition usually occurring in the elderly. It rarely occurs before age 30. Men seem to be affected more frequently than women.

CAUSES

Throughout adult life, bones are continually being remodeled. Small amounts of old bone are removed and new bone is laid down in its place. Generally, this is a well-balanced process with little net gain or loss of bone. Paget's disease results from the excessive removal of old bone followed by the formation of new bone that is laid down in a very haphazard fashion. This newly formed bone is not constructed as well as normal bone and therefore tends to be weaker.

Paget's disease can affect only one bone or many bones. The bones most commonly involved are the pelvis, spine, the bones of the legs, and the skull. Most people with Paget's disease have no symptoms. Often the disease is detected inadvertently by the doctor finding an abnormal blood test result or an abnormal bone X ray, when these tests had been ordered for unrelated reasons. If symptoms should occur, the most common complaints are pain and deformity of the bones. Problems associated with involvement of the skull include hearing loss, ringing in the ears, and vertigo. Back pain can be severe and bones involved with Paget's disease are more likely to break than normal bones. Other serious complications include damage to nerves and the spinal cord by the excessive growth of abnormal bone in the skull and spine.

THERAPY

The main goals of therapy for Paget's disease are to relieve pain, maintain function, and prevent serious complications. Most people with this condition do not require any treatment or may only need occasional medication for pain such as aspirin, acetaminophen, or one of the nonsteroidal anti-inflammatory drugs. For patients requiring more than only occasional pain medication, the primary treatments available are calcitonin and etidronate disodium. Both medications work by slowing the bone remodeling process. The effectiveness of these treatments is usually determined by monitoring for improvement in symptoms and evaluation of blood tests. Surgery may be required in selected patients to relieve compression on nerves or the spinal cord by the diseased bone.

OUTLOOK

Paget's disease varies greatly from person to person. Some individuals are completely without symptoms and require no treatment while others suffer serious complications of the disease. There is currently no means available to prevent Paget's disease.

CONDITION: **PAGET'S DISEASE OF BONE**

CATEGORY: **PARATHYROID HORMONE**

GENERIC (CHEMICAL) NAME	BRAND (TRADE) NAME	DOSAGE FORMS AND STRENGTHS
Calcitonin	CALCIMAR CIBACALCIN	Vials: 200 I.U. per ml (2 ml) Syringes: 0.5 mg

DRUG PROFILE

The hormone calcitonin is given by injection to treat Paget's disease of bone. Calcimar is also used to treat postmenopausal osteoporosis (in conjunction with a prescribed diet) and hypercalcemia (too much calcium in the blood.).

In Paget's disease, bone metabolism—that is, the cycle of breaking down and building up of bone—is accelerated to an abnormal degree. This drug works by reducing the transfer of calcium from the bone to the bloodstream, slowing down bone metabolism, and helping to prevent the loss of bone mass in osteoporosis.

BEFORE USING THIS DRUG

Let your doctor know *IF*

You have ever had allergic reactions or other problems with ■ calcitonin.

You have ever had any of the following medical problems: ■ allergies.

You are taking any of the following medicines: ■ calcium-containing preparations ■ vitamin D.

SPECIAL RESTRICTIONS WHILE TAKING THIS DRUG

FOOD AND DRUG INTERACTIONS

Foods and Beverages	If you are taking this drug for osteoporosis, your doctor may prescribe a diet to help maintain healthy bones, which you should follow carefully. Such a diet is usually high in calcium and vitamin D; if it is difficult for you to include enough calcium and/or vitamin D in your diet, your doctor may suggest that you take supplements. Do not take these supplements without guidance from your doctor.
	If you are taking this drug for hypercalcemia, your doctor will probably advise you to limit your intake of calcium and vitamin D.

No special restrictions on other drugs, alcohol use, or smoking.

DAILY LIVING

Examinations or Tests	It is important for you to keep all appointments with your doctor so that your progress can be checked. Periodic blood and urine tests, as well as X rays may be required while you are taking this drug.
	A small percentage of the population is allergic to calcitonin; if your doctor suspects you fall into this category, you may be given a skin test before the drug is prescribed.
Other Precautions	This product is designed for self-injection. Be sure to follow package instructions carefully and call your doctor if you have any questions about the technique.

If the solution is discolored or contains particles, it should not be used. Examine each vial or syringe before use to make sure that it is colorless and clear.

Helpful Hints	*For cibacalcin only:* If side effects such as nausea and flushing are a problem, administration of your daily dose at bedtime should help. Side effects generally improve with continued therapy; if they persist or worsen, let your doctor know.
Exertion and Exercise	Check with your doctor concerning the type of physical activity you can do. Some people with Paget's disease may be susceptible to fractures.

No special restriction on driving, sun exposure, or exposure to excessive heat or cold.

POSSIBLE SIDE EFFECTS

Although this list of adverse effects may seem somewhat intimidating, keep in mind that some are quite rare. Of course, should these or any other problems arise while you are on medication, it is always a good idea to consult your doctor.

IF YOU DEVELOP	WHAT TO DO
difficulty in breathing ■ swelling of tongue or throat ■ fainting	**Urgent** Get in touch with your doctor immediately.
flushing of face, ears, hands, or feet ■ swelling, redness, or pain at injection site ■ rash or hives ■ nausea or vomiting	**May be serious** Check with your doctor as soon as possible.

loss of appetite ■ diarrhea ■ stomach or abdominal pain ■ increased frequency of urination ■ chills ■ weakness ■ feeling of fullness in chest ■ headache ■ shortness of breath ■ stuffy nose ■ tender palms and soles ■ metallic taste ■ tingling or burning sensations in hands or feet ■ dizziness

if symptoms are disturbing, let your doctor know.

STORAGE INSTRUCTIONS

Cibacalcin should be stored in a cool (less than 77° F) place (not in a bathroom medicine cabinet). Reconstituted solution must be used within six hours. Calcimar should be refrigerated, using caution to prevent the solution from freezing. Discard the solution if it becomes discolored or cloudy.

STOPPING OR INTERRUPTING THERAPY

Take this medicine exactly as instructed by your doctor. If you are taking calcitonin for Paget's disease, it may take several months before you notice improvement. Do not stop taking this drug without talking to your doctor. Missed doses: If you are taking one dose a day, take the missed dose as soon as you remember and resume your regular schedule; if you do not remember until the following day, skip the missed dose and resume your regular schedule. If you are taking one dose every other day, take the missed dose as soon as you remember and resume your regular schedule; if you do not remember until the following day (the alternate day), take the missed dose, skip the following day, and so on. If you are taking one dose three times a week, take the missed dose the following day and then take each injection a day later than scheduled for the rest of the week. Resume your regular schedule the following week. Do not take two doses at the same time. When you no longer need to take this drug, your doctor will give you directions on how to taper off gradually.

CONDITION: **PAGET'S DISEASE OF BONE**

CATEGORY: **BONE METABOLISM INHIBITORS**

GENERIC (CHEMICAL) NAME	BRAND (TRADE) NAME	DOSAGE FORMS AND STRENGTHS
Etidronate disodium	DIDRONEL	Tablets: 200, 400 mg

DRUG PROFILE

Etidronate is given to treat Paget's disease of bone and to prevent and treat heterotopic ossification (a kind of abnormal bone growth) which can occur following surgery for hip replacement or spinal cord injury. In both of these conditions, bone metabolism—that is, the cycle of breaking down and building up of bone—is accelerated to an abnormal degree. This drug is thought to act directly on the bone, slowing down bone metabolism.

BEFORE USING THIS DRUG

Let your doctor know *IF*

You have ever had allergic reactions or other problems with ■ etidronate.

You have ever had any of the following medical problems: ■ kidney disease ■ heart failure ■ intestinal or bowel disease ■ bone fractures, especially of the arm or leg ■ high blood levels of calcium or vitamin D.

You are taking the following medicine: ■ calcitonin.

SPECIAL RESTRICTIONS WHILE TAKING THIS DRUG

FOOD AND DRUG INTERACTIONS

Food and Beverages	Your doctor may prescribe a diet to help maintain healthy bones, which you should follow carefully. Such a diet is usually high in calcium and vitamin D; if it is difficult for you to include enough calcium and/or vitamin D in your diet, your doctor may suggest that you take supplements.
	However, the medicine should be taken on an empty stomach, at least two hours before or after a meal, along with a clear liquid such as black coffee, tea, juice, or water. Within two hours of your dose of

etidronate, it is especially important to avoid calcium-containing foods such as milk or other dairy products, vitamins with mineral supplements high in calcium, magnesium, or iron, or antacids that contain magnesium, aluminum or calcium.

No special restrictions on other drugs, alcohol use, or smoking.

DAILY LIVING

Examinations or Tests	It is important for you to keep all appointments with your doctor so that your progress can be checked. Periodic blood and urine tests, as well as X rays may be required while you are taking this drug.
Other Precautions	If you will be undergoing diagnostic X-ray tests using radioactive dye, let your doctor know that you are taking this drug, as etidronate has been known to interfere with the results of such tests. This medicine may cause stomach upset. If this persists, let your doctor know, as your dosage may need to be adjusted.
Exercise	Check with your doctor concerning the type of physical activity you can do. Some people with Paget's disease may be susceptible to fractures.

No special restrictions on driving, sun exposure, or exposure to excessive heat or cold.

POSSIBLE SIDE EFFECTS

Although this list of adverse effects may seem somewhat intimidating, keep in mind that some are quite rare. Of course, should these or any other problems arise while you are on medication, it is always a good idea to consult your doctor.

IF YOU DEVELOP	WHAT TO DO
bone pain ■ bone fracture ■ rash or hives ■ itching	**May be serious** Check with your doctor as soon as possible.
diarrhea ■ loose stools ■ black, tarry stools ■ nausea or vomiting ■ upset stomach	If symptoms are disturbing or persist, let your doctor know.

STORAGE INSTRUCTIONS

Store in a cool, dark place (not in a bathroom medicine cabinet).

STOPPING OR INTERRUPTING THERAPY

It may be one to three months before you notice the effects of this medicine, but you should continue to take it exactly as instructed. If you miss a dose, take it as soon as possible. If it is almost time for your next dose, skip the missed dose and resume your regular schedule. Do not take two doses at the same time. This drug may be used intermittently. It is important to take this drug only when directed by your doctor.

SPECIAL CONSIDERATIONS FOR THOSE OVER SIXTY-FIVE

None.

Chapter 6
Sleep Disorders
and Emotional Problems

INSOMNIA

As we get older, one of our most common complaints is poor sleep. Approximately one-half of people over sixty years of age report symptoms due to sleep disturbance. It takes longer to fall asleep, and we awaken more often during the night, are not as refreshed on arising in the morning, and are sleepy during the day. Studies done in sleep laboratories confirm these complaints. Older people spend more time in lighter sleep and have shorter periods of deeper sleep. While older people sleep less at night, they nap more during the day. Because insomnia is more common in this age group, older people use more sleeping pills.

CAUSES

For some, sleep becomes an elusive goal night after night. In fact, doctors estimate that one out of every five people who come to see them has some difficulty sleeping. Much of this difficulty is due to stress, such as that caused by family problems, job pressures, the loss of a job, or the death of a loved one. These stressful emotions are physically arousing; they make us more vigilant, less able to assume the relaxed state that permits sleep to begin and to progress normally. As a result, we sleep less, plagued with symptoms of insomnia at just those times when we may need more sleep.

Emotions aren't the only things that cause insomnia. It may be something that's more concrete, such as a bedroom that's too warm or too cold, too noisy, or too dry or an unfamiliar sleeping environment, such as a hospital. Lack of exercise can make it hard to get to sleep. Such medical disorders as peptic ulcer, asthma, angina, and insulin-dependent diabetes may produce insomnia. The pain of arthritis or other medical conditions may sometimes be so acute that it hinders sleep. In addition, some medicines, such as those for high blood pressure and Parkinson's disease or those that have a stimulating effect, can interfere with your normal sleeping pattern. If you are undergoing diuretic therapy, you may find your nights interrupted by visits to the bathroom. (This may also occur if you drink too much fluid too soon before retiring.)

DIAGNOSIS

The term *insomnia* covers several kinds of sleep problems, including these:
• Difficulty in falling asleep—lying in bed and tossing and turning, trying unsuccessfully to sleep.
• Broken sleep—repeatedly waking during the night.
• Early morning awakening—waking earlier than you want and being unable to go back to sleep before getting up for the day.

TREATMENT

• Have a medical checkup. Insomnia is a symptom that something may be wrong—something physical or psychological or both.

- Start an exercise program. Regular, moderate exercise is helpful for those of us who lead basically sedentary lives. Late afternoon or early evening is the best time to exercise—never just before bedtime.
- Try a light snack of high protein foods (eg, turkey, beef, cheese or milk) right before bedtime.
- Take a warm (not hot) shower or bath just before getting into bed; warmth relaxes muscles.
- Make sure the bedroom is quiet and at a comfortable temperature. Strategic placement of curtains or change in lighting from global to spot may be helpful. Ear plugs or background noise from a fan or bland noise from a radio may also be useful.
- Learn to associate the bed/bedroom only with sleep; avoid using the bedroom for nonsleep activities such as reading, eating, or watching TV.
- If your blankets cling together and your hair is full of static electricity, use a vaporizer or small room humidifier to add moisture to the air.
- Avoid daytime napping if you have trouble sleeping at night.
- Avoid coffee, tea, cola drinks, and cigarettes, especially in the evening. Lowering your caffeine (or nicotine) intake may be enough to "cure" your insomnia. Spicy foods or too much fluid in the evening may contribute to insomnia because of indigestion or having to get up to urinate.
- Some people cope with insomnia by using alcohol—but alcohol is not a good sedative. Even if you initially fall asleep easily, you're likely to wake up in the middle of the night unable to go back to sleep.
- If your insomnia is caused by a particularly stressful—but temporary—situation, your doctor may prescribe a sleep-inducing drug for a short period. If a sleeping pill is felt to be necessary, shorter-acting drugs (oxazepam, lorazepam, temazepam) at low doses are preferred for older patients. See the drug charts on pages 580–594 for detailed information about these medicines. Drugs from the antihistamine family are sometimes prescribed for brief insomnia. Avoid alcohol completely if you're taking sleeping pills.
- Learn about normal changes in sleep throughout a person's life. Discuss your sleep pattern with your doctor to find out if you do have insomnia and to identify factors that contribute to it. Your doctor may be able to recommend relaxation techniques to help you fall asleep.

OUTLOOK

The key to solving a sleep problem is to find the cause. Physical problems as well as emotional concerns may cause sleeplessness, so the first step to a good night's sleep is a visit to your doctor. Steps you can take yourself to relieve insomnia include exercising regularly, taking a warm bath and/or eating a light snack before bed, and ensuring comfortable surroundings. Sleep-inducing drugs are a temporary solution for short-term problems and may help you get back into the pattern of sleeping through the night.

Caution: Some drugs in this section may affect pregnancy or fetal development. Check with your doctor if this concerns you.

CONDITION: **INSOMNIA**

CATEGORY: **HYPNOTICS (BENZODIAZEPINES)**

GENERIC (CHEMICAL) NAME	BRAND (TRADE) NAME	DOSAGE FORMS AND STRENGTHS
Alprazolam	XANAX	Tablets: 0.25, 0.5, 1, 2 mg
Clorazepate dipotassium	TRANXENE T-TAB TRANXENE-SD	Tablets: 3.75, 7.5, 15 mg Tablets: 11.25, 22.5 mg
Chlordiazepoxide hydrochloride	LIBRITABS LIBRIUM	Tablets: 5, 10, 25 mg Capsules: 5, 10, 25 mg
Clonazepam	KLONOPIN	Tablets: 0.5, 1, 2 mg
Diazepam	VALIUM VALRELEASE	Tablets: 2, 5, 10 mg Controlled-release capsules: 15 mg
Estazolam	PROSOM	Tablets: 1, 2 mg
Flurazepam	DALMANE	Capsules: 15, 30 mg
Lorazepam	ATIVAN	Tablets: 0.5, 1, 2 mg
Oxazepam	SERAX	Capsules: 10, 15, 30 mg Tablets: 15 mg

Prazepam	CENTRAX	Capsules: 5, 10, 20 mg
		Tablets: 10 mg
Quazepam	DORAL	Tablets: 7.5, 15 mg
Temazepam	RESTORIL	Capsules: 15, 30 mg
Triazolam	HALCION	Tablets: 0.125, 0.25 mg

DRUG PROFILE

Benzodiazepines are used to treat a number of conditions, including anxiety, insomnia, muscle spasm, and seizures. Exactly how these drugs work is a matter of some debate. However, what they all seem to have in common is that they reduce nerve cell activity in those areas of the central nervous system (CNS) and peripheral nervous system (PNS) thought to be responsible for the experience of anxiety and muscular tension. The benzodiazepines most often used as sleep-inducing drugs are flurazepam (Dalmane), temazepam (Restoril), triazolam (Halcion), oxazepam (Serax), estazolam (Prosom), and quazepam (Doral). Low doses of short-acting agents, such as oxazepam (Serax) or lorazepam (Ativan), are preferred over long-acting drugs, such as diazepam (Valium), flurazepam (Dalmane), or chlordiaz-epoxide (Librium). Alprazolan (Xanax) may be used to treat panic disorder in older people.

BEFORE USING THIS DRUG

Let your doctor know *IF*

You have ever had allergic reactions or other problems with ■ any benzodiazepines ■ tartrazine (FD&C Yellow Dye No. 5) (contained in Serax tablets) ■ aspirin.

You have ever had any of the following medical problems: ■ seizures ■ asthma or other lung disease ■ kidney disease ■ liver disease ■ depression or any other serious mental illness ■ myasthenia gravis ■ porphyria ■ glaucoma.

You are taking any of the following medicines: ■ other benzodiazepines ■ medicine for seizures ■ sleep medicines ■ tranquilizers ■ muscle relaxants ■ medicine for depression ■ narcotics or other prescription pain-killers ■ medicine for hay fever, coughs, or colds ■ antihistamines ■ medicine for ulcers ■ Antabuse (used in treatment of alcoholism) ■ antibiotics ■ levodopa (medicine for Parkinson's disease) ■ anticoagulants (blood thinners) ■ appetite supressants.

SPECIAL RESTRICTIONS WHILE TAKING THIS DRUG

FOOD AND DRUG INTERACTIONS

Other Drugs	Do not take any other drugs, including over-the-counter (OTC) drugs, before checking with your doctor. This drug increases the effect of other drugs that depress the central nervous system, such as antihistamines; medicine for hay fever, allergies, or colds; other sleep medicines; tranquilizers; narcotics or other prescription pain-killers; muscle relaxants; and medicine for seizures.
Foods and Beverages	Excessive consumption of caffeine (found in coffee, tea, cola drinks, cocoa, chocolate) may aggravate symptoms of anxiety and counteract the calming effects of benzodiazepines.
Alcohol	Avoid alcohol, another central nervous system depressant, while taking benzodiazepines; this combination can be dangerous.
Smoking	Cigarette smoking may reduce the effect of benzodiazepines. If you smoke, try to stop or at least cut down.

DAILY LIVING

Driving	This drug may cause drowsiness or loss of alertness. Be careful when driving, operating household appliances, or doing any other tasks that require alertness until you know how this drug affects you.

Examinations or Tests	It is important for you to keep all appointments with your doctor so that your progress can be checked. If you are on long-term therapy for prevention of seizures, periodic blood and urine tests may be required. If you are taking this type of medicine for anxiety or insomnia, ask your doctor every few weeks if you need to keep taking it.
Other Precautions	Taking this medicine more often or for a longer period of time than prescribed by your doctor may make it habit-forming. If you suspect that this medicine is not working, do not increase the dose but check with your doctor.
	Tell any doctor or dentist you consult that you are taking any of these drugs, especially if you will be undergoing any type of surgery.
Helpful Hints	Swallow the controlled-release capsules whole—do not break, crush, or chew them.

No special restrictions on exertion and exercise, sun exposure, or exposure to excessive heat or cold.

POSSIBLE SIDE EFFECTS

Although this list of adverse effects may seem somewhat intimidating, keep in mind that some are quite rare. Of course, should these or any other problems arise while you are on medication, it is always a good idea to consult your doctor.

IF YOU DEVELOP

difficulty in speech ■ confusion ■ severe drowsiness or weakness ■ difficulty in walking ■ difficulty in breathing

WHAT TO DO

Urgent Get in touch with your doctor immediately.

---

depression ■ hallucinations ■ sleeplessness ■ uncontrollable movements of the body, mouth, or cheek ■ excitement ■ agitation ■ nervousness ■ irritability ■ talkativeness ■ restlessness ■ anxiety ■ nightmares ■ fainting ■ personality changes ■ tiredness or weakness ■ tremors ■ rage ■ burning or prickling feeling ■ irregular or fast heartbeat ■ flushing ■ increased sweating ■ shortness of breath ■ sores in mouth or throat ■ rash, hives, or itching ■ bleeding or bruising ■ sore throat or fever ■ yellowing of eyes or skin

May be serious Check with your doctor as soon as possible.

With clonazepam only: abnormal eye movements ■ movement difficulties ■ glassy eyes ■ memory problems ■ hysteria ■ muscle pain or weakness ■ tightness in chest ■ runny nose ■ uncontrollable bowel movements ■ swelling of ankles or face ■ swollen lymph glands ■ changes in skin color

After you STOP taking this medicine: anxiety ■ sleeplessness ■ depression ■ clumsiness ■ tremors ■ loss of appetite ■ diarrhea ■ vomiting ■ stomach or muscle cramps ■ irritability ■ memory problems ■ personality changes ■ seizures ■ hallucinations ■ increased sweating drowsiness ■ dizziness or light-headedness ■ "high" feeling ■ vivid dreams ■ clumsiness or poor balance ■ headache ■ blurred or double vision or other visual disturbances ■ stomach cramps or pain ■ constipation ■ diarrhea ■ nausea or vomiting ■ dry mouth ■ increased thirst ■ increased salivation ■ increased production of phlegm in lungs ■ difficulty in urination ■ urinary frequency ■ urinary retention ■ incontinence ■ hiccups ■ increase or decrease in appetite ■ weight gain or loss ■ swelling of tongue ■ bitter or metallic taste in mouth ■ increased or diminished sex drive ■ breast swelling in men ■ increased eye sensitivity to light

With clonazepam only: heartburn ■ hair loss

If symptoms are disturbing or persist, let your doctor know.

STORAGE INSTRUCTIONS

Store in a cool, dark place (not in a bathroom medicine cabinet).

STOPPING OR INTERRUPTING THERAPY

Take this medicine exactly as prescribed by your doctor. Do not suddenly discontinue taking this medicine, since uncomfortable and potentially serious withdrawal reactions may occur (see "Possible Side Effects"). Your doctor will advise you how to reduce your dosage gradually and safely. If you miss a dose, take it as soon as possible. If it is not within an hour of the scheduled time of the missed dose, skip it and resume your regular schedule. Do not take two doses at the same time.

SPECIAL CONSIDERATIONS FOR THOSE OVER SIXTY-FIVE

Because older people may be especially prone to the side effects of benzodiazepines (particularly, drowsiness, difficulty in walking, confusion, agitation, and excitement), doctors may start people over sixty-five on a lower dosage.

CONDITION: **INSOMNIA**

CATEGORY: **HYPNOTICS (BARBITURATES)**

GENERIC (CHEMICAL) NAME	BRAND (TRADE) NAME	DOSAGE FORMS AND STRENGTHS
Butabarbital sodium	BUTICAPS BUTISOL Sodium	Capsules: 15, 30 mg Elixir: 30 mg per tsp Tablets: 15, 30, 50, 100 mg
Mephobarbital	MEBARAL	Tablets: 32, 50, 100 mg
Pentobarbital and Pentobarbital sodium	NEMBUTAL	Capsules: 50, 100 mg Elixir: 18.2 mg pentobarbital equivalent to 20 mg pentobarbital sodium per tsp Rectal suppositories: 30, 60, 120, 200 mg
Phenobarbital	Available from many manufacturers	Capsules: 16 mg Controlled-release capsules: 65 mg Elixir: 15, 20 mg per tsp Tablets: 8, 16, 32, 65, 100 mg
Secobarbital sodium	SECONAL	Capsules: 50, 100 mg

DRUG PROFILE

Barbiturates are only rarely used to treat insomnia and to relieve anxiety or nervousness. Although it is not understood exactly how the barbiturates work, some experts believe that these drugs act on the part of the brain responsible for wakefulness.

Barbiturates have a relatively high propensity for interactions with other drugs. Infrequently, they may cause agitation instead of relieving anxiety and nervousness. They are also associated with daytime drowsiness and morning "hangover." Doctors usually prefer not to prescribe these drugs for older people, since other drugs are both safer and more effective.

BEFORE USING THIS DRUG

Let your doctor know *IF*

You have ever had allergic reactions or other problems with ■ any barbiturates ■ tartrazine (FD&C Yellow Dye No. 5) (contained in Buticaps, Butisol, and Nembutal) ■ aspirin.

You have ever had any of the following medical problems: ■ asthma or other lung disease ■ kidney disease ■ liver disease ■ mental illness ■ porphyria ■ overactive thyroid ■ high or low blood pressure ■ drug abuse, including alcoholism.

You are taking any of the following medicines: ■ any medicine containing alcohol ■ antihistamines ■ medicine for hay fever, coughs, or colds ■ muscle relaxants ■ narcotics or other prescription pain-killers ■ medicine for seizures ■ medicine for depression ■ anticoagulants (blood thinners).

SPECIAL RESTRICTIONS WHILE TAKING THIS DRUG

FOOD AND DRUG INTERACTIONS

Other Drugs	Do not take any other drugs, including over-the-counter (OTC) drugs, before checking with your doctor. This drug increases the effect of other drugs that depress the central nervous system, such as antihistamines; medicine for hay fever, allergies, or colds; other sleep medicines; tranquilizers; narcotics or other prescription pain-killers; muscle relaxants; and medicine for seizures.
Alcohol	Avoid alcohol, another central nervous system depressant, while taking this drug; this combination can be very dangerous.

Smoking	Smoking may reduce the effectiveness of this drug. If you smoke, try to stop or at least cut down.

No special restrictions on foods and beverages.

DAILY LIVING

Driving	This drug may cause drowsiness or loss of alertness. Be careful when driving, operating household appliances, or doing any other tasks that require alertness until you know how this drug affects you.
Examinations or Tests	It is important for you to keep all appointments with your doctor so that your progress can be checked. Ask your doctor every couple of months if you need to keep taking this medicine.
Other Precautions	Taking this medicine more often or for a longer period of time than prescribed by your doctor may make it habit-forming. If you suspect that this medicine is not working, do not increase the dose, but check with your doctor.
	Tell any doctor or dentist you consult that you are taking this drug, especially if you will be undergoing any type of surgery.
	If you accidentally take an overdose, go to an emergency room immediately.
Helpful Hints	The controlled-release capsules should be swallowed whole—without chewing, breaking, or crushing.
	If you have been storing the suppository form of this medicine in a warm place, it may be too soft to use. Put it in the refrigerator for half an hour or run cold water over the wrapped suppository before use.

No special restrictions on exertion or exercise, sun exposure, or exposure to excessive heat or cold.

POSSIBLE SIDE EFFECTS

Although this list of adverse effects may seem somewhat intimidating, keep in mind that some are quite rare. Of course, should these or any other problems arise while you are on medication, it is always a good idea to consult your doctor.

IF YOU DEVELOP

cold, clammy skin ■ slow or fast heartbeat ■ chest pain ■ confusion ■ slurred speech ■ wheezing or other difficulty in breathing ■ loss of balance ■ fever ■ severe headache ■ swelling of the tip of the penis ■ pain in urination

WHAT TO DO

Urgent Get in touch with your doctor immediately.

---

bleeding (including nosebleed or bleeding lip sores) or bruising ■ muscle or joint pain ■ any other unusual pain ■ scaly, red skin ■ yellowing of eyes or skin ■ rash or hives ■ mouth sores ■ swelling of face or lips ■ red, itching, or swollen eyes ■ stuffy nose ■ depression ■ agitation ■ excitement ■ hallucinations ■ extreme tiredness

May be serious Check with your doctor as soon as possible.

---

clumsiness ■ staggering ■ dizziness or light-headedness ■ drowsiness ■ "hangover" feeling ■ anxiety ■ nightmares ■ sleeplessness ■ irritability ■ constipation ■ diarrhea ■ nausea or vomiting

After you STOP taking this medicine: increased dreaming ■ nightmares ■ sleeplessness

If symptoms are disturbing or persist, let your doctor know.

STORAGE INSTRUCTIONS

Store in a cool, dark place (not in a bathroom medicine cabinet). If your medicine is in a liquid form, make sure that it does not freeze. Suppositories should be stored in the refrigerator.

STOPPING OR INTERRUPTING THERAPY

Do not suddenly discontinue taking this drug, since dangerous withdrawal reactions (for example, seizures) may occur. Your doctor will advise you on how to reduce your dosage gradually. Take this medicine exactly as prescribed by your doctor. If you miss a dose, take it as soon as possible. If it is almost time for your next dose, skip the missed dose and resume your regular schedule. Do not take two doses at the same time.

SPECIAL CONSIDERATIONS FOR THOSE OVER SIXTY-FIVE

Because older people may be especially prone to the side effects of barbiturates (particularly, excitement, depression, and confusion), doctors rarely prescribe these drugs to people over the age of sixty-five.

CONDITION: **INSOMNIA**

CATEGORY: **HYPNOTICS (NONBARBITURATES)**

GENERIC (CHEMICAL) NAME	BRAND (TRADE) NAME	DOSAGE FORMS AND STRENGTHS
Chloral hydrate	NOCTEC	Capsules: 250, 500 mg Syrup: 500 mg per tsp

DRUG PROFILE

Chloral hydrate is a sleep-inducing medicine. The way this drug works is not completely understood, but many experts believe that it acts on the part of the brain that controls sleeping and waking. Chloral hydrate, unlike some other sedatives, is usually not associated with worsening of insomnia after it is discontinued. It is inexpensive, has few side effects, and is considered a safe choice for older people when nondrug measures fail.

BEFORE USING THIS DRUG

Let your doctor know *IF*

You have ever had allergic reactions or other problems with ■ chloral hydrate.

You have ever had any of the following medical problems: ■ heart disease ■ liver disease ■ kidney disease ■ porphyria ■ ulcers ■ depression or other mental illness ■ drug abuse, including alcoholism.

You are taking any of the following medicines: ■ other sleep medicines ■ tranquilizers ■ any medicine containing alcohol ■ medicine for high blood pressure ■ antihistamines ■ medicine for hay fever, coughs, or colds ■ muscle relaxants ■ narcotics or other prescription pain-killers ■ medicine for Parkinson's disease ■ medicine for seizures ■ barbiturates ■ medicine for depression ■ anticoagulants (blood thinners).

SPECIAL RESTRICTIONS WHILE TAKING THIS DRUG

FOOD AND DRUG INTERACTIONS

Other Drugs	Do not take any other drugs, including over-the-counter (OTC) drugs, before checking with your doctor. This drug increases the effect of other drugs that depress the central nervous system, such as antihistamines; medicine for hay fever, allergies, or colds; other sleep medicines; tranquilizers; narcotics or other prescription pain-killers; muscle relaxants; and medicine for seizures.
Alcohol	Avoid alcohol, another central nervous system depressant, while taking chloral hydrate; this combination can be dangerous.
Smoking	Smoking may reduce the effectiveness of this drug. If you smoke, try to stop or at least cut down.

No special restrictions on foods and beverages.

DAILY LIVING

Driving	This drug will probably cause drowsiness or loss of alertness. Do not drive, operate household appliances, or do any other tasks that require alertness until you know how this drug affects you.
Examinations or Tests	Ask your doctor every few months if you need to keep taking this drug.
Other Precautions	Taking this medicine more often or for a longer period of time than prescribed by your doctor may make it habit-forming. If you suspect that this medicine is not working, do not increase the dose, but check with your doctor.
	If you accidentally take an overdose, get in touch with your doctor immediately.
Helpful Hints	If your medicine is in capsule form, swallow it whole without chewing, crushing, or breaking it. Taking the capsules with a full glass of water or other liquid lessens the chance of stomach upset.
	Some people find the taste of the syrup unpleasant. To improve the taste and lessen the chance of upset stomach, mix your dose with water, juice, or other liquids.

No special restrictions on exertion and exercise, sun exposure, or exposure to excessive heat or cold.

POSSIBLE SIDE EFFECTS

Although this list of adverse effects may seem somewhat intimidating, keep in mind that some are quite rare. Of course, should these or any other problems arise while you are on medication, it is always a good idea to consult your doctor.

IF YOU DEVELOP	WHAT TO DO
confusion ■ loss of balance ■ paranoia (unreasonable suspiciousness) ■ irregular or slow heartbeat ■ difficulty in swallowing ■ severe drowsiness ■ continued nausea and vomiting ■ difficulty in breathing ■ severe weakness ■ low body temperature	**Urgent** Get in touch with your doctor immediately.
rash or hives ■ blisters ■ purplish or brownish-red spots on skin ■ sleepwalking ■ hallucinations ■ extreme agitation or excitement	**May be serious** Check with your doctor as soon as possible.
nausea or vomiting ■ diarrhea ■ stomach pain ■ unpleasant taste in mouth ■ general ill feeling ■ clumsiness ■ drowsiness ■ dizziness, or light-headedness ■ headache ■ "hangover" feeling ■ nightmares	If symptoms are disturbing or persist, let your doctor know.

STORAGE INSTRUCTIONS

Store in a cool, dark place (not in a bathroom medicine cabinet). If your medicine is in a liquid form, make sure that it does not freeze.

STOPPING OR INTERRUPTING THERAPY

Take this medicine exactly as prescribed by your doctor. If you have been using chloral hydrate for six months or longer, suddenly stopping the drug may result in serious withdrawal effects. Your doctor will advise you on how to reduce your dosage gradually. If you miss a dose, take it as soon as possible. If it is almost time for your next dose, skip the missed dose and resume your regular schedule. Do not take two doses at the same time.

SPECIAL CONSIDERATIONS FOR THOSE OVER SIXTY-FIVE

Because older people may be especially prone to the side effects of sleep medicines (particularly, drowsiness, confusion, agitation, and clumsiness), doctors may start people over sixty-five on a lower dosage.

EMOTIONAL AND BEHAVIOR DISORDERS

Virtually all of us have experienced the worry, uneasiness, and panic that characterize anxiety. Some people become so anxious that they think they're "going crazy" or "losing" their mind. Others fear that something awful is about to happen and experience exaggerated feelings of doom. These emotions are often associated with frightening physical symptoms as well; difficulty in breathing, pounding heart, dizziness, chest tightness, choking sensation, increased sweating, "jitters," insomnia, and nightmares are just some of them.

Some anxiety is normal, but when it becomes so extreme that it interferes with day-to-day living, it's time to get some help.

FORMS OF ANXIETY

Generalized anxiety disorder is a vague, persistent feeling that something is wrong. People suffering from generalized anxiety feel worried and on edge all the time. They find concentration and decision making difficult. They can't sleep well at night and feel fatigued during the day. The disorder is often accompanied by physical problems, such as chest pain and blurred vision, that have no apparent cause. In an effort to find relief, sufferers tend to go from doctor to doctor looking for a cure.

Panic attacks are sudden episodes of severe anxiety and fear that can be mistaken for heart attacks because of the accompanying physical symptoms. These may begin in old age.

Phobias are extreme anxieties that focus on a specific place, activity, or object (eg, snakes or elevators).

Some people who experience severe panic attacks may limit normal activities such as shopping, going to the movies, driving, or visiting friends to avoid the frightening symptoms of such attacks when they're away from home. When their activities become so restricted that they won't leave home at all, they're said to be suffering from *agoraphobia*, a fear of public places. Some people experience an obsessive-compulsive disorder. They are affected with repetitive thoughts or compulsive behavior, such as excessive handwashing or checking to see if the door is locked, or the stove is off. Occasionally this set of behavior or thoughts can be so bothersome that a person may be unable to work or leave the house.

CAUSES

Just as anxiety takes different forms, it has different causes. Physical problems such as heart conditions, endocrine disorders (such as an overactive or underactive thyroid), and neurologic and respiratory diseases can all cause feelings of anxiety. Other culprits include caffeine, alcohol withdrawal, certain vitamin deficiencies, and drug side effects. Anxiety may also be a prominent feature of depression.

Physical changes that occur as we get older may also provoke a good deal of anxiety. Some people become anxious because their hearing or sight becomes less sharp with age, others because of hair loss or prominent wrinkles. Not surprisingly, anxiety is also provoked by changes in lifestyle; financial strain; housing difficulties; failing health; and the loss of a spouse, family member, or close friend.

DIAGNOSIS

Because the condition can be caused by so many different physical and emotional factors, your doctor will do a complete physical examination and will also want to know exactly what prescription and over-the-counter drugs you're taking.

TREATMENT

If a medical problem is at the root of anxiety, treating the condition often relieves the anxious feelings.

If a specific situation caused the anxiety, just talking about the upsetting event may be enough to alleviate the symptoms.

If the anxiety isn't caused by physical problems or a specific event, your doctor may prescribe a medicine to relieve the anxiety, ease the physical symptoms it causes, and help you sleep at night. For detailed information on drugs commonly used to treat anxiety, see the charts on pages 597–615. As a rule, antianxiety agents should only be used when symptoms are intense and disruptive. Shorter-acting benzodiazepines (oxazepam, lorazepam, alprazolam) are preferred for older people and are usually only prescribed for several weeks. Your doctor may prescribe them for a longer period of time for disruptive chronic anxiety.

Antidepressant drugs (pages 618–647) are also often prescribed for anxiety disorders, especially for obsessive-compulsive disorders and panic disorders.

OUTLOOK

Some anxiety is part of living. However, if anxiety gets out of hand and becomes distressing, it can be relieved. Anxiety stemming from a physical illness often resolves itself once the illness is treated. Anxiety that is caused by a specific event can often be put into perspective by talking about it with a doctor or counselor. Anxiety for which no cause can be determined can now be eased by the use of one of several drugs.

Caution: Some drugs in this section may affect pregnancy or fetal development. Check with your doctor if this concerns you.

CONDITION: **ANXIETY**

CATEGORY: **ANTIANXIETY AGENTS (BENZODIAZEPINES)**

GENERIC (CHEMICAL) NAME	BRAND (TRADE) NAME	DOSAGE FORMS AND STRENGTHS
Alprazolam	XANAX	Tablets: 0.25, 0.5, 1, 2 mg
Chlorazepate dipotassium	TRANXENE T-TAB TRANXENE-SD	Tablets: 3.75, 7.5, 15 mg Tablets: 11.25, 22.5 mg
Chlordiazepoxide hydrochloride	LIBRITABS LIBRIUM	Tablets: 5, 10, 25 mg Capsules: 5, 10, 25 mg
Clonazepam	KLONOPIN	Tablets: 0.5, 1, 2 mg
Diazepam	VALIUM VALRELEASE	Tablets: 2, 5, 10 mg Controlled-release capsules: 15 mg
Halazepam	PAXIPAM	Tablets: 20, 40 mg
Lorazepam	ATIVAN	Tablets: 0.5, 1, 2 mg
Oxazepam	SERAX	Capsules: 10, 15, 30 mg Tablets: 15 mg
Prazepam	CENTRAX	Capsules: 5, 10, 20 mg

DRUG PROFILE

Benzodiazepines are used to treat a number of conditions, including anxiety, insomnia, muscle spasm, and seizures. Exactly how these drugs work is a matter of some debate. They seem to reduce nerve cell activity in those areas of the central nervous system (CNS) and peripheral nervous system (PNS) thought to be responsible for the experience of anxiety and muscular tension. The benzodiazepines most often used as antianxiety agents are alprazolam (Xanax), chlorazepate (Tranxene T-TAB, Tranxene-SD), chlordiazepoxide (Libritabs, Librium), diazepam (Valium, Valrelease), lorazepam (Ativan), oxazepam (Serax), and prazepam (Centrax). Low doses of short-acting agents, such as oxazepam or lorazepam, are preferred over long-acting drugs, such as diazepam, flurazepam, or chlordiazepoxide, for older people.

For complete information on these drugs, see pages 580–585.

CONDITION: **ANXIETY**

CATEGORY: **ANTIANXIETY AGENTS (NONBENZODIAZEPINES)**

GENERIC (CHEMICAL) NAME	BRAND (TRADE) NAME	DOSAGE FORMS AND STRENGTHS
Meprobamate	EQUANIL	Tablets: 200, 400 mg
	MILTOWN	Tablets: 200, 400 mg
	MILTOWN 600	Tablets: 600 mg
	MEPROSPAN	Sustained-action capsules: 200, 400 mg

DRUG PROFILE

Meprobamate is rarely used to relieve short-term anxiety, including anxiety associated with such disorders as phobias and panic attacks. The way this drug works is not completely understood, though it is believed to act on the area of the brain that is the center of the emotions. This drug is rarely prescribed to the elderly since other agents are safer and more effective.

BEFORE USING THIS DRUG

Let your doctor know *IF*

You have ever had allergic reactions or other problems with ■ meprobamate ■ carbromal ■ carisoprodol ■ tartrazine (FD&C Yellow Dye No. 5) (contained in Equanil tablets) ■ aspirin.

You have ever had any of the following medical problems: ■ seizures ■ kidney disease ■ liver disease ■ porphyria.

You are taking any of the following medicines: ■ other tranquilizers ■ sleep medicines ■ medicine for depression ■ narcotics or other prescription pain-killers ■ antihistamines ■ medicine for hay fever, coughs, or colds ■ medicine for seizures ■ medicine for Parkinson's disease ■ muscle relaxants ■ barbiturates.

SPECIAL RESTRICTIONS WHILE TAKING THIS DRUG

FOOD AND DRUG INTERACTIONS

Other Drugs	Do not take any other drugs, including over-the-counter (OTC) drugs, before checking with your doctor. This drug increases the effect of other drugs that depress the central nervous system, such as antihistamines; medicine for hay fever, allergies, or colds; sleep medicines; tranquilizers; narcotics or other prescription pain-killers; muscle relaxants; and medicine for seizures.
Alcohol	Avoid alcohol, another central nervous system depressant, while taking this drug; this combination can be dangerous.
Smoking	Smoking may reduce the effectiveness of this drug. If you smoke, try to stop or at least cut down.

No special restrictions on foods and beverages.

DAILY LIVING

Driving	Meprobamate may cause drowsiness or loss of alertness. Be careful when driving, operating household appliances, or doing any other tasks that require alertness until you know how this drug affects you.

Examinations or Tests	It is important for you to keep all appointments with your doctor so that your progress can be checked. Ask your doctor every few weeks if you need to keep taking this drug.
Other Precautions	Taking this medicine more often or for a longer period of time than prescribed by your doctor may make it habit-forming. If you suspect that the drug is not working, do not increase the dose, but check with your doctor.
	Tell any doctor or dentist you consult that you are taking this drug, especially if you will be undergoing any type of surgery.
	If you accidentally take an overdose, go to an emergency room immediately.

No special restrictions on exertion and exercise, sun exposure, or exposure to excessive heat or cold.

POSSIBLE SIDE EFFECTS

Although this list of adverse effects may seem somewhat intimidating, keep in mind that some are quite rare. Of course, should these or any other problems arise while you are on medication, it is always a good idea to consult your doctor.

IF YOU DEVELOP

extreme drowsiness or weakness ■ difficulty in breathing ■ slurred speech ■ loss of balance ■ sore throat ■ fever ■ chills ■ bleeding or bruising ■ fainting ■ decreased urination ■ irregular, slow, or fast heartbeat

WHAT TO DO

Urgent Get in touch with your doctor immediately.

rash, hives, or itching ■ blisters ■ purplish or brownish-red spots on skin ■ agitation ■ excitement ■ tingling, burning, or prickling sensations ■ "high" feeling ■ swelling of feet or ankles ■ swollen glands ■ stomach pain	**May be serious** Get in touch with your doctor immediately.
clumsiness ■ headache ■ blurred vision or other visual disturbances ■ diarrhea ■ drowsiness ■ dizziness or light-headedness ■ nausea or vomiting ■ tiredness ■ loss of appetite	If symptoms are disturbing or persist, let your doctor know.

STORAGE INSTRUCTIONS

Store in a cool, dark place (not in a bathroom medicine cabinet).

STOPPING OR INTERRUPTING THERAPY

Take this medicine exactly as prescribed by your doctor. *Do not suddenly discontinue taking this medicine, since potentially serious withdrawal reactions may occur.* Your doctor will advise you how to reduce your dosage gradually. If you miss a dose, take it as soon as possible. If it is almost time for your next dose, skip the missed dose and resume your regular schedule. Do not take two doses at the same time.

SPECIAL CONSIDERATIONS FOR THOSE OVER SIXTY-FIVE

Because older people may be especially prone to the side effects of meprobamate, doctors only rarely prescribe this drug to those over the age of sixty-five.

CONDITION: **ANXIETY**

CATEGORY: **ANTIANXIETY AGENTS (NONBENZODIAZEPINES)**

GENERIC (CHEMICAL) NAME	BRAND (TRADE) NAME	DOSAGE FORMS AND STRENGTHS
Buspirone hydrochloride	BUSPAR	Tablets: 5, 10 mg

DRUG PROFILE

Buspirone is used to relieve short-term anxiety as well as certain anxiety disorders. The way this drug works is not completely understood. It differs from other antianxiety drugs such as the benzodiazepines in that it causes less sedation and does not cause muscle relaxation.

BEFORE USING THIS DRUG

Let your doctor know *IF*

You have ever had allergic reactions or other problems with ■ buspirone.

You have ever had any of the following medical problems: ■ kidney disease ■ liver disease ■ drug abuse.

You are taking any of the following medicines: ■ other tranquilizers ■ sleep medicines ■ medicine for depression ■ narcotics or other prescription pain-killers ■ antihistamines ■ medicine for hay fever, coughs, and colds ■ medicine for seizures ■ medicine for Parkinson's disease ■ muscle relaxants ■ barbiturates ■ anticoagulants (blood thinners) ■ digoxin or digitalis (heart medicine).

SPECIAL RESTRICTIONS WHILE TAKING THIS DRUG

FOOD AND DRUG INTERACTIONS

Other Drugs	Do not take any other drugs, including over-the-counter (OTC) drugs, before checking with your doctor. This drug increases the effect of other drugs that depress the central nervous system, such as antihistamines; medicine for hay fever, allergies, or colds; sleep medicines; tranquilizers; narcotics or other prescription pain-killers; muscle relaxants; and medicine for seizures.
Alcohol	Avoid alcohol, another central nervous system depressant, while taking this drug; this combination can be dangerous.

No special restrictions on foods and beverages or smoking.

DAILY LIVING

Driving	Buspirone may cause dizziness or drowsiness. Be careful when driving, operating household appliances, or doing any other tasks that require alertness until you know how this drug affects you.
Examinations or Tests	It is important for you to keep all appointments with your doctor so that your progress can be checked. Ask your doctor every several weeks if you need to keep taking this drug.
Other Precautions	Take this medicine exactly as instructed; it may take one to two weeks before you see any improvement in your symptoms.
	Tell any doctor or dentist you consult that you are taking this drug, especially if you will be undergoing any type of surgery.
	If you accidentally take an overdose, go to an emergency room immediately.

No special restrictions on exertion and exercise, sun exposure, or exposure to excessive heat or cold.

POSSIBLE SIDE EFFECTS

Although this list of adverse effects may seem somewhat intimidating, keep in mind that some are quite rare. Of course, should these or any other problems arise while you are on medication, it is always a good idea to consult your doctor.

IF YOU DEVELOP

extreme dizziness or drowsiness ■ persistent nausea or vomiting ■ severe stomach pain ■ unusually small pupils

WHAT TO DO

Urgent Get in touch with your doctor immediately.

chest pain ■ confusion ■ depression ■ sore throat ■ fever ■ fast or pounding heartbeat ■ numbness, tingling, weakness, or pain in hands and feet ■ fainting ■ slow heartbeat ■ swelling of hands or feet ■ high blood pressure ■ muscle pain, cramps or weakness ■ slowed reaction time ■ clumsiness ■ problems with balance	**May be serious** Get in touch with your doctor immediately.
restless or nervousness ■ dizziness ■ light-headedness ■ drowsiness ■ trouble concentrating ■ headache ■ nausea or vomiting ■ dry mouth ■ upset stomach ■ diarrhea ■ ringing in ears ■ sleep-lessness ■ nightmares or vivid dreams ■ tiredness or weakness ■ rash ■ increased sweating or "clamminess" ■ runny nose	If symptoms are disturbing or persist, let your doctor know.

STORAGE INSTRUCTIONS

Store in a cool, dark place (not in a bathroom medicine cabinet).

STOPPING OR INTERRUPTING THERAPY

Take this medicine exactly as prescribed by your doctor. Your doctor will advise you how to reduce your dosage gradually. If you miss a dose, take it as soon as possible. If it is almost time for your next dose, skip the missed dose and resume your regular schedule. Do not take two doses at the same time.

SPECIAL CONSIDERATIONS FOR THOSE OVER SIXTY-FIVE

Buspirone has not been specifically studied in patients age sixty-five or older; however no unusual problems have been identified in elderly patients at this time.

CONDITION: **ANXIETY**

CATEGORY: **ANTIANXIETY AGENTS (ANTIHISTAMINES)**

GENERIC (CHEMICAL) NAME	BRAND (TRADE) NAME	DOSAGE FORMS AND STRENGTHS
Hydroxyzine hydrochloride	ATARAX	Syrup: 10 mg per tsp Tablets: 10, 25, 50, 100 mg
Hydroxyzine pamoate	VISTARIL	Capsules: 25, 50, 100 mg Suspension: 25 mg per tsp

DRUG PROFILE

When you are exposed to a substance to which you are allergic, a chemical called *histamine* is released into the bloodstream and produces the itchy, watery eyes, runny nose, and rashes that are typical of an allergic reaction. Antihistamines work by blocking the action of histamine. They are used to treat allergies as well as to relieve the symptoms of a cold. Hydroxyzine is also used to treat anxiety. Exactly how it works to relieve anxiety is not completely understood.

For complete information on this drug, see pages 753–758.

CONDITION: **EMOTIONAL AND BEHAVIOR DISORDERS**
CATEGORY: **ANTIPSYCHOTICS (NEUROLEPTICS)**

GENERIC (CHEMICAL) NAME	BRAND (TRADE) NAME	DOSAGE FORMS AND STRENGTHS
Acetophenazine	TINDAL	Tablets: 20 mg
Chlorpromazine hydrochloride	THORAZINE	Tablets: 10, 25, 50, 100, 200 mg Concentrate: 30, 100 mg per ml Controlled-release capsules: 30, 75, 150, 200, 300 mg Rectal suppositories: 25, 100 mg Syrup: 10 mg per tsp
Chlorprothixene	TARACTAN	Tablets: 10, 25, 50, 100 mg Concentrate: 100 mg per tsp
Fluphenazine hydrochloride	PROLIXIN	Tablets: 1, 2.5, 5, 10 mg Concentrate: 5 mg per ml Elixir: 2.5 mg per tsp
	PERMITIL	Tablets: 2.5, 5, 10 mg Concentrate: 5 mg per ml
Haloperidol	HALDOL	Tablets: 0.5, 1, 2, 5, 10, 20 mg Concentrate: 2 mg per ml
Loxapine	LOXITANE	Capsules: 5, 10, 25, 50 mg Concentrate: 25 mg per ml
Mesoridazine	SERENTIL	Tablets: 10, 25, 50, 100 mg Concentrate: 25 mg per ml
Molindone	MOBAN	Tablets: 5, 10, 25, 50, 100 mg Concentrate: 20 mg per ml

Perphenazine	TRILAFON	Tablets: 2, 4, 8, 16 mg Concentrate: 16 mg per tsp
Prochlorperazine	COMPAZINE	Tablets: 5, 10, 25 mg Controlled-release capsules: 10, 15, 30 mg Rectal suppositories: 2.5, 5, 25 mg Syrup: 5 mg per tsp
Promazine	SPARINE	Tablets: 25, 50, 100 mg
Thiethylperazine maleate*	TORECAN	Tablets: 10 mg Rectal suppositories: 10 mg
Thioridazine hydrochloride	MELLARIL	Tablets: 10, 15, 25, 50, 100, 150, 200 mg Concentrate: 30, 100 mg per ml Suspension: 25, 100 mg per tsp
Thiothixene	NAVANE	Capsules: 1, 2, 5, 10, 20 mg Concentrate: 5 mg per 5 ml
Trifluoperazine hydrochloride	STELAZINE	Tablets: 1, 2, 5, 10 mg Concentrate: 10 mg per ml

*Thiethylperazine is only used to relieve nausea and vomiting and not to treat emotional disorders. It is listed here because of its many similarities to the other phenothiazines discussed in this chart.

DRUG PROFILE

Neuroleptics are used to treat a variety of very severe emotional disorders, including severe anxiety, agitation, or psychosis. These drugs are not used to treat simple anxiety. Some neuroleptic drugs (prochlorperazine, thiethylperazine, and chlorpromazine) at very low doses are also used to treat nausea and vomiting. These drugs are thought to work by inhibiting the action of dopamine, a chemical messenger, in the part of the brain that is the seat of the emotions as well as in the zone of the brain that controls nausea and vomiting.

BEFORE USING THIS DRUG

Let your doctor know *IF*

You have ever had allergic reactions or other problems with ■ any phenothiazines ■ tartrazine (FD&C Yellow Dye No. 5) ■ aspirin.

You have ever had any of the following medical problems: ■ seizures ■ anemia or other blood disease ■ asthma or other lung disease ■ respiratory tract infection, such as pneumonia ■ liver disease ■ kidney disease ■ heart or blood vessel disease ■ glaucoma ■ enlarged prostate ■ urinary problems ■ Parkinson's disease.

You are taking any of the following medicines: ■ medicine for seizures ■ antacids ■ appetite suppressants ■ medicine for high blood pressure ■ medicine for asthma ■ medicine for Parkinson's disease ■ medicine for depression ■ beta-blockers ■ antihistamines ■ medicine for hay fever, coughs, or colds ■ barbiturates ■ narcotics or other prescription pain-killers ■ sleep medicines ■ tranquilizers ■ cimetidine (medicine for ulcers) ■ Antabuse (used in the treatment of alcoholism) ■ medicine for nausea or vomiting ■ antibiotics ■ anti-coagulants (blood thinners) ■ medicine for irregular heartbeat.

You are often exposed to extreme heat or cold or to organophosphate insecticides (eg, if you work in a plant that manufactures this type of pesticide).

SPECIAL RESTRICTIONS WHILE TAKING THIS DRUG

FOOD AND DRUG INTERACTIONS

Other Drugs	Do not take any other drugs, including over-the-counter (OTC) drugs, before checking with your doctor. This drug increases the effects of other drugs that depress the central nervous system, such as antihistamines; medicine for hay fever, allergies, or colds; sleep medicines; other tranquilizers; narcotics or other prescription pain-killers; muscle relaxants; and medicine for seizures.
Alcohol	Avoid alcohol, another central nervous system depressant, while taking this drug; the combination can be dangerous.

Smoking	Smoking may reduce the effectiveness of this drug. If you smoke, try to stop or at least cut down.

No special restrictions on foods and beverages.

DAILY LIVING

Driving	These drugs may cause drowsiness or loss of alertness. Be careful when driving, operating household appliances, or doing any other tasks that require alertness until you know how this drug affects you.
Exertion and Exercise	This drug may cause you to sweat less than normally. Sweating is your body's natural way of cooling down, and not sweating enough can be dangerous. Use caution not to become overheated when you exercise or exert yourself.
Sun Exposure	Your skin may become more sensitive to sunlight and more likely to develop a sunburn while you are taking this drug. It is a good idea to avoid too much sun and to apply a sunscreen to exposed skin surfaces before going outdoors.
Excessive Heat	See "Exertion and Exercise"; use caution during hot weather, since overexertion may result in heat stroke. Avoid extremely hot baths or saunas.
Excessive Cold	This drug may disturb your body's ability to regulate its temperature; use care during very cold weather and make sure all exposed parts are well covered. Also, do not swim in extremely cold water.
Examinations or Tests	It is important for you to keep all appointments with your doctor so that your progress can be checked.

Other Precautions	Tell any doctor or dentist you consult that you are taking this drug, especially if you will be undergoing any type of surgery.

Helpful Hints	Drink plenty of liquids, particularly water and fruit juices, while taking this drug.
	Taking this drug with food or a glass of water will lessen the chance of upset stomach.
	If you have been storing the suppository form of this medicine in a warm place, it may be too soft to use. Put it in the refrigerator for half an hour or run cold water over the wrapped suppository before use.
	If you are taking a controlled-release form, swallow the capsule or tablet whole without crushing, breaking, or chewing it.
	You may feel dizzy, light-headed, or faint when starting out on this type of drug. This should disappear in a few weeks or so. Getting up slowly from a reclining or sitting position should help.
	If your mouth or throat feels dry, chewing sugarless gum or sucking ice chips or sugarless hard candy will help.

POSSIBLE SIDE EFFECTS

Although this list of adverse effects may seem somewhat intimidating, keep in mind that some are quite rare. The most common side effects of these drugs are sleepiness, sudden faintness or falling when getting up from a reclining or sitting position, muscle stiffness, and slowness of movement. Of course, should these or any other problems arise while you are on medication, it is always a good idea to consult your doctor.

IF YOU DEVELOP	**WHAT TO DO**
seizures ■ difficulty in breathing ■ increased sweating ■ incontinence ■ fainting ■ severe muscle stiffness ■ extreme tiredness or weakness ■ irregular or fast heartbeat ■ swelling in throat ■ yellowing of eyes or skin ■ fever	**Urgent** Get in touch with your doctor immediately.
cough ■ body aches ■ sore throat ■ blurred vision or other visual disturbances ■ dilated pupils, or other changes in pupil size ■ slurred speech ■ rigid facial expression ■ spasms of neck, back, feet, or other parts of the body ■ uncontrollable movements of the tongue, face, mouth, or jaw ■ shuffling walk ■ twisting of body ■ tremors ■ restlessness ■ agitation ■ jitters ■ inability to sit still ■ sleeplessness ■ swelling of hands or feet ■ urinary retention ■ rigidness ■ posture changes ■ difficulty in speech ■ difficulty in swallowing ■ drooling or excessive salivation ■ slow, monotonous speech ■ protrusion of tongue ■ slow movements or inability to move	**May be serious** Check with your doctor as soon as possible.
constipation ■ diarrhea ■ decreased sweating ■ drowsiness ■ dizziness, light-headedness, or fainting, especially when getting up from a reclining or sitting position ■ male sexual problems ■ increased skin sensitivity to sunlight ■ headache ■ anxiety ■ "high" feeling ■ depression ■ weakness ■ reddened skin, rash, or hives ■ loss of appetite ■ upset stomach ■ increased appetite ■ weight gain ■ breast pain or swelling in men and women ■ darkening or whitening of mouth membranes ■ loosened teeth ■ cracked lips and corners of mouth ■ tongue discoloration	If symptoms are disturbing or persist, let your doctor know.

STORAGE INSTRUCTIONS

Store in a cool, dark place (not in a bathroom medicine cabinet). If your medicine is in a liquid form, make sure that it does not freeze. Suppositories should be stored in the refrigerator.

STOPPING OR INTERRUPTING THERAPY

Take this medicine exactly as prescribed by your doctor; it may take several weeks before you see an effect. Do not suddenly discontinue taking this medicine, since this may result in withdrawal reactions (abnormal movements). Your doctor will advise you on how to reduce your dosage gradually. If you miss a dose, take it as soon as possible. If it is almost time for your next dose, skip the missed dose and resume your regular schedule. Do not take two doses at the same time.

SPECIAL CONSIDERATIONS FOR THOSE OVER SIXTY-FIVE

Because older people may be especially susceptible to the side effects of the neuroleptics, doctors may start people over sixty-five on a lower dosage.

CONDITION: **EMOTIONAL AND BEHAVIORAL DISORDERS**

CATEGORY: **ANTIPSYCHOTICS (NEUROLEPTICS)**

GENERIC (CHEMICAL) NAME	BRAND (TRADE) NAME	DOSAGE FORMS AND STRENGTHS
Clozapine	CLOZARIL	Tablets: 25, 100 mg

DRUG PROFILE

The mechanism by which clozapine exerts its effect is unknown, but it is believed to work by inhibiting the action of dopamine, a chemical messenger, in the brain.

BEFORE USING THIS DRUG

Let your doctor know *IF*

You have ever had allergic problems with ■ clozapine.

You have had any of the following medical problems: ■ severe depression ■ blood disorders ■ high or low blood pressure ■ abnormal heart rhythm ■ glaucoma ■ liver disease ■ kidney disease ■ epilepsy ■ enlarged prostate gland ■ gastrointestinal problems.

You are taking any of the following medicines: ■ alcohol ■ drugs that depress the nervous system (eg, barbiturates, benzodiazepines, antihistamines, prescription pain medicines, medicine for seizures, sleeping medicines, cold and hay fever medicine) ■ tricyclic antidepressants ■ amphotericin B ■ medicine for overactive thyroid ■ medicines for the treatment of cancer or leukemia (azathioprine, chlorambucil, cyclophosphamide, interferon, flucytosine, mercaptopurine, methotrexate, plicamycin) ■ zidovudine ■ chloramphenicol ■ lithium ■ blood thinners (warfarin, heparin).

SPECIAL RESTRICTIONS WHILE TAKING THIS DRUG

FOOD AND DRUG INTERACTIONS

Other Drugs	Do not take any other drugs, including over-the-counter (OTC) medicine before checking with your doctor. This medicine will add to the effects of central nervous system depressants (medicines that slow down the nervous system). Some examples of these medicines include: antihistamines; sleeping medicines; cold, flu, and hay fever medicines; prescription pain medicines.
Alcohol	This medicine will add to the effects of alcohol. Avoid taking alcohol while you are using this medicine.
Smoking	Smoking may reduce the effectiveness of this drug. If you smoke, try to stop or at least cut down.

No special restrictions on food and beverages.

DAILY LIVING

Driving	This drug may cause drowsiness or blurred vision. Be careful when driving, operating household appliances, or doing other tasks that require alertness until you know how this drug affects you.

Examinations and Tests	This medicine can only be prescribed in quantities sufficient for a seven-day supply. You must have your blood tested each week in order to receive a new seven-day supply. It is, therefore, extremely important that you have your blood tests done weekly and that your doctor check your progress at regular weekly visits.
Other Precautions	Tell any doctor or dentist you consult you are taking this drug, especially if you will be undergoing any type of surgery or spinal X ray.
Helpful Hints	You may feel dizzy, light-headed, or faint while taking this drug. Getting up slowly from a reclining or sitting position should help. This drug may also cause dryness of the mouth. For temporary relief, chewing sugarless gum or sucking on sugarless candy or bits of ice may help. This medicine is not available through all pharmacies. Your doctor will advise you where this medicine can be obtained in your area.

No special restrictions on exertion and exercise, or exposure to excessive heat and cold.

POSSIBLE SIDE EFFECTS

Although this list of adverse effects may seem somewhat intimidating, keep in mind that some are quite rare. Of course, should these or any other problems arise while you are on medication, it is always a good idea to consult your doctor.

IF YOU DEVELOP	WHAT TO DO
fast or irregular heart beat ■ fever ■ dizziness ■ fainting ■ constant headache ■ chills ■ convulsions ■ difficult or rapid breathing ■ increased sweating ■ loss of bladder control ■ severe muscle stiffness ■ sore throat ■ sores, ulcers, or white spots on lips or in mouth ■ unusual bleeding or bruising ■ unusual tiredness or weakness ■ unusually pale skin	**Urgent** Get in touch with your doctor.
blurred vision ■ confusion ■ nervousness ■ irritability ■ anxiety ■ restlessness or a need to keep moving ■ slowness of movement ■ severe muscle stiffness ■ decreased sexual ability ■ trouble sleeping ■ difficulty in urinating ■ increased sweating ■ lip smacking or puckering of lips ■ puffing of cheeks ■ rapid or wormlike movements of tongue ■ uncontrolled chewing movements ■ uncontrolled movements of arms and legs ■ severe drowsiness ■ hallucinations ■ increased watering of the mouth	**May be serious** Check with your doctor as soon as possible.
constipation ■ light-headedness ■ drowsiness ■ moderate headache ■ nausea or vomiting ■ unusual weight gain ■ abdominal discomfort ■ dryness of mouth	If symptoms are disturbing or persist, let your doctor know.

STORAGE INSTRUCTIONS

Store in a cool, dry, dark place (not in a bathroom medicine cabinet).

STOPPING OR INTERRUPTING THERAPY

Take this medicine exactly as prescribed by your doctor. Do not suddenly discontinue taking this medicine. If you miss a dose, take it as soon as possible. If it is almost time for your next dose, skip the missed dose and resume your regular schedule. Do not take two doses at the same time.

SPECIAL CONSIDERATIONS FOR THOSE OVER SIXTY-FIVE

Older people taking this drug may be more prone to develop confusion or excitement or experience dizziness or fainting. Thus doctors may start people over sixty-five on a lower dose.

DEPRESSION

All of us have depressed moods or feel "blue" about certain events or circumstances such as a serious illness, financial difficulties, the need to move from a familiar home to a new community, or the death of someone close. These are normal feelings that tend to ease with the passage of time. This kind of minor depression is sometimes called reactive depression because it's a reaction to a specific event. It usually doesn't require any medical treatment.

In some cases, the depression isn't relieved with time. In other instances, a depression occurs for no apparent reason and is severe enough to interfere with normal daily function. Such depressions are much more serious and may call for medical treatment.

Depression is the most common emotional disorder of older people. The first episode of depression most often occurs between ages fifty and sixty in women and fifty-five and sixty-five in men. Frequently, there is a history of depression in the family.

CAUSES

According to current scientific thinking, depression may be caused by a chemical imbalance in the brain. Although emotional factors can trigger a depressive episode, diseases or drugs may also be responsible. Depression is known to accompany such illnesses as diabetes, thyroid disease, Parkinson's disease, influenza, hepatitis, and viral pneumonia. Certain cancers and rheumatoid arthritis can also depress mood. Unwanted side effects of some drugs—such as alcohol, sedatives, and some blood pressure medicines—may cause depressive symptoms.

DIAGNOSIS

Depression is a painful emotional experience. Typical symptoms of depression include weight loss, loss of appetite and energy, fatigue, and feelings of profound helplessness and hopelessness. Waking early in the morning (3:00 to 5:00 a.m.) and being unable to fall back to sleep, frequent or unexplained crying spells, and a loss of interest in people or pleasurable activities are other common signs. Depression may also wear the mask of a physical illness, such as a gastrointestinal problem, chest pain, or muscle or bone pain. In reality, depression is the underlying problem.

In another kind of depression, known as manic depression, there are extreme mood swings; periods of profound despair alternate with periods of intense animation and excitement.

Because depression may result from such a variety of conditions and can masquerade as many other problems, your doctor will do a thorough physical examination, including an electrocardiogram (ECG), blood pressure readings, and blood and urine tests. To further aid in the diagnosis, your doctor will inquire exactly which over-the-counter and prescription medicines you're taking. Your doctor will also conduct a diagnostic interview. This discussion of your problems and feelings will help differentiate true depression from grief, mourning, or dementia. True depression can be identified by the signs and symptoms described earlier.

TREATMENT

Fortunately, depression can be treated successfully with currently available techniques and medicines. If the depression is caused by drugs or by interactions of drugs, your doctor may discontinue a drug you don't really need or substitute one drug for another. Very often, this is all that's necessary to solve the problem. If the depression is related to a physical illness, treating the illness may lift the depression.

Your doctor may also prescribe an antidepressant that can help improve your mood. There are several kinds of antidepressant drugs, some of which are just recently available. All of them act on the areas of the brain that determine mood and probably affect substances in brain tissue that transmit nerve impulses. For a detailed description of these drugs, including their side effects, refer to the drug charts on pages 618–647.

In addition to prescribing medicine for your depression, your doctor may suggest that you talk over your feelings with a trained professional. Often, this will help you find ways to deal with the psychological factors that contribute to depression.

OUTLOOK

Depression can be a serious illness, but most people who suffer from this emotional disorder can be helped. In some cases, changing or foregoing certain medicines is enough. In others, treating a previously undetected medical condition will relieve the depression. In still others, an antidepressant medicine, perhaps combined with psychotherapy, is the suitable treatment approach.

The sense of hopelessness and helplessness that is an integral part of depression often prevents people from seeking help. But now that effective treatments are available, there is no longer any need to live with the pain of depression.

CONDITION: **DEPRESSION**

CATEGORY: **CYCLIC ANTIDEPRESSANTS**

GENERIC (CHEMICAL) NAME	BRAND (TRADE) NAME	DOSAGE FORMS AND STRENGTHS
Amitriptyline	ELAVIL	Tablets: 10, 25, 50, 75, 100, 150 mg
	ENDEP	Tablets: 25, 50, 75, 100, 150 mg
Amoxapine	ASENDIN	Tablets: 25, 50, 100, 150 mg
Desipramine hydrochloride	NORPRAMIN	Tablets: 10, 25, 50, 75, 100, 150 mg
	PERTOFRANE	Capsules: 25, 50 mg
Doxepin hydrochloride	SINEQUAN	Capsules: 10, 25, 50, 75, 100, 150 mg Concentrate: 10 mg per ml
Imipramine hydrochloride	TOFRANIL TOFRANIL-PM	Tablets: 10, 25, 50 mg Capsules: 75, 100, 125, 150 mg
Fluoxetine	PROZAC	Capsules: 20 mg
Maprotiline hydrochloride	LUDIOMIL	Tablets: 25, 50, 75 mg
Nortriptyline hydrochloride	AVENTYL	Capsules: 10, 25 mg Solution: 10 mg per tsp
	PAMELOR	Capsules: 10, 25, 50, 75 mg Solution: 10 mg per tsp

Protriptyline hydrochloride	VIVACTIL	Tablets: 5, 10 mg

Trimipramine maleate	SURMONTIL	Capsules: 25, 50, 100 mg

DRUG PROFILE

The cyclic antidepressants are used to treat depressive illnesses and to relieve the anxiety and nervousness that may accompany these problems. According to one widely held theory, severe depression stems at least in part from having low levels of certain chemical messengers in the brain. These drugs may alleviate depression by increasing the amounts of chemical messengers available to the brain. Some of these drugs are too strong to be used in the elderly (eg, amoxapine and imipramine) except in very rare circumstances.

BEFORE USING THIS DRUG

Let your doctor know *IF*

You have ever had allergic reactions or other problems with ■ any cyclic antidepressants ■ trazodone ■ tartrazine (FD&C Yellow Dye No. 5) (contained in Norpramin and Tofranil) ■ aspirin.

You have ever had any of the following medical problems: ■ other mental illness ■ heart disease, including heart attack, chest pain, and abnormal heart rhythms ■ alcoholism ■ asthma or other lung disease ■ seizures ■ difficulty in urination ■ enlarged prostate ■ glaucoma ■ kidney disease ■ liver disease ■ high or low blood pressure ■ overactive or underactive thyroid.

You are taking any of the following medicines: ■ other medicine for depression ■ antihistamines ■ medicine for hay fever, coughs, or colds ■ barbiturates ■ medicine for seizures ■ medicine for Parkinson's disease ■ narcotics or other prescription pain-killers ■ tranquilizers ■ sleep medicines ■ medicine for a thyroid condition ■ medicine for asthma ■ methylphenidate (medicine for narcolepsy) ■ anticoagulants (blood thinners) ■ male or female hormones ■ cimetidine (medicine for ulcers) ■ Antabuse (used in treatment of alcoholism) ■ furazolidone (antibiotic) ■ muscle relaxants ■ medicine for high blood pressure ■ calcium blockers (eg, diltiazem, nifedipine, verapamil, etc.) ■ digitalis (medicine for heart failure) ■ lithium.

SPECIAL RESTRICTIONS WHILE TAKING THIS DRUG

FOOD AND DRUG INTERACTIONS

Other Drugs	Do not take any other drugs, including over-the-counter (OTC) drugs, before checking with your doctor. This drug increases the effects of other drugs that depress the central nervous system, such as antihistamines; medicine for hay fever, allergies, or colds; sleep medicines; tranquilizers; narcotics or other prescription pain-killers; muscle relaxants; and medicine for seizures.
Alcohol	Avoid alcohol, another central nervous system depressant, while taking this drug; this combination may cause drowsiness and reduce the effectiveness of this medicine.
Smoking	Smoking may reduce the effectiveness of this medicine. If you smoke, try to stop or at least cut down.

No special restrictions on foods and beverages.

DAILY LIVING

Driving	This drug may cause drowsiness or loss of alertness. Be careful—especially during the first two to four weeks of therapy—when driving, operating household appliances, or doing any other tasks that require alertness until you know how this drug affects you.
Exertion and Exercise	This drug may cause you to sweat less than normally. Sweating is your body's natural way of cooling down, and not sweating enough can be dangerous. Use caution not to become overheated when you exercise or exert yourself.

Sun Exposure	Your skin may become more sensitive to sunlight and more likely to develop a sunburn while you are taking this drug. It is a good idea to avoid too much sun and to apply a sunscreen to exposed skin surfaces before going outdoors.
Excessive Heat	See "Exertion and Exercise"; use caution during hot weather, since overexertion may result in heat stroke. Avoid extremely hot baths or saunas.
Examinations or Tests	It is important for you to keep all appointments with your doctor so that your progress can be checked. Periodic electrocardiograms and blood or urine tests may be required.
Other Precautions	Tell any doctor or dentist you consult that you are taking this drug, especially if you will be undergoing any type of surgery.
Helpful Hints	You may feel dizzy, light-headed, or faint when first starting out on this drug. This should disappear in a few weeks or so. Getting up slowly from a reclining or sitting position should help.
	If your mouth or throat feels dry, chewing sugarless gum or sucking ice chips or sugarless hard candy will help.
	If this medicine causes upset stomach, ask your doctor whether you can take it with food.

No special restrictions on excessive cold.

POSSIBLE SIDE EFFECTS

Although this list of adverse effects may seem somewhat intimidating, keep in mind that some are quite rare. Of course, should these or any other problems arise while you are on medication, it is always a good idea to consult your doctor.

IF YOU DEVELOP	WHAT TO DO
collapse ■ seizures ■ hallucinations ■ agitation ■ difficulty in breathing ■ irregular, slow, or fast heartbeat ■ yellowing of the eyes or skin	**Urgent** Get in touch with your doctor immediately.
blurred vision ■ confusion ■ inability to concentrate ■ inability to sit still ■ personality changes ■ tremors ■ constipation ■ slurred speech ■ eye pain ■ fainting ■ nervousness ■ restlessness ■ excitement ■ flushing ■ chills ■ swollen glands ■ difficulty in urination ■ shuffling walk ■ sleeplessness ■ rigid facial expression ■ irritability ■ hair loss ■ sore throat or fever ■ swelling of face or tongue ■ nightmares ■ ringing in ears ■ numbness or tingling sensations ■ worsening of depression ■ "high" feeling ■ difficulty in swallowing ■ difficulty in speech ■ rash, hives, or itching ■ reddened skin or other skin changes *For amoxapine only:* painful ejaculation *For fluoxetine only*: decreased eating ■ weight loss	**May be serious** Check with your doctor as soon as possible.

drowsiness ■ dry mouth or throat ■ stuffy nose ■ headache ■ nausea or vomiting ■ tiredness or weakness ■ dizziness or light-headedness, especially when getting up from a reclining or sitting position ■ increased appetite ■ loss of appetite ■ weight gain ■ unpleasant taste in mouth ■ fatigue ■ diarrhea ■ increased sweating ■ increased skin sensitivity to sunlight ■ increased or diminished sex drive ■ male impotence ■ swelling of testicles ■ swelling of breasts in men and women ■ upset stomach ■ heartburn ■ stomach cramps ■ black tongue

After you STOP taking this medicine: restlessness ■ inability to sit still ■ anxiety ■ chills ■ runny nose ■ general feeling of unwellness ■ muscle ache ■ headache ■ dizziness ■ nausea or vomiting ■ worsening of depression ■ sleeplessness

If symptoms are disturbing or persist, let your doctor know.

STORAGE INSTRUCTIONS

Store in a cool, dark place (not in a bathroom medicine cabinet). If your medicine is in a liquid form, make sure that it does not freeze.

STOPPING OR INTERRUPTING THERAPY

Take this medicine exactly as prescribed by your doctor; it may take several weeks before you see an effect. Do not suddenly discontinue taking this medicine. Your doctor will advise you on how to reduce your dosage gradually. For a week after you stop taking a cyclic antidepressant, continue to follow the precautions listed in this chart, since some of the drug will still be in your body. If you miss a dose, take it as soon as possible. If it is almost time for your next dose, skip the missed dose and resume your regular schedule. Do not take two doses at the same time.

SPECIAL CONSIDERATIONS FOR THOSE OVER SIXTY-FIVE

Because older people may be more prone to side effects of cyclic antidepressants (specifically—confusion, inability to concentrate, tremors, drowsiness, dry mouth, and difficulty in urination), doctors may start people over sixty-five on a lower dosage and build it up gradually over a period of weeks.

CONDITION: **OBSESSIVE-COMPULSIVE DISORDER**
CATEGORY: **CYCLIC ANTIDEPRESSANT**

GENERIC (CHEMICAL) NAME	BRAND (TRADE) NAME	DOSAGE FORMS AND STRENGTHS
Clomipramine	ANAFRANIL	Capsules: 25, 50, 75 mg

DRUG PROFILE

Clomipramine is used to treat obsessive-compulsive illness. It is believed to work by inhibiting the action of chemical substances produced in the brain.

BEFORE USING THIS DRUG

Let your doctor know *IF*

You have ever had allergic problems with ■ tricyclic antidepressants ■ trazodone.

You have had any of the following medical problems: ■ other mental illnesses ■ heart disease ■ heart attack ■ chest pain ■ abnormal heart rhythm ■ alcoholism ■ asthma or other lung disease ■ seizures ■ difficulty in urination ■ enlarged prostrate ■ glaucoma ■ thyroid disease ■ kidney disease ■ liver disease ■ high or low blood pressure.

You are taking any of the following medicines: ■ MAO inhibitors (phenylzine, tranylcypromine, isocarboxazid) and other medicines for depression ■ medicine for seizures ■ medicine for high blood pressure ■ haloperidol (Haldol) ■ methylphenidate (Ritalin) ■ cimetidine (Tagamet) ■ blood thinners (warfarin) ■ phenobarbital ■ fluoxetine (Prozac) ■ digoxin ■ furazolidine (antibiotic).

SPECIAL RESTRICTIONS WHILE TAKING THIS DRUG

FOOD AND DRUG INTERACTIONS

Other Drugs	Do not take any other drugs, including over-the-counter (OTC) drugs, before checking with your doctor. This drug increases the effects of other drugs that depress the central nervous system, such as antihistamines; medicine for hay fever, allergies, or colds; sleep medicines; tranquilizers; narcotics or other prescription pain-killers; muscle relaxants; and medicine for seizures.
Alcohol	Avoid alcohol, another central nervous system depressant, while taking this drug; this combination may cause drowsiness and reduce the effectiveness of this medicine.
Smoking	Smoking may reduce the effectiveness of this medicine. If you smoke, try to stop or at least cut down.

No special restrictions on foods and beverages.

DAILY LIVING

Driving	This drug may cause drowsiness or loss of alertness. Be careful—especially during the first two to four weeks of therapy—when driving, operating household appliances, or doing any other tasks that require alertness until you know how this drug affects you.
Exertion and Exercise	This drug may cause you to sweat less than normal. Sweating is your body's natural way of cooling down, and not sweating enough can be dangerous. Use caution not to become overheated when you exercise or exert yourself.

Sun Exposure	Your skin may become more sensitive to sunlight and more likely to develop a sunburn while you are taking this drug. It is a good idea to avoid too much sun and to apply a sunscreen to exposed skin surfaces before going out.
Examinations or Tests	It is important for you to keep all appointments with your doctor so that your progress can be checked. Periodic blood, urine, and stool cultures may be required.
Other Precautions	Tell any doctor or dentist you consult that you are taking this drug, especially if you will be undergoing any surgery or diagnostic procedure. This medicine may cause seizures. Discuss this side effect with your doctor.
Helpful Hints	You may feel dizzy, light-headed, or faint when first starting on this drug. This should disappear in a few weeks or so. Getting up slowly from a reclining or sitting position should help.
	If your mouth or throat feels dry, chewing sugarless gum or sucking ice chips or sugarless hard candy will help.
	If this medicine causes an upset stomach, ask your doctor whether you can take it with food.

No special restrictions on excessive heat or cold.

POSSIBLE SIDE EFFECTS

Although this list of adverse effects may seem somewhat intimidating, keep in mind that some are quite rare. Of course, should these or any other problems arise while you are on medication, it is always a good idea to consult your doctor.

IF YOU DEVELOP

severe drowsiness ■ loss of consciousness ■ confusion ■ agitation ■ difficulty in breathing ■ seizures ■ irregular heart beat ■ fever with increased sweating ■ hallucinations

WHAT TO DO

Urgent Get in touch with your doctor.

blurred vision ■ inability to concentrate ■ inability to sit still ■ personality changes ■ tremors ■ constipation ■ slurred speech ■ eye pain ■ fainting ■ nervousness ■ restlessness ■ excitement ■ chills ■ flushing ■ swollen glands ■ difficulty in urinating ■ shuffling walk ■ sleeplessness ■ rigid facial expression ■ irritability ■ hair loss ■ sore throat or fever ■ swelling of face or tongue ■ nightmares ■ ringing in ears ■ numbness or tingling sensations ■ worsening of depression ■ "high" feeling ■ difficulty in swallowing ■ difficulty in speech ■ rash, hives, or itching ■ reddened skin or other skin changes

May be serious Check with your doctor immediately.

drowsiness ■ dry mouth or throat ■ stuffy nose ■ headache ■ nausea or vomiting ■ tiredness or weakness ■ dizziness or light-headedness, especially when getting up from a reclining or sitting position ■ increase or loss in appetite ■ weight gain ■ unpleasant taste in mouth ■ fatigue ■ diarrhea ■ increased sweating ■ increased skin sensitivity to sunlight ■ change in sexual drive ■ male impotence ■ swelling of testes ■ swelling of breasts in men and women ■ upset stomach ■ heartburn ■ stomach cramps

After you STOP taking this medicine: restlessness ■ inability to sit still ■ anxiety ■ chills ■ runny nose ■ general feeling of being sick ■ muscle ache ■ headache ■ dizziness ■ nausea or vomiting ■ worsening of depression

If symptoms are disturbing or persist, let your doctor know.

STORAGE INSTRUCTIONS

Store in a cool, dark place (not in a bathroom medicine cabinet).

STOPPING OR INTERRUPTING THERAPY

Take this medicine exactly as prescribed by your doctor; it may take several weeks (usually two to three weeks, but sometimes six to eight weeks) before you see an effect. Do not suddenly discontinue taking this medicine. Your doctor will advise you on how to reduce your dosage gradually. For a week after you stop taking this medicine, continue to follow the precautions listed in this chart, since some of the drug will still be in your body. If you miss a dose take it as soon as possible. If it is almost time for your next dose, skip the missed dose and resume your regular schedule. Do not take two doses at the same time.

SPECIAL CONSIDERATIONS FOR THOSE OVER SIXTY-FIVE

Because older people may be more prone to side effects of cyclic antidepressants (specifically—confusion, blurred vision, dry mouth, difficulty in urination, inability to concentrate, tremors, and drowsiness), doctors may start people over sixty-five on a lower dosage and build it up gradually over a period of weeks.

CONDITION: **DEPRESSION**

CATEGORY: **OTHER ANTIDEPRESSANTS**

GENERIC (CHEMICAL) NAME	BRAND (TRADE) NAME	DOSAGE FORMS AND STRENGTHS
Trazodone hydrochloride	DESYREL	Tablets: 50, 100, 150, 300 mg

DRUG PROFILE

Trazodone is used to treat acute depression that occurs with or without anxiety. According to one widely held theory, severe depression stems at least in part from having low levels of certain chemical messengers in the brain. This drug may alleviate depression by increasing the amounts of chemical messengers available to the brain.

BEFORE USING THIS DRUG

Let your doctor know *IF*

You have ever had allergic reactions or other problems with ■ trazodone.

You have ever had any of the following medical problems: ■ heart disease, including heart attack or abnormal heart rhythms ■ kidney disease ■ liver disease ■ high or low blood pressure ■ alcoholism ■ anemia.

You are taking any of the following medicines: ■ other medicine for depression ■ medicine for high blood pressure ■ antihistamines ■ medicine for hay fever, coughs, or colds ■ barbiturates ■ medicine for seizures (especially phenytoin) ■ medicine for Parkinson's disease ■ narcotics or other prescription pain-killers ■ tranquilizers ■ sleep medicines ■ muscle relaxants ■ digoxin or digitalis (heart medicines).

You are undergoing electroconvulsive shock therapy.

SPECIAL RESTRICTIONS WHILE TAKING THIS DRUG

FOOD AND DRUG INTERACTIONS

Other Drugs	Do not take any other drugs, including over-the-counter (OTC) drugs, before checking with your doctor. This drug increases the effects of other drugs that depress the central nervous system, such as antihistamines; medicine for hay fever, allergies, or colds; sleep medicines; tranquilizers; narcotics or other prescription pain-killers; muscle relaxants; and medicine for seizures.
Alcohol	Avoid alcohol, another central nervous system depressant, while taking this drug; the combination can be dangerous.
Smoking	Smoking may reduce the effectiveness of this medicine. If you smoke, try to stop or at least cut down.

No special restrictions on foods and beverages.

DAILY LIVING

Driving	This drug may cause drowsiness or blurred vision. Be careful when driving, operating household appliances, or doing any other tasks that require alertness until you know how this drug affects you.
Sun Exposure	Your skin may become more sensitive to sunlight and more likely to develop a sunburn while you are taking this drug. It is a good idea to avoid too much sun and to apply a sunscreen to exposed skin surfaces before going outdoors.

Excessive Heat	Use caution during hot weather since this drug may make you more sensitive to extremely hot temperatures. Avoid extremely hot baths or saunas.
Excessive Cold	You may be more sensitive to extreme cold while taking this drug.
Examinations or Tests	It is important for you to keep all appointments with your doctor so that your progress can be checked.
Other Precautions	Tell any doctor or dentist you consult that you are taking this drug, especially if you will be undergoing any type of surgery.
Helpful Hints	You may feel dizzy, light-headed, or faint while taking this drug. Getting up slowly from a reclining or sitting position should help.

For maximum benefit, take this medicine shortly after eating a meal or snack. In addition to getting more of the medicine into your bloodstream, this will lessen the chance of dizziness or light-headedness.

If this medicine makes you feel drowsy, let your doctor know; you may be able to take most of your daily dose at bedtime.

If your mouth or throat feels dry, chewing sugarless gum or sucking ice chips or sugarless hard candy will help. |

No special restrictions on exertion and exercise.

POSSIBLE SIDE EFFECTS

Although this list of adverse effects may seem somewhat intimidating, keep in mind that some are quite rare. Of course, should these or any other problems arise while you are on medication, it is always a good idea to consult your doctor.

IF YOU DEVELOP	WHAT TO DO
seizures ■ difficulty in breathing ■ prolonged or inappropriate penile erection ■ fainting ■ chest pain ■ irregular, slow, or fast heartbeat ■ sore throat or fever	**Urgent** Get in touch with your doctor immediately.
confusion ■ clumsiness ■ anger or hostility ■ agitation ■ excitement ■ restlessness ■ nervousness ■ inability to concentrate ■ memory problems ■ difficulty in speech ■ hallucinations ■ personality changes ■ "high" feeling ■ inability to sit still ■ muscle twitches ■ rash or hives ■ tingling or prickling sensations ■ blood in urine ■ difficulty in urination ■ urinary frequency	**May be serious** Check with your doctor as soon as possible.
blurred or double vision ■ dizziness or light-headedness, especially when getting up from a reclining or sitting position ■ drowsiness ■ dry mouth ■ headache ■ full or heavy feeling in head ■ nausea or vomiting ■ constipation ■ diarrhea ■ gas ■ muscle aches ■ tiredness ■ general ill feeling ■ sleeplessness ■ unpleasant taste in mouth ■ increased salivation ■ increased appetite ■ weight gain ■ acne ■ increased skin sensitivity to sunlight ■ swelling of skin ■ stuffy nose ■ increased sweating or clammy feeling ■ eye pain ■ ringing in ears ■ change in sexual drive ■ male impotence ■ problems with ejaculation in males	If symptoms are disturbing or persist, let your doctor know.

STORAGE INSTRUCTIONS

Store in a cool, dark place (not in a bathroom medicine cabinet).

STOPPING OR INTERRUPTING THERAPY

Take this medicine exactly as prescribed by your doctor; it may take several weeks before you see an effect. If you miss a dose, take it as soon as possible. If it is within four hours of your next dose, skip the missed dose and resume your regular schedule. Do not take two doses at the same time. Do not suddenly discontinue taking this medicine. Your doctor will advise you on how to reduce your dosage gradually.

SPECIAL CONSIDERATIONS FOR THOSE OVER SIXTY-FIVE

Because older people may be more prone to side effects of trazodone (especially drowsiness, dizziness, confusion, visual disturbances, dry mouth, and constipation), doctors may start people over sixty-five on a lower dosage.

CONDITION: **DEPRESSION**

CATEGORY: **MAO INHIBITORS**

GENERIC (CHEMICAL) NAME	BRAND (TRADE) NAME	DOSAGE FORMS AND STRENGTHS
Isocarboxazid	MARPLAN	Tablets: 10 mg
Phenelzine sulfate	NARDIL	Tablets: 15 mg
Tranylcypromine sulfate	PARNATE	Tablets: 10 mg

DRUG PROFILE

MAO (monoamine oxidase) activity increases after age forty-five. This enzyme is responsible for the breakdown of chemical messengers to the brain; reduced levels of these messengers may affect mood in older people. MAO inhibitors are used to treat severe depression. They block the action of monoamine oxidase, which, in turn, increases the levels of the messengers in the brain.

BEFORE USING THIS DRUG

Let your doctor know *IF*

You have ever had allergic reactions or other problems with ■ tranylcypromine, isocarboxazid, phenelzine sulfate, or any other MAO inhibitor drug ■ pargyline hydrochloride (medicine for high blood pressure).

You have ever had any of the following medical problems: ■ drug abuse, including alcohol and cocaine ■ heart disease, including angina (chest pain), coronary artery disease, and heart attack ■ diabetes ■ seizures ■ severe or frequent headaches ■ high blood pressure ■ kidney disease ■ liver disease ■ mental illness ■ overactive thyroid ■ Parkinson's disease ■ stroke ■ glaucoma ■ pheochromocytoma (adrenal gland tumor) ■ asthma or other lung disease ■ anemia ■ angioneurotic edema (accumulation of excess fluid under the skin, often associated with hives, redness, or purplish or brownish-red spots).

You are taking any of the following medicines ■ other medicine for depression (within the past two weeks) ■ medicine for diabetes ■ medicine for high blood pressure ■ medicine for asthma ■ diuretics (water pills) ■ medicine for Parkinson's disease ■ medicine for seizures ■ barbiturates ■ muscle relaxants ■ antihistamines ■ medicine for hay fever, coughs, or colds ■ appetite suppressants ■ narcotics or other prescription pain-killers ■ sleep medicines ■ any medicine containing alcohol ■ any medicine containing caffeine ■ amphetamines ■ methylphenidate (medicine for narcolepsy) ■ Antabuse (used in treatment of alcoholism) ■ tranquilizers ■ fluoxetine (within two weeks) ■ buspirone (within two weeks) ■ clomipramine (within two weeks).

You are receiving electroconvulsive shock therapy.

SPECIAL RESTRICTIONS WHILE TAKING THIS DRUG

FOOD AND DRUG INTERACTIONS

Other Drugs	Do not take any other drugs, including over-the-counter (OTC) drugs, before checking with your doctor. OTC drugs that may interact adversely with this drug include those used for colds, coughs, hay fever, and appetite suppression, as well as drugs containing caffeine.

Foods and Beverages	The combination of MAO inhibitors and food or beverages that contain tyramine or tryptophan can result in serious problems. Foods to avoid include cheese (Cheddar, Camembert, Stilton, or processed cheese), sour cream, yogurt, liver (especially chicken liver), pickled herring, canned figs, raisins, bananas, avocados, soy sauce, meat tenderizers, fava beans, cured meats (eg, bologna, sausage, and salami), and yeast or meat extracts. Also, avoid large quantities of cocoa, coffee, tea, and cola beverages. Ask your doctor to provide you with a full list of foods to avoid; also, let your doctor know if you are on any special kind of diet. Continue to avoid the above foods and beverages for two weeks after stopping therapy with an MAO inhibitor.
Alcohol	Imported beer and Chianti wine are especially dangerous. Some alcoholic beverages are acceptable; ask your doctor if you can drink alcohol.

No special restrictions on smoking.

DAILY LIVING

Driving	MAO inhibitors may cause drowsiness or loss of alertness. Be careful when driving, operating household appliances, or doing any other tasks that require alertness until you know how this drug affects you.
Examinations or Tests	It is important for you to keep all appointments with your doctor so that your progress can be checked. Periodic blood and urine tests may be required.

Other Precautions	Tell any doctor or dentist you consult that you are taking this drug, especially if you will be undergoing any type of surgery or radiologic diagnostic test.
Helpful Hints	You may feel dizzy, light-headed, or faint while taking this drug. Getting up slowly from a reclining or sitting position should help. If you become extremely dizzy, lie down until you feel better. If you continue to experience these symptoms, let your doctor know.

No special restrictions on exertion and exercise, sun exposure, or exposure to excessive heat or cold.

POSSIBLE SIDE EFFECTS

Although this list of adverse effects may seem somewhat intimidating, keep in mind that some are quite rare. Of course, should these or any other problems arise while you are on medication, it is always a good idea to consult your doctor.

IF YOU DEVELOP

severe headache ■ stiff or sore neck ■ chest pain ■ irregular, slow, or fast heartbeat ■ nausea or vomiting ■ excessive sweating with clammy skin ■ chills or fever ■ increased eye sensitivity to light ■ confusion ■ incoherence ■ difficulty in breathing ■ seizures ■ personality changes ■ hallucinations ■ jaw spasms or difficulty in opening mouth ■ body spasms

WHAT TO DO

Urgent Get in touch with your doctor immediately.

severe dizziness, light-headedness, or fainting
■ dilated pupils ■ swelling of feet or legs ■ agitation
■ nervousness ■ clumsiness ■ rash ■ purplish or
brownish-red spots ■ aggravation of glaucoma
■ aching joints ■ diarrhea ■ pounding heartbeat
■ yellowing of eyes or skin ■ changes in pupil size

After you STOP taking this medicine: restlessness
■ anxiety ■ confusion ■ hallucinations ■ depression
■ weakness ■ diarrhea ■ headache

May be serious Check with your doctor as soon as possible.

blurred vision or other visual disturbances
■ constipation ■ difficulty in urination ■ numbness,
tingling, or pain in hands or feet ■ tremors
■ dizziness or light-headedness, especially when
getting up from a reclining or sitting position
■ headache ■ drowsiness ■ dry mouth ■ weight gain
■ fatigue ■ restlessness ■ sleeplessness ■ male impotence ■ loss of appetite ■ flushing ■ urinary frequency ■ weakness ■ increased appetite ■ stomach
pain

If symptoms are disturbing or persist, let your doctor know.

STORAGE INSTRUCTIONS

Store in a cool, dark place (not in a bathroom medicine cabinet).

STOPPING OR INTERRUPTING THERAPY

Take this medicine exactly as prescribed by your doctor. Do not suddenly discontinue taking this medicine. Your doctor will advise you on how to reduce your dosage
gradually. If you miss a dose, take it as soon as possible. If it is within two hours of
your next dose, skip the missed dose and resume your regular schedule. Do not
take two doses at the same time. For two weeks after stopping this drug, continue to
follow the precautions listed in this chart, since some of the drug will still be in your
body.

SPECIAL CONSIDERATIONS FOR THOSE OVER SIXTY-FIVE

None.

CONDITION: **DEPRESSION**

CATEGORY: **ANTIDEPRESSANTS (COMBINATIONS)**

GENERIC (CHEMICAL) NAME	BRAND (TRADE) NAME	DOSAGE FORMS AND STRENGTHS
Chlordiazepoxide and amitriptyline hydrochloride	LIMBITROL LIMBITROL DS	Tablets: 5 mg chlordiazepoxide and 12.5 mg amitriptyline Tablets: 10 mg chlordiazepoxide and 25 mg amitriptyline

DRUG PROFILE

This drug—a combination of a benzodiazepine (chlordiazepoxide) and an antidepressant (amitriptyline)—is used to treat depressive illnesses and to relieve the anxiety and nervousness that may accompany these illnesses. According to one widely held theory, severe depression stems at least in part from having low levels of certain chemical messengers in the brain. Antidepressants may alleviate depression by increasing the amounts of chemical messengers available to the brain. Since amitriptyline is a very strong antidepressant, this drug is rarely used in the elderly.

BEFORE USING THIS DRUG

Let your doctor know *IF*

You have ever had allergic reactions or other problems with ■ any benzodiazepines ■ any cyclic antidepressants ■ trazodone.

You have ever had any of the following medical problems: ■ other mental illness ■ alcoholism ■ asthma or other lung disease ■ seizures ■ difficulty in urination ■ enlarged prostate ■ glaucoma ■ heart disease, including heart attack, chest pain, and abnormal heart rhythms ■ kidney disease ■ liver disease ■ high or low blood pressure ■ overactive thyroid ■ myasthenia gravis ■ porphyria.

You are taking any of the following medicines: ■ other medicine for depression ■ any benzodiazepines ■ antihistamines ■ medicine for hay fever, coughs, or colds ■ barbiturates ■ medicine for seizures ■ medicine for Parkinson's disease ■ narcotics or other prescription pain-killers ■ tranquilizers ■ sleep medicines ■ medicine for a thyroid condition ■ medicine for asthma ■ methylphenidate (medicine for narcolepsy) ■ anticoagulants (blood thinners) ■ male or female hormones ■ cimetidine (medicine for ulcers) ■ Antabuse (used in treatment of alcoholism) ■ medicine for arthritis ■ antacids ■ medicine for high blood pressure ■ digoxin or digitalis (heart medicines) ■ antibiotics ■ medicine for tuberculosis ■ muscle relaxants ■ beta-blockers (eg, propranolol, atenolol, metoprolol).

You are receiving electroconvulsive shock therapy.

SPECIAL RESTRICTIONS WHILE TAKING THIS DRUG

FOOD AND DRUG INTERACTIONS

Other Drugs	Do not take any other drugs, including over-the-counter (OTC) drugs, before checking with your doctor. This drug increases the effect of other drugs that depress the central nervous system, such as antihistamines; medicine for hay fever, allergies, or colds; sleep medicines; tranquilizers; narcotics or other prescription pain-killers; muscle relaxants; and medicine for seizures.
Alcohol	Avoid alcohol, another central nervous system depressant, while taking this drug; the combination can be dangerous.
Smoking	Smoking may reduce the effectiveness of this drug. If you smoke, try to stop or at least cut down.

No special restrictions on foods and beverages.

DAILY LIVING

Driving	This drug may cause drowsiness or loss of alertness. Be careful when driving, operating household appliances, or doing any other tasks that require alertness until you know how this drug affects you.
Exertion and Exercise	This drug may cause you to sweat less than normally. Sweating is your body's natural way of cooling down, and not sweating enough can be dangerous. Use caution not to become overheated when you exercise or exert yourself.
Sun Exposure	Your skin may become more sensitive to sunlight and more likely to develop a sunburn while you are taking this drug. It is a good idea to avoid too much sun and to apply a sunscreen to exposed skin surfaces before going outdoors.
Excessive Heat	See "Exertion and Exercise"; use caution during hot weather, since overexertion may result in heat stroke. Avoid extremely hot baths or saunas.
Examinations or Tests	It is important for you to keep all appointments with your doctor so that your progress can be checked. Periodic electrocardiograms and blood or urine tests may be required.
Other Precautions	Do not take more of this medicine or take it for a longer period of time than prescribed. If you suspect that this drug is not working, do not increase the dosage, but check with your doctor.
	Tell any doctor or dentist you consult that you are taking this drug, especially if you will be undergoing any type of surgery.

Helpful Hints	You may feed dizzy, light-headed, or faint when first starting out on this drug. This should disappear in a few weeks or so. Getting up slowly from a reclining or sitting position should help. If your mouth or throat feels dry, chewing sugarless gum or sucking ice chips or sugarless hard candy will help. If this medicine causes upset stomach, ask your doctor whether you can take it with food.

No special restrictions on exposure to excessive cold.

POSSIBLE SIDE EFFECTS

Although this list of adverse effects may seem somewhat intimidating, keep in mind that some are quite rare. Of course, should these or any other problems arise while you are on medication, it is always a good idea to consult your doctor.

IF YOU DEVELOP	WHAT TO DO
confusion ■ severe drowsiness or weakness ■ staggering ■ difficulty in breathing ■ collapse ■ seizures ■ hallucinations ■ sore throat or fever ■ yellowing of eyes or skin	**Urgent** Get in touch with your doctor immediately.

depression ■ sleeplessness ■ uncontrollable movements of the body, mouth, or cheek ■ excitement ■ nervousness ■ irritability ■ talkativeness ■ restlessness ■ inability to sit still ■ inability to concentrate ■ anxiety ■ nightmares ■ fainting ■ personality changes ■ tremors ■ rage ■ burning or prickling sensation ■ irregular or fast heartbeat ■ flushing ■ increased sweating ■ shortness of breath ■ tiredness or weakness ■ sores in mouth or throat ■ rash, hives, or itching ■ bleeding or bruising ■ eye pain

After you STOP taking this medicine: anxiety ■ sleeplessness ■ depression ■ loss of appetite ■ increased sweating ■ diarrhea ■ nausea or vomiting ■ irritability ■ memory problems ■ clumsiness ■ tremors ■ stomach or muscle cramps ■ personality changes ■ seizures ■ hallucinations ■ restlessness ■ chills ■ runny nose ■ general ill feeling ■ muscle ache ■ headache ■ dizziness ■ hair loss ■ ringing in ears ■ numbness or tingling sensations ■ worsening of depression ■ twisting of torso

May be serious Check with your doctor as soon as possible.

---

drowsiness ■ dizziness or light-headedness, especially when getting up from a reclining or sitting position ■ "high" feeling ■ vivid dreams ■ clumsiness or poor balance ■ headache ■ blurred or double vision or other visual disturbances ■ stomach cramps or pain ■ constipation ■ diarrhea ■ nausea or vomiting ■ upset stomach ■ dry mouth or throat ■ increased thirst ■ increased salivation ■ increased phlegm production in lungs ■ difficulty in urination ■ urinary frequency or other urinary problems ■ hiccups ■ increase or decrease in appetite ■ weight gain or loss ■ swelling of face or tongue ■ bitter or metallic taste in mouth ■ change in sex drive ■ male impotence ■ swelling of breasts in men and women ■ increased skin sensitivity to sunlight ■ stuffy nose ■ swelling of testicles ■ black tongue ■ heartburn

If symptoms are disturbing or persist, let your doctor know.

STORAGE INSTRUCTIONS

Store in a cool, dark place (not in a bathroom medicine cabinet).

STOPPING OR INTERRUPTING THERAPY

Take this medicine exactly as prescribed by your doctor; it may take several weeks before you see an effect. Do not suddenly discontinue taking this medicine. Your doctor will advise you on how to reduce your dosage gradually. If you miss a dose, take it as soon as possible. If it is almost time for your next dose, skip the missed dose and resume your regular schedule. Do not take two doses at the same time. For a week after you stop taking this medicine, continue to follow the precautions listed in this chart, since some of the drug will still be in your body.

SPECIAL CONSIDERATIONS FOR THOSE OVER SIXTY-FIVE

Because older people may be more prone to side effects of this drug, doctors rarely prescribe this drug to people over the age of sixty-five.

CONDITION: **MANIC DEPRESSION**
CATEGORY: **ANTIDEPRESSANT AND ANTIMANIC DRUGS**

GENERIC (CHEMICAL) NAME	BRAND (TRADE) NAME	DOSAGE FORMS AND STRENGTHS
Lithium carbonate	ESKALITH	Capsules: 300 mg Tablets: 300 mg
	ESKALITH CR	Controlled-release tablets: 450 mg
	LITHOBID	Controlled-release tablets: 300 mg
	LITHONATE	Capsules: 300 mg
	LITHOTABS	Tablets: 300 mg

Lithium citrate	CIBALITH-S	Syrup: 8 milliequivalents (equivalent to 300 mg lithium carbonate) per tsp

DRUG PROFILE

Lithium is used to treat manic-depressive illness—severe mood swings between an excited, "high," or irritable state and a state of extreme depression. It is sometimes added to an antidepressant drug to treat depressions that persist. It is not known exactly how this drug produces its therapeutic effect.

BEFORE USING THIS DRUG

Let your doctor know *IF*

You have ever had allergic reactions or other problems with ■ lithium.

You have ever had any of the following medical problems: ■ diabetes ■ difficulty in urination ■ seizures ■ heart disease, including abnormal heart rhythms ■ kidney disease ■ thyroid disease ■ Parkinson's disease ■ recent infection ■ high blood pressure.

You are taking any of the following medicines: ■ other medicine for depression ■ medicine for asthma ■ medicine for arthritis (NSAIDs) ■ diuretics ■ appetite suppressants ■ medicine for thyroid disease ■ baking soda ■ antacids ■ antibiotics ■ tranquilizers ■ medicine for mental illness ■ medicine for diabetes ■ medicine for seizures ■ muscle relaxants ■ narcotics or other prescription pain-killers ■ medicine to make the urine less acidic ■ verapamil (calcium blocker) ■ any medicine containing caffeine ■ salt pills ■ medicine for high blood pressure ■ ACE inhibitors (eg, captopril, enalapril, lisinopril) ■ any medicine containing caffeine ■ salt pills.

You are undergoing electroconvulsive shock therapy.

SPECIAL RESTRICTIONS WHILE TAKING THIS DRUG

FOOD AND DRUG INTERACTIONS

Other Drugs	Do not take any other drugs, including over-the-counter (OTC) drugs, before checking with your doctor.
Foods and Beverages	It is important for you to drink plenty of liquids (two and a half to three quarts a day) while you are taking this medicine. If you become ill and develop fever, vomiting, or diarrhea, be sure to drink more liquids to supplement the fluids you are losing. Let your doctor know if you are on any type of special diet.

No special restrictions on alcohol use or smoking.

DAILY LIVING

Driving	This drug may cause drowsiness or loss of alertness. Be careful when driving, operating household appliances, or doing any other tasks that require alertness until you know how this drug affects you.
Exertion and Exercise	The loss of fluids and salt from your body can cause a dangerous buildup of lithium in your body. Use caution while exercising or exerting yourself, and drink fluids to replace those lost by sweating.
Excessive Heat	See above; use caution during hot weather, and drink fluids to replace those lost by sweating. Avoid extremely hot baths or saunas.
Examinations or Tests	It is important for you to keep all appointments with your doctor so that your progress can be checked. Blood and urine tests are required during lithium

therapy in order to check the level of lithium in the blood and to evaluate its effects on various organs, especially the thyroid gland and kidneys.

Other Precautions	Tell any doctor or dentist you consult that you are taking this drug, especially if you will be undergoing any type of surgery. If you become ill and develop fever, excessive sweating, diarrhea, or vomiting, let your doctor know immediately. The loss of fluid can result in a dangerous buildup of lithium in your body.
Helpful Hints	If you are taking the controlled-release capsules, swallow them whole without breaking, crushing, or chewing. If your mouth or throat feels dry, chewing sugarless gum or sucking ice chips or sugarless hard candy will help.

No special restrictions on sun exposure or exposure to excessive cold.

POSSIBLE SIDE EFFECTS

Although this list of adverse effects may seem somewhat intimidating, keep in mind that some are quite rare. Of course, should these or any other problems arise while you are on medication, it is always a good idea to consult your doctor.

IF YOU DEVELOP

diarrhea ■ drowsiness ■ muscle weakness ■ vomiting ■ tremors ■ clumsiness ■ confusion ■ seizures ■ delirium ■ blackouts ■ difficulty in moving ■ severe dizziness ■ incontinence ■ fainting ■ severe muscle twitching ■ jerky or writhing movements ■ irregular or fast heartbeat

WHAT TO DO

Urgent Get in touch with your doctor immediately.

difficulty in breathing ■ tiredness ■ weight gain ■ swelling of neck, wrist, feet, or lower legs ■ hair loss ■ headache ■ memory problems ■ inability to concentrate ■ dulled senses ■ rigidity ■ difficulty in speech ■ confusion ■ restlessness ■ blurred vision	**May be serious** Check with your doctor as soon as possible.
increased thirst ■ nausea ■ stomach pain ■ bloating ■ mild tremors or muscle twitching ■ rash or dry skin ■ numbness in skin ■ skin ulcers ■ inflammation of the hair follicles ■ acne ■ thinning of hair or change in hair texture ■ stomach discomfort ■ increased urination ■ unpleasant taste in mouth ■ dry mouth ■ weight loss	If symptoms are disturbing or persist, let your doctor know.

STORAGE INSTRUCTIONS

Store in a cool, dark place (not in a bathroom medicine cabinet). If your medicine is in a liquid form, make sure that it does not freeze.

STOPPING OR INTERRUPTING THERAPY

Take this medicine exactly as prescribed by your doctor; it may take several weeks before you see an effect. If you miss a dose, take it as soon as possible. If it is within two hours (with the regular-acting form) or six hours (with the controlled-release form) of your next dose, skip the missed dose and resume your regular schedule. Do not take two doses at the same time.

SPECIAL CONSIDERATIONS FOR THOSE OVER SIXTY-FIVE

Because older people may be especially susceptible to the side effects of lithium, doctors may start people over sixty-five on a lower dosage.

Chapter 7
Diet, Nutrition, and Health Maintenance

NUTRITIONAL DEFICIENCIES

For a variety of reasons, older people tend to eat less. With a reduced intake of total daily food, there is an increased need to maintain adequate intake of essential nutrients, such as vitamins and minerals. Older persons must make sure that their meal provides a greater quantity of essential nutrients for a given quantity of food than when they were younger. If this is not possible then the older person must use nutrient supplementation to ensure an adequate daily intake of essential nutrients.

Maintaining proper intake of nutrients can be a particular challenge for people with a chronic illness, such as heart disease, diabetes, hypertension, or cancer. These conditions can further increase the body's need for certain vitamins and minerals. Surgery, stress, digestive problems such as constipation, and alcohol abuse are other factors that make it especially important to consume ample amounts of these nutrients.

Taking vitamin or mineral supplements is not always the best answer for maintaining an adequate nutrient intake. They are sometimes not effective for certain individuals and, occasionally, the supplements may interfere with the effectiveness of certain prescription drugs. Also, taking megadoses of certain vitamins and minerals can cause problems on their own. Some vitamins at high doses may also have toxic effects. The question of what, if any, supplements to take should be discussed with your doctor as part of your overall health care.

By maintaining a proper diet, you can contribute to your overall health and minimize the quantity of nutrient supplements you may have to take. To maintain a healthy and nutritional diet you should do the following: (a) eat a variety of foods, (b) eat foods that contain adequate amounts of starch and fiber, (c) avoid too much fat, saturated fat, and cholesterol, (d) avoid too much sodium, (e) maintain a desirable weight, (f) if you drink alcoholic beverages, do so in moderation.

SOURCES AND RECOMMENDED DOSES OF CRITICAL NUTRIENTS

The recommended daily allowances (RDA) for older people are estimations based on studies that were carried out in young adults. Current research indicates that nutrient requirements change with age and in the future more accurate RDAs for older people will be developed. Until then, the RDAs that are presented here are adequate and give one a good idea of the older person's nutrient requirements.

Iron is a mineral that, in general, is rarely deficient in the older person. Despite advertisements to the contrary, which would have us believe that all older people are deficient in iron ("iron-poor blood" is the slogan), the older person has a higher amount of iron stored in the body than does a young person. Studies have shown that the iron content in the diet of most older people is adequate. Foods that are good sources of iron are red meats, liver, soybeans, and fortified bread.

Calcium is the nutrient in which older people, especially women, are most likely to be deficient. As we age, our bodies absorb calcium less efficiently. A lack of calcium has been linked to osteoporosis—the gradual loss of bone tissue—which weakens the bones and makes them more vulnerable to fracture (see also pages 557–559). In some people the problem is a low calcium intake, but in others the problem is poor absorption of calcium. Everyone, regardless of age, should consume at least 800 milligrams (mg) of calcium a day. Women who have passed menopause should get 1,500 mg of calcium a day. Foods that are rich in calcium include milk (whole or skim), yogurt, cheese, greens, and sardines and canned salmon with the bones. Alternatively, your doctor may recommend that you take a calcium supplement, such as calcium carbonate or calcium gluconate.

Vitamin D is another nutrient crucial for healthy bones. Proper amounts of this vitamin can prevent or even reverse osteomalacia, a weakening of the bones that can lead to bone fractures. A quart of fortified milk a day, plus fifteen minutes of sunshine twice a week, will probably give you all the vitamin D you need (400–600 International Units [IU] per day). In addition to milk, fish oils and deep-sea fish are good sources of vitamin D. (If you suspect that you may not be getting enough vitamin D, discuss this with your doctor.) However, because vitamin D is stored in the body, too much of a good thing may be toxic. Avoid high-dose vitamin D supplements—some contain as much as 50,000 IU and should not be taken.

Zinc is important for maintaining the body's immune system and its ability to heal wounds. Red meat, liver, fish, and dark poultry are all good sources of this mineral. Supplements are usually not necessary, but people who have chronic illnesses or serious infections might benefit from supplements as prescribed by a doctor. High doses of zinc can cause diarrhea and nausea.

Consuming adequate amounts of vitamin A in foods may help to prevent some forms of cancer, but there is no evidence that large doses of this vitamin can reverse visual or skin problems, as many people believe. Too much vitamin A can actually do damage. For example, 50,000 IU or more per day can cause bone disease, liver disease, hair loss, drowsiness, and itching. The recommended daily intake is 5,000 IU. Carrots, sweet potatoes, spinach, and liver are good sources of this vitamin.

Beware of any "miracle products" promoted to prevent aging. In general, it's a good idea to check with your doctor before taking any product that contains more than one to two times the recommended daily allowance.

OUTLOOK

As we age, our nutritional requirements change, and a diet that once supplied us with plentiful nutrients may no longer be adequate for our needs. Some minor menu modifications are usually enough to make up the difference, though the use of vitamin and mineral supplements is sometimes helpful. The most important thing to remember is that eating well is important to living well, and that as we grow older, we can learn to do both better.

CONDITION: **NUTRITIONAL DEFICIENCIES**

CATEGORY: **VITAMINS**

GENERIC (CHEMICAL) NAME	BRAND (TRADE) NAME	DOSAGE FORMS AND STRENGTHS
Vitamins A, B_1, B_2, B_6, B_{12}, C, E, niacin, pantothenic acid, biotin, folic acid, iron, chromium, magnesium, manganese, copper, zinc	BERROCA Plus	Tablets
Vitamins A, B_1, B_2, B_6, B_{12}, C, E, niacinamide, pantothenic acid, folic acid, zinc, magnesium, manganese	VICON Forte	Capsules

This type of drug is available both by prescription and over the counter under a variety of brand names and dosage forms.

DRUG PROFILE

Multivitamins are used as nutritional supplements in people with inadequate diets. They are also used in people recovering from surgery or in those with medical conditions (such as severe illness or injury or overactive thyroid) for which nutritional requirements are increased. Those with conditions in which the body is unable to absorb enough essential nutrients or excretes excessive nutrients, those who abuse alcohol, and those whose chronic use of certain medicines results in specific nutrient deficiencies may also need multivitamins.

BEFORE USING THIS DRUG

Let your doctor know *IF*

You have ever had any of the following medical problems: ■ severe vitamin deficiency ■ anemia ■ Parkinson's disease ■ any other chronic disease.

You are taking any of the following medicines: ■ levodopa (medicine for Parkinson's disease) ■ diuretics (water pills) ■ laxatives ■ medicine for seizures ■ medicine for high cholesterol ■ isoniazid (medicine for tuberculosis) ■ tetracycline.

SPECIAL RESTRICTIONS WHILE TAKING THIS DRUG

FOOD AND DRUG INTERACTIONS

Other Drugs	Many drugs affect vitamin requirements. Let your doctor know about any other drugs you are taking, including over-the-counter (OTC) drugs.
Foods and Beverages	Before prescribing a vitamin supplement, your doctor will probably evaluate your diet and make specific recommendations, which you should follow carefully.
Alcohol	Excessive alcohol intake may cause depletion of vitamins. It may also prevent the body from absorbing a vitamin supplement.
Smoking	Smokers have lower levels of vitamin C in their blood. But a small supplement (40 mg/day—the amount contained in a glass of orange juice) should be sufficient to meet this extra need. However, taking vitamins does not protect against the other harmful effects of smoking.

DAILY LIVING

No special restrictions on driving, exertion and exercise, sun exposure, or exposure to excessive heat or cold.

POSSIBLE SIDE EFFECTS

Although this list of adverse effects may seem somewhat intimidating, keep in mind that some are quite rare. Of course, should these or any other problems arise while you are on medication, it is always a good idea to consult your doctor.

IF YOU DEVELOP	WHAT TO DO
flushing (from large doses of niacin) ■ headache ■ confusion ■ weakness ■ rash or hives ■ heart disturbances ■ increased thirst ■ increased urination ■ indigestion ■ kidney stones	**Urgent** Get in touch with your doctor immediately.
nausea, vomiting, or other digestive disorders	**May be serious** Check with your doctor as soon as possible.

STORAGE INSTRUCTIONS

Store in a cool, dark place (not in a bathroom medicine cabinet).

STOPPING OR INTERRUPTING THERAPY

Try to remember to take this supplement every day. If you should miss a day, skip the missed dose and resume your regular schedule.

SPECIAL CONSIDERATIONS FOR THOSE OVER SIXTY-FIVE

Vitamin toxicity is more apt to occur in older people (see "Possible Side Effects" for symptoms).

CONDITION: **NUTRITIONAL DEFICIENCIES**

CATEGORY: **VITAMINS**

GENERIC (CHEMICAL) NAME	BRAND (TRADE) NAME	DOSAGE FORMS AND STRENGTHS

Vitamins B_1, B_2, B_6, B_{12}, C, niacin, pantothenic acid, folic acid

This type of drug is available both by prescription and over the counter under a variety of brand names and dosage forms.

DRUG PROFILE

Vitamin B complex and vitamin B complex with C are used as nutritional supplements in people with inadequate diets. They are also used in people recovering from surgery or in those with medical conditions (such as severe illness or injury or overactive thyroid) for which nutritional requirements are increased. Those with conditions in which the body is unable to absorb enough essential nutrients or excretes excessive nutrients, those who abuse alcohol, and those whose use of certain medicines results in specific nutrient deficiencies may also need multivitamins.

BEFORE USING THIS DRUG

Let your doctor know *IF*

You have ever had allergic reactions or other problems with ■ vitamin C.

You have ever had any of the following medical problems: ■ anemia ■ any serious or chronic medical condition.

You are taking any of the following medicines: ■ medicine for seizures ■ sulfasalazine (medicine for inflammatory bowel disease) ■ aspirin ■ isoniazid (medicine for tuberculosis) ■ penicillamine (medicine for arthritis) ■ aluminum hydroxide (antacid) ■ medicine for ulcers (eg, cimetidine, ranitidine, etc.) ■ levodopa or carbidopa (medicine for Parkinson's disease).

SPECIAL RESTRICTIONS WHILE TAKING THIS DRUG

FOOD AND DRUG INTERACTIONS

Other Drugs	Many drugs affect vitamin requirements. Let your doctor know about any other drugs you are taking, including over-the-counter (OTC) drugs.
Foods and Beverages	Before prescribing a vitamin supplement, your doctor will probably evaluate your diet and make specific recommendations, which you should follow carefully.
Alcohol	Excessive alcohol intake may cause depletion of vitamins. It may also prevent the body from absorbing a vitamin supplement.
Smoking	Smokers have lower levels of vitamin C in their blood, but a small supplement (40 mg/day—the amount contained in a glass of orange juice) should be sufficient to meet this extra need. However, taking vitamins does not protect against the other harmful effects of smoking.

DAILY LIVING

No special restrictions on driving, exertion and exercise, sun exposure, or exposure to excessive heat or cold.

POSSIBLE SIDE EFFECTS

Although this list of adverse effects may seem somewhat intimidating, keep in mind that some are quite rare. Of course, should these or any other problems arise while you are on medication, it is always a good idea to consult your doctor.

IF YOU DEVELOP	WHAT TO DO
skin redness ■ rash or itching ■ difficulty in breathing	**Urgent** Get in touch with your doctor immediately.
nausea or vomiting ■ flushing ■ diarrhea ■ kidney stones	**May be serious** Check with your doctor as soon as possible.

STORAGE INSTRUCTIONS

Store in a cool, dark place (not in a bathroom medicine cabinet).

STOPPING OR INTERRUPTING THERAPY

Try to remember to take this supplement every day. If you should miss a day, skip the missed dose and resume your regular schedule.

SPECIAL CONSIDERATIONS FOR THOSE OVER SIXTY-FIVE

None.

CONDITION: **NUTRITIONAL DEFICIENCIES**

CATEGORY: **VITAMINS**

GENERIC (CHEMICAL) NAME	BRAND (TRADE) NAME	DOSAGE FORMS AND STRENGTHS
Vitamin B_{12} (cyanocobalamin)		

This drug is available both by prescription and over the counter under a variety of brand names and dosage forms.

DRUG PROFILE

Vitamin B_{12} (cyanocobalamin) is involved in the production of red blood cells and is important in maintaining healthy nerves. This nutritional supplement is used to treat people with severe deficiency, those with certain metabolic disorders, and those with conditions in which the body is unable to absorb this vitamin from food.

BEFORE USING THIS DRUG

Let your doctor know *IF*

You have ever had any of the following medical problems: ■ heart disease ■ Leber's disease (atrophy of the optic nerve) ■ pernicious anemia ■ stomach or intestinal problems.

You are taking any of the following medicines: ■ folic acid ■ vitamin C ■ aspirin or aspirinlike medicine ■ medicine for seizures ■ prednisone (corticosteroid) ■ neomycin, chloramphenicol, or aminoglycosides (antibiotics) ■ cholestyramine (medicine for high cholesterol) ■ medicine for ulcers (eg, cimetidine, ranitidine, etc.).

You are undergoing cobalt irradiation of the small intestine.

SPECIAL RESTRICTIONS WHILE TAKING THIS DRUG

FOOD AND DRUG INTERACTIONS

No special restrictions on other drugs, foods and beverages, alcohol use, or smoking.

DAILY LIVING

Examinations or Tests	It is important for you to keep all doctor or laboratory appointments so that your doctor can check on your progress.
Other Precautions	Vitamin B_{12} is often taken by people who do not need it. If you are anemic, it is important that the cause of anemia be determined before B_{12} therapy is started.

No special restrictions on driving, exertion and exercise, sun exposure, or exposure to excessive heat or cold.

POSSIBLE SIDE EFFECTS

It is unlikely that any side effects will occur with this supplement.

STORAGE INSTRUCTIONS

Store in a cool, dark place (not in a bathroom medicine cabinet).

STOPPING OR INTERRUPTING THERAPY

If you should miss a dose, skip the missed dose and resume your regular schedule.

SPECIAL CONSIDERATIONS FOR THOSE OVER SIXTY-FIVE

None.

CONDITION: **NUTRITIONAL DEFICIENCIES**

CATEGORY: **VITAMINS**

GENERIC (CHEMICAL) NAME	BRAND (TRADE) NAME	DOSAGE FORMS AND STRENGTHS
Niacin	NICOBID	Controlled-release capsules: 125, 250, and 500 mg

This drug is available both by prescription and over the counter under a variety of brand names and dosage forms.

DRUG PROFILE

Niacin helps the body break down food so that it can be used for energy. This type of supplement is used to prevent or treat niacin deficiency, or pellagra. Niacin is also used to lower blood levels of fats and cholesterol.

BEFORE USING THIS DRUG

Let your doctor know *IF*

You have ever had allergic reactions or other problems with ■ niacin or niacinamide.

You have ever had any of the following medical problems: ■ diabetes ■ ulcer ■ gout ■ liver disease ■ gallbladder disease ■ glaucoma.

You are taking any of the following medicines: ■ isoniazid (medicine for tuberculosis) ■ medicine for cancer.

SPECIAL RESTRICTIONS WHILE TAKING THIS DRUG

FOOD AND DRUG INTERACTIONS

Foods and Beverages	Before prescribing vitamin supplements, your doctor will probably evaluate your diet and make specific recommendations, which you should follow carefully.
Alcohol	Alcohol abuse commonly causes niacin deficiency.

No special restrictions on other drugs or smoking.

DAILY LIVING

Precautions	If you have diabetes, be aware that this medicine may affect blood-sugar levels. If you notice any change when testing sugar levels in your blood or urine, let your doctor know.

Helpful Hints	Swallow the capsule whole—without chewing, crushing, or breaking. If the capsule is too large for you, try swallowing it with a spoonful of jelly.
	If this medicine upsets your stomach, taking it with milk, meals, or snacks should help.

No special restrictions on driving, exertion and exercise, sun exposure, or exposure to excessive heat or cold.

POSSIBLE SIDE EFFECTS

Although this list of adverse effects may seem somewhat intimidating, keep in mind that some are quite rare. Of course, should these or any other problems arise while you are on medication, it is always a good idea to consult your doctor.

IF YOU DEVELOP

flushing (especially of the face and neck) or feeling of warmth ■ dizziness or fainting ■ fast heartbeat ■ itching ■ "burning" sensation, stinging, or tingling of skin ■ dry skin or skin color changes ■ bloating or gas ■ headache ■ nausea or vomiting ■ heartburn ■ diarrhea ■ hunger pangs or other stomach pain ■ worsening of stomach ulcer ■ yellowing of eyes or skin ■ worsening of diabetes ■ visual disturbances ■ nervousness ■ vasovagal attacks (paleness, nausea, increased sweating, slow heartbeat, faintness) ■ gout

WHAT TO DO

If symptoms are disturbing or persist, let your doctor know.

STORAGE INSTRUCTIONS

Store in a cool, dark place (not in a bathroom medicine cabinet).

STOPPING OR INTERRUPTING THERAPY

If you should miss a dose, skip the missed dose and resume your regular schedule.

SPECIAL CONSIDERATIONS FOR THOSE OVER SIXTY-FIVE

None.

CONDITION: **NUTRITIONAL DEFICIENCIES**
CATEGORY: **VITAMINS**

GENERIC (CHEMICAL) NAME	BRAND (TRADE) NAME	DOSAGE FORMS AND STRENGTHS
Folic acid		

This drug is available both by prescription and over the counter under a variety of brand names and dosage forms.

DRUG PROFILE

Folic acid helps produce red blood cells. This supplement is used to treat certain types of anemia that may be the result of disease, alcoholism, drug therapy, or kidney dialysis.

BEFORE USING THIS DRUG

Let your doctor know *IF*

You have ever had any of the following medical problems: ■ seizures ■ malnutrition ■ long illness or serious injury ■ anemia (hemolytic or pernicious) ■ alcoholism ■ chronic diarrhea ■ intestinal disease ■ liver disease.

You are taking any of the following medicines: ■ tetracycline ■ chloramphenicol ■ aspirin ■ antacids ■ anti-inflammatory drugs ■ diuretics (water pills) ■ sulfasalazine (medicine for inflammatory bowel disease) ■ phenytoin (medicine for seizures).

SPECIAL RESTRICTIONS WHILE TAKING THIS DRUG

FOOD AND DRUG INTERACTIONS

Foods and Beverages	Before prescribing vitamin supplements, your doctor will probably evaluate your diet and make specific recommendations, which you should follow carefully.
Alcohol	Alcohol abuse is a leading cause of folic acid deficiency.
Smoking	Some scientists believe that folic acid may have anticancer properties; however, taking vitamins does not protect against the harmful effects of smoking.

No special restrictions on other drugs.

DAILY LIVING

No special restrictions on driving, exertion and exercise, sun exposure, or exposure to excessive heat or cold.

POSSIBLE SIDE EFFECTS

It is unlikely that any side effects will occur with this supplement.

STORAGE INSTRUCTIONS

Store in a cool, dark place (not in a bathroom medicine cabinet).

STOPPING OR INTERRUPTING THERAPY

Try to remember to take this supplement every day. If you should miss a day, skip the missed dose and resume your regular schedule.

SPECIAL CONSIDERATIONS FOR THOSE OVER SIXTY-FIVE

None.

CONDITION: **NUTRITIONAL DEFICIENCIES**
CATEGORY: **VITAMINS**

GENERIC (CHEMICAL) NAME	BRAND (TRADE) NAME	DOSAGE FORMS AND STRENGTHS
Vitamin D (calcitriol)	ROCALTROL	Capsules: 0.25, 0.5 mcg

DRUG PROFILE

Calcitriol is a synthetic form of vitamin D and is used when the body does not absorb enough of this vitamin. This may occur in people with medical conditions like rickets, osteomalacia, and osteoporosis; those undergoing kidney dialysis; those taking certain drugs; or in homebound people who do not get enough sunlight. Vitamin D regulates the metabolism of calcium and phosphorus, which are primary components of bone.

BEFORE USING THIS DRUG

Let your doctor know *IF*

You have ever had any of the following medical problems: ■ milk intolerance ■ kidney disease, including kidney stones ■ heart disease ■ sarcoidosis ■ disease of the parathyroid gland ■ bone disease ■ liver disease ■ intestinal problems.

You are taking any of the following medicines: ■ thiazide diuretics (water pills) ■ cholestyramine or colestipol (medicine for high cholesterol) ■ corticosteroids ■ antacids containing magnesium ■ calcium blockers (eg, diltiazem, nifedipine, verapamil) ■ laxatives ■ antibiotics ■ sucralfate (medicine for ulcers) ■ medicine for seizures ■ heart medicine (digoxin, etc.) ■ mineral oil.

SPECIAL RESTRICTIONS WHILE TAKING THIS DRUG

FOOD AND DRUG INTERACTIONS

Foods and Beverages	Before prescribing vitamin supplements, your doctor will probably evaluate your diet and make specific recommendations, which you should follow carefully.
	It is important to drink plenty of fluids while you are taking this supplement.
Alcohol	Alcohol will not cause vitamin D deficiency unless you have a malabsorption condition or advanced liver disease.
Smoking	Smoking increases the risk of osteoporosis. You should not smoke, particularly if you are being treated for bone disease.

No special restrictions on other drugs.

DAILY LIVING

Examinations or Tests	It is important for you to keep all doctor and laboratory appointments so that your progress can be checked. Depending on what you are being treated for, periodic blood and urine tests may be required to determine your body levels of vitamin D, calcium, and phosphorus.
Other Precautions	Take this supplement exactly as instructed. Vitamin D toxicity develops very rapidly if excess doses are taken.

No special restrictions on driving, exertion and exercise, sun exposure, or exposure to excessive heat or cold.

POSSIBLE SIDE EFFECTS

Although this list of adverse effects may seem somewhat intimidating, keep in mind that some are quite rare. Of course, should these or any other problems arise while you are on medication, it is always a good idea to consult your doctor.

IF YOU DEVELOP	WHAT TO DO
severe stomach pain ■ seizures ■ irregular heartbeat	**Urgent** Get in touch with your doctor immediately.
weakness ■ headache ■ dizziness ■ drowsiness ■ constipation ■ ringing in ears ■ nausea or vomiting ■ dry mouth ■ metallic taste ■ clumsiness ■ mood or mental changes ■ muscle or bone pain ■ increased urination or need to urinate at night ■ increased thirst ■ loss of appetite or weight loss ■ eye irritation ■ stomach cramps or pain ■ fever ■ decreased sex drive ■ rash or itching ■ increased sensitivity of eyes to light	**May be serious** Check with your doctor as soon as possible.

STORAGE INSTRUCTIONS

Store in cool, dark place (not in a bathroom medicine cabinet).

STOPPING OR INTERRUPTING THERAPY

Try to remember to take this supplement every day. If you should miss a day, skip the missed dose and resume your regular schedule.

SPECIAL CONSIDERATIONS FOR THOSE OVER SIXTY-FIVE

Older people are particularly prone to developing vitamin D toxicity (see "Possible Side Effects" for symptoms).

CONDITION: **NUTRITIONAL DEFICIENCIES**

CATEGORY: **VITAMINS**

GENERIC (CHEMICAL) NAME	BRAND (TRADE) NAME	DOSAGE FORMS AND STRENGTHS
Vitamin K_4 (menadiol sodium diphosphate)	SYNKAYVITE	Tablets: 5 mg
Vitamin K_1 (phytonadione)	MEPHYTON	Tablets: 5 mg

DRUG PROFILE

Vitamin K promotes certain substances in the body that help blood clot. Your doctor will prescribe vitamin K if your body is having trouble absorbing it from your regular diet because of a medical condition or because you are taking certain drugs (antibiotics, quinidine, quinine, or aspirin). Vitamin K is also used to treat certain types of bleeding disorders.

BEFORE USING THIS DRUG

Let your doctor know *IF*

You have ever had any of the following medical conditions: ■ liver disease ■ cystic fibrosis ■ prolonged diarrhea ■ intestinal problems.

You are taking any of the following medicines: ■ anticoagulants (blood thinners) ■ mineral oil or other laxatives ■ aspirin or aspirinlike medicine ■ antibiotics ■ medicine for high cholesterol ■ vitamin E.

SPECIAL RESTRICTIONS WHILE TAKING THIS DRUG

FOOD AND DRUG INTERACTIONS

Other Drugs	Many drugs affect the absorption of vitamin K. Let your doctor know about all other drugs you are taking, including over-the-counter (OTC) drugs.

No special restrictions on foods and beverages, alcohol use, or smoking.

DAILY LIVING

Examinations or Tests	It is important for you to keep all appointments with your doctor so that your progress can be checked. Periodic blood tests are usually required.
Other Precautions	Tell any doctor or dentist you consult that you are taking vitamin K, especially if you will be undergoing any type of surgery.

No special restrictions on driving, exertion and exercise, sun exposure, or exposure to excessive heat or cold.

POSSIBLE SIDE EFFECTS

Although this list of adverse effects may seem somewhat intimidating, keep in mind that some are quite rare. Of course, should these or any other problems arise while you are on medication, it is always a good idea to consult your doctor.

IF YOU DEVELOP

abnormal bleeding ■ abnormal clotting ■ skin rash

WHAT TO DO

Urgent Get in touch with your doctor immediately.

STORAGE INSTRUCTIONS

Store in a cool, dark place (not in a bathroom medicine cabinet).

STOPPING OR INTERRUPTING THERAPY

If you are taking vitamin K for bleeding disorders, keep your doctor informed about any change from your usual dosage schedule.

SPECIAL CONSIDERATIONS FOR THOSE OVER SIXTY-FIVE

Older people are particularly prone to developing vitamin K toxicity (see "Possible Side Effects" for symptoms).

CONDITION: **NUTRITIONAL DEFICIENCIES**

CATEGORY: **POTASSIUM SUPPLEMENTS**

GENERIC (CHEMICAL) NAME	BRAND (TRADE) NAME	DOSAGE FORMS AND STRENGTHS
Potassium chloride	KAOCHLOR SF 10%	Liquid: 20 mEq per tbsp
	KLOR-CON 8	Controlled-release tablets: 600 mg (8 mEq)
	KAON-CI	Controlled-release tablets: 500 mg (6.7 mEq)
	KAON-CL-10	Controlled-release tablets: 750 mg (10 mEq)
	KLOR-CON 10	Controlled-release tablets: 750 mg (10 mEq)
	KLOTRIX	Controlled-release tablets: 750 mg (10 mEq)
	K-TAB	Controlled-release tablets: 750 mg (10 mEq)
	K-DUR 10	Controlled-release tablets: 750 mg (10 mEq)
	TEN-K	Controlled-release tablets: 750 mg (10 mEq)
	K-DUR 20	Controlled-release tablets: 1500 mg (20 mEq)
	K-LOR	Powder: 15, 20 mEq per packet
	KLOR-CON	Powder: 20, 25 mEq per packet
	K-LYTE-CL	Effervescent tablet: 25 mEq
	K-LEASE	Controlled-release tablets: 750 mg (10 mEq)
	MICRO-K	Controlled-release capsules: 600 mg (8 mEq)
	MICRO-K LS	Powder: 20 mEq per packet
	MICRO-K 10	Controlled-release capsules: 750 mg (10 mEq)
	K-NORM	Controlled release capsules: 750 mg (10 mEq)
	SLOW-K	Controlled-release tablets: 600 mg (8 mEq)

DRUG PROFILE

Potassium supplements are used to prevent and treat the lack of potassium, a vital element in the body, when this lack cannot be made up by diet. Hypokalemia (lack of potassium) occurs in various medical conditions or with the administration of potassium-depleting drugs such as some diuretics (see pages 28–40).

BEFORE USING THIS DRUG

Let your doctor know *IF*

You have ever had allergic reactions or other problems with ■ any form of potassium.

You have ever had any of the following medical problems: ■ heart disease ■ muscle problems or congenital muscle disease ■ kidney disease ■ urinary problems ■ intestinal blockage or motility (movement) problems ■ diabetes.

You are taking any of the following medicines: ■ any potassium-containing medicines or supplements ■ appetite suppressants ■ decongestants ■ aminophylline, oxtriphylline, or theophylline (medicine for asthma) ■ laxatives ■ baking soda ■ flecainide or mexilitine (medicine for abnormal heart rhythms) ■ medicine for diabetes ■ diuretics (water pills) ■ digoxin or digitalis (heart medicines) ■ ACE inhibitors (captopril, enalapril, lisinopril) ■ beta-blockers (eg, propranolol, atenolol, metoprolol).

SPECIAL RESTRICTIONS WHILE TAKING THIS DRUG

FOOD AND DRUG INTERACTIONS

Other Drugs	Many drugs interact with potassium supplements. Let your doctor know about all other drugs you are taking, including over-the-counter (OTC) drugs.
Foods and Beverages	Too much potassium can be harmful. Let your doctor know if you use salt substitutes or if you drink low-salt milk, as these substances contain potassium.

Alcohol	It is all right to drink alcohol in small amounts while taking this supplement.

No special restrictions on smoking.

DAILY LIVING

Exertion and Exercise	Some potassium-deficient people may experience cramps or weakness after exercise due to additional potassium lost through sweating.
Sun Exposure/ Excessive Heat	Some potassium-deficient people may experience cramps, weakness, irregular heartbeat, and other signs of dehydration due to additional potassium loss through sweating.
Examinations or Tests	It is important for you to keep all appointments with your doctor so that your progress can be checked. Periodic blood and urine tests may be required.
Helpful Hints	If you are taking a soluble granule or powder, dissolve the medicine in at least four ounces of cold water or juice. Wait until the mixture has stopped fizzing before drinking.
	Controlled-release tablets or capsules should be swallowed whole without crushing or chewing. Take each dose with a full glass of water immediately after meals or with food to prevent nausea, vomiting, or upset stomach.
	If you have trouble swallowing tablets or capsules, let your doctor know.
	Some tablets can be broken or added to water before swallowing, and some can be broken and the contents mixed with soft food.

Some special tablets have a wax base that passes into the stool after the potassium is absorbed.

No special restrictions on driving or exposure to excessive cold.

POSSIBLE SIDE EFFECTS

Although this list of adverse effects may seem somewhat intimidating, keep in mind that some are quite rare. Of course, should these or any other problems arise while you are on medication, it is always a good idea to consult your doctor.

IF YOU DEVELOP	WHAT TO DO
numbness or tingling in hands or feet ■ tiredness or weakness ■ confusion ■ irregular heartbeat ■ heaviness of limbs ■ cold, grayish skin ■ dizziness ■ difficulty in breathing ■ vomiting ■ diarrhea ■ stomach pain ■ black, tarry stools ■ bloody rectal discharge ■ severe vomiting ■ skin rash	**Urgent** Get in touch with your doctor immediately.
nausea or stomach discomfort	If symptoms are disturbing or persist, let your doctor know.

STORAGE INSTRUCTIONS

Store in a cool, dark place (not in a bathroom medicine cabinet).

STOPPING OR INTERRUPTING THERAPY

If you miss a dose, take it as soon as possible. If it is not within two hours of the missed dose, skip it and resume your regular schedule.

SPECIAL CONSIDERATIONS FOR THOSE OVER SIXTY-FIVE

The side effects of dehydration (signaled by irregular heartbeat or weakness), nausea, and vomiting are particularly serious in older people.

SMOKING

Until fairly recently, smoking was considered a bad habit—but one that anyone could control with a little willpower. Recent evidence has shown, however, that cigarette smoking is a stubborn form of drug addiction; the smoker has a true physical dependence on nicotine, the active ingredient in tobacco. In fact, nicotine is probably one of the most addictive drugs used in our society.

Nicotine is a stimulant, leading to an increase in heart rate and blood pressure and the narrowing of blood vessels. In addition, the nicotine in tobacco smoke reaches the brain within ten seconds of inhaling it. If the amount of nicotine contained in a single cigarette were injected directly into the bloodstream rather than being absorbed through the lungs, it would paralyze the centers in the brain controlling breathing and cause death.

Nicotine is not the only culprit in cigarette smoke. *Tar*—the short name for the condensed solid particles in smoke—contains several thousand chemicals that have been implicated in a number of diseases. Among the chemicals are hydrocarbons, phenols, and ketones; the corrosive gases hydrogen cyanide and nitrogen oxide; and carbon monoxide. The presence of carbon monoxide interferes with oxygen delivery to the brain, heart, and other tissues.

WHY YOU SHOULD QUIT

We are all familiar with the link between cigarette smoking and lung cancer. The risk of lung cancer is ten times greater for a smoker than for a nonsmoker. But smoking has also been identified as a major cause, or at least a contributing factor, in many other forms of cancer. In total, three out of every ten cancer deaths can be attributed to the use of tobacco. Cigarette smoking also takes its toll in terms of heart disease, as well as such lung diseases as emphysema and chronic bronchitis.

These are compelling arguments not to start smoking—but what about stopping? Hasn't the damage been done after years of inhaling all the dangerous components of cigarette smoke? Isn't it too late?

A growing body of evidence shows that even people in their sixties and seventies who have smoked since adolescence can benefit substantially from giving it up. For example, if a man who has smoked a half pack to one pack of cigarettes a day all his life quits smoking at age sixty-five, he will add two years to his life expectancy. If he has smoked more than two packs a day, the gain will be four years. (This information is based on a study of more than one million people who were studied over a twenty-year period.) A more recent study of more than two thousand five hundred people between the ages of sixty-five and seventy-four showed that stopping smoking substantially decreases the death rate from coronary heart disease. In a study of more than forty thousand British doctors (the majority of them middle-aged or older), it was found that within two and a half years, the lung cancer rate was cut in half in the group that stopped smoking. Clearly, even older people can achieve substantial health benefits—and increased odds of living longer—from stopping smoking.

BUT HOW DO I STOP?

It's hard to stop smoking. Some smokers seem to be able to do so without much trouble, but most people go through a period of withdrawal that includes agitation, nausea, headache, and other physical symptoms. Drowsiness and the persistent inability to concentrate are other common complaints. These symptoms usually abate within ten days to two weeks, but sometimes they last longer than that.

If you really decide to stop and feel that you need something more than will power, your doctor may prescribe nicotine polacrilex (Nicorette), a nicotine chewing gum. (See the chart on pages 677–680.) Each piece of gum delivers about the same amount of nicotine as a cigarette. Nicorette relieves the craving for nicotine and relieves the withdrawal symptoms that so often cause people to start smoking again.

Using Nicorette is most helpful when it's combined with a program to eliminate the psychological dependency on cigarette smoking. This involves, for example, learning other ways to relax, cope with stress, and handle boredom. Once this is achieved, the next goal is to withdraw from all sources of nicotine—including Nicorette. Research has shown that a comprehensive treatment program, including the use of nicotine gum and group counseling, is more successful than reliance on the gum alone.

Questions have been raised about the safety of Nicorette in older people who may suffer from a chronic lung problem or cerebrovascular or cardiovascular disease. Currently, it is up to the doctor to weigh the risks of short-term (three to six months) exposure to the low levels of nicotine contained in the gum against the risks of continued smoking—long-term exposure to nicotine, carbon monoxide, and carcinogens.

A number of other treatments can help people stop smoking. These include such behavior-modification techniques as rapid smoking. This consists of having the person inhale his or her own cigarette smoke every six seconds until he or she no longer wants to take another puff; as part of this approach, the doctor or therapist teaches alternative coping skills to replace smoking. Recent studies have shown that rapid smoking therapy poses no particular danger for older people, including those who have heart and lung ailments. In fact, it produces no greater physiologic changes than does smoking at a regular rate.

Smokenders, which involves behavior modification in a group format similar to that of Alcoholics Anonymous, is a ten-week program that is believed to have a success rate of about 25 percent (though whether this is permanent abstinence is unknown). The American Cancer Society (ACS) also offers a program, known as Fresh Start, to help people stop smoking. It is a four-session, group program that is led by former smokers who understand well the difficulties of quitting. Videotapes and audiotapes of the ACS program, which uses behavioral and other techniques, are also available. They can be purchased at commercial outlets. (For more information on Fresh Start, call your local ACS office.) Other approaches to quitting smoking include acupuncture and hypnosis, as well as self-help manuals for those who prefer doing it on their own.

OUTLOOK

Smoking is the number one preventable cause of premature death and disability in this country—and an addiction that's hard to break. But more than thirty million Americans have quit; you can too. It may be difficult, but it's not impossible. The benefits, a healthy and longer life, make it worthwhile.

CONDITION: **SMOKING**

CATEGORY: **SMOKING DETERRENTS**

GENERIC (CHEMICAL) NAME	BRAND (TRADE) NAME	DOSAGE FORMS AND STRENGTHS
Nicotine polacrilex	NICORETTE	Chewing gum: nicotine polacrilex equivalent to 2 mg nicotine per piece of gum

DRUG PROFILE

This drug, which comes in the form of chewing gum, is used as part of a medically supervised behavior-modification program to stop smoking for people who have a strong physical dependence on nicotine. The drug is absorbed through the lining of the cheek into the bloodstream and helps reduce nicotine withdrawal symptoms.

BEFORE USING THIS DRUG

Let your doctor know *IF*

You have ever had allergic reactions or other problems with ■ nicotine.

You have ever had any of the following medical problems: ■ angina (chest pain) ■ heart attack ■ abnormal heart rhythms ■ disease of the blood vessels ■ high blood pressure ■ temporomandibular (jaw muscle) joint disease (TMJ) ■ dental problems ■ inflammation of the vocal cords ■ stomach ulcer ■ heartburn ■ diabetes ■ overactive thyroid ■ pheochromocytoma (adrenal gland tumor) ■ gout.

You are taking any of the following medicines: ■ aminophylline, oxtriphylline, or theophylline (medicine for asthma) ■ medicine containing caffeine ■ decongestants ■ medicine for migraine or vascular headaches ■ pentazocine or propoxyphene (prescription pain-killers) ■ beta-blockers (eg, propranolol, atenolol, metoprolol) ■ medicine for high blood pressure ■ nitrates (medicine for angina) ■ sulfinpyrazone (medicine for gout) ■ ergoloid mesylate (vasodilator) ■ imipramine (medicine for depression) ■ furosemide (diuretic).

You wear dentures.

SPECIAL RESTRICTIONS WHILE TAKING THIS DRUG

FOOD AND DRUG INTERACTIONS

Other Drugs | Stopping smoking may change the body's response to drugs. Let your doctor know about all other drugs you are taking, including over-the-counter (OTC) drugs.

Smoking | You must stop smoking completely when you start using this drug. In addition, you may not use any other form of tobacco, such as chewing tobacco.

No special restrictions on foods and beverages or alcohol use.

DAILY LIVING

Other Precautions | Read the accompanying pamphlet carefully; your doctor may want you to chew one piece of the gum in the office to make sure you have mastered the technique.

To use: When you feel the urge to smoke, chew one piece of gum slowly until you can taste it or until you feel a tingling sensation in your mouth. Resume chewing when the taste or sensation disappears. Adverse effects from this drug usually subside after the first few days of use.

Your doctor will probably warn you that you may experience withdrawal symptoms after stopping this drug, such as craving for tobacco, irritability, anxiety, restless ness, impatience, depression, inability to concentrate, hostility, headache, drowsiness, and upset stomach.

Overdose may occur if too many pieces are chewed in rapid succession or if the gum is chewed too fast. If overdose occurs (see "Possible Side Effects" for symptoms) or if a child should accidentally chew the gum, call your doctor or a poison control center immediately.

If dental problems or damage to your dental work occurs, stop use of this drug and check with your doctor or dentist.

Helpful Hints	If your mouth feels dry or irritated, sucking hard sugarless candy in between pieces of gum will help.

No special restrictions on driving, exertion and exercise, sun exposure, or exposure to excessive heat or cold.

POSSIBLE SIDE EFFECTS

Although this list of adverse effects may seem somewhat intimidating, keep in mind that some are quite rare. Of course, should these or any other problems arise while you are on medication, it is always a good idea to consult your doctor.

IF YOU DEVELOP

signs of overdose: cold sweat; hearing problems; visual disturbances; confusion; extreme weakness; fainting; dizziness; difficulty in breathing; seizures; weak, irregular pulse; diarrhea

WHAT TO DO

Urgent Get in touch with your doctor immediately.

light-headedness or dizziness ■ nausea or vomiting ■ upset stomach ■ loss of appetite ■ heartburn ■ mouth or throat irritation ■ sleeplessness ■ irritability ■ headache ■ ringing in ears ■ palpitations ■ gas ■ belching ■ laxative effect ■ constipation ■ flushing ■ aching jaw muscles ■ hiccups ■ increased salivation ■ hoarseness ■ dry mouth ■ cough ■ sneezing

If symptoms are disturbing or persist, let your doctor know.

STORAGE INSTRUCTIONS

Store in a cool, dark place (not in a bathroom medicine cabinet).

STOPPING OR INTERRUPTING THERAPY

Use this drug exactly as instructed by your doctor and the pamphlet that accompanies the chewing gum. Your doctor will probably direct you to cut down on the gum gradually to avoid withdrawal symptoms.

SPECIAL CONSIDERATIONS FOR THOSE OVER SIXTY-FIVE

Older people may be especially sensitive to the adverse effects of this drug.

Chapter 8
Hormonal Disorders

DIABETES MELLITUS

From the sugar in your tea to last night's spaghetti, all sugars and starchy foods eventually break down in your body, in part to glucose, a form of carbohydrate. Glucose supplies a major amount of the body's fuel; it travels through the blood and readily enters cells to give them the energy they need. When diabetes mellitus ("sugar diabetes") complicates the picture, glucose has trouble entering the cells that need it, causing an energy crisis. In addition, glucose builds up to high levels in the blood, where it can cause further trouble.

CAUSES

Two types of illnesses account for the vast majority of cases of diabetes. In insulin-dependent diabetes (IDDM), a person loses the ability to make the hormone insulin. Insulin is the key that unlocks the cells and permits glucose to enter. Without insulin, body cells literally starve for glucose, even as this sugar rises to higher and higher levels in the blood. A person with IDDM must take daily insulin injections to survive.

Non-insulin-dependent diabetes (NIDDM) is most common in older people. In NIDDM, the body produces less than the amount of insulin required for glucose to enter the cells, and the cells show resistance to insulin's action.

IDDM most often develops in childhood or adolescence, which is why it used to be called juvenile-onset diabetes. NIDDM generally occurs in people over forty. Most NIDDM diabetics are overweight. If you've recently developed diabetes, chances are it is NIDDM—this is the form of diabetes we will focus on here.

Many people, doctors included, mistakenly think of NIDDM as a mild form of the disease. However, NIDDM can cause some serious complications. In the short run (especially during times of illness or stress), high blood-sugar levels can lead to diabetic coma, which can be fatal if not treated quickly in a hospital. And, over the years, NIDDM, like IDDM, can lead to conditions as varied as infection, nerve impairment, kidney disease, cataract formation, and changes in the retina of the eye that impair vision. It can also contribute (along with other factors, such as high blood pressure, high blood fat levels, and smoking) to heart disease, stroke, and gangrene of the feet and legs.

Fortunately, proper control and care of diabetes can practically eliminate problems like diabetic coma. And most authorities believe that working to keep blood-sugar levels close to normal may help prevent many long-term complications as well.

DIAGNOSIS

Extreme thirst, urinary frequency, and unusual hunger are the three "classic" symptoms of diabetes—if you have these symptoms, diabetes will be the first thing to come to a doctor's mind. However, the classic symptoms do not always occur in people with non-insulin-dependent diabetes. Sometimes more subtle signs—such as confusion, constant fatigue, blurred vision, or cuts that take unusually long to heal—are the only outward indications of the disease. Or there may be no symptoms at all, with the first sign of trouble being an unusually high glucose level in a routine blood or urine test.

In any event, once diabetes is suspected, your doctor may use one or more blood tests to confirm the diagnosis. Your doctor may want to perform a fasting blood-sugar test, in which a blood sample will be taken in the morning, before you've eaten anything.

TREATMENT

If you are diagnosed as having NIDDM, the first course of action is to try to control blood sugar through diet and exercise alone. Dietary needs vary, so you'll need to work out a diet plan individually with your doctor or dietitian. Appropriate diet will successfully control diabetes in about one-half of older diabetics.

Lifestyle Changes   In general, a healthy diet for a person with diabetes includes a variety of food groups, derives most of its calories from whole-grain starchy foods, and is low in fats (especially saturated fats and cholesterol). Sugary foods, of course, need to be restricted. In addition, four out of five people with NIDDM need to lose weight, so there's a good chance your diet will be designed to cut calories.

Losing weight improves your body's ability to use its own insulin effectively to lower blood sugar.

Exercise is also essential in treating NIDDM. Aerobic exercise, the kind that gets your heart and lungs pumping, lowers blood sugar by burning glucose, and it can contribute to needed weight loss. Moreover, regular aerobic exercise, like weight loss, conditions your body cells to be more receptive to insulin and therefore to take glucose in from the blood with less of a struggle. Routine eye care and increased care of feet and nails are also standard practice.

Medicine—The Next Step   If diet and exercise don't succeed in keeping your blood sugar at desired levels, medicine is the next option. Insulin is one choice, and some doctors consider it the first choice. However, most doctors prefer to try an oral diabetes medicine first (see the chart on pages 685–689). Approximately 60–70 percent of older diabetics requiring medicine control their diabetes with oral medicines. Oral diabetes medicines are *not* substitutes for diet and exercise; to be most effective, they should be an addition to a treatment plan that already includes diet and exercise.

Insulin—There If You Need It   If an oral diabetes medicine fails to lower blood sugar adequately, you can count on daily injections of insulin to do the job. About 30 percent of older diabetics require insulin sometime in the course of their disease. If you do need to take insulin injections, you will need to eat your meals regularly and always carry some form of sugary food with you to treat low blood sugar (hypoglycemia) if it occurs. Signs of hypoglycemia include sweating, fainting, feeling very hot, weakness, tremors, unsteadiness, hunger, blurred vision, slurred speech, headache, tingling in feet or hands, seizures, nervousness, shakiness, and a general feeling of being sick. Your doctor will review and perhaps stop certain medicines such as beta-blocking agents (used for hypertension, angina, and other diseases of the heart) that may hide these warning signals when treatment for diabetes begins.

Keeping an Eye on Things In addition to following your diet and exercise routine and taking medicine if necessary, your doctor may also want you to test your urine or blood for glucose regularly. Urine tests are less accurate than self-performed blood tests, but they can be useful as a general indication that blood sugar is rising too high.

OUTLOOK

The list of tools for helping people with diabetes normalize their blood-sugar levels has grown tremendously in the last decade. By making the best use of these tools, doctors hope to prevent the long-term complications of the disease. Meanwhile, techniques for treating those complications if they occur have also improved; the most dramatic has been the perfection of laser treatments to prevent vision loss from diabetes-related eye disease.

Through such techniques as manipulating the immune system and transplanting insulin-making cells, researchers are looking at ways of preventing or curing insulin-dependent diabetes. And continuing research into how cells use insulin may lead to improved oral medicines for NIDDM.

CONDITION: **DIABETES MELLITUS**

CATEGORY: **ORAL ANTIDIABETIC AGENTS (SULFONYLUREAS)**

GENERIC (CHEMICAL) NAME	BRAND (TRADE) NAME	DOSAGE FORMS AND STRENGTHS
Acetohexamide	DYMELOR	Tablets: 250, 500 mg
Chlorpropamide	DIABINESE	Tablets: 100, 250 mg
Glipizide	GLUCOTROL	Tablets: 5, 10 mg
Glyburide	DIAβETA MICRONASE	Tablets: 1.25, 2.5, 5 mg Tablets: 1.25, 2.5, 5 mg
Tolazamide	RONASE TOLINASE	Tablets: 100, 250, 500 mg Tablets: 100, 250, 500 mg
Tolbutamide	ORINASE	Tablets: 250, 500 mg

DRUG PROFILE

These drugs, known collectively as sulfonylureas, are used to lower blood-glucose (sugar) levels in people with non-insulin-dependent diabetes (NIDDM) that is not controlled by diet alone. These agents are thought to work by stimulating the pancreas to produce insulin, a hormone that helps the body break down glucose for energy. They may also work by reducing the resistance to insulin.

BEFORE USING THIS DRUG

Let your doctor know *IF*

You have ever had allergic reactions or other problems with ■ any sulfonylureas ■ sulfonamides (sulfa drugs) ■ thiazide diuretics (water pills).

You have ever had any of the following medical problems: ■ porphyria ■ underactive pituitary gland ■ Addison's disease (underactive adrenal glands) ■ thyroid disease ■ kidney disease ■ liver disease ■ heart disease ■ recent severe infection.

You are taking any of the following medicines: ■ any other medicine for diabetes, including insulin or other sulfonylureas ■ anticoagulants (blood thinners) ■ medicine for asthma ■ medicine for seizures ■ aspirin or aspirinlike medicine ■ nonsteroidal anti-inflammatory agents ■ medicine for gout ■ diuretics, especially thiazide diuretics ■ sulfonamides (sulfa drugs) ■ medicine for depression ■ beta-blockers (eg, propranolol, atenolol, metoprolol, etc.) ■ medicine for ulcers (cimetidine or ranitidine) ■ calcium blockers (eg, diltiazem, nifedipine, verapamil, etc.) ■ estrogens ■ thyroid hormones ■ corticosteroids ■ tranquilizers ■ medicine for nausea or vomiting ■ androgens (male sex hormones) ■ nicotinic acid ■ isoniazid (medicine for tuberculosis) ■ antibiotics ■ clofibrate (medicine for high cholesterol) ■ medicine for high blood pressure ■ digoxin or digitalis (heart medicines) ■ appetite suppressants ■ barbiturates ■ any medicine containing alcohol ■ medicine to make the urine more or less acidic.

SPECIAL RESTRICTIONS WHILE TAKING THIS DRUG

FOOD AND DRUG INTERACTIONS

Other Drugs	It is a good idea to check with your doctor before taking any other medicines. Many drugs affect the way these drugs work. Let your doctor know about any other drugs you are taking, including over-the-counter (OTC) drugs.
Foods and Beverages	It is important to follow your doctor's diet recommendations. Do not skip meals. You may be advised to go on a weight-reduction diet.

Alcohol	Drinking alcohol while taking this drug may cause you to become hypoglycemic (to have low blood sugar). Some of these drugs, when combined with alcohol, may make you very sick. Avoid alcohol unless your doctor has approved its use.
Smoking	Smoking may worsen your medical condition. If you smoke, try to stop, or at least cut down.

DAILY LIVING

Exertion and Exercise	Appropriate exercise is an important part of the management of diabetes. Ask your doctor about an exercise program for you. Keep in mind that severe or prolonged exercise can sometimes result in hypoglycemia, so be careful not to overexert yourself.
Sun Exposure	Your skin may become more sensitive to sunlight and more likely to develop a sunburn while you are taking this drug. It is a good idea to avoid too much sun and to apply a sunscreen to exposed skin surfaces before going outdoors.
Examinations or Tests	It is very important for you to keep all appointments with your doctor so that your progress and reactions to therapy can be checked. Your doctor may instruct you to perform tests at home for sugar in blood or urine. If you are being switched from insulin to a sulfonylurea, you may be asked to perform a urine ketone test as well.
Other Precautions	Tell any doctor or dentist you consult that you are taking any of these drugs, especially if you will be undergoing any type of surgery.

If you become sick with a fever, let your doctor know; your body is under added stress when fighting off an infection, and you may need insulin to maintain blood sugar at normal levels. Also, let your doctor know if you are unable to eat because of severe nausea or vomiting.

You should keep something sweet with you (a piece of candy, for example) to eat immediately if you become hypoglycemic. Also, you should check your blood-sugar levels if you experience symptoms of hypoglycemia.

If you experience upset stomach with a sulfonylurea, let your doctor know; it may be possible to reduce your dosage.

No special restrictions on driving or exposure to excessive heat or cold.

POSSIBLE SIDE EFFECTS

Although this list of adverse effects may seem somewhat intimidating, keep in mind that some are quite rare. Not all of these effects have been reported with all sulfonylureas. Of course, should these or any other problems arise while you are on medication, it is always a good idea to consult your doctor.

IF YOU DEVELOP

signs of hypoglycemia: increased sweating; fainting; feeling very hot; weakness; tremors; unsteadiness; hunger; blurred vision; slurred speech; headache; tingling in feet or hands; seizures; nervousness; shakiness; pale, moist skin; pounding heart; rapid breathing; and a general ill feeling

WHAT TO DO

Urgent Get in touch with your doctor immediately, after first drinking a glass of orange juice or eating some candy.

rash, hives, itching, skin redness, or other skin problems ■ bleeding or bruising ■ sore throat or fever ■ yellowing of eyes or skin ■ pale stools ■ dark urine ■ severe diarrhea ■ confusion ■ nausea or vomiting ■ loss of appetite ■ depression ■ dizziness	**May be serious** Check with your doctor as soon as possible.
full feeling ■ heartburn ■ diarrhea ■ headache ■ increased skin sensitivity to sunlight ■ upset stomach ■ stomach cramps ■ constipation ■ weakness or tiredness ■ tingling or prickling feeling ■ drowsiness ■ gas ■ taste changes	If symptoms are disturbing or persist, let your doctor know.

STORAGE INSTRUCTIONS

Store in a cool, dark place (not in a bathroom medicine cabinet).

STOPPING OR INTERRUPTING THERAPY

If you miss a dose of this medicine, take it as soon as possible. If it is almost time for your next dose, skip the missed dose and resume your regular schedule. Do not take two doses at the same time.

SPECIAL CONSIDERATIONS FOR THOSE OVER SIXTY-FIVE

Older people are more prone to developing hypoglycemia with these drugs, particularly at night and especially if you are thin. Doctors may want to start people over sixty-five on a lower dosage and check their progress often.

THYROID DISEASE

Just as a conductor sets a proper tempo for a musical performance, your thyroid gland helps set the tempo for daily life. When the thyroid works properly, your many bodily processes, such as your heartbeat, digestion, and metabolism, all function at their optimum speeds. But when thyroid problems develop, it can seem as if the body's conductor has gone out of control, causing the body's tempo to speed up or slow down abnormally.

Problems with the thyroid—a butterfly-shaped gland perched around the windpipe in the neck—become somewhat more common in older persons. About one in fourteen elderly individuals have some form of thyroid disease. They also tend to be more common in women. Fortunately, though, the treatments for most thyroid conditions are very effective.

CAUSES

Your thyroid influences metabolic rate by means of several hormones it secretes into the bloodstream. The two main ones are T-4 (thyroxine) and T-3 (triiodothyronine). The gland varies its secretion of thyroid hormones in response to a number of chemical messages. In particular, another gland, the pituitary, strongly influences thyroid activity by secreting or withholding a substance called thyroid-stimulating hormone (TSH). This elaborate system of chemical checks and balances helps ensure that the body gets only as much thyroid hormone as it needs.

Thyroid disease can result if this series of controls goes awry. Some thyroid diseases are caused when the body's immune system mistakenly attacks the gland. Others may develop as a side effect of other diseases. Often, the cause of thyroid disease cannot be found.

Regardless of the cause, however, the result is generally either an overactive or an underactive gland. If you have an overactive thyroid (*hyperthyroidism*), your thyroid gland is usually enlarged (goiter) and you may experience such symptoms as fast heartbeat, increased sweating, high blood pressure, agitation, difficulty in sleeping, diarrhea, and bulging eyes. You may also find that you lose weight no matter how much you eat. However, about 40 percent of older people with hyperthyroidism do not experience an enlarged thyroid gland, nervousness, increased sweating, fast heartbeat, or bulging eyes. Instead, older patients may show such symptoms as abnormal heart rhythm, congestive heart failure, muscle wasting, poor appetite, and fatigue.

Symptoms of an underactive thyroid (*hypothyroidism*) are much the opposite. You may experience constant fatigue, a slow pulse, a feeling of coldness, constipation, coarse hair and puffy skin, slowness of movement, and mental dullness. People with an underactive thyroid often have high levels of lipids (fats) in the blood and can be at greater risk of developing atherosclerosis.

An enlarged thyroid gland, or goiter, can occur in a variety of thyroid conditions, both hyperthyroid and hypothyroid. Sometimes a goiter can develop even though there is no change in thyroid activity at all. Unless a goiter grows very large, it is seldom harmful in itself, though the condition that gave rise to it may need treatment. Iodine deficiency, once a major cause of goiters, is now rare in the United States.

Another possible thyroid problem is the growth of nodules, or lumps, on the gland. "Hot" thyroid nodules actively produce thyroid hormone and can contribute to hyperthyroidism; "cold" nodules produce no thyroid hormone. Thyroid nodules deserve special attention because they can sometimes become cancerous.

DIAGNOSIS

Symptoms can be useful in detecting thyroid trouble, but they can also be deceiving. In particular, many of the signs of hypothyroidism can look a great deal like the normal signs of aging. Fortunately, doctors have a wide range of tests at their disposal to help them diagnose thyroid problems.

Measurements of T-4 and T-3 in the blood are often the most direct evidence of an over- or underactive thyroid. In addition, the doctor will probably measure TSH. In hypothyroidism, TSH levels are high.

TREATMENT

In older persons, thyroid problems are most likely to involve an underactive gland. Treatment generally consists of replacing the missing thyroid hormones with oral thyroid supplements. Most doctors prescribe a drug called levothyroxine sodium, which is a synthetic form of T-4.

Oral thyroid hormone is generally taken once a day in the morning. Your doctor will probably start you on a low dose and increase it gradually over a period of several weeks. To work properly, it must be taken consistently over a long period of time. It should start improving some symptoms, such as fatigue, in a matter of weeks. Other symptoms will take longer to correct. To learn more about this type of treatment, check the drug chart on pages 693–696.

If you have an overactive thyroid, there are a number of treatments your doctor may initiate. Two medicines, propylthiouracil and methimazole, work directly on the thyroid gland to inhibit the secretion of thyroid hormone. Depending on the specific condition you have, it may be necessary for you to take these oral drugs for many years, or your doctor may tell you to discontinue their use once your thyroid activity is back to normal.

A more direct treatment approach is to partially destroy an overactive thyroid gland by using radioactive iodine. This highly effective treatment usually has to be done only once.

About half the time, it turns an overactive thyroid into an underactive one—still a plus, since hypothyroidism is much easier to control (using thyroid hormone tablets) than is hyperthyroidism.

Several medicines are commonly used in hyperthyroid states. Beta-blockers can be very effective in controlling a number of the consequences of hyperthyroidism, such as high blood pressure and rapid heart rate. Less frequently, oral iodide can be used to quickly return thyroid levels to normal by blocking the release of thyroid hormone from the gland.

Finally, surgical removal of part or all of a diseased thyroid gland is sometimes necessary, especially in the case of thyroid cancer or a dangerously enlarged goiter. If the entire thyroid must be taken out, the shortage of thyroid hormone can, again, easily be corrected with thyroid hormone tablets.

OUTLOOK

The number and range of thyroid tests continue to increase, making it easier for specialists to diagnose or rule out thyroid disease in the face of confusing symptoms. Meanwhile, doctors are becoming more adept at using such tools as medicine or radiation to make appropriate changes in thyroid functioning. As the trend toward more precise monitoring and control of thyroid activity continues, we can expect it to become easier and easier for doctors to keep the body running at a satisfying tempo. And it will be easier for people who have a thyroid condition to achieve a satisfying tempo in their daily lives.

CONDITION: **HYPOTHYROIDISM**

CATEGORY: **THYROID HORMONES**

GENERIC (CHEMICAL) NAME	BRAND (TRADE) NAME	DOSAGE FORMS AND STRENGTHS
Levothyroxine sodium	LEVOTHROID	Tablets: 0.025, 0.05, 0.075, 0.1, 0.125, 0.15, 0.175, 0.2, 0.3 mg
	SYNTHROID	Tablets: 0.025, 0.05, 0.075, 0.088, 0.1, 0.112, 0.125, 0.15, 0.175, 0.2, 0.3 mg
Liothyronine sodium	CYTOMEL	Tablets: 5, 25, 50 mcg
Liotrix	EUTHROID	Tablets: ½, 1, 2, 3 gr
Thyroglobulin	PROLOID	Tablets: 30, 60, 90, 120, 180 mg
Thyroid, desiccated	ARMOUR THYROID	Tablets: 15, 30, 60, 90, 120, 180, 240, 300 mg

DRUG PROFILE

Replacement thyroid hormones are prescribed when the thyroid gland does not produce enough natural thyroid hormone. This condition is called hypothyroidism, and it may occur spontaneously or as the result of thyroid removal, either by surgery or radiation therapy. Depending on the exact preparation used, your symptoms of thyroid deficiency should gradually disappear.

BEFORE USING THIS DRUG

Let your doctor know *IF*

You have ever had allergic reactions or other problems with ■ any thyroid medicines ■ pork products ■ corn ■ milk products (contained in levothyroxine) ■ tartrazine (FD&C Yellow Dye No. 5) (contained in Synthroid and some strengths of Euthroid).

You have ever had any of the following medical problems: ■ overactive thyroid ■ diabetes ■ heart disease, including heart attack and angina (chest pain) ■ high blood pressure ■ kidney disease ■ underactive adrenal gland or pituitary gland.

You are taking any of the following medicines: ■ anticoagulants (blood thinners) ■ beta-blockers (eg, propranolol, atenolol, metoprolol, etc.) ■ medicine for depression ■ digoxin or digitalis (heart medicines) ■ medicine for asthma containing adrenaline, ephedrine, or isoproterenol ■ cholestyramine, colestipol (medicine for high cholesterol) ■ medicine for diabetes ■ estrogens (female hormones) ■ androgens (male hormones) ■ corticosteroids ■ aspirin or aspirinlike medicine ■ phenylbutazone (medicine for arthritis) ■ tranquilizers ■ sleep medicines ■ narcotics or other prescription pain-killers ■ diet pills ■ amiodarone (medicine for abnormal heart rhythm).

SPECIAL RESTRICTIONS WHILE TAKING THIS DRUG

FOOD AND DRUG INTERACTIONS

No special restrictions on other drugs, foods and beverages, alcohol use, or smoking.

DAILY LIVING

Exertion and Exercise | In some kinds of heart disease, thyroid medicine may cause chest pain or shortness of breath when you exert yourself. If you have ever had any kind of heart disease, let your doctor know, and discuss what type of exercise and how much of it is safe for you.

Examinations or Tests	It is important for you to keep all appointments for laboratory or blood tests, since these tests will help your doctor adjust your dosage.
Other Precautions	Tell any doctor or dentist you consult that you are taking this medicine, especially if you will be undergoing any type of surgery.
	If you have diabetes, the dosage of your diabetes medicine may need to be adjusted while you are on thyroid hormone therapy. Your doctor may give you special instructions on testing your blood or urine for sugar.

No special restrictions on driving, sun exposure, or exposure to excessive heat or cold.

POSSIBLE SIDE EFFECTS

Although this list of adverse effects may seem somewhat intimidating, keep in mind that some are quite rare. Of course, should these or any other problems arise while you are on medication, it is always a good idea to consult your doctor.

IF YOU DEVELOP	WHAT TO DO
chest pain ■ irregular or fast heartbeat ■ shortness of breath ■ rash or hives ■ increased sweating ■ nervousness ■ sensitivity to heat	**Urgent** Get in touch with your doctor immediately.
increase in appetite ■ diarrhea ■ nausea or vomiting ■ tremors ■ headache ■ sleeplessness ■ fever ■ stomach cramps ■ weight loss	**May be serious** Check with your doctor as soon as possible.

STORAGE INSTRUCTIONS

Store in a cool, dark place (not in a bathroom medicine cabinet).

STOPPING OR INTERRUPTING THERAPY

If you have had thyroid surgery, you may need to take this medicine for the rest of your life. Do not stop taking this medicine without first checking with your doctor. If you miss a dose, take it as soon as possible. If it is almost time for your next dose, skip the missed dose and resume your regular schedule. Do not take two doses at the same time.

SPECIAL CONSIDERATIONS FOR THOSE OVER SIXTY-FIVE

Older people are often more sensitive to the effects of thyroid medicines. Doctors may start people over sixty-five on a low dosage and gradually increase the amount until it reaches a level that is effective. Older patients require a lower total dosage.

Chapter 9
Disorders of the
Respiratory System

RESPIRATORY INFECTIONS

THE COMMON COLD

It's been said that if you don't treat a cold, it'll last seven days, and that if you do take care of it, you'll be well in a week.

Colds are caused by viruses—lots of them. Doctors have identified more than one hundred sixty different types of viruses, which explains why you can catch so many colds in a lifetime. The immunity you develop to one type of cold virus doesn't help protect you against the other one hundred fifty-nine.

Cold viruses are spread through the air, from sneezing and coughing—we've known that for years. But what's now being shown is that cold viruses are often spread through hand-to-hand contact. For example, if you handle a phone or a glass that has been used by somebody with a cold, your chances of catching a cold rise sharply.

Colds often start slowly with that little tickle in the back of the throat. Within a few hours, your eyes begin to water, and you start sneezing and feeling congested. Within a day or two, you may develop a dry, hacking cough.

Treatment The diagnosis of a cold is not difficult. Doctors look at the season and the symptoms and prescribe accordingly. Although there's no cure for the cold, a variety of medicines can help you feel better while you're recovering.

Antihistamines, which are frequently used to relieve allergy symptoms, can help cold sufferers feel better by drying up the excess amounts of mucus that a cold produces. Decongestants shrink swollen blood vessels in the nose and the sinuses, thus clearing the passages to make breathing easier. Antihistamines and decongestants are also found in combination form. All three types of products are available over the counter, with somewhat stronger formulations available by prescription (see the drug charts on pages 703–705).

Analgesics, or pain-killers, such as aspirin or acetaminophen, can help you feel better during a cold by relieving fever, headache, and muscular pain. To help you cough up mucus or to quiet the cough so that you can get a good night's sleep, a cough suppressant may be prescribed (see the drug charts on pages 729–742).

Some over-the-counter pills for colds combine all these ingredients, serving as a kind of shotgun approach to cold symptoms.

Outlook Since time immemorial, people with colds have been told to stay warm, take it easy, and drink plenty of fluids. Fruit juices and hot drinks like tea and soups thin the mucus, making breathing easier. Studies have shown that chicken soup, which was called *Bubbiemycetin* by the *New England Journal of Medicine*, actually does make people feel better. The therapeutic benefit of chicken soup has been attributed to a combination of the steam, the liquid, the protein content, and maybe a little love.

Simple colds are self-limiting, and people usually feel better within a few days. However, a cold can sometimes develop into a more serious problem, such as acute sinusitis or acute bronchitis.

ACUTE SINUSITIS

The sinuses are nothing but trouble. No one knows their exact function, and we only notice them when they become infected.

Technically, the sinuses are hollow spaces in the bones of the face. There are four pairs of sinuses around the nose and eyes, all of which connect to the nasal passages by a narrow duct. Both the duct and the sinus cavities are lined with cilia, tiny little hairlike filaments that sweep mucus, as well as particles of dirt and bacteria, out of the nose and down the throat, finally to be destroyed in the stomach.

Trouble starts when a cold virus seemingly paralyzes the cilia. Mucus and bacteria accumulate in the sinuses, causing infection. As the cold runs its course, the trapped mucus causes pressure and facial pain, as well as headache, especially when a person bends over. Coming in the middle of a bad cold, such symptoms are a good sign of acute sinus infection. However, since they also signal an allergy, or even a dental infection, it may be necessary for the doctor to confirm the diagnosis by taking X rays

of the face from different angles. Normally, the sinus bones appear hollow and empty on an X ray, but if there's an infection, an accumulation of mucus and fluid will make the sinuses seem filled and solid.

Treatment If your symptoms and X rays all point to acute sinusitis, antibiotics and decongestants are called for. Antibiotics (see the drug charts on pages 706–729), given for ten days to two weeks, are necessary to knock out the bacterial infection. Your doctor may recommend that you take a decongestant to help drain the nasal passages (see section on colds). He or she may also suggest that you take an over-the-counter analgesic such as aspirin (see the drug charts on pages 748–749), acetaminophen, or ibuprofen (see the drug chart on page 750) to relieve sinus headache.

Outlook Most of the symptoms of even a bad sinus infection can be cleared up within a week. If acute sinusitis is not taken care of, you can develop chronic sinusitis that reappears over months or even years.

ACUTE BRONCHITIS

While most colds clear up within a week, some can develop into bronchitis—an inflammation of the bronchi, or air tubes, in the lungs. The hallmarks of bronchitis are an exhausting cough and fever. Usually, the cough produces thick, yellowish mucus, but many people can have a dry, hacking cough. Bronchitis can also follow a bout of influenza. Your doctor will usually rely on your description of your symptoms and a physical exam to make the diagnosis of bronchitis, though he or she may order a chest X ray to rule out pneumonia.

Treatment Although the cough of bronchitis is annoying and exhausting, doctors are reluctant to give medicine simply to still the cough reflex. The cough is an automatic reflex that helps the body clear airways of secretions and obstructions. Generally, coughs are divided into two types—productive coughs that bring up mucus and nonproductive, or dry, coughs.

Productive coughs should not be discouraged, inasmuch as bringing up mucus helps clear infection. Dry coughs should actually be made more productive to help rid the body of bacteria-laden phlegm. Expectorant drugs are sometimes prescribed to do just this—loosen mucus, though there is no evidence that these drugs actually work. If a cough is keeping you awake at night, your doctor may prescribe a cough suppressant (see the drug charts on pages 729–742). These products often contain codeine, which acts by blocking the nerve signals in the brain that trigger the cough reflex.

Outlook With proper medicine, acute bronchitis due to influenza or a bad cold should clear up within ten days to two weeks. However, if you suffer from chronic bronchitis and are a smoker, you may take longer to recover from the acute infection.

INFLUENZA

Each winter, along with snow, New Year's Eve, and football, comes the flu. The influenza season starts in late November and continues until March. During these months, up to 60 percent of people develop cough, high fever, and body ache, the classic trio of flu symptoms.

Influenza is not hard to diagnose. The symptoms, the season, and a physical exam will usually give the doctor the information he or she needs.

Prevention In most cases, flu means about a week of discomfort and time lost from work and other activities. But if you're over sixty-five, especially if you have a chronic health problem such as chronic lung disease, asthma, heart disease, or diabetes, the flu can develop into a serious form of pneumonia. Individuals with sarcoidosis or those who have recently undergone an organ transplant or are being treated for cancer by drug therapy are at risk as well.

Thus, with influenza, the best offense is a good defense. Medical authorities, such as the American College of Physicians, the Centers for Disease Control, and the American Geriatric Society, strongly recommend an annual flu vaccination (see the drug chart on pages 745–747) to protect against the current flu virus.

Unlike vaccinations for such other common viral diseases as measles or chickenpox, where a single shot confers long-lasting protection, flu shots must be given each year. The flu virus changes slightly from year to year, so the immunity you have against one type may not protect you against another.

The best time for the shot is in the early fall to allow the body to build up enough immunity in time for the flu season. The shots are safe and up to 80 percent protective in older people. Even in those cases where flu does develop, it is usually far milder than if you hadn't been immunized at all.

Treatment If the flu does strike, bed rest, aspirin or acetaminophen (see the drug charts on pages 748–749), fluids, and the appropriate cough medicine (see the drug charts on pages 729–742) will relieve symptoms until the disease runs its course. Unless bronchitis or pneumonia develops, there is usually no need for antibiotics.

In addition to these time-honored flu remedies, there is a drug that relieves symptoms and speeds recovery from some strains of influenza. Called amantadine, this medicine works by interfering with the replication and growth of the flu virus (see the drug chart on page 747–748). To be effective, amantadine must be given twenty-four to forty-eight hours after the onset of flu symptoms. The added benefit of amantadine is that it lessens the spread of disease to friends and family.

Short-lived side effects of amantadine are usually limited to insomnia and light-headedness. This drug also can be given to prevent influenza during an epidemic, but must be taken for four to six weeks to confer protection. Frequently, it is given to people with chronic illnesses as well as to older residents of nursing homes and hospitals to boost vaccination immunity.

Outlook The acute stages of influenza usually last a week to ten days. It may take another week to feel fully well and energetic. If the flu symptoms persist, or actually worsen after a week, it's a good idea to check with your doctor.

PNEUMOCOCCAL PNEUMONIA

While a variety of bacteria can cause pneumonia, most cases are due to a tiny organism called the pneumococcus. Each year, more than half a million people develop pneumococcal pneumonia, and nearly half of them are over the age of sixty.

Prevention Fortunately, there is a safe and effective vaccine that can protect adults against pneumococcal pneumonia (see the drug chart on pages 743–745). Only one shot of the vaccine is needed to confer permanent immunity.

Treatment If pneumococcal pneumonia does occur, its hallmark is severe chest pain in combination with fever; a dry, hacking cough; headache; and body ache. If a person who has had influenza or a cold develops these symptoms, a doctor might well suspect pneumonia and do further tests to confirm the diagnosis. He or she may look for the pneumococcus bacteria in the sputum that the person coughs up and do a chest X ray as well.

People with pneumococcal pneumonia are usually hospitalized and treated with antibiotics to reduce infection and with strong analgesics to relieve the chest pain. In addition, doctors can prescribe oxygen to help breathing and intravenous fluids to guard against dehydration.

VIRAL PNEUMONIA

Viral pneumonia is less serious than pneumococcal pneumonia but is still an important health problem during the winter months. It often begins with coldlike symptoms of sore throat, sneezing, and nasal congestion but soon develops into chest pains and a bad cough. By listening to the chest with a stethoscope the doctor can hear the characteristic rumbles called *rales* that are typical of pneumonia.

Treatment Bed rest, fluids, and a cough suppressant (see the drug charts on pages 729–742) are usually all that's required for recovery. Some doctors prescribe antibiotics (see the drug charts on pages 706–729) to prevent secondary infections such as bronchitis or bacterial pneumonia.

Caution: Some drugs in this section may affect pregnancy or fetal development. Check with your doctor if this concerns you.

CONDITION: **RESPIRATORY INFECTIONS**

CATEGORY: **ANTIHISTAMINES AND ANTIHISTAMINE-DECONGESTANT COMBINATIONS**

GENERIC (CHEMICAL) NAME	BRAND (TRADE) NAME	DOSAGE FORMS AND STRENGTHS
Azatadine maleate	OPTIMINE	Tablets: 1 mg
Clemastine fumarate	TAVIST	Syrup: 0.5 mg per tsp Tablets: 1, 2 mg
Chlorpheniramine maleate	CHLOR-TRIMETON	Sustained-release tablets: 8, 12 mg Tablets: 4 mg
Dexchlorpheniramine maleate	POLARAMINE	Controlled-release tablets: 4, 6 mg Syrup: 2 mg per tsp Tablets: 2 mg
Diphenhydramine hydrochloride	BENADRYL BENADRYL 25	Capsules: 25, 50 mg Elixir: 12.5 mg per tsp Capsules: 25 mg Tablets: 25 mg
Hydroxyzine hydrochloride	ATARAX	Syrup: 10 mg per tsp Tablets: 10, 25, 50, 100 mg
Hydroxyzine pamoate	VISTARIL	Capsules: 25, 50, 100 mg Suspension: 25 mg per tsp
Promethazine hydrochloride	PHENERGAN	Rectal suppositories: 12.5, 25, 50 mg Syrup: 6.25, 25 mg per tsp Tablets: 12.5, 25, 50 mg

Tripelennamine hydrochloride	PBZ	Elixir: tripelennamine citrate equivalent to 25 mg tripelennamine hydrochloride per tsp
		Tablets: 25, 50 mg
	PBZ-SR	Controlled-release tablets: 100 mg
Phenylpropanolamine hydrochloride and chlorpheniramine maleate	DEHIST	Controlled-release capsules: 75 mg phenylpropanolamine hydrochloride and 8 mg chlorpheniramine maleate

Many brands of antihistamines and antihistamine-decongestant combinations are sold over the counter as well.

DRUG PROFILE

When you are exposed to a substance to which you are allergic, a chemical called histamine is released into the bloodstream and produces the itchy, watery eyes; runny nose; and rashes that are typical of an allergic reaction. Antihistamines work by blocking the action of histamine. They are used to treat allergies as well as to relieve the symptoms of a cold. Antihistamines are sometimes combined in the same preparation with a decongestant, such as phenylpropanolamine. Phenylpropanolamine is thought to work by constricting blood vessels in the respiratory tract, shrinking the swollen membranes so that you are less congested and can breathe more easily. Hydroxyzine is also used to treat anxiety. Exactly how it works to relieve anxiety is not completely understood.

For complete information on these drugs, see pages 753–758.

CONDITION: **RESPIRATORY INFECTIONS**

CATEGORY: **ANTIHISTAMINES**

GENERIC (CHEMICAL) NAME	BRAND (TRADE) NAME	DOSAGE FORMS AND STRENGTHS
Astemizole	HISMANAL	Tablets: 10 mg
Terfenadine	SELDANE	Tablets: 60 mg

DRUG PROFILE

When you are exposed to a substance to which you are allergic, a chemical called histamine is released into the bloodstream and produces the itchy, watery eyes; runny nose; and rashes that are typical of an allergic reaction. Antihistamines block the action of histamine and are used to treat the symptoms of allergies, especially such seasonal allergies as hay fever.

For complete information on this drug, see pages 759–763.

CONDITION: **RESPIRATORY INFECTIONS**

CATEGORY: **ANTIBIOTICS (TETRACYCLINES)**

GENERIC (CHEMICAL) NAME	BRAND (TRADE) NAME	DOSAGE FORMS AND STRENGTHS
Demeclocycline hydrochloride	DECLOMYCIN	Capsules: 150 mg Tablets: 150, 300 mg
Doxycycline	VIBRAMYCIN	Capsules: 50, 100 mg Suspension: 25 mg per tsp Syrup: 50 mg per tsp
	VIBRATABS	Tablets: 100 mg
Minocycline	MINOCIN	Capsules: 50,100 mg Suspension: 50 mg per tsp Tablets: 50, 100 mg
Oxytetracycline	TERRAMYCIN	Capsules: 250 mg
Tetracycline hydrochloride	ACHROMYCIN V	Capsules: 250, 500 mg Suspension: 125 mg per tsp
	PANMYCIN	Capsules: 250 mg
	ROBITET	Capsules: 250, 500 mg
	SUMYCIN	Capsules: 250, 500 mg Tablets: 250, 500 mg

This type of drug is available under other brand names as well.

DRUG PROFILE

Tetracyclines are antibiotics that are used to treat a wide variety of bacterial infections, including skin eruptions and bronchitis and pneumonia. These antibiotics suppress the growth of the bacteria by interfering with their manufacture of protein.

BEFORE USING THIS DRUG

Let your doctor know *IF*

You have ever had any allergic reactions or other problems with ■ any tetracyclines.

You have ever had any of the following medical problems: ■ liver disease ■ kidney disease ■ diabetes ■ systemic lupus erythematosus ■ pancreas disease ■ myasthenia gravis ■ asthma, allergies, or hay fever.

You are taking any of the following medicines: ■ antacids ■ calcium supplements ■ iron supplements ■ any medicine containing magnesium, aluminum, or zinc ■ baking soda ■ penicillin ■ anticoagulants (blood thinners) ■ medicine for diarrhea ■ medicine to make the urine less acidic ■ methotrexate (medicine for cancer, severe rheumatoid arthritis, or severe psoriasis) ■ heart medicine (digoxin).

SPECIAL RESTRICTIONS WHILE TAKING THIS DRUG

FOOD AND DRUG INTERACTIONS

Other Drugs	Antacids containing calcium or magnesium; calcium, zinc, and iron supplements; and antidiarrheal preparations interfere with the absorption of this drug. Allow one to three hours between the time you take tetracycline and the time you take any of these substances.
Foods and Beverages	Some food (especially certain dairy products) interferes with the absorption of this drug. To avoid this interaction, it is best to take this drug on an empty stomach, at least one hour before or two hours after meals. This does not apply to doxycycline or minocycline.

No special restrictions on alcohol use or smoking.

DAILY LIVING

Driving	Minocycline may cause dizziness and drowsiness. If you are taking minocycline, be careful when driving, operating household appliances, or doing any other tasks that require alertness until you know how this drug affects you.
Sun Exposure	You are more likely to get a sunburn while taking this medicine. Therefore, it is a good idea to avoid too much sun while you are taking this medicine. If you feel a tingling or burning sensation on your hands, feet, or nose or any other unusual reaction after being exposed to the sun, let your doctor know right away.
Examinations or Tests	It is important for you to keep all appointments with your doctor, even if you feel well, so that your progress can be checked. If you are on long-term tetracycline therapy, periodic blood and urine tests are usually required.
Other Precautions	Tell any doctor or dentist you consult that you are taking this drug, especially if you will be undergoing any type of surgery. This drug causes tooth staining if given to children younger than fourteen.
Helpful Hints	This drug should be taken with a full glass of water. If this drug upsets your stomach, ask your doctor if it may be taken with food.

No special restrictions on exposure to excessive heat or cold.

POSSIBLE SIDE EFFECTS

Although this list of adverse effects may seem somewhat intimidating, keep in mind that some are quite rare. Of course, should these or any other problems arise while you are on medication, it is always a good idea to consult your doctor.

IF YOU DEVELOP

fever ■ severe diarrhea ■ difficulty in breathing ■ headache ■ joint pain ■ loose or discolored nails ■ worsening of any skin cuts ■ tingling and burning of hands, feet, or nose (after sun exposure) ■ tongue inflammation or discoloration ■ sore throat ■ hoarseness ■ blurred vision

With democycline only: increased urination ■ extreme thirst ■ extreme fatigue or weakness

WHAT TO DO

May be serious Check with your doctor as soon as possible.

cramps ■ diarrhea ■ bulky, loose stools ■ loss of appetite ■ gas ■ indigestion ■ difficulty in swallowing ■ rash, hives, or itching ■ nausea or vomiting ■ change in skin color ■ skin flushing ■ vaginal discharge ■ itching or swelling in the rectal or genital area ■ increased skin sensitivity to sunlight

With minocycline only: light-headedness or dizziness ■ drowsiness ■ tiredness ■ clumsiness

If symptoms are disturbing or persist, let your doctor know.

STORAGE INSTRUCTIONS

Store in a cool, dark place (not in a bathroom medicine cabinet). If your medicine is in a liquid form, make sure that it does not freeze. If the color, appearance, or taste of the medicine changes, or if the expiration date has passed, discard it immediately. If you are uncertain whether your medicine is all right, consult your pharmacist or doctor.

STOPPING OR INTERRUPTING THERAPY

Tetracyclines should be taken without interruption for the full length of time prescribed by your doctor even if you begin to feel better. This will ensure that the infection clears up completely and that your symptoms don't return. If after several days of therapy, your symptoms either do not improve or worsen, contact your doctor. If you miss a dose, take it as soon as possible. If it is almost time for your next dose, space the next two doses half the time apart they would usually be (for instance, if you were taking two doses a day twelve hours apart, space the missed dose and the next dose five to six hours apart).

SPECIAL CONSIDERATIONS FOR THOSE OVER SIXTY-FIVE

None.

CONDITION: **RESPIRATORY INFECTIONS**

CATEGORY: **ANTIBIOTICS (ERYTHROMYCINS)**

GENERIC (CHEMICAL) NAME	BRAND (TRADE) NAME	DOSAGE FORMS AND STRENGTHS
Erythromycin	E-MYCIN	Tablets: 250, 333 mg
	ERYC	Capsules: 125, 250 mg
	ERY-TAB	Tablets: 250, 333, 500 mg
	PCE	Tablets: 333, 500 mg
Erythromycin estolate	ILOSONE	Capsules: 250 mg
		Chewable tablets: 125, 250 mg
		Drops: 100 mg per ml
		Suspension: 125, 250 mg per tsp
		Tablets: 500 mg
Erythromycin ethylsuccinate	E.E.S.	Chewable tablets: 200 mg
		Drops: 100 mg per 2.5 ml

		Suspension: 200, 400 mg per tsp
		Suspension granules: 200 mg per tsp
		Tablets: 400 mg
	E-MYCIN E	Suspension: 200, 400 mg per tsp
	WYAMYCIN E	Suspension: 200, 400 mg per tsp
Erythromycin stearate	ERYTHROCIN Stearate	Tablets: 250, 500 mg
	WYAMYCIN S	Tablets: 250, 500 mg

This type of drug is available under other brand names as well.

DRUG PROFILE

Erythromycins are antibiotics that are used to treat a variety of bacterial infections, including such respiratory tract infections as bronchitis and pneumonia. These drugs suppress the growth of the bacteria and keep them from multiplying by blocking the bacteria's ability to manufacture protein.

BEFORE USING THIS DRUG

Let your doctor know *IF*

You have ever had allergic reactions or other problems with ■ any erythromycins.

You have ever had the following medical problem: ■ liver disease.

You are taking any of the following medicines: ■ other antibiotics ■ theophylline (medicine for asthma) ■ carbamazepine (medicine for seizures) ■ anticoagulants (blood thinners) ■ corticosteroids ■ digoxin or digitalis (heart medicines) ■ cyclosporine.

SPECIAL RESTRICTIONS WHILE TAKING THIS DRUG

FOOD AND DRUG INTERACTIONS

No special restrictions on other drugs, foods and beverages, alcohol use, or smoking.

DAILY LIVING

Examinations or Tests	It is important for you to keep all appointments with your doctor, even if you feel well, so that your progress can be checked.
Other Precautions	While you are taking this drug, you may develop fungal infections of the mouth, anus, or vagina. Let your doctor know if you develop itching, burning, soreness, or general irritation in the anal or vaginal area; a white vaginal discharge; or a white coating on the inside of your mouth.
Helpful Hints	This drug is best taken with a full glass of water on an empty stomach unless otherwise directed by your doctor.
	Chewable tablets should be chewed or crushed before swallowing; do not swallow them whole. Capsules or coated tablets should be swallowed whole.

No special restrictions on driving, exertion and exercise, sun exposure, or exposure to excessive heat or cold.

POSSIBLE SIDE EFFECTS

Although this list of adverse effects may seem somewhat intimidating, keep in mind that some are quite rare. Of course, should these or any other problems arise while you are on medication, it is always a good idea to consult your doctor.

IF YOU DEVELOP	WHAT TO DO
severe stomach pain or cramps ■ dark urine ■ pale stools ■ extreme tiredness or weakness ■ yellowing of eyes or skin ■ vomiting, with blood ■ bloody stools	**Urgent** Get in touch with your doctor immediately.
hearing loss	**May be serious** Check with your doctor as soon as possible.
diarrhea ■ nausea or vomiting ■ upset stomach ■ heartburn ■ loss of appetite ■ sore mouth or tongue ■ rash, hives, or itching ■ itching in the vaginal or anal area	If symptoms are disturbing or persist, let your doctor know.

STORAGE INSTRUCTIONS

Store in a cool, dark place (not in a bathroom medicine cabinet). If your medicine is in a liquid form, make sure that it does not freeze.

STOPPING OR INTERRUPTING THERAPY

Erythromycins should be taken without interruption for the full length of time prescribed by your doctor, even if you begin to feel better. This will ensure that the infection clears up completely and that your symptoms do not return. If you miss a dose, take it as soon as possible and resume your regular schedule. If it is almost time for your next dose, double that next dose.

SPECIAL CONSIDERATIONS FOR THOSE OVER SIXTY-FIVE

None.

CONDITION: **RESPIRATORY INFECTIONS**

CATEGORY: **ANTIBIOTICS (PENICILLINS)**

GENERIC (CHEMICAL) NAME	BRAND (TRADE) NAME	DOSAGE FORMS AND STRENGTHS
Amoxicillin	AMOXIL	Capsules: 250, 500 mg Chewable tablets: 125, 250 mg Suspension: 125, 250 mg per tsp
	LAROTID	Capsules: 250, 500 mg Suspension: 125, 250 mg per tsp
	POLYMOX	Capsules: 250, 500 mg Suspension: 125, 250 mg per tsp
	TRIMOX	Capsules: 250, 500 mg Suspension: 125, 250 mg per tsp
Ampicillin	AMCILL	Capsules: 250, 500 mg Suspension: 125, 250 mg per tsp
	OMNIPEN	Capsules: 250, 500 mg Suspension: 125, 250 mg per tsp
	POLYCILLIN	Capsules: 250, 500 mg Suspension: 125, 250, 500 mg per tsp
	TOTACILLIN	Capsules: 250, 500 mg Suspension: 125, 250 mg per tsp
Bacampicillin hydrochloride	SPECTROBID	Suspension: 125 mg per tsp Tablets: 400 mg

Carbenicillin indanyl sodium	GEOCILLIN	Tablets: 382 mg
Cloxacillin sodium	TEGOPEN	Capsules: 250, 500 mg Solution: 125 mg per tsp
Cyclacillin	CYCLAPEN-W	Suspension: 125, 250 mg per tsp Tablets: 250, 500 mg
Nafcillin sodium	UNIPEN	Capsules: 250 mg Solution: 250 mg per tsp Tablets: 500 mg
Oxacillin sodium	PROSTAPHLIN	Capsules: 250, 500 mg Solution: 250 mg per tsp
Penicillin G potassium	PENTIDS	Tablets: 125, 250, 500 mg
Penicillin V potassium	LEDERCILLIN VK	Solution: 125, 250 mg per tsp Tablets: 250, 500 mg
	PEN•VEE•K	Solution: 125, 250 mg per tsp Tablets: 250, 500 mg
	V-CILLIN K	Solution: 125, 250 mg per tsp Tablets: 125, 250, 500 mg

This type of drug is available under other brand names as well.

DRUG PROFILE

Penicillins are antibiotics that are used to treat a wide variety of bacterial infections, including infections of the ear, nose, and throat and such respiratory tract infections as bronchitis and pneumonia. Penicillins suppress the growth of bacteria by interfering with the bacteria's ability to form new protective cell walls.

BEFORE USING THIS DRUG

Let your doctor know *IF*

You have ever had allergic reactions or other problems with ■ any penicillins ■ procaine (an anesthetic or heart drug) ■ cephalosporins or griseofulvin (antibiotics) ■ penicillamine (medicine for arthritis) ■ tartrazine (FD&C Yellow Dye No. 5) ■ aspirin ■ any other medicine.

You have ever had any of the following medical problems: ■ any allergy ■ bleeding problems ■ kidney disease ■ liver disease ■ stomach or intestinal problems.

You are taking any of the following medicines: ■ any other medicine for infection (antibiotics) ■ medicine for gout ■ medicine for arthritis ■ medicine for seizures ■ anticoagulants (blood thinners) ■ Antabuse (used in treatment of alcoholism) ■ aspirin or aspirinlike medicine ■ triamterene, spironolactone, or amiloride (potassium-sparing diuretics) ■ medicine for high cholesterol ■ medicine for diarrhea.

SPECIAL RESTRICTIONS WHILE TAKING THIS DRUG

FOOD AND DRUG INTERACTIONS

Other Drugs	If you need to take medicine for diarrhea, check with your doctor. Penicillin, when taken with medicine for diarrhea, may make the diarrhea more severe. If you are taking the drug colestipol for high cholesterol, take your dose of penicillin at least one hour before or four hours after your dose of colestipol.
Foods and Beverages	If you are taking penicillin G, do not drink any acidic juices (eg, orange, grapefruit, tomato) for at least an hour before and after you take your medicine. Such juices may reduce the effect of this type of penicillin.

No special restrictions on alcohol use or smoking.

DAILY LIVING

Examinations or Tests

It is important for you to keep all appointments with your doctor, even if you feel well, so that your progress can be checked. If you are on long-term penicillin therapy, periodic blood and urine tests may be required.

Other Precautions

Tell any doctor or dentist you consult that you are taking this drug, especially if you will be undergoing any type of surgery.

People with diabetes may find that this drug causes false results in urine-sugar tests. Check with your doctor to see if you need another kind of diabetes medicine or if you should use a different kind of test.

While you are taking this drug, you may develop fungal infections of the mouth, anus, or vagina. Let your doctor know if you develop itching, burning, soreness, or general irritation in the anal or vaginal area, a white vaginal discharge, or a white coating on the inside of your mouth.

Helpful Hints

This drug is best taken with a full glass of water on an empty stomach unless otherwise directed by your doctor.

Chewable tablets should be chewed or crushed before swallowing; do not swallow them whole.

No special restrictions on driving, exertion and exercise, sun exposure, or exposure to excessive heat or cold.

POSSIBLE SIDE EFFECTS

Although this list of adverse effects may seem somewhat intimidating, keep in mind that some are quite rare. Of course, should these or any other problems arise while you are on medication, it is always a good idea to consult your doctor.

IF YOU DEVELOP	WHAT TO DO
difficulty in breathing ■ fever or chills ■ severe dizziness or fainting ■ tightness in throat ■ severe stomach cramps ■ severe diarrhea ■ rash or hives ■ purplish or brownish-red spots on skin ■ extreme tiredness or weakness ■ seizures ■ bleeding or bruising ■ extreme thirst ■ blood in urine or other urine changes ■ difficulty in urination ■ swelling of face or ankles ■ yellowing of eyes or skin ■ pale stools ■ bluish tinge to the skin ■ severe nausea and vomiting ■ excessive sweating	**Urgent** Get in touch with your doctor immediately.
itching ■ general ill feeling ■ bone or muscle pain ■ swollen lymph glands ■ rapid weight loss	**May be serious** Check with your doctor as soon as possible.
mild diarrhea or loose stools ■ gas ■ nausea or vomiting ■ upset stomach ■ sore mouth ■ sore tongue or black, hairy tongue ■ stomach cramps ■ headache ■ dizziness	If symptoms are disturbing or persist, let your doctor know.

STORAGE INSTRUCTIONS

Store in a cool, dark place (not in a bathroom medicine cabinet). If your medicine is in a liquid form, make sure that it does not freeze.

STOPPING OR INTERRUPTING THERAPY

Penicillins should be taken without interruption for the full length of time prescribed by your doctor, even if you begin to feel better. This will ensure that the infection clears up completely and that your symptoms do not return. If you miss a dose, take it as soon as possible and resume your regular schedule. If it is almost time for your next dose, double that next dose.

SPECIAL CONSIDERATIONS FOR THOSE OVER SIXTY-FIVE

Older people may be more prone to developing diarrhea while taking amoxicillin, ampicillin, bacampicillin, and cyclacillin.

CONDITION: **RESPIRATORY INFECTIONS**
CATEGORY: **ANTIBIOTICS (CEPHALOSPORINS)**

GENERIC (CHEMICAL) NAME	BRAND (TRADE) NAME	DOSAGE FORMS AND STRENGTHS
Cefaclor	CECLOR	Capsules: 250, 500 mg Suspension: 125, 187, 250, 375 mg per tsp
Cefadroxil	DURICEF	Capsules: 500 mg Suspension: 125, 250, 500 mg per tsp Tablets: 1 g
	ULTRACEF	Capsules: 500 mg Suspension: 125, 250 mg per tsp Tablets: 1 g
Cefixime	SUPRAX	Suspension: 100 mg per tsp Tablets: 200, 400 mg
Cefuroxime	CEFTIN	Tablets: 125, 250, 500 mg
Cephalexin	KEFLEX	Capsules: 250, 500 mg Suspension: 125, 250 mg per tsp Drops: 100 mg per ml
	KEFLET	Tablets: 250, 500 mg Tablets: 1 g
Cephalexin Hcl	KEFTAB	Tablets: 250, 500 mg

Cephradine	ANSPOR	Capsules: 250, 500 mg Suspension: 125, 250 mg per tsp
	VELOSEF	Capsules: 250, 500 mg Suspension: 125, 250 mg per tsp

This type of drug is available under other brand names as well.

DRUG PROFILE

Cephalosporins are antibiotics that are used to treat a wide variety of bacterial infections, including such upper respiratory tract infections as bronchitis and pneumonia. These drugs work by interfering with the bacteria's ability to multiply and to form new protective cell walls.

BEFORE USING THIS DRUG

Let your doctor know *IF*

You have ever had any allergic reactions or other problems with ▪ any cephalosporins ▪ any penicillins ▪ any other antibiotics ▪ penicillamine (medicine for arthritis) ▪ any other medicine.

You have ever had any of the following medical problems: ▪ stomach or intestinal problems, especially colitis ▪ kidney disease ▪ liver disease ▪ bleeding disorders.

You are taking any of the following medicines: ▪ medicine for diarrhea ▪ probenicid (medicine for gout) ▪ any medicine containing alcohol ▪ anticoagulants (blood thinners) ▪ any other antibiotics.

SPECIAL RESTRICTIONS WHILE TAKING THIS DRUG

FOOD AND DRUG INTERACTIONS

Other Drugs	If you need to take medicine for diarrhea, check with your doctor. Cephalosporins, when taken with medicine for diarrhea, may make the diarrhea more severe.

Alcohol	Avoid alcohol while on cephalosporin therapy. The combination of alcohol and some cephalosporins may cause flushing, headache, shortness of breath, nausea, vomiting, dizziness, fainting, chest pain, and irregular or fast heartbeat.

No special restrictions on foods and beverages or smoking.

DAILY LIVING

Examinations or Tests	It is important for you to keep all appointments with your doctor, even if you feel well, so that your progress can be checked.
Other Precautions	People with diabetes may find that this drug causes false results in urine-sugar tests. Check with your doctor to see if you need another kind of diabetes medicine or if you should use a different kind of test. While you are taking this drug, you may develop fungal infections of the mouth, anus, or vagina. Let your doctor know if you develop itching, burning, soreness, or general irritation in the anal or vaginal area; a white vaginal discharge; or a white coating on the inside of your mouth.
Helpful Hints	Take this medicine with a full glass of water on an empty stomach. If it causes upset stomach, speak to your doctor to see if you can take it with meals or snacks.

No special restrictions on driving, exertion and exercise, sun exposure, or exposure to excessive heat or cold.

POSSIBLE SIDE EFFECTS

Although this list of adverse effects may seem somewhat intimidating, keep in mind that some are quite rare. Of course, should these or any other problems arise while you are on medication, it is always a good idea to consult your doctor.

IF YOU DEVELOP	WHAT TO DO
severe stomach cramps ■ severe diarrhea ■ fever or chills ■ extreme weakness or fatigue ■ excessive thirst ■ swelling in any part of the body	**Urgent** Get in touch with your doctor immediately.
joint pain ■ rapid weight loss ■ difficulty in urination or defecation	**May be serious** Check with your doctor as soon as possible.
mild diarrhea ■ upset stomach ■ nausea or vomiting ■ stomach pain ■ sore mouth or tongue ■ heartburn ■ skin redness, rash, hives, itching, or other skin problems	If symptoms are disturbing or persist, let your doctor know.

STORAGE INSTRUCTIONS

Store in a cool, dark place (not in a bathroom medicine cabinet). If your medicine is in a liquid form, make sure that it does not freeze.

STOPPING OR INTERRUPTING THERAPY

Cephalosporins should be taken without interruption for the full length of time prescribed by your doctor, even if you begin to feel better. This will ensure that the infection clears up completely and that your symptoms don't return. If you miss a dose, take it as soon as possible and resume your regular schedule. If it is almost time for your next dose, double that next dose.

SPECIAL CONSIDERATIONS FOR THOSE OVER SIXTY-FIVE

Because this drug is excreted by the kidneys, and kidney function commonly decreases with age, doctors may start people over sixty-five on a lower dosage.

CONDITION: **RESPIRATORY INFECTIONS**
CATEGORY: **ANTIBIOTICS (QUINOLONES)**

GENERIC (CHEMICAL) NAME	BRAND (TRADE) NAME	DOSAGE FORMS AND STRENGTHS
Ciprofloxacin hydrochloride	CIPRO	Tablets: 250, 500, 750 mg
Ofloxacin	FLOXIN	Tablets 200, 300, 400 mg

DRUG PROFILE

Ciprofloxacin and ofloxacin are antibiotics used to treat a variety of bacterial infections. These include such respiratory tract infections as bronchitis and pneumonia as well as urinary tract infections. These drugs kill bacteria by interfering with the bacteria's genetic material.

BEFORE USING THIS DRUG

Let your doctor know *IF*

You have ever had allergic reactions or other problems with ■ ciprofloxacin ■ ofloxacin ■ nalidixic acid ■ norfloxacin.

You have ever had any of the following medical problems: ■ kidney disease ■ liver disease ■ epilepsy (seizures) ■ spinal cord or brain disease, including hardening of the arteries in the brain.

You are taking any of the following medicines: ■ theophylline ■ antacids ■ probenecid (medicine for gout) ■ sucralfate (medicine for ulcers).

SPECIAL RESTRICTIONS WHILE TAKING THIS DRUG

FOOD AND DRUG INTERACTIONS

Other Drugs	Antacids containing aluminum or magnesium interfere with the absorption of this drug. Allow two hours between the time you take this medicine and the time you take this kind of antacid.

No special restrictions on foods and beverages, alcohol use, or smoking.

DAILY LIVING

Driving	These medicines may cause drowsiness, light-headedness, or vision disturbances. Be careful when driving, operating household appliances, or doing any other tasks that require alertness until you know how this drug affects you.
Sun Exposure	You are more likely to get a sunburn while taking this medicine. Therefore, it is a good idea to avoid too much sun while you are taking this medicine. If you feel a tingling or burning sensation on your hands, feet, or nose or any other unusual reaction after being exposed to the sun, let your doctor know right away.
Examinations or Tests	It is important for you to keep all appointments with your doctor, even if you feel well, so that your progress can be checked. Blood and urine tests may be required.

Other Precautions

Tell any doctor or dentist you consult that you are taking these drugs.

While you are taking these drugs, you may develop fungal infections of the mouth, anus, or vagina. Let your doctor know if you develop itching, burning, soreness, or general irritation in the anal or vaginal area; a white vaginal discharge; or a white coating on the inside of your mouth.

Helpful Hints

It is best to take ofloxacin on an empty stomach, that is, one hour before or two hours after a meal. Make sure you drink plenty of water—several glasses a day in addition to your regular liquid intake—in order to avoid urinary side effects. However ciprofloxacin may be taken without regard to meals.

No special restrictions on exertion and exercise or exposure to excessive heat or cold.

POSSIBLE SIDE EFFECTS

Although this list of adverse effects may seem somewhat intimidating, keep in mind that some are quite rare. Of course, should these or any other problems arise while you are on medication, it is always a good idea to consult your doctor.

IF YOU DEVELOP

shakiness ■ restlessness ■ seizures ■ light-headedness ■ dizziness ■ confusion ■ hallucinations ■ blurred vision or other vision problems ■ headache ■ increased sensitivity of skin to sunlight ■ difficulty swallowing ■ mood/behavior changes ■ swelling of eyes, face, neck, lips, hands ■ trouble breathing ■ shortness of breath ■ bronchospasm ■ hoarseness ■ lower back pain ■ blood in urine, or pain when urinating

WHAT TO DO

Urgent Get in touch with your doctor immediately.

nausea or vomiting ■ abdominal or stomach pain
■ diarrhea ■ drowsiness ■ pain or stiffness in joints
■ rash, itching, or reddened skin ■ sleeplessness
■ unpleasant taste

If symptoms are disturbing
or persist, let your doctor
know.

STORAGE INSTRUCTIONS

Store in a cool, dark place (not in a bathroom medicine cabinet).

STOPPING OR INTERRUPTING THERAPY

Take this drug without interruption for the full length of time prescribed by your doctor, even if you begin to feel better. This will ensure that the infection clears up completely and that your symptoms do not return. If you miss a dose, take it as soon as possible. If it is almost time for your next dose, skip the missed dose and resume your regular schedule. Do not take two doses at the same time.

SPECIAL CONSIDERATIONS FOR THOSE OVER SIXTY-FIVE

Because this drug is excreted by the kidney, and some elderly patients may have decreased kidney function, doctors may start certain older patients at a lower dosage of this drug.

CONDITION: **RESPIRATORY INFECTIONS**

CATEGORY: **OTHER ANTIBIOTICS**

GENERIC (CHEMICAL) NAME	BRAND (TRADE) NAME	DOSAGE FORMS AND STRENGTHS
Clindamycin hydrochloride	CLEOCIN HCl	Capsules: 75, 150, 300 mg

DRUG PROFILE

Clindamycin is used to treat bacterial infections, including such infections of the respiratory tract as strep throat and pneumonia. This drug suppresses the growth of bacteria and keeps them from multiplying by blocking the bacteria's ability to manufacture cell protein.

BEFORE USING THIS DRUG

Let your doctor know *IF*

You have ever had allergic reactions or other problems with ■ clindamycin ■ lincomycin ■ tartrazine (FD&C Yellow Dye No. 5) ■ aspirin.

You have ever had any of the following medical problems: ■ kidney disease ■ liver disease ■ stomach or intestinal problems ■ myasthenia gravis.

You are taking any of the following medicines: ■ other antibiotics ■ medicine for diarrhea ■ narcotics or other prescription pain-killers.

SPECIAL RESTRICTIONS WHILE TAKING THIS DRUG

FOOD AND DRUG INTERACTIONS

Other Drugs	If you need to take medicine for diarrhea, check with your doctor. Clindamycin, when taken with medicine for diarrhea, may make the diarrhea more severe.

No special restrictions on foods and beverages, alcohol use, or smoking.

DAILY LIVING

Examinations or Tests	It is important for you to keep all appointments with your doctor, even if you feel well, so that your progress can be checked. If you are on long-term therapy or if you have liver or kidney disease, periodic blood and urine tests may be required.
Other Precautions	Tell any doctor or dentist you consult that you are taking this drug, especially if you will be undergoing any type of surgery.

While you are taking this drug, you may develop fungal infections of the mouth, anus, or vagina. Let your doctor know if you develop itching, burning, soreness, or general irritation in the anal or vaginal area; a white vaginal discharge; or a white coating on the inside of your mouth.

| Helpful Hints | Take this medicine with a full glass of water to avoid irritating the esophagus. |

No special restrictions on driving, exertion and exercise, or exposure to excessive heat or cold.

POSSIBLE SIDE EFFECTS

Although this list of adverse effects may seem somewhat intimidating, keep in mind that some are quite rare. Of course, should these or any other problems arise while you are on medication, it is always a good idea to consult your doctor.

IF YOU DEVELOP	WHAT TO DO
stomach pain or cramps ■ severe diarrhea ■ severe nausea and vomiting ■ fever ■ extreme thirst ■ extreme weakness ■ yellowing of the eyes or skin	**Urgent** Get in touch with your doctor immediately.
rapid weight loss ■ joint pain ■ difficulty in urination or defecation ■ loss of appetite	**May be serious** Check with your doctor as soon as possible.
diarrhea ■ gas or bloating ■ rash or itching ■ itching in genital or anal area	If symptoms are disturbing or persist, let your doctor know.

STORAGE INSTRUCTIONS

Store in a cool, dark place (not in a bathroom medicine cabinet).

STOPPING OR INTERRUPTING THERAPY

Clindamycin should be taken without interruption for the full length of time prescribed by your doctor, even if you begin to feel better. This will ensure that the infection clears up completely and that your symptoms do not return. If you miss a dose, take it as soon as possible and resume your regular schedule. If it is almost time to take your next dose, double that next dose.

SPECIAL CONSIDERATIONS FOR THOSE OVER SIXTY-FIVE

Older people who are very ill can be particularly susceptible to such side effects of clindamycin as diarrhea.

CONDITION: **COUGH**

CATEGORY: **COUGH SUPPRESSANTS**

GENERIC (CHEMICAL) NAME	BRAND (TRADE) NAME	DOSAGE FORMS AND STRENGTHS
Benzonatate	TESSALON	Capsules: 100 mg

DRUG PROFILE

Benzonatate is used to treat the dry cough associated with acute infections including the common cold, bronchitis, and pneumonia, as well as such chronic conditions as emphysema, bronchial asthma, and tuberculosis. This drug works by inhibiting the cough reflex, both in the brain center that stimulates coughing and in the nerves of the respiratory tract.

BEFORE USING THIS DRUG

Let your doctor know *IF*

You have ever had allergic reactions or other problems with ■ benzonatate.

You are taking any of the following medicines: ■ any local anesthetics.

SPECIAL RESTRICTIONS WHILE TAKING THIS DRUG

FOOD AND DRUG INTERACTIONS

No special restrictions on other drugs, foods and beverages, alcohol use, or smoking.

DAILY LIVING

Examinations or Tests	It is important for you to keep all appointments with your doctor so that your progress can be checked.
Helpful Hints	Swallow the capsules whole. They contain an anesthetic that could make your mouth and throat temporarily numb and cause choking if you chew or crush them.
Driving	This drug may cause drowsiness or dizziness. Be careful driving until you know how this medicine affects you.

No special restrictions on exertion and exercise, sun exposure, or exposure to excessive heat or cold.

POSSIBLE SIDE EFFECTS

Although this list of adverse effects may seem somewhat intimidating, keep in mind that some are quite rare. Of course, should these or any other problems arise while you are on medication, it is always a good idea to consult your doctor.

IF YOU DEVELOP	WHAT TO DO
convulsions ■ restlessness ■ tremors	**Urgent** Get in touch with your doctor immediately.

numbness in chest	**May be serious** Check with your doctor as soon as possible.
headache ■ drowsiness ■ dizziness ■ rash or itching ■ stuffy nose ■ constipation ■ upset stomach ■ nausea ■ eye irritation ■ chills	If symptoms are disturbing or persist, let your doctor know.

STORAGE INSTRUCTIONS

Store in a cool, dark place (not in a bathroom medicine cabinet).

STOPPING OR INTERRUPTING THERAPY

Benzonatate should be taken without interruption for the full length of time prescribed by your doctor. If you miss a dose, take it as soon as possible. If it is almost time for your next dose, skip the missed dose and resume your regular schedule. Do not take two doses at the same time.

SPECIAL CONSIDERATIONS FOR THOSE OVER SIXTY-FIVE

None.

CONDITION: **COUGH**

CATEGORY: **COUGH SUPPRESSANTS**

GENERIC (CHEMICAL) NAME	BRAND (TRADE) NAME	DOSAGE FORMS AND STRENGTHS
Hydrocodone bitartrate and homatropine methylbromide	HYCODAN	Syrup: 5 mg hydrocodone bitartrate and 1.5 mg homatropine methylbromide per tsp Tablets: 5 mg hydrocodone bitartrate and 1.5 mg homatropine methylbromide

DRUG PROFILE

This combination drug is used to treat coughs. Hydrocodone inhibits the cough reflex in the brain center that stimulates coughing, dries the membranes of the respiratory tract, and thins out the mucus in the respiratory tract so that it can be coughed up more easily. Homatropine also has a drying effect on the respiratory tract.

BEFORE USING THIS DRUG

Let your doctor know *IF*

You have ever had allergic reactions or other problems with ■ hydrocodone ■ homatropine ■ atropine ■ belladonna.

You have ever had any of the following medical problems: ■ head injury ■ seizures ■ asthma or other lung disease ■ enlarged prostate ■ urinary problems ■ glaucoma ■ kidney disease ■ liver disease ■ abnormal heart rhythms ■ alcoholism ■ colitis or other intestinal problems ■ underactive thyroid ■ gallbladder disease.

You are taking any of the following medicines: ■ medicine for glaucoma ■ antihistamines ■ medicine for seizures ■ barbiturates ■ muscle relaxants ■ tranquilizers ■ sleep medicines ■ medicine for depression ■ narcotics or other prescription pain-killers ■ cimetidine (medicine for ulcers).

SPECIAL RESTRICTIONS WHILE TAKING THIS DRUG

FOOD AND DRUG INTERACTIONS

Other Drugs	Do not take any other drugs, including over-the-counter (OTC) drugs, before checking with your doctor. This medicine increases the effect of drugs that depress the central nervous system, such as antihistamines; medicine for hay fever, allergies, or colds; sleep medicines; tranquilizers; narcotics or other prescription pain-killers; muscle relaxants; and medicine for seizures.
Alcohol	This drug increases the effect of alcohol, a central nervous system depressant. Avoid alcohol unless your doctor has approved its use.

No special restrictions on foods and beverages or smoking.

DAILY LIVING

Driving

This drug may cause drowsiness, light-headedness, or dizziness, as well as loss of alertness and coordination. Be careful when driving, operating household appliances, or doing any other tasks that require alertness until you know how this drug affects you.

Examinations or Tests

It is important for you to keep all appointments with your doctor so that your progress can be checked.

Other Precautions

Tell any doctor or dentist you consult that you are taking this drug, especially if you will be undergoing any type of surgery.

Taking this medicine more often or for a longer period of time than prescribed by your doctor may make it habit-forming. If you accidentally take an overdose of this medicine, call your doctor or go to an emergency room immediately.

Helpful Hints

You may vomit or feel nauseated when you first start taking this drug. If this happens, lie down until you feel better. You also may experience dizziness or light-headedness, especially when getting up from a reclining or sitting position. Getting up slowly may help prevent this.

No special restrictions on exertion and exercise, sun exposure, or exposure to excessive heat or cold.

POSSIBLE SIDE EFFECTS

Although this list of adverse effects may seem somewhat intimidating, keep in mind that some are quite rare. Of course, should these or any other problems arise while you are on medication, it is always a good idea to consult your doctor.

IF YOU DEVELOP

difficulty in breathing ■ severe dizziness ■ severe drowsiness ■ blurred vision or other visual disturbances ■ agitation ■ delirium ■ extreme restlessness or nervousness ■ slow heartbeat ■ severe weakness ■ seizures ■ confusion ■ hallucinations ■ swelling of face

eye pain ■ rash, hives, or itching ■ depression ■ sleeplessness ■ faintness ■ ringing in the ears ■ fast heartbeat ■ shallow breathing ■ stomach pain

dizziness or light-headedness, especially when getting up from a reclining or sitting position ■ constipation ■ drowsiness ■ nausea or vomiting ■ flushing or warm feeling ■ sexual problems ■ difficulty in urination or decreased urination ■ increased sweating ■ dry mouth

WHAT TO DO

Urgent Get in touch with your doctor immediately.

May be serious Check with your doctor as soon as possible.

If symptoms are disturbing or perist, let your doctor know.

STORAGE INSTRUCTIONS

Store in a cool, dark place (not in a bathroom medicine cabinet). If your medicine is in a liquid form, make sure that it does not freeze.

STOPPING OR INTERRUPTING THERAPY

If you have been taking this medicine for three weeks or more, do not abruptly stop taking it; you must cut down on your dosage gradually in order to avoid the side effects that occur when this drug is abruptly stopped. Your doctor will advise you on how to reduce your dosage gradually. If you miss a dose, take it as soon as possible. If it is almost time for your next dose, skip the missed dose and resume your regular schedule. Do not take two doses at the same time.

SPECIAL CONSIDERATIONS FOR THOSE OVER SIXTY-FIVE

Older people may be more susceptible to such side effects of this medicine as breathing problems, confusion, agitation, or drowsiness.

CONDITION: **COUGH**

CATEGORY: **COUGH SUPPRESSANTS**

GENERIC (CHEMICAL) NAME	BRAND (TRADE) NAME	DOSAGE FORMS AND STRENGTHS
Hydrocodone and chlorpheniramine	TUSSIONEX	Suspension: 10 mg hydrocodone and 8 mg chlorpheniramine per tsp

DRUG PROFILE

This combination drug is used to treat the cough associated with acute infections, including the common cold, bronchitis, and pneumonia, as well as such chronic conditions as emphysema, bronchial asthma, and tuberculosis. Hydrocodone inhibits the cough reflex in the brain center that stimulates coughing, while chlorpheniramine, an antihistamine, dries out the mucous secretions in the lungs and provides a mild sedative effect.

BEFORE USING THIS DRUG

Let your doctor know *IF*

You have ever had any allergic reactions or other problems with ■ hydrocodone ■ any antihistamines.

You have ever had any of the following medical problems: ■ head injury ■ seizures ■ asthma or other lung disease ■ enlarged prostate ■ urinary problems ■ glaucoma ■ kidney disease ■ liver disease ■ abnormal heart rhythms ■ high blood pressure ■ overactive or underactive thyroid ■ alcoholism ■ colitis or other intestinal problems ■ gallbladder disease.

You are taking any of the following medicines: ■ medicine for glaucoma ■ antihistamines ■ medicine for hay fever, allergies, or colds ■ medicine for seizures ■ barbiturates ■ muscle relaxants ■ tranquilizers ■ sleep medicines ■ medicine for depression ■ narcotics or other prescription pain-killers ■ cimetidine (medicine for ulcers) ■ appetite suppressants ■ medicine for cancer ■ medicine for abnormal heart rhythms ■ medicine for high blood pressure.

SPECIAL RESTRICTIONS WHILE TAKING THIS DRUG

FOOD AND DRUG INTERACTIONS

Other Drugs	Do not take any other drugs, including over-the-counter (OTC) drugs, before checking with your doctor. This medicine increases the effect of drugs that depress the central nervous system, such as antihistamines; medicine for hay fever, allergies, or colds; sleep medicines; tranquilizers; narcotics or other prescription pain-killers; muscle relaxants; and medicines for seizures.
Alcohol	This drug increases the effect of alcohol, a central nervous system depressant. Avoid alcohol unless your doctor has approved its use.

No special restrictions on foods and beverages or smoking.

DAILY LIVING

Driving	This drug may cause drowsiness, light-headedness, or dizziness, as well as loss of alertness and coordination. Be careful when driving, operating household appliances, or doing any other tasks that require alertness until you know how this drug affects you.
Examinations or Tests	It is important for you to keep all appointments with your doctor so that your progress can be checked.

Other Precautions	Tell any doctor or dentist you consult that you are taking this medicine, especially if you will be undergoing any type of surgery.
	Taking this medicine more often or for a longer period of time than prescribed by your doctor may make it habit-forming. If you accidentally take an overdose of this medicine, call your doctor or go to an emergency room immediately.
Helpful Hints	You may vomit or feel nauseated when you first start taking this medicine. If this happens, lie down until you feel better. You may also experience dizziness or light-headedness, especially when getting up from a reclining or sitting position. Getting up slowly will help prevent this.
	Shake the suspension well before taking your prescribed dose. This is a special long-acting suspension that must not be mixed with other fluids or medicines. Mixing it may change how the medicine is absorbed.

No special restrictions on exertion and exercise, sun exposure, or exposure to excessive heat or cold.

POSSIBLE SIDE EFFECTS

Although this list of adverse effects may seem somewhat intimidating, keep in mind that some are quite rare. Of course, should these or any other problems arise while you are on medication, it is always a good idea to consult your doctor.

IF YOU DEVELOP	WHAT TO DO
difficulty in breathing ■ severe dizziness ■ severe drowsiness ■ blurred vision or other visual disturbances ■ extreme restlessness or nervousness ■ delirium ■ slow heartbeat ■ severe weakness ■ seizures ■ clammy skin ■ unsteadiness or clumsiness ■ hallucinations ■ dilated pupils ■ confusion ■ difficulty in speech ■ difficulty in swallowing ■ irritability ■ tremors ■ tightness in chest	**Urgent** Get in touch with your doctor immediately.
facial itching ■ rash, hives, or itching ■ depression ■ sleeplessness ■ faintness ■ irregular or fast heartbeat ■ sore throat or fever ■ bleeding or bruising ■ tiredness	**May be serious** Check with your doctor as soon as possible.
dizziness or light-headedness, especially when getting up from a reclining or sitting position ■ constipation ■ drowsiness ■ nausea or vomiting ■ flushing or warm feeling ■ male impotence ■ difficulty in urination ■ decreased urination ■ increased sweating ■ thickened phlegm ■ dry or stuffy nose ■ increased skin sensitivity to sunlight ■ nightmares ■ loss of appetite ■ upset stomach ■ diarrhea ■ chills ■ ringing in the ears or other hearing problems	If symptoms are disturbing or persist, let your doctor know.

STORAGE INSTRUCTIONS

Store in a cool, dark place (not in a bathroom medicine cabinet). If your medicine is in a liquid form, make sure that it does not freeze.

STOPPING OR INTERRUPTING THERAPY

If you have been taking this medicine for three weeks or more, do not abruptly stop taking it; you must cut down on your dosage gradually in order to avoid the side effects that occur when this drug is abruptly stopped. Your doctor will advise you on how to reduce your dosage gradually. If you miss a dose, take it as soon as possible. If it is almost time for your next dose, skip the missed dose and resume your regular schedule. Do not take two doses at the same time.

SPECIAL CONSIDERATIONS FOR THOSE OVER SIXTY-FIVE

Because older people are more sensitive to the effects of this drug, as well as less able to metabolize it, doctors may start people over sixty-five on a lower dosage.

CONDITION: **COUGH**

CATEGORY: **COUGH SUPPRESSANTS**

GENERIC (CHEMICAL) NAME	BRAND (TRADE) NAME	DOSAGE FORMS AND STRENGTHS
Codeine		Tablets: 15, 30, 60 mg

DRUG PROFILE

Codeine is prescribed to relieve a cough associated with colds, influenza, or hay fever. It suppresses coughing by acting directly on the cough center of the brain. It is an ingredient in a large number of products used for cough control.

BEFORE USING THIS DRUG

Let your doctor know *IF*

You have ever had allergic reactions or other problems with ■ codeine (or narcotic-type drugs) ■ any prescription pain-killers.

You have ever had any of the following medical problems: ■ head injury ■ brain disease ■ stomach or intestinal problems ■ seizures ■ asthma or other lung disease ■ enlarged prostate ■ urinary problems ■ heart disease ■ kidney disease ■ liver disease ■ underactive thyroid.

You are taking any of the following medicines: ■ antibiotics ■ anticoagulants (blood thinners) ■ barbiturates ■ antihistamines ■ medicine for hay fever, coughs, or colds ■ diuretics or other high blood pressure medicine ■ medicine for abnormal heart rhythms ■ medicine for depression ■ bromocriptine or other medicine for Parkinson's disease ■ medicine for diarrhea, stomach spasms, or cramps ■ metoclopramide (medicine for nausea and vomiting) ■ muscle relaxants

■ naltrexone (medicine for opiate abuse) ■ narcotics or other prescription pain-killers ■ medicine for seizures ■ sleep medicines ■ tranquilizers.

SPECIAL RESTRICTIONS WHILE TAKING THIS DRUG

FOOD AND DRUG INTERACTIONS

Other Drugs	Do not take any other drugs, including over-the-counter (OTC) drugs, before checking with your doctor. This drug increases the effect of drugs that depress the central nervous system, such as antihistamines; medicine for hay fever, allergies, or colds; sleep medicines; tranquilizers; narcotics or other prescription pain-killers; muscle relaxants; and medicine for seizures.
Alcohol	This drug increases the effect of alcohol, a central nervous system depressant. Avoid alcohol while taking this drug.

No special restrictions on foods and beverages or smoking.

DAILY LIVING

Driving	This drug may cause drowsiness, light-headedness, or dizziness as well as loss of alertness and coordination. Be careful when driving, operating household appliances, or doing any other tasks that require alertness until you know how this drug affects you.
Examinations or Tests	It is important for you to keep all appointments with your doctor so that your progress can be checked.
Other Precautions	Tell any doctor or dentist you consult that you are taking this drug, especially if you will be undergoing any type of surgery.

Taking this medicine more often or for a longer period of time than prescribed by your doctor may make it habit-forming. If you have been taking this medicine for a few weeks and you think that it is no longer working as well as it did before, do not increase your dose, but check with your doctor.

If you continue to have a cough for more than seven days or you have a high fever, rash, headache, or sore throat with your cough, let your doctor know.

Helpful Hints

You may vomit or feel nauseated when you first start taking this medicine. If this happens, lie down until you feel better. You may also experience dizziness or light-headedness, especially when getting up from a reclining or sitting position. Getting up slowly will help prevent this.

No special restrictions on exertion and exercise, sun exposure, or exposure to excessive heat or cold.

POSSIBLE SIDE EFFECTS

Although this list of adverse effects may seem somewhat intimidating, keep in mind that some are quite rare. Of course, should these or any other problems arise while you are on medication, it is always a good idea to consult your doctor.

IF YOU DEVELOP

seizures ■ severe dizziness ■ severe drowsiness ■ difficulty in breathing ■ severe weakness ■ extreme restlessness or nervousness ■ low blood pressure ■ slow heart rate ■ cold, clammy skin ■ severe confusion

WHAT TO DO

Urgent Get in touch with your doctor immediately.

confusion ■ hallucinations ■ depression ■ "high" feeling or other mood change ■ irregular or fast heartbeat ■ rash, hives, or itching ■ swelling of face ■ ringing or buzzing in ears ■ shortness of breath ■ jerky movements, twitching, or tremors	**May be serious** Get in touch with your doctor as soon as possible.
dizziness or light-headedness, especially when getting up from a reclining or sitting position ■ drowsiness ■ constipation ■ nausea or vomiting	If symptoms are disturbing or persist, let your doctor know.

STORAGE INSTRUCTIONS

Store in a cool, dark place (not in a bathroom medicine cabinet). If your medicine is in a liquid form, make sure that it does not freeze.

STOPPING OR INTERRUPTING THERAPY

If you have been taking this medicine for several weeks or more, do not abruptly stop taking it; you must cut down on your dosage gradually in order to avoid the side effects that occur when this drug is abruptly stopped. Your doctor will advise you on how to reduce your dosage gradually. If you are taking this medicine according to a regular schedule and you miss a dose, take it as soon as possible. If it is almost time for your next dose, skip the missed dose and resume your regular schedule. Do not take two doses at the same time.

SPECIAL CONSIDERATIONS FOR THOSE OVER SIXTY-FIVE

Older people may be more susceptible to such side effects of this medicine as breathing problems.

CONDITION: **PNEUMOCOCCAL PNEUMONIA**

CATEGORY: **VACCINES**

GENERIC (CHEMICAL) NAME	BRAND (TRADE) NAME	DOSAGE FORMS AND STRENGTHS
Pneumococcal vaccine	PNEUMOVAX 23	Injection: 25 mcg
	PNU-IMUNE 23	Injection: 25 mcg

DRUG PROFILE

This vaccine is given to prevent pneumococcal pneumonia. It is often recommended for people over the age of sixty-five and for people who have chronic illnesses or are undergoing cancer chemotherapy. Other people who may face a higher risk of pneumonia include those who live in closed groups in which infection can easily spread (such as nursing homes) or in communities experiencing a pneumonia epidemic. The vaccine consists of extract from the pneumonia bacteria, which, when injected, causes the body to form antibodies against pneumonia.

BEFORE USING THIS DRUG

Let your doctor know *IF*

You have ever had any of the following medical problems: ■ Hodgkin's disease (cancer of the lymph nodes) ■ heart disease ■ lung disease ■ infection of the respiratory tract, including pneumonia ■ recent fever ■ any recent infection ■ a disease of the immune system.

You are taking any of the following medicines: ■ medicine for cancer ■ medicine that suppresses the immune system ■ corticosteroids (prednisone, cortisone).

You have recently been given a flu vaccine.

You have ever been given a vaccine for pneumonia.

SPECIAL RESTRICTIONS WHILE TAKING THIS DRUG

FOOD AND DRUG INTERACTIONS

No special restrictions on other drugs, foods and beverages, alcohol use, or smoking.

DAILY LIVING

Examinations or Tests	If you have a serious heart or lung condition, your doctor may want to check you regularly after you receive this vaccine.
Other Precautions	You may experience redness, soreness, swelling, or formation of a hard spot at the site of injection. This should disappear in a few days.

No special restrictions on driving, exertion and exercise, sun exposure, or exposure to excessive heat or cold.

POSSIBLE SIDE EFFECTS

Although this list of adverse effects may seem somewhat intimidating, keep in mind that some are quite rare. Of course, should these or any other problems arise while you are on medication, it is always a good idea to consult your doctor.

IF YOU DEVELOP

wheezing or difficulty in breathing ■ faintness ■ skin eruptions ■ fast heartbeat

WHAT TO DO

Urgent Get in touch with your doctor immediately.

fever ■ redness, soreness, swelling, or formation of a hard spot at the injection site ■ weakness ■ muscle or joint pain ■ headache ■ increased eye sensitivity to light ■ chills ■ nausea ■ rash	If symptoms are disturbing or persist, let your doctor know.

SPECIAL CONSIDERATIONS FOR THOSE OVER SIXTY-FIVE

None.

CONDITION: **INFLUENZA**

CATEGORY: **VACCINES**

GENERIC (CHEMICAL) NAME	BRAND (TRADE) NAME	DOSAGE FORMS AND STRENGTHS
Influenza virus vaccine	INFLUENZA VIRUS VACCINE, TRIVALENT	Injection: 15 mcg
	FLUOGEN	Injection: 15 mcg
	FLUZONE	Injection: 15 mcg
	FLUZONE-A	Injection: 15 mcg

DRUG PROFILE

This vaccine is given to prevent influenza, or flu. It is often recommended for people over the age of sixty-five, for heavy smokers, and for people with such medical problems as certain types of heart conditions, lung disease, or kidney disease. It is also often recommended for people who live in closed groups in which infection can easily spread (such as people in nursing homes), or for those who come into contact with many unvaccinated people (such as those in a public health or service job).

BEFORE USING THIS DRUG

Let your doctor know *IF*

You have ever had allergic reactions or other problems with ■ chicken or chicken eggs.

You have ever had any of the following medical problems: ■ Guillain-Barré syndrome ■ any nerve disorder ■ heart disease ■ lung disease ■ infection of the respiratory tract ■ blood vessel disease ■ cancer ■ recent fever ■ any recent infection.

You are taking any of the following medicines: ■ anticoagulants (blood thinners) ■ theophylline (medicine for asthma) ■ medicine for cancer ■ corticosteroids ■ medicine for seizures.

You have recently been given any other vaccine.

SPECIAL RESTRICTIONS WHILE TAKING THIS DRUG

FOOD AND DRUG INTERACTIONS

No special restrictions on other drugs, foods and beverages, alcohol use, or smoking.

DAILY LIVING

Examinations or Tests	If you have a serious heart or lung condition, your doctor may want to check you regularly after you receive this vaccine.
Other Precautions	You may experience soreness, redness, or formation of a hard spot at the site of injection. This should disappear in a few days.

No special restrictions on driving, exertion and exercise, sun exposure, or exposure to excessive heat or cold.

POSSIBLE SIDE EFFECTS

Although this list of adverse effects may seem somewhat intimidating, keep in mind that some are quite rare. Of course, should these or any other problems arise while you are on medication, it is always a good idea to consult your doctor.

IF YOU DEVELOP	WHAT TO DO
difficulty in breathing ■ rash or hives	**Urgent** Get in touch with your doctor immediately.
fever ■ redness, soreness, swelling, or formation of a hard spot at the injection site ■ general ill feeling ■ headache ■ muscle or joint pain	If symptoms are disturbing or persist, let your doctor know.

SPECIAL CONSIDERATIONS FOR THOSE OVER SIXTY-FIVE

None.

CONDITION: **INFLUENZA**

CATEGORY: **ANTIVIRAL AGENTS**

GENERIC (CHEMICAL) NAME	BRAND (TRADE) NAME	DOSAGE FORMS AND STRENGTHS
Amantadine hydrochloride	SYMMETREL	Capsules: 100 mg Syrup: 50 mg per tsp

DRUG PROFILE

Amantadine is used to treat Parkinson's disease and other movement disorders. Many experts think that the rigidity, shaking, and walking disturbances associated with these conditions result from a deficiency of a chemical called dopamine in the brain. Amantadine makes more dopamine available to the brain, thereby helping restore the chemical balance that regulates the nervous system. This drug is sometimes used along with levodopa or other medicine for Parkinson's disease. Amantadine is also used to treat influenza. It works by interfering with the ability of the influenza virus to multiply.

For complete information on this drug, see pages 309–312.

CONDITION: **RESPIRATORY INFECTIONS**

CATEGORY: **ANALGESICS**

GENERIC (CHEMICAL) NAME	BRAND (TRADE) NAME	DOSAGE FORMS AND STRENGTHS

Aspirin and other salicylate drugs

Aspirin and other salicylate drugs are available over the counter under a variety of brand names, dosage forms, and strengths. Some of these preparations have a special coating to help protect the lining of the stomach against possible irritation. Because of the importance of salicylate drugs in the treatment of chronic pain, even though they are most often nonprescription drugs, they are included in this book for reader reference.

For complete information on this drug, see pages 471–475.

DRUG PROFILE

Aspirin and other drugs in the salicylate family are used to relieve pain, inflammation, and fever. Large doses are used to treat symptoms of arthritis and rheumatism such as swelling, stiffness, and joint pain. Aspirin and other salicylates are thought to control pain and swelling by blocking the production of naturally occurring triggers of pain and inflammation, called prostaglandins. These drugs also relieve fever by changing the way the body regulates its temperature.

CONDITION: **RESPIRATORY INFECTIONS**

CATEGORY: **ANALGESICS**

GENERIC (CHEMICAL) NAME	BRAND (TRADE) NAME	DOSAGE FORMS AND STRENGTHS
Acetaminophen	Regular Strength ANACIN-3	Tablets: 325 mg
	Maximum Strength ANACIN-3	Caplets: 500 mg Tablets: 500 mg
	Aspirin-free ARTHRITIS PAIN FORMULA	Tablets: 500 mg
	Extra Strength DATRIL	Caplets: 500 mg Tablets: 500 mg
	PANADOL	Capsules: 500 mg Tablets: 500 mg
	Maximum Strength ST. JOSEPH Aspirin-Free	Tablets: 500mg
	Regular Strength TYLENOL	Caplets: 325 mg Tablets: 325 mg
	Extra-Strength TYLENOL	Caplets: 500 mg Gelcaps: 500 mg Liquid: 500 mg per tbsp Tablets: 500 mg

DRUG PROFILE

Acetaminophen is used to relieve fever and pain. It is thought to work by blocking pain centers in the central nervous system and by resetting the body's thermostat to its normal temperature.

For complete information on this drug, see pages 476–478.

CONDITION: **RESPIRATORY INFECTIONS**

CATEGORY: **ANALGESICS**

GENERIC (CHEMICAL) NAME	BRAND (TRADE) NAME	DOSAGE FORMS AND STRENGTHS
Ibuprofen	ADVIL (OTC)	Tablets: 200 mg
	MOTRIN	Tablets: 300, 400, 600, 800 mg
	MOTRIN IB (OTC)	Tablets: 200 mg
		Caplets: 200 mg
	NUPRIN (OTC)	Tablets: 200 mg
	RUFEN	Tablets: 400, 600, 800 mg

DRUG PROFILE

Nonsteroidal anti-inflammatory drugs, or NSAIDs, help relieve swelling, stiffness, joint pain, and inflammation in the long-term treatment of arthritis. These drugs are thought to act by blocking the production of naturally occurring pain and inflammation triggers called prostaglandins.

For complete information on this drug, see pages 524–530.

ALLERGIC RHINITIS

If you think you've got a cold that just won't quit—complete with drippy nose, teary eyes, and nonstop sneezing, you might actually be suffering from a condition known as allergic rhinitis. This means that an abnormal sensitivity reaction, an allergy, has caused the mucous membranes lining your nose to become inflamed. The symptoms are very much like those of a cold, but colds generally run their course in a week or so, while allergic symptoms hang on for several weeks or even months. Another difference is that the sore throat, fever, and muscle aches that often accompany a cold are not part of an allergy attack.

The tendency to have allergies is genetic, passed from parent to child. An allergy generally appears for the first time during adolescence, but it can begin earlier or later, striking people of any age. While more than fifteen million Americans have allergies of one kind or another, about six million have allergic rhinitis, meaning that the reaction is confined to the nose.

CAUSES

An allergic reaction occurs when the body mistakes a harmless substance like pollen or animal dander for an invader, or antigen, and mounts a defense against it. The body defends itself by producing antibodies, which are designed to neutralize the antigen. The antigen and antibody lock together in combat. In response to the binding of the antigen and antibody, a chemical called histamine is released, which causes the swelling and itching.

The substance that most often sets off an episode of allergic rhinitis is pollen, from trees or grass in the spring and from ragweed in the late summer or early fall. Ragweed allergy is sometimes referred to as hay fever. The tiny mites that float in house dust, the microscopic flakes of dry skin shed into the air by household pets, or the mold spores spewed into the atmosphere by air-conditioning systems are a few of the other substances that can also set off allergy attacks. A person who is sensitive to one substance can subsequently become sensitive to others.

TREATMENT

Preventing an allergy attack by avoiding the allergen is the best strategy. If you're allergic to animal fur, for example, it's not hard to figure out how to stay away from it (though if you're an animal lover, you might not want to). People allergic to pollens should stay indoors as much as possible, with windows closed and air-conditioners running, during their allergy seasons. Their rooms should be cleaned regularly; bedrooms, especially, should be free of knickknacks, books, and other dust collectors. (This also applies to people who are allergic to house dust.) Down comforters are not for people allergic to feathers, nor is a cashmere sweater ideal for the individual whose nose tickles at the mere mention of wool.

But you can't completely avoid your allergens, so if your allergic reaction is troublesome enough, you will probably need some medicine to relieve your symptoms. The kinds of drugs generally used for allergy include antihistamines and decongestants. Corticosteroids, administered as a topical nasal spray, can also be very effective in treating this condition. They block the allergic reaction and reduce inflammation. Further information on all these medicines can be found in the drug charts on page 763. A relatively new prescription drug used to treat chronic allergies is cromolyn sodium (brand names, Intal and Nasalcrom).

OUTLOOK

Medical therapy generally provides relief to sufferers of allergic rhinitis. But in some cases, no medicines seem to do the job, or their side effects prove worse than the dripping and sneezing of an allergic attack. Your doctor may then refer you to an allergist, who can do skin tests to determine the precise sources of your symptoms and, if your condition is severe enough, administer a series of allergy shots to desensitize your system.

Caution: Some drugs in this section may affect pregnancy or fetal development. Check with your doctor if this concerns you.

CONDITION: **ALLERGIC RHINITIS**

CATEGORY: **ANTIHISTAMINES AND ANTIHISTAMINE-DECONGESTANT COMBINATIONS**

GENERIC (CHEMICAL) NAME	BRAND (TRADE) NAME	DOSAGE FORMS AND STRENGTHS
Azatadine maleate	OPTIMINE	Tablets: 1 mg
Clemastine fumarate	TAVIST TAVIST-1	Tablets: 2.68 mg Tablets: 1.34 mg
Clemastine fumarate with phenylpropa-nolamine	TAVIST D	Tablets: 1.34 mg clemastine 75 mg phenylpropanolamine
Chlorpheniramine maleate	CHLOR-TRIMETON	Sustained-release tablets: 8, 12 mg Tablets: 4 mg
Dexchlorpheniramine maleate	POLARAMINE	Controlled-release tablets: 4, 6 mg Syrup: 2 mg per tsp Tablets: 2 mg
Diphenhydramine hydrochloride	BENADRYL BENADRYL 25	Capsules: 25, 50 mg Elixir: 12.5 mg per tsp Capsules: 25 mg Tablets: 25 mg
Hydroxyzine	ATARAX VISTARIL	Syrup: 10 mg per tsp Tablets: 10, 25, 50, 100 mg Capsules: 25, 50, 100 mg Suspension: 25 mg per tsp

Promethazine hydrochloride	PHENERGAN	Rectal suppositories: 12.5, 25, 50 mg Syrup: 6.25, 25 mg per tsp Tablets: 12.5, 25, 50 mg
Tripelennamine hydrochloride	PBZ	Elixir: tripelennamine citrate equivalent to 25 mg tripelennamine hydrochloride per tsp Tablets: 25, 50 mg
	PBZ-SR	Controlled-release tablets: 100 mg
Phenylpropanolamine hydrochloride and chlorpheniramine maleate	DEHIST	Controlled-release capsules: 75 mg phenylpropanolamine hydrochloride and 8 mg chlorpheniramine maleate

Many brands of antihistamines and antihistamine-decongestant combinations are sold over the counter as well.

DRUG PROFILE

When you are exposed to a substance to which you are allergic, a chemical called histamine is released into the bloodstream and produces the itchy, watery eyes; runny nose; and rashes that are typical of an allergic reaction. Antihistamines work by blocking the action of histamine. They are used to treat allergies as well as to relieve the symptoms of a cold. Antihistamines are sometimes combined in the same preparation with a decongestant, such as phenylpropanolamine. Phenylpropanolamine is thought to work by constricting blood vessels in the respiratory tract, shrinking the swollen membranes so that you are less congested and can breathe more easily. Hydroxyzine is also used to treat anxiety. Exactly how it works to relieve anxiety is not completely understood.

BEFORE USING THIS DRUG

Let your doctor know *IF*

You have ever had allergic reactions or other problems with ■ any antihistamines or decongestants ■ amphetamines ■ medicine for asthma.

You have ever had any of the following medical problems: ■ asthma or other lung disease ■ enlarged prostate ■ urinary problems or difficulty in urination ■ glaucoma ■ epilepsy or other seizure disorders ■ high blood pressure ■ overactive thyroid.

With medicine containing a decongestant only: ■ diabetes ■ ulcers.

You are taking any of the following medicines: ■ any other antihistamines ■ medicine for Parkinson's disease ■ medicine for seizures ■ aspirin or aspirinlike medicine ■ medicine for arthritis ■ medicine for cancer ■ antibiotics ■ digoxin or digitalis (heart medicines) ■ medicine for abnormal heart rhythms ■ barbiturates ■ muscle relaxants ■ medicine for hay fever, coughs, or colds ■ narcotics or other prescription pain-killers ■ sleep medicines ■ tranquilizers ■ medicine for depression ■ medicine for high blood pressure ■ appetite suppressants ■ medicine for asthma.

SPECIAL RESTRICTIONS WHILE TAKING THIS DRUG

FOOD AND DRUG INTERACTIONS

Other Drugs	Do not take any other drugs, including over-the-counter (OTC) drugs, before checking with your doctor. This medicine increases the effect of drugs that depress the central nervous system, such as other antihistamines; medicine for hay fever, allergies, or colds; sleep medicines; tranquilizers; narcotics or other prescription pain-killers; muscle relaxants; and medicine for seizures.
	Antihistamines may mask ringing in the ears caused by aspirin. Let your doctor know if you are taking aspirin or aspirinlike medicine.

Alcohol	Antihistamines increase the effect of alcohol, a central nervous system depressant. Avoid alcohol unless your doctor has approved its use.

No special restrictions on foods and beverages or smoking.

DAILY LIVING

Driving	This drug may cause dizziness, drowsiness, weakness, or blurred vision. Be careful when driving, operating household appliances, or doing any other tasks that require alertness until you know how this drug affects you.
Other Precautions	Tell any doctor or dentist you consult that you are taking this drug, especially if you will be undergoing any type of surgery. If you are going to be tested for allergies, tell the doctor in charge that you are taking this drug, since it affects the results of allergy tests.
Helpful Hints	If this drug upsets your stomach, taking it with food, milk, or water should help. If your mouth or throat feels dry, chewing sugarless gum or sucking ice chips or sugarless hard candy will help. This drug may sometimes cause insomnia, which can be avoided by taking your last dose several hours before bedtime; check with your doctor about the best dosing schedule for you. If you have been storing the suppository form of this medicine, it may be too soft to use. Put it in the refrigerator for half an hour or run cold water over the wrapped suppository before use.

No special restrictions on exertion and exercise, sun exposure, or exposure to excessive heat or cold.

POSSIBLE SIDE EFFECTS

Although this list of adverse effects may seem somewhat intimidating, keep in mind that some are quite rare. Of course, should these or any other problems arise while you are on medication, it is always a good idea to consult your doctor.

IF YOU DEVELOP

seizures ■ unsteadiness or clumsiness ■ severe drowsiness ■ fainting ■ flushing ■ hallucinations ■ difficulty in breathing ■ dilated pupils ■ sleeplessness ■ confusion ■ difficulty in speech ■ difficulty in swallowing ■ nervousness or restlessness ■ irritability ■ excitement or other mood changes ■ muscle weakness ■ tremors ■ tightness of chest ■ irregular or fast heartbeat

WHAT TO DO

Urgent Get in touch with your doctor immediately.

---

sore throat or fever ■ bleeding or bruising ■ tiredness

May be serious Check with your doctor as soon as possible.

---

drowsiness ■ dizziness ■ thickening phlegm ■ blurred or double vision or other visual disturbances ■ pain or difficulty in urination ■ urinary frequency ■ dry mouth or throat ■ dry or stuffy nose ■ increased skin sensitivity to sunlight ■ nightmares ■ rash ■ loss of appetite ■ upset stomach ■ constipation ■ diarrhea ■ nausea or vomiting ■ male impotence ■ chills ■ increased sweating ■ ringing in the ears or other hearing problems

If symptoms are disturbing or persist, let your doctor know.

With phenylpropanolamine only: headache

STORAGE INSTRUCTIONS

Store in a cool, dark place (not in a bathroom medicine cabinet). If your medicine is in a liquid form, make sure that it does not freeze. Suppositories should be stored in the refrigerator.

STOPPING OR INTERRUPTING THERAPY

This drug should be taken without interruption for the full length of time prescribed by your doctor. If you miss a dose, take it as soon as possible. If it is almost time for your next dose, skip the missed dose and resume your regular schedule. Do not take two doses at the same time.

SPECIAL CONSIDERATIONS FOR THOSE OVER SIXTY-FIVE

Older people taking this drug may be more prone to develop confusion, difficulty in urination, dizziness, drowsiness, fainting, visual disturbances, fever, or dry mouth. Nightmares, restlessness, and irritability are also more apt to occur in those over sixty-five.

CONDITION: **ALLERGIC RHINITIS**

CATEGORY: **ANTIHISTAMINES**

GENERIC (CHEMICAL) NAME	BRAND (TRADE) NAME	DOSAGE FORMS AND STRENGTHS
Astemizole	HISMANAL	Tablets: 10 mg
Terfenadine	SELDANE	Tablets: 60 mg
Terfenadine with pseudoephedrine	SELDANE-D	Tablets: 60 mg terfenadine 120 mg pseudoephedrine

DRUG PROFILE

When you are exposed to a substance to which you are allergic, a chemical called histamine is released into the bloodstream and produces the itchy, watery eyes; runny nose; and rashes that are typical of an allergic reaction. Terfenadine and astemizole, antihistamines, block the action of histamine and are used to treat the symptoms of allergies, especially such seasonal allergies as hay fever.

BEFORE USING THIS DRUG

Let your doctor know *IF*

You have ever had allergic reactions or other problems with ■ any antihistamines.

You have ever had any of the following medical problems: ■ asthma or other lung disease ■ liver disease ■ enlarged prostate ■ glaucoma ■ urinary problems or difficulty in urination.

You are taking any of the following medicines: ■ any other antihistamines.

With terfenadine only: ■ antibiotics ■ medicine for Parkinson's disease ■ medicine for stomach spasms or cramps ■ medicine for arthritis ■ aspirin or aspirinlike medicine ■ medicine for cancer ■ medicine for high blood pressure ■ medicine for abnormal heart rhythms ■ tranquilizers ■ medicine for depression ■ medicine for seizures ■ narcotics or other prescription pain-killers ■ sleep medicines

■ medicine for hay fever, coughs, or colds ■ metyrosine (medicine for adrenal gland tumor) ■ muscle relaxants ■ paromomycin (medicine for amebic infection). ■ ketoconazole (medicine for fungal infection).

SPECIAL RESTRICTIONS WHILE TAKING THIS DRUG

FOOD AND DRUG INTERACTIONS

Other Drugs	Do not take any other drugs, including over-the-counter (OTC) drugs, before checking with your doctor.
	Antihistamines may mask ringing in the ears caused by aspirin. Let your doctor know if you are taking aspirin or apirinlike medicine.
With terfenadine only:	*This medicine may increase the effect of drugs that depress the central nervous system, such as other antihistamines; medicine for hay fever, allergies, or colds; sleep medicines; tranquilizers, narcotics or other prescription pain-killers; muscle relaxants; and medicine for seizures. However, such problems occur to a lesser extent with this antihistamine than with other antihistamines.*
Food and Beverages	Astemizole should be taken on an empty stomach, at least two hours before or after a meal.
Alcohol	This drug increases the effect of alcohol, a central nervous system depressant. Avoid alcohol unless your doctor has approved its use.

No special restrictions on smoking.

DAILY LIVING

Driving	Although this drug rarely causes drowsiness, antihistamines may cause dizziness, drowsiness, weakness, or blurred vision in some individuals. Be careful when driving, operating household appliances, or doing any other tasks that require alertness until you know how this drug affects you.
Other Precautions	Tell any doctor or dentist you consult that you are taking this medicine, especially if you will be undergoing any type of surgery.
	If you are going to be tested for allergies, tell the doctor in charge that you are taking this drug, since it affects the results of allergy tests.
Helpful Hints	If your mouth or throat feels dry, chewing sugarless gum or sucking on ice chips or sugarless candy may be helpful.
	For Terfenadine: If terfenadine upsets your stomach, taking it with food, milk, or water should help.

No special restrictions on exertion and exercise, sun exposure, or exposure to excessive heat or cold.

POSSIBLE SIDE EFFECTS

Although this list of adverse effects may seem somewhat intimidating, keep in mind that some are quite rare. Of course, should these or any other problems arise while you are on medication, it is always a good idea to consult your doctor.

IF YOU DEVELOP	**WHAT TO DO**
seizures ■ unsteadiness or clumsiness ■ severe drowsiness ■ fainting ■ flushing ■ hallucinations ■ confusion ■ difficulty in breathing ■ sleeplessness	**Urgent** Get in touch with your doctor immediately.
sore throat or fever ■ bleeding or bruising ■ tiredness ■ excitement ■ nervousness or restlessness ■ irritability ■ depression ■ sensitivity to light ■ rash ■ abnormal or irregular heart rhythm ■ itching ■ swelling of face, arms, and legs ■ rash	**May be serious** Check with your doctor as soon as possible.
blurred vision or other visual disturbances ■ pain or difficulty in urination ■ dizziness ■ dry mouth or throat ■ dry or stuffy nose ■ loss of appetite ■ nightmares ■ ringing in the ears or other hearing problems ■ fast heartbeat ■ upset stomach or stomach pain ■ nausea or vomiting ■ increased sweating ■ drowsiness ■ thickening phlegm ■ hair loss ■ anxiety ■ insomnia ■ cold sweats ■ headache *With astemizole only:* increased appetite ■ weight gain ■ red, irritated eyes ■ nosebleed ■ muscle or joint aches	If symptoms are disturbing or persist, let your doctor know.

STORAGE INSTRUCTIONS

Store in a cool, dark place (not in a bathroom medicine cabinet).

STOPPING OR INTERRUPTING THERAPY

This drug should be taken without interruption for the full length of time prescribed by your doctor. If you miss a dose, take it as soon as possible. If it is almost time for your next dose, skip the missed dose, and resume your regular schedule. Do not take two doses at the same time.

SPECIAL CONSIDERATIONS FOR THOSE OVER SIXTY-FIVE

Terfenadine and astemizole have been in widespread use for only a short period of time, and the full extent of their effects in older people is not yet known. Astemizole has a long duration of action and its effect may last even longer in older people.

CONDITION: **ALLERGIC RHINITIS**

CATEGORY: **CORTICOSTEROIDS**

GENERIC (CHEMICAL) NAME	BRAND (TRADE) NAME	DOSAGE FORMS AND STRENGTHS
Beclomethasone dipropionate	BECLOVENT	Inhaler: 42 mcg per inhalation
	BECONASE	Nasal inhaler: 42 mcg per inhalation
	BECONASE AQ	Nasal spray: 42 mcg per inhalation
	VANCENASE	Nasal inhaler: 42 mcg per inhalation
	VANCENASE AQ	Nasal spray: 42 mcg per inhalation
	VANCERIL Inhaler	Inhaler: 42 mcg per inhalation

DRUG PROFILE

Inhaled corticosteroids such as beclomethasone are used as long-term therapy to prevent asthma attacks. They work by shrinking the swollen membranes of the respiratory tract, allowing the lungs to take in more air and making the flow of air easier. Inhaled steroids are sometimes used along with inhaled bronchodilators such as albuterol or terbutaline (see the charts on pages 775–779).

Beclomethasone is also available as a nasal spray to be inhaled through the nose to treat nasal inflammation from allergies and to prevent recurrence of surgically removed nasal polyps.

For complete information on this drug, see pages 779–783.

CONDITION: **ALLERGIC RHINITIS**

CATEGORY: **MAST-CELL INHIBITORS**

GENERIC (CHEMICAL) NAME	BRAND (TRADE) NAME	DOSAGE FORMS AND STRENGTHS
Cromolyn sodium	NASALCROM	Solution: 40 mg cromolyn sodium per ml

DRUG PROFILE

Cromolyn nasal solution is used to prevent and treat symptoms of allergic rhinitis such as sneezing, itching, and runny nose.

For complete information on this drug see page 784–787.

ASTHMA

If you have asthma, you're probably all too familiar with its symptoms—the coughing, the struggle for breath, the wheezing and whistling as air rushes through tightened passages in your lungs. But you may be less aware of what causes these sometimes disabling symptoms to occur.

In asthma, a chronic condition that can occur for the first time even after the age of fifty, the muscles of the bronchioles—the tubes that carry air back and forth from the lungs—tighten. This causes the bronchioles to narrow, go into spasm, and fill with mucus. The coughing and rattling sounds in the chest that accompany asthma result from the accumulation of mucus. Because of the narrowing of the bronchial passages, some of the air that has delivered its oxygen content and that should be exhaled is stuck in the lungs, and fresh air cannot be properly inhaled. Asthmatic breathing is hard physical work.

CAUSES

The tendency for muscles in the airways to go into spasm is hereditary and is sometimes related to allergies to pollen, dust, pet dander, mold spores, or particular foods, such as eggs or milk. In other people, the airways may be supersensitive to cold air, smoke (including cigarette smoke), smog, lint, chalk dust, or chemical fumes. Sometimes, a respiratory infection can bring on an asthma attack. Physical exercise is an-

other common trigger of asthmatic symptoms.

The role of emotional pressure in causing asthma is debatable, though many experts believe that the existing illness is worsened by any form of stress. One thing is certain: The breathing problems caused by an attack of asthma and the ongoing frustration of being an asthmatic can lead to a lot of anxiety and emotional strain.

DIAGNOSIS

To determine whether your asthmatic symptoms can be caused by such diseases as chronic bronchitis, emphysema, or heart failure, your doctor may perform tests to rule out these problems. An important guide to an accurate assessment of your condition is your history of symptoms, especially if the attacks are worse during allergy seasons. Because of the genetic component to asthma, your doctor will also inquire whether anyone in your family is or has been allergic or asthmatic.

To confirm the diagnosis, your doctor may also perform blood tests and measurements of your ability to exhale air. One of the characteristics of asthma is that the airway obstruction is eased by a class of medicines called bronchodilators, which open the bronchial tubes. The doctor may therefore use this kind of medicine as a diagnostic tool before deciding whether it's an appropriate treatment for your condition.

TREATMENT

Although the large array of drugs available for asthma may seem confusing, there are actually only a few basic types. None can cure the asthma, but they may relieve its symptoms. In deciding what kind of medicine you should take and the proper dosage, your doctor will consider a number of factors, including the frequency and severity of your asthma attacks.

The most widely used preparations for treating asthma are bronchodilators. They relax the muscles that have tightened around the bronchioles and reduce the swelling of the mucous membranes. These drugs are available in tablet, liquid, and aerosol form. More information on bronchodilators can be found in the drug charts on pages 771–779.

If bronchodilators don't stop your attacks, your doctor may prescribe a corticosteroid in aerosolized or oral form (described in the drug charts on pages 779–783). These medicines must be used under close medical supervision, since they can produce severe side effects. Some people need these drugs only occasionally, while others require long-term steroid therapy.

Antihistamines may be prescribed as well because they help dry up the accumulated mucus in the lungs. Other available measures are aimed at stopping asthma attacks before they begin. For example, if your particular allergy is identified through skin tests or other diagnostic procedures, you may be given allergy injections to decrease your sensitivity—and the severity of your asthmatic condition. If you smoke, you should do everything possible to stop and also stay away from people who smoke.

Your bedroom should be scrupulously cleaned on a regular basis with a damp mop (avoid using a vacuum cleaner because it can send dust particles back into the air). If possible, have someone else do the cleaning, and don't enter the room until at least an hour after the cleaning has been finished. Avoid sleeping with a feather pillow, and get rid of such dust collectors as thick rugs, heavy drapes, and knickknacks. You may even have to find a new home for your dog or cat.

If cold air triggers your attacks, keep your mouth and nose covered with a scarf when you go outdoors in cold weather. If a particular food seems to contribute to your asthmatic symptoms, exclude it from your diet.

OUTLOOK

Most of the time, asthma can be managed by control of the environment, preventive medicine, and medicines that relieve the attacks. Sometimes, however, an attack of asthma can be so severe that you require hospitalization, where respiratory help is available and medicine can be given in the most effective manner.

It's important to remember that, while asthma is not a psychosomatic disease, it can produce emotional problems involving the affected individual as well as other family members. Emotional support is an important part of the overall treatment plan, making it easier for everyone involved to live with asthma.

CHRONIC BRONCHITIS

You may not consider a cough anything to worry about, but if you're told that it's a result of bronchitis, you should take it seriously.

Bronchitis is an inflammation of the bronchial tubes, the passages that bring air into the lungs. When the tubes are inflamed, either because of an infection or persistent irritation, they produce a heavy secretion of mucus. The coughing that is characteristic of bronchitis is the body's attempt to clear the mucus. If not properly treated, this condition can cause further health complications, especially in older people.

CAUSES

Bronchitis is characterized as either acute or chronic. (For a discussion of acute bronchitis see pages 699–700.) An acute attack is generally caused by a virus but may be caused by bacteria. Typically, a head cold becomes a chest cold, or a case of the flu lingers and starts to affect your bronchial tubes. A bronchial cough may be accompanied by fever, aches and pains, and difficulty in breathing. Usually this type of bronchitis lasts about ten days. But it can lead to a more serious disorder—one that extends deeper into the lungs—if not treated promptly.

Chronic bronchitis keeps you coughing up mucus almost every day for months at a time, year after year, especially during cold weather. Its most common cause is cigarette smoking, which irritates the bronchial lining. Air pollution and the development of respiratory illnesses in childhood may predispose you to developing chronic bronchitis as an adult. In some cases, a series of attacks of acute bronchitis or chronic allergic asthma leads to chronic bronchitis. A rare condition known as alpha-antitrypsin deficiency may result in chronic bronchitis.

Periodically, the bronchitis may get so bad that you are breathless, have even more frequent coughing spells, and bring up pus along with the mucus. The danger of chronic bronchitis is that it can make you vulnerable to pneumonia.

TREATMENT

It's especially important for older people to seek medical help whenever they have breathing difficulty or coughing spells. Before making the diagnosis of bronchitis, your doctor will perform tests that rule out heart disease, lung infections, cancer, and other disorders that may produce the symptoms typical of bronchitis. A chest X ray certainly will be part of your exam. Your doctor may ask you to breathe into a tube as a way of measuring how seriously your airways are obstructed; if your breathing is severely impaired, you may need to have oxygen at home. Specially designed exercises may also be recommended to improve your ability to breathe.

The treatment of acute bronchitis generally includes staying indoors if the weather is cold, avoiding fatigue, and drinking plenty of fluids. If you're a smoker, you'll be told to give it up, at least while you're ill, because airways cannot heal if they're constantly irritated. Expectorant drugs are sometimes prescribed to loosen mucus, though there is no evidence that these drugs actually work. Antibiotics are not routinely prescribed, as acute bronchitis is generally caused by a virus. However, some doctors prescribe them to older people to eliminate the risk of serious bacterial infection resulting from lowered resistance. See the drug charts on pages 791–797 for further information.

If you have chronic bronchitis, you'll be told to stop smoking altogether, even when you feel fine. This will help prevent further damage to your bronchial airways. A vaporizer may come in handy (for acute as well as chronic sufferers) because the steam can help relieve the chest congestion. And you're almost certain to be given a prescription for an antibiotic, especially if your airways are se-verely obstructed. You may also be put on a bronchodilator, a drug class covered in the charts on pages 771–779. If you don't feel somewhat better within three or four days of starting medicine, a corticosteroid may be added to your drug therapy. (See the drug charts on pages 779–783.) This is usually given in cases in which the person is sick enough to be hospitalized.

OUTLOOK

Bronchitis should not be dismissed as "just an annoying cough" that will go away. It can do serious damage if left untreated. But effective treatment *is* available. If you let your doctor know about any breathing trouble or coughing spells you experience, you'll be less likely to cough the winter away.

Caution: Some drugs in this section may affect pregnancy or fetal development. Check with your doctor if this concerns you.

EMPHYSEMA

Emphysema is a long-term illness in which breathing becomes increasingly difficult over the years. Known also as chronic obstructive pulmonary disease (COPD), it most often strikes men and women between the ages of fifty and the late seventies.

Normally, the oxygen in the air we breathe passes through the walls of air sacs in the lungs, called alveoli, and into the small blood vessels of the lungs. At the same time, carbon dioxide passes out of the blood vessels, into the air sacs, and then up through the bronchial tubes so that it can be exhaled. But in emphysema, the lungs' small airways are damaged, and the walls of the alveoli rupture. Therefore, less oxygen and carbon dioxide can move back and forth. In fact, some of the carbon dioxide gets stuck in the lungs, preventing the inhalation of fresh air.

CAUSES

Emphysema is a disease that would hardly exist if people didn't smoke cigarettes. Generally, years and years of smoking lead to the rupture of the alveoli, and continued smoking only worsens this life-threatening condition. Sometimes, other factors come into play. For example, genetic factors, exposure to industrial chemicals over a long period of time, other diseases of the lungs, and the physical stress of certain occupations may all contribute to the development of emphysema.

DIAGNOSIS

The main symptom of emphysema is difficulty in breathing, which may become so severe that you feel as if you're suffocating. You may have to puff in order to move enough air in and out of your lungs. All this straining will cause muscles in your chest to over-expand, giving your chest a barrel shape. Your neck and shoulder muscles may also become over-developed because of the effort it takes to breathe. Even with all that extra effort, you may not get enough air, and your skin may take on a blue tone because of oxygen deprivation.

Chronic bronchitis usually precedes emphysema, and you may have the persistent wet cough of that disease, as well. For some people, the cough is more severe than the breathing difficulty. During a respiratory infection, the symptoms of emphysema often become worse, and wheezing and shortness of breath occur.

To determine the cause of your breathing difficulties, your doctor will take a medical history and perform a physical examination, paying special attention to your chest sounds. As part of the exam, you'll probably be asked to blow into a device that provides a measurement of your ability to exhale. Blood tests, sputum analysis, and a chest X ray will also aid the doctor in arriving at a correct diagnosis.

TREATMENT

Therapy is aimed at easing your breathing and slowing the rate at which damage occurs. Your doctor is likely to prescribe a bronchodilator, which relieves the tightening of the bronchial tubes and loosens mucus. (See the drug charts on pages 771–779.) Your treatment may also include use of a portable oxygen tank to help prevent oxygen deprivation.

First and foremost, people with emphysema should stop smoking. They should also avoid areas of air pollution. Respiratory infections can worsen your problems, so stay away from people with such contagious diseases as influenza. If you have been exposed, your doctor might prescribe antibiotics for you to take as a preventive measure.

Being unable to breathe can cause a great deal of emotional stress, and emotional stress can increase difficulty in breathing. Many people with emphysema become depressed and angry; they may also feel frustrated that there is currently no cure for their illness. Such medicines as tranquilizers and antidepressants are often prescribed to help relieve those feelings and to enhance the effectiveness of treatment.

OUTLOOK

Emphysema is an irreversible condition that can lead to such other problems as pulmonary hypertension and heart failure. (Be sure to tell your doctor if your ankles begin to swell or your breathing problems suddenly become much worse—these are possible signals of complications.) Keep in mind, however, that there have been significant advances in the treatment of emphysema and that continuing research will undoubtedly lead to even more effective therapeutic approaches. Meanwhile, follow your current treatment plan, and don't hesitate to seek help if you feel emotionally overwhelmed by the effects of your illness.

CONDITION: **ASTHMA, BRONCHITIS, AND EMPHYSEMA**
CATEGORY: **BRONCHODILATORS (THEOPHYLLINE AND RELATED DRUGS)**

GENERIC (CHEMICAL) NAME	BRAND (TRADE) NAME	DOSAGE FORMS AND STRENGTHS
Theophylline	Available under a number of brand names and dosage forms and strengths.*	
Oxtriphylline	CHOLEDYL	Syrup: 50 mg per tsp Elixir: 100 mg per tsp Tablets: 100, 200 mg
	CHOLEDYL SA	Controlled-release tablets: 400, 600 mg
Oxtriphylline and guaifenesin	BRONDECON	Elixir: 100 mg oxtriphylline and 50 mg guaifenesin per tsp Tablets: 200 mg oxtriphylline and 100 mg guaifenesin

*Common brand names for theophylline include BRONKODYL, CONSTANT-T, DURAPHYL, ELIXICON, ELIXOPHYLLIN, QUIBRON-T, RESPBID, SLO-BID, SLO-PHYLLIN, SOMOPHYLLIN-T, THEO-24, THEO-DUR, THEOBID, THEOLAIR, THEOPHYL, and UNIPHYL.

DRUG PROFILE

Theophylline and its relative, oxtriphylline, are used to treat the wheezing, cough, and breathing problems associated with bronchial asthma, chronic bronchitis, and emphysema. They work by relaxing the muscles of the respiratory tract, allowing the lungs to take in more air and making the flow of air easier. These drugs also increase the supply of blood to the lungs. Guaifenesin is an expectorant—it thins and loosens the mucus in the lungs so that it can be coughed up more easily.

BEFORE USING THIS DRUG

Let your doctor know *IF*

You have ever had allergic reactions or other problems with ∎ theophylline ∎ oxtriphylline ∎ caffeine ∎ theobromine.

With Brondecon only: ∎ guaifenesin.

You have ever had any of the following medical problems: ∎ other respiratory infections, including influenza ∎ heart disease or any disease of the blood vessels ∎ stomach problems ∎ ulcers ∎ liver disease ∎ kidney disease ∎ overactive thyroid ∎ diabetes ∎ glaucoma ∎ high blood pressure ∎ abnormal heart rhythms ∎ diarrhea.

You are taking any of the following medicines: ∎ other medicine for respiratory problems ∎ medicine for gout ∎ antibiotics ∎ medicine for seizures ∎ medicine for tuberculosis ∎ barbiturates ∎ appetite suppressants ∎ beta-blockers ∎ calcium blockers ∎ lithium (medicine for depression) ∎ medicine for diarrhea ∎ influenza vaccine ∎ cimetidine or ranitidine (medicine for ulcers) ∎ diuretics ∎ tranquilizers ∎ muscle relaxants ∎ drugs for thyroid disease ∎ sleep medicines ∎ baking soda.

SPECIAL RESTRICTIONS WHILE TAKING THIS DRUG

FOOD AND DRUG INTERACTIONS

Other Drugs	Because many other drugs interact with this drug, check with your doctor before taking any other medicine, including over-the-counter (OTC) drugs. Also, tell your doctor if you are planning to be vaccinated for influenza.
Foods and Beverages	Limit your intake of foods and beverages that contain caffeine, such as cocoa, chocolate, coffee, tea, and colas. These may add to the stimulant effects of this drug. Also, cut down on charcoal-broiled foods because they decrease the effectiveness of this drug.

Smoking	Tell your doctor if you smoke or have given up smoking within the last two years. Your dosage may need to be adjusted accordingly.

No special restrictions on alcohol use.

DAILY LIVING

Examinations or Tests	It is important for you to keep all appointments with your doctor so that your progress can be checked. Periodic blood tests are usually required to keep track of how much of this drug is in your body.
Other Precautions	Taking this medicine more often or for a longer period of time than prescribed by your doctor may make you more prone to developing side effects. If you develop diarrhea, fever, or flulike symptoms (cough, fever, or body aches), contact your doctor. Your dosage may need to be adjusted. Do not switch brands or dosage forms without consulting your doctor. Tell any doctor or dentist you consult that you are taking this medicine, especially if you will be undergoing any type of surgery.
Helpful Hints	Make sure you take this drug in regularly spaced doses exactly as instructed by your doctor, in order to maintain a constant level of medicine in your blood. For maximum benefit, take the tablets and liquid form of this medicine with a glass of water on an empty stomach (half an hour before or two hours after meals).

If this drug causes upset stomach, taking it with an antacid should help.

Both the regular and controlled-release tablets should be swallowed whole, without chewing or crushing.

No special restrictions on driving, exertion and exercise, sun exposure, or exposure to excessive heat or cold.

POSSIBLE SIDE EFFECTS

Although this list of adverse effects may seem somewhat intimidating, keep in mind that some are quite rare. Of course, should these or any other problems arise while you are on medication, it is always a good idea to consult your doctor.

IF YOU DEVELOP

behavior changes ■ frequent vomiting ■ fever ■ ringing in ears ■ irregular heartbeat ■ muscle twitching ■ vomiting, with blood or vomit that looks like coffee grounds ■ excessive sweating ■ seizures ■ rapid, shallow breathing ■ bloody or black, tarry stools ■ tremors ■ confusion

WHAT TO DO

Urgent Get in touch with your doctor immediately.

---

dizziness ■ headache ■ urinary frequency ■ stomach pain or cramps ■ sleeplessness ■ fast heartbeat ■ flushing ■ rash or hives

May be serious Check with your doctor as soon as possible.

---

diarrhea ■ nausea or vomiting ■ loss of appetite ■ nervousness or restlessness ■ irritability

If symptoms are disturbing or persist, let your doctor know.

STORAGE INSTRUCTIONS

Store in a cool, dark place (not in a bathroom medicine cabinet). If your medicine is in a liquid form, make sure that it does not freeze.

STOPPING OR INTERRUPTING THERAPY

Take this medicine exactly as prescribed by your doctor. If you miss a dose, take it as soon as possible. If it is almost time for your next dose, skip the missed dose and resume your regular schedule. Do not take two doses at the same time.

SPECIAL CONSIDERATIONS FOR THOSE OVER SIXTY-FIVE

Older people, especially men, may be more prone to side effects. Doctors may want to monitor them especially closely and check their blood levels of this drug to make sure they are receiving the correct dosage. This drug can cause urinary frequency, particularly in women, and this may be an important problem for those over sixty-five.

CONDITION: ASTHMA, BRONCHITIS, AND EMPHYSEMA

CATEGORY: BRONCHODILATORS (BETA-AGONISTS)

GENERIC (CHEMICAL) NAME	BRAND (TRADE) NAME	DOSAGE FORMS AND STRENGTHS
Albuterol	PROVENTIL Inhaler	Inhaler: 90 mcg per inhalation
	VENTOLIN Inhaler	Inhaler: 90 mcg per inhalation
Albuterol sulfate	PROVENTIL	Repetabs: 4 mg Solution: 0.5% Syrup: 2 mg per tsp Tablets: 2, 4 mg
	VENTOLIN	Rotacaps: 200 mcg Syrup: 2 mg per tsp Tablets: 2, 4 mg
Bitolterol mesylate	TORNALATE	Inhaler: 370 mcg per inhalation
Isoetharine hydrochloride	BRONKOMETER BRONKOSOL	Inhaler: 340 mcg per inhalation Inhalation solution: 1%

Metaproterenol sulfate	ALUPENT	Inhalation solution: 0.4%, 0.6%, 5%
		Metered-dose inhaler: 0.65 mg per inhalation
		Syrup: 10 mg per tsp
		Tablets: 10, 20 mg
	METAPREL	Inhalation solution: 5%
		Metered-dose inhaler: 0.65 mg per inhalation
		Syrup: 10 mg per tsp
		Tablets: 10, 20 mg
Pirbuterol	MAXAIR	Inhaler: 200 mcg per inhalation
Terbutaline sulfate	BRETHAIRE	Inhaler: 200 mcg per inhalation
	BRETHINE	Tablets: 2.5, 5 mg
	BRICANYL	Tablets: 2.5, 5 mg

DRUG PROFILE

Beta-agonists are used to treat the bronchial spasm and wheezing associated with asthma, bronchitis, and emphysema. These drugs work by relaxing the muscles of the respiratory tract, allowing the lungs to take in more air and making the flow of air easier. The inhalant form of albuterol is also used to prevent bronchial spasm triggered by exercise.

BEFORE USING THIS DRUG

Let your doctor know *IF*

You have ever had allergic reactions or other problems with ■ albuterol ■ bitolterol ■ isoetharine ■ metaproterenol ■ pirbuterol ■ terbutaline ■ medicines with a stimulant effect (amphetamines, ephedrine, isoproterenol, and phenylpropanolamine).

You have ever had any of the following medical problems: ■ diabetes ■ heart disease, including abnormal heart rhythms ■ high blood pressure ■ overactive thyroid ■ enlarged prostate ■ seizures.

You are taking any of the following medicines: ■ medicine for asthma ■ beta-blockers ■ medicine for depression ■ appetite suppressants ■ medicine for Parkinson's disease ■ medicine for high blood pressure ■ nitrates (medicine for chest pain) ■ any medicine containing caffeine ■ antihistamines ■ medicine for hay fever or other allergies (including nose drops or nose sprays) ■ thyroid hormones ■ digoxin or digitalis (heart medicines).

SPECIAL RESTRICTIONS WHILE TAKING THIS DRUG

FOOD AND DRUG INTERACTIONS

Other Drugs	Do not take any other drugs, including over-the-counter (OTC) drugs, before checking with your doctor. Drugs that may add to the stimulant effects of this drug include appetite suppressants, medicine containing caffeine, decongestants, and some medicines for allergies or colds. If you are also using an inhalant corticosteroid, allow fifteen minutes between the use of the corticosteroid and this drug.
Smoking	Smoking aggravates any kind of lung disease. If you smoke, try to stop or at least cut down.

No special restrictions on foods and beverages or alcohol use.

DAILY LIVING

Examinations or Tests	It is important for you to keep all appointments with your doctor so that your progress can be checked.
Other Precautions	Taking this medicine more often or for a longer period of time than prescribed by your doctor may make you more prone to developing side effects. If this medicine fails to relieve your symptoms or if your condition worsens, call your doctor immediately.

| Helpful Hints | If your mouth or throat feels dry, rinse your mouth with water after each dose. |

No special restrictions on driving, exertion and exercise, sun exposure, or exposure to excessive heat or cold.

POSSIBLE SIDE EFFECTS

Although this list of adverse effects may seem somewhat intimidating, keep in mind that some are quite rare. Of course, should these or any other problems arise while you are on medication, it is always a good idea to consult your doctor.

IF YOU DEVELOP	WHAT TO DO
chest pain or tight feeling in chest ■ pounding heartbeat ■ rapid, shallow breathing ■ wheezing ■ seizures	**Urgent** Get in touch with your doctor immediately.
severe dizziness ■ muscle cramps ■ irregular or fast heartbeat ■ excitement ■ irritability ■ tremors ■ increased sweating ■ dilated pupils ■ weakness ■ nosebleed ■ severe headache *For albuterol only:* rash ■ itching ■ difficulty breathing ■ swelling in mouth or throat	**May be serious** Check with your doctor as soon as possible.
nervousness or restlessness ■ headache ■ nausea or vomiting ■ unusual taste in mouth ■ heartburn ■ dry mouth or throat ■ cough ■ sleeplessness ■ increased appetite ■ dizziness or light-headedness	If symptoms are disturbing or persist, let your doctor know.

STORAGE INSTRUCTIONS

Store tablets, capsules, and all liquids in a cool, dark place (not in a bathroom medicine cabinet). Do not allow the inhalant to freeze. Store inhalation canister at room temperature and discard it after using the labeled quantity of inhalations.

STOPPING OR INTERRUPTING THERAPY

Take this medicine exactly as prescribed by your doctor. If you miss a dose, take it as soon as possible. If it is almost time for your next dose, skip the missed dose and resume your regular schedule. Do not take two doses at the same time.

SPECIAL CONSIDERATIONS FOR THOSE OVER SIXTY-FIVE

Older people may be more prone to the side effects of this drug. Doctors will probably start people over sixty-five on a lower than normal dosage and check them regularly. This drug can cause urinary frequency, particularly in women, and this may be an important problem for those over sixty-five.

CONDITION: **ASTHMA, BRONCHITIS, AND EMPHYSEMA**
CATEGORY: **CORTICOSTEROIDS**

GENERIC (CHEMICAL) NAME	BRAND (TRADE) NAME	DOSAGE FORMS AND STRENGTHS
Beclomethasone dipropionate	BECLOVENT	Inhaler: 42 mcg per inhalation
	VANCERIL Inhaler	Inhaler: 42 mcg per inhalation
Triamcinolone acetonide	AZMACORT	Inhaler: 100 mcg per inhalation

DRUG PROFILE

Inhaled corticosteroids such as beclomethasone are used as long-term therapy to prevent asthma attacks. They work by shrinking the swollen membranes of the respiratory tract, allowing the lungs to take in more air and making the flow of air easier. Inhaled steroids are sometimes used along with inhaled bronchodilators such as albuterol or terbutaline (see the charts on pages 775–779).

BEFORE USING THIS DRUG

Let your doctor know *IF*

You have ever had allergic reactions or other problems with ■ any corticosteroids ■ aerosol sprays.

You have ever had any of the following medical problems: ■ colitis or diverticulitis ■ diabetes ■ bone disease, such as osteoporosis ■ recent fungal infection ■ glaucoma ■ heart disease ■ disease of the blood vessels ■ herpes eye infection ■ any viral infection, such as chickenpox ■ high blood pressure ■ kidney disease ■ liver disease ■ myasthenia gravis ■ stomach ulcer ■ stomach cramps ■ tuberculosis ■ underactive thyroid ■ mental illness ■ seizures ■ recent infection of the mouth, throat, or lungs ■ high cholesterol.

You are taking any of the following medicines: ■ any other medicine for asthma antibiotics ■ digoxin or digitalis (heart medicines) ■ medicine for abnormal heart rhythms ■ diuretics ■ medicine for high blood pressure ■ medicine for inflammation, such as medicine for arthritis (including aspirin or aspirinlike medicine) ■ insulin or other medicine for diabetes ■ anticoagulants (blood thinners) ■ medicine for Parkinson's disease ■ phenobarbital ■ medicine for seizures ■ estrogens (female hormones) ■ thiazides or furosemide (potassium-depleting diuretics) ■ medicine for myasthenia gravis.

You have recently had a vaccination.

SPECIAL RESTRICTIONS WHILE TAKING THIS DRUG

FOOD AND DRUG INTERACTIONS

Other Drugs

Corticosteroids interact with many other drugs. Do not take any other drugs, including over-the-counter (OTC) drugs, before checking with your doctor.

If you are also using a bronchodilator inhaler, use the bronchodilator first and allow at least five minutes between the use of the bronchodilator and the beclomethasone inhaler.

Corticosteroids may affect how your body absorbs medicine for diabetes, and your dosage may need to be adjusted.

Tell your doctor if you are planning to receive any kind of vaccine.

Foods and Beverages	As this drug may deplete your body of calcium and potassium, your doctor may recommend a diet rich in these minerals. You may also be advised to go on a low-salt diet.
Smoking	Smoking aggravates any kind of lung disease. If you smoke, try to stop or at least cut down.

No special restrictions on alcohol use.

DAILY LIVING

Examinations or Tests	It is important for you to keep all appointments with your doctor so that your progress can be checked. If you are on long-term therapy with this drug, your doctor may want to perform periodic blood and urine tests.
Other Precautions	Tell any doctor or dentist you consult that you are taking this medicine, especially if you will be undergoing any type of surgery.

Taking this medicine more often or for a longer period of time than prescribed by your doctor may make you more prone to developing side effects. If this medicine fails to relieve your symptoms or if your condition worsens, call your doctor immediately.

You should also inform your doctor if you are undergoing some sort of unusual stress or if you develop a respiratory infection.

You may become more prone to fungal infections of the mouth and throat while using a corticosteroid inhaler. Let your doctor know if you develop signs of such an infection (white patches in the mouth or throat). You may also have a sore throat and hoarseness. Gargling with salt water or a special mouthwash prescribed by your doctor after each use and cleaning the inhaler daily should help prevent these effects.

No special restrictions on driving, exertion and exercise, sun exposure, or exposure to excessive heat or cold.

POSSIBLE SIDE EFFECTS

Although this list of adverse effects may seem somewhat intimidating, keep in mind that some are quite rare. Of course, should these or any other problems arise while you are on medication, it is always a good idea to consult your doctor.

IF YOU DEVELOP

stomach pain ■ dizziness or faintness ■ fever ■ muscle or joint pain or weakness ■ nausea or vomiting ■ difficulty in breathing ■ tiredness ■ weight loss ■ slow or fast heartbeat ■ palpitations ■ swelling of mouth or tongue ■ difficulty in speech ■ seizures ■ loss of appetite ■ pain in urination ■ urinary frequency

After you STOP taking this medicine: loss of appetite or weight loss ■ nausea or vomiting ■ drowsiness ■ headache ■ fever ■ joint or muscle pain ■ skin problems ■ dizziness ■ depression

WHAT TO DO

Urgent Get in touch with your doctor immediately.

back, hip, or rib pain ■ acne ■ increased sweating ■ hair growth ■ rash, hives, or other skin changes ■ bruising ■ depression or other mood changes ■ nervousness or restlessness ■ bloody stools ■ bloating ■ halos around lights or other visual disturbances ■ wounds that take a long time to heal ■ swelling of hands, feet, or ankles ■ diarrhea ■ constipation ■ reactivation of an ulcer ■ any lung or throat infection ■ white patches in mouth or throat ■ skin redness ■ hoarseness or sore throat ■ dry mouth ■ swelling of face ■ "high" feeling ■ headache ■ eye pain ■ decreased vision	**May be serious** Check with your doctor as soon as possible.
indigestion ■ bloating ■ increased appetite ■ weight gain ■ eruptions on mouth or lips ■ sleeplessness ■ cough	If symptoms are disturbing or persist, let your doctor know.

STORAGE INSTRUCTIONS

Store inhalant canister at room temperature and discard it after you have used the labeled quantity of inhalations.

STOPPING OR INTERRUPTING THERAPY

Take this medicine exactly as prescribed by your doctor. Inhaled corticosteroids need to be used at regular intervals to be effective; it may be one to four weeks before you notice improvement of your symptoms. If you miss a dose, take it as soon as possible. If it is almost time for your next dose, skip the missed dose and resume your regular schedule. Do not take two doses at the same time.

SPECIAL CONSIDERATIONS FOR THOSE OVER SIXTY-FIVE

Long-term use of corticosteroids may cause gradual bone loss; this can be serious in older people—particularly women, who are vulnerable to osteoporosis.

CONDITION: **ASTHMA**

CATEGORY: **MAST-CELL INHIBITORS**

GENERIC (CHEMICAL) NAME	BRAND (TRADE) NAME	DOSAGE FORMS AND STRENGTHS
Cromolyn sodium	INTAL Capsules INTAL Inhaler INTAL Nebulizer Solution	Capsules: 20 mg Inhaler: 800 mcg per inhalation Ampuls: 20 mg per 2 ml

DRUG PROFILE

Cromolyn sodium is given to prevent attacks in patients with chronic asthma. This drug may also be prescribed to prevent asthma attacks that occur in response to specific stimuli such as exercise, cold dry air, environmental pollutants, animal dander, and drugs such as aspirin.

It is important to note that the use of cromolyn sodium is a preventive measure; this drug is NOT helpful against an asthma attack already in progress.

BEFORE USING THIS DRUG

Let your doctor know *IF*

You have ever had allergic reactions or other problems with ■ cromolyn sodium

Capsules only: ■ lactose (milk sugar).

Aerosol only: ■ aerosol sprays.

You have ever had any of the following medical problems: ■ liver disease ■ kidney disease ■ heart disease ■ abnormal heart rhythms.

You are taking any of the following medicines: ■ other medicine for asthma.

SPECIAL RESTRICTIONS WHILE TAKING THIS DRUG

FOOD AND DRUG INTERACTIONS

Other Drugs	If you are also taking corticosteroids for your asthma, continue to do so unless your doctor instructs you to stop. If you are using a bronchodilator inhaler, use it first and wait five minutes before your dose of cromolyn sodium. If you have any questions about this, check with your doctor.
Smoking	Smoking aggravates any kind of lung disease. If you smoke, try to stop or at least cut down.

No special restrictions on foods and beverages or alcohol use.

DAILY LIVING

Examinations or Tests	It is important for you to keep all appointments with your doctor so that your progress can be checked.
Other Precautions	Tell any doctor or dentist you consult that you are taking this medicine, especially if you will be undergoing any type of surgery. Taking this medicine more often or for a longer period of time than prescribed by your doctor may make you more prone to developing side effects. If this medicine fails to relieve your symptoms or if your condition worsens, call your doctor immediately. You should also inform your doctor if you are undergoing some sort of unusual stress, or if you develop a respiratory infection or a serious illness.

Cromolyn sodium is used to PREVENT asthma attacks. If used while an attack is already in progress, this drug may actually make symptoms worse.

Cough, sore throat, or hoarseness may occur while you are taking this medicine. Gargling and rinsing with water or simply drinking a glass of water before and/or after your dose of cromolyn sodium may help.

Helpful Hints

For the aerosol spray: Follow directions carefully and be sure to keep the spray away from the eye area.

For the capsules: These come with their own special inhaler unit. Remember that several deep inhalations may be necessary to completely empty a capsule. At least once a week, the unit should be washed in warm water and then dried thoroughly.

For the solution: Use a power- (NOT hand-) operated nebulizer with an adequate flow rate and a suitable face mask or mouthpiece. If you have any questions about this, check with your doctor.

No special restrictions on driving, exertion and exercise, sun exposure, or exposure to excessive heat or cold.

POSSIBLE SIDE EFFECTS

Although this list of adverse effects may seem somewhat intimidating, keep in mind that some are quite rare. Of course, should these or any other problems arise while you are on medication, it is always a good idea to consult your doctor.

IF YOU DEVELOP	WHAT TO DO
increased wheezing ■ difficulty breathing ■ tightness in chest ■ chest pain ■ dizziness ■ headache ■ nausea or vomiting ■ difficulty swallowing ■ chills ■ sweating ■ rash, hives, or itching ■ swelling of lips and eyes ■ difficult, painful, or frequent urination ■ swelling or pain in joints ■ muscle pain or weakness ■ coughing up blood from the lungs ■ severe skin irritation	**May be serious** Check with your doctor as soon as possible.
cough ■ hoarseness ■ throat irritation ■ dry mouth or throat ■ stuffy nose ■ sneezing, watery eyes ■ unpleasant taste ■ skin sensitivity to the sun ■ inflammation or pain in many muscles ■ bloody nose	If symptoms are disturbing or persist, let your doctor know.

STORAGE INSTRUCTIONS

Store the capsules and solution in a cool, dark place (not in a bathroom medicine cabinet). Do not allow the ampuls or inhalant to freeze. Store the inhaler at room temperature.

STOPPING OR INTERRUPTING THERAPY

Take this medicine exactly as prescribed by your doctor. This medicine needs to be used at regular intervals to be effective; it may take two to four weeks before you experience the full benefits. Your doctor will give you instructions on how to taper off gradually. If you miss a dose, take it as soon as possible, and space the rest of your doses for that day at even intervals. Do not take two doses at the same time.

SPECIAL CONSIDERATIONS FOR THOSE OVER SIXTY-FIVE

None.

CONDITION: **ASTHMA, BRONCHITIS, AND EMPHYSEMA**
CATEGORY: **BRONCHODILATORS**

GENERIC (CHEMICAL) NAME	BRAND (TRADE) NAME	DOSAGE FORMS AND STRENGTHS
Ipratropium bromide	ATROVENT	Inhaler: 18 mcg per inhalation

DRUG PROFILE

Ipratropium bromide is used to prevent or control wheezing, cough, and breathing problems associated with lung diseases such as chronic bronchitis and emphysema. This drug works by relaxing the muscles of the respiratory tract, allowing the lungs to take in more air and making the flow of air easier.

It is important to note that ipratropium is a preventive measure and not used to treat acute symptoms when a fast-acting medicine is needed.

BEFORE USING THIS DRUG

Let your doctor know *IF*

You have ever had allergic reactions or other problems with ■ ipratropium ■ atropine ■ hyoscyamine ■ scopolamine ■ belladonna ■ aerosol sprays.

You have ever had any of the following medical problems: ■ bladder disease ■ enlarged prostate ■ difficulty urinating ■ glaucoma.

You are taking any of the following medicines: ■ other medicine for respiratory problems ■ eye medicine.

SPECIAL RESTRICTIONS WHILE TAKING THIS DRUG

FOOD AND DRUG INTERACTIONS

Other Drugs	If you are using a corticosteroid or cromolyn sodium inhaler, use the ipratropium inhaler first and wait five minutes before your dose of corticosteroid or cromolyn sodium.
	If you are using another bronchodilator (beta agonist) inhaler, use it first and wait five minutes before your dose of ipratropium bromide. If you have any questions, check with your doctor.
Smoking	Smoking aggravates any kind of lung disease. If you smoke, try to stop or at least cut down.

No special restrictions on foods and beverages or alcohol use.

DAILY LIVING

Examinations or Tests	It is important for you to keep all appointments with your doctor so that your progress can be checked.
Other Precautions	Tell any doctor or dentist you consult that you are taking this medicine, especially if you will be undergoing any type of surgery.
	Taking this medicine more often or for a longer period of time than prescribed by your doctor may make you more prone to developing side effects.
	Ipratropium bromide is used to PREVENT symptoms. If used while an attack is already in progress, this drug may actually make symptoms worse.

If you should accidentally get some of the aerosol in your eyes, be aware that temporary blurring of vision may occur.

Helpful Hints

If your mouth or throat feels dry, chewing sugarless gum or sucking ice chips or sugarless hard candy will help. If dryness persists for more than two weeks, consult your doctor or dentist.

No special restrictions on driving, exertion and exercise, sun exposure, or exposure to excessive heat or cold.

POSSIBLE SIDE EFFECTS

Although this list of adverse effects may seem somewhat intimidating, keep in mind that some are quite rare. Of course, should these or any other problems arise while you are on medication, it is always a good idea to consult your doctor.

IF YOU DEVELOP	WHAT TO DO
increased wheezing	**Urgent** Get in touch with your doctor immediately.
mouth or lip sores ■ skin rash or hives	**May be serious** Get in touch with your doctor as soon as possible.
cough ■ throat irritation ■ dry mouth or throat ■ nausea ■ upset stomach ■ headache ■ dizziness ■ nervousness ■ blurred vision or other vision changes ■ trouble sleeping ■ tiredness or weakness ■ rapid or pounding heartbeat ■ trembling ■ metallic or unpleasant taste ■ stuffy nose ■ constipation ■ eye pain ■ flushing	If symptoms are disturbing or persist, let your doctor know.

STORAGE INSTRUCTIONS

Store in a cool, dark place (not in a bathroom medicine cabinet). Do not allow your medicine to freeze.

STOPPING OR INTERRUPTING THERAPY

Take this medicine exactly as prescribed by your doctor. If you miss a dose, take it as soon as possible. If it is almost time for your next dose, skip the missed dose and resume your regular schedule. Do not take two doses at the same time.

SPECIAL CONSIDERATIONS FOR THOSE OVER SIXTY-FIVE

None.

CONDITION: **BRONCHITIS**

CATEGORY: **ANTIBIOTICS (TETRACYCLINES)**

GENERIC (CHEMICAL) NAME	BRAND (TRADE) NAME	DOSAGE FORMS AND STRENGTHS
Demeclocycline hydrochloride	DECLOMYCIN	Capsules: 150 mg Tablets: 150, 300 mg
Doxycycline	VIBRAMYCIN	Capsules: 50, 100 mg Suspension: 25 mg per tsp Syrup: 50 mg per tsp
	VIBRATABS	Tablets: 100 mg
Methacycline hydrochloride	RONDOMYCIN	Capsules: 150, 300 mg
Minocycline	MINOCIN	Capsules: 50,100 mg Suspension: 50 mg per tsp Tablets: 50, 100 mg

| Oxytetracycline | TERRAMYCIN | Capsules: 250 mg |
| | | Tablets: 250 mg |

Tetracycline hydrochloride	ACHROMYCIN V	Capsules: 250, 500 mg
		Suspension: 125 mg per tsp
	PANMYCIN	Capsules: 250 mg
	ROBITET	Capsules: 250, 500 mg
	SUMYCIN	Capsules: 250, 500 mg
		Tablets: 250, 500 mg

This type of drug is available under other brand names as well.

DRUG PROFILE

Tetracyclines are antibiotics that are used to treat a wide variety of bacterial infections, including skin eruptions and bronchitis and pneumonia. These antibiotics suppress the growth of the bacteria by interfering with their manufacture of protein.

For complete information on these drugs, see pages 706–710.

CONDITION: **BRONCHITIS**

CATEGORY: **ANTIBIOTICS (ERYTHROMYCINS)**

GENERIC (CHEMICAL) NAME	BRAND (TRADE) NAME	DOSAGE FORMS AND STRENGTHS
Erythromycin	E-MYCIN	Tablets: 250, 333 mg
	ERYC	Capsules: 250 mg
	ERY-TAB	Tablets: 250, 333, 500 mg
	PCE	Tablets: 333, 500 mg

Erythromycin estolate	ILOSONE	Capsules: 250 mg
		Chewable tablets: 125, 250 mg
		Drops: 100 mg per ml
		Suspension: 125, 250 mg per tsp
		Tablets: 500 mg
Erythromycin ethylsuccinate	E.E.S.	Chewable tablets: 200 mg
		Drops: 100 mg per 2.5 ml
		Suspension: 200, 400 mg per tsp
		Suspension granules: 200 mg per tsp
		Tablets: 400 mg
	WYAMYCIN E	Suspension: 200, 400 mg per tsp
Erythromycin stearate	ERYTHROCIN Stearate	Tablets: 250, 500 mg
	WYAMYCIN S	Tablets: 250, 500 mg

This type of drug is available under other brand names as well.

DRUG PROFILE

Erythromycins are antibiotics that are used to treat a variety of bacterial infections, including such respiratory tract infections as bronchitis and pneumonia. These drugs suppress the growth of the bacteria and keep them from multiplying by blocking the bacteria's ability to manufacture protein.

For complete information on these drugs, see pages 710–713.

CONDITION: **BRONCHITIS**

CATEGORY: **ANTIBIOTICS (PENICILLINS)**

GENERIC (CHEMICAL) NAME	BRAND (TRADE) NAME	DOSAGE FORMS AND STRENGTHS
Amoxicillin	AMOXIL	Capsules: 250, 500 mg Chewable tablets: 125, 250 mg Suspension: 125, 250 mg per tsp
	LAROTID	Capsules: 250, 500 mg Suspension: 125, 250 mg per tsp
	POLYMOX	Capsules: 250, 500 mg Suspension: 125, 250 mg per tsp
	TRIMOX	Capsules: 250, 500 mg Suspension: 125, 250 mg per tsp
Ampicillin	AMCILL	Capsules: 250, 500 mg Suspension: 125, 250 mg per tsp
	OMNIPEN	Capsules: 250, 500 mg Suspension: 125, 250 mg per tsp
	POLYCILLIN	Capsules: 250, 500 mg Suspension: 125, 250, 500 mg per tsp
	TOTACILLIN	Capsules: 250, 500 mg Suspension: 125, 250 mg per tsp
Bacampicillin hydrochloride	SPECTROBID	Suspension: 125 mg per tsp Tablets: 400 mg
Carbenicillin indanyl sodium	GEOCILLIN	Tablets: 382 mg

Cloxacillin sodium	TEGOPEN	Capsules: 250, 500 mg Solution: 125 mg per tsp
Cyclacillin	CYCLAPEN-W	Suspension: 125, 250 mg per tsp Tablets: 250, 500 mg
Nafcillin sodium	UNIPEN	Capsules: 250 mg Solution: 250 mg per tsp Tablets: 500 mg
Oxacillin sodium	PROSTAPHLIN	Capsules: 250, 500 mg Solution: 250 mg per tsp
Penicillin G potassium	PENTIDS	Tablets: 125, 250, 500 mg Solution: 250 mg per tsp
Penicillin V potassium	LEDERCILLIN VK	Solution: 125, 250 mg per tsp Tablets: 250, 500 mg
	PEN•VEE•K	Solution: 125, 250 mg per tsp Tablets: 250, 500 mg
	V-CILLIN K	Solution: 125, 250 mg per tsp Tablets: 125, 250, 500 mg

This type of drug is available under other brand names as well.

DRUG PROFILE

Penicillins are antibiotics that are used to treat a wide variety of bacterial infections, including infections of the ear, nose, and throat and such respiratory tract infections as bronchitis and pneumonia. Penicillins suppress the growth of bacteria by interfering with the bacteria's ability to form new protective cell walls.

For complete information on these drugs, see pages 714–718.

CONDITION: **BRONCHITIS**

CATEGORY: **ANTIBIOTICS (CEPHALOSPORINS)**

GENERIC (CHEMICAL) NAME	BRAND (TRADE) NAME	DOSAGE FORMS AND STRENGTHS
Cefaclor	CECLOR	Capsules: 250, 500 mg Suspension: 125, 187, 250, 375 mg per tsp
Cefadroxil	DURICEF	Capsules: 500 mg Suspension: 125, 250, 500 mg per tsp Tablets: 1 g
	ULTRACEF	Capsules: 500 mg Suspension: 125, 250 mg per tsp Tablets: 1 g
Cefixime	SUPRAX	Suspension: 100 mg per tsp Tablets: 200, 400 mg
Cefuroxime	CEFTIN	Tablets: 125, 250, 500 mg
Cephalexin	KEFLEX	Capsules: 250, 500 mg Suspension: 125, 250 mg per tsp Drops: 100 mg per ml
	KEFLET	Tablets: 250, 500 mg Tablets: 1 g
Cephalexin hydrochloride	KEFTAB	Tablets: 250, 500 mg

Cephradine	ANSPOR	Capsules: 250, 500 mg
		Suspension: 125, 250 mg per tsp
	VELOSEF	Capsules: 250, 500 mg
		Suspension: 125, 250 mg per tsp

This type of drug is available under other brand names as well.

DRUG PROFILE

Cephalosporins are antibiotics that are used to treat a wide variety of bacterial infections, including such upper respiratory tract infections as bronchitis and pneumonia. These drugs work by interfering with the bacteria's ability to multiply and to form new protective cell walls.

For complete information on these drugs, see pages 719–722.

TUBERCULOSIS

We tend to think of tuberculosis (TB) as a disease of the past—until it strikes us or someone we know. Its incidence is declining, but every year thousands of Americans are diagnosed as having an active case of TB. The most likely candidates for the white plague, as it has been called, are people forty-five and older. To understand why requires a brief review of the origins of this disorder.

TB is an infection that usually lodges in the lungs, though it can also affect other organs. Its cause is invasion of the body by a bacillus, a rod-shaped type of bacteria. In many cases, the body's own immune system fights back successfully, walling off the bacteria and keeping them inactive for years or even decades.

In the first half of this century, TB was a major public health hazard, affecting people of all ages. In many people, however, the disease has remained dormant. But with aging, their immune systems might have been weakened by other diseases, by immunosuppressive medicines, or just by getting older; the bacteria are thus able to break free and multiply, causing widespread damage in the lungs. Such a scenario is common to most people now being diagnosed as victims of TB—they are older people who were probably infected long ago.

DIAGNOSIS

The classic symptoms of TB are fatigue, fever, night sweats, weight loss, chronic wet cough, and blood in the mucus that is coughed up. But in older people, the symptoms are often more subtle—a slight cough, a little fever, and a general feeling of unwellness. Sometimes this decline in health is wrongly attributed to emotional depression or to the natural aging process. This kind of decline is *not* a normal part of the aging process but a signal that medical help is needed.

During your visit to the doctor, you will be asked to provide a detailed medical history. At that time, if you think you were ever infected with TB, or even just exposed to it, you should make a point of explaining the circumstances to your doctor.

If your doctor suspects that TB is the reason for your discomfort, you will probably be injected with a substance that causes a skin reaction if you have, or have ever had, a TB infection. This procedure, known as a tuberculin skin test, may have to be done twice in order to get an accurate result.

If you test positive, a chest X ray will be taken to check for the presence of TB-caused abnormalities in your lungs. These are signs of an active case of TB. A sputum sample may also be collected for analysis. If your doctor has reason to believe that the bacillus has invaded other body systems, you may be hospitalized for more comprehensive testing.

TREATMENT

Modern medicine has produced a real revolution in the treatment of TB. The sanitariums where TB patients used to stay isolated while they rested, breathed fresh air, and hoped to get well no longer exist. Instead, people with TB take a combination of antiTB drugs that can stop the infectious stage of the disease in two to four weeks. (See the drug charts on pages 800–806 for more information on these medicines.) Bed rest is not generally necessary, and even during the initial period of drug therapy, hospitalization and isolation are not always required.

The most effective drug can, however, have some very serious side effects, especially if the person is alcoholic, has vision problems, or suffers from kidney or liver disease. In those cases, substitute medicines are prescribed. Whatever drugs are prescribed, the doctor may insist on monthly office visits, with sputum and urine analyses and periodic chest X rays, to be sure the drugs are working without damaging vulnerable organs.

Your doctor may also want to test members of your family and other people you have been close to for possible TB infection. If they test positive, they will be instructed to take the anti-TB medicine also, as a preventive measure.

OUTLOOK

If your system is able to handle the most effective antiTB drugs, and if you take them conscientiously as your doctor orders, you can expect to return to at least some of your normal activities within a month. In as little as nine months, your TB may be completely cured. But if you have drug-resistant bacteria or have to use second-choice medicines because you react adversely to the faster-acting drugs, your treatment period could stretch to twice that long.

You may have to return for checkups on a regular basis for six months to a year after you've stopped taking medicines. If, during that time, there are no signs of reactivation of TB, you may consider yourself not only cured but also out of danger of recurrence.

CONDITION: **TUBERCULOSIS**

CATEGORY: **ANTITUBERCULOSIS DRUGS**

GENERIC (CHEMICAL) NAME	BRAND (TRADE) NAME	DOSAGE FORMS AND STRENGTHS
Isoniazid	INH	Tablets: 300 mg
	LANIAZID	Syrup: 50 mg per tsp
		Tablets: 50, 100 mg
	TEEBACONIN	Tablets: 50, 100, 300 mg

DRUG PROFILE

Isoniazid is used to treat tuberculosis or prevent it from developing in people who have a positive tuberculin skin test. This drug arrests the growth of the tuberculosis bacteria.

BEFORE USING THIS DRUG

Let your doctor know *IF*

You have ever had allergic reactions or other problems with ■ isoniazid or any other medicine for tuberculosis ■ niacin (vitamin B_3).

You have ever had any of the following medical problems: ■ alcoholism ■ kidney disease ■ liver disease ■ diabetes ■ seizures.

You are taking any of the following medicines: ■ other medicine for tuberculosis ■ antacids ■ anticoagulants (blood thinners) ■ medicine for seizures ■ antibiotics ■ niacin (vitamin B_3) ■ sleep medicines ■ tranquilizers ■ corticosteroids ■ Antabuse (used in treating alcoholism) ■ theophylline (medicine for asthma) ■ aspirin ■ vitamin B_6 (pyridoxine).

SPECIAL RESTRICTIONS WHILE TAKING THIS DRUG

FOOD AND DRUG INTERACTIONS

Other Drugs	Allow at least one hour between taking isoniazid and any antacid containing aluminum.
Foods and Beverages	In rare circumstances, certain foods with a large amount of tyramine or histamine (eg, certain cheeses [Swiss], fish [tuna], etc.) may cause a reaction if eaten while taking isoniazid. Check with your doctor if foods cause headaches, palpitations, sweating, flushing, light-headedness, diarrhea or itching.
Alcohol	Avoid alcohol while taking this medicine. Alcohol decreases the effect of this drug, and liver problems may develop as a result of this combination.
Smoking	Smoking aggravates any kind of lung disease. If you smoke, try to stop or at least cut down.

No special restrictions on foods and beverages.

DAILY LIVING

Examinations or Tests	It is important for you to keep all appointments with your doctor so that your progress can be checked. Periodic eye examinations may be required.
Other Precautions	Tell any doctor or dentist you consult that you are taking this drug, especially if you will be undergoing any type of surgery.
	If you have diabetes, be aware that this drug may affect the results of urine-sugar tests. Do not change the dose of your diabetes medicine, but check with your doctor.

Your doctor will probably recommend that you take vitamin B_6 (pyridoxine) along with your daily dose of this drug; vitamin B_6 helps reduce the side effects of this drug.

| Helpful Hints | If this medicine upsets your stomach, taking it with food should help. Or instead, you may take an antacid, but allow at least one hour between the antacid and your dose of this drug. |

No special restrictions on driving, exertion and exercise, sun exposure, or exposure to excessive heat or cold.

POSSIBLE SIDE EFFECTS

Although this list of adverse effects may seem somewhat intimidating, keep in mind that some are quite rare. Of course, should these or any other problems arise while you are on medication, it is always a good idea to consult your doctor.

IF YOU DEVELOP	WHAT TO DO
blurred vision ■ eye pain ■ general ill feeling ■ slurred speech ■ hallucinations ■ difficulty in breathing ■ extreme tiredness or weakness ■ clumsiness or unsteadiness ■ loss of appetite ■ pain, numbness, or tingling in hands or feet ■ seizures ■ muscle twitching ■ personality changes ■ nausea or vomiting ■ fever ■ rash ■ swollen lymph glands	**Urgent** Get in touch with your doctor immediately.
dark urine ■ yellowing of eyes or skin ■ ringing in ears ■ memory problems ■ euphoria ■ dizziness ■ upset stomach	**May be serious** Check with your doctor as soon as possible.

dry mouth ∎ male breast swelling	If symptoms are disturbing or persist, let your doctor know.

STORAGE INSTRUCTIONS

Store in a cool, dark place (not in a bathroom medicine cabinet).

STOPPING OR INTERRUPTING THERAPY

This medicine should be taken without interruption for the full length of time prescribed by your doctor, even if you begin to feel better. You may have to take isoniazid for one to two years to clear up your tuberculosis infection. It is very important not to miss any doses. If you do miss a dose, take it as soon as possible. If it is almost time for your next dose, skip the missed dose and resume your regular schedule. Do not take two doses at the same time.

SPECIAL CONSIDERATIONS FOR THOSE OVER SIXTY-FIVE

None.

CONDITION: **TUBERCULOSIS**

CATEGORY: **ANTITUBERCULOSIS DRUGS**

GENERIC (CHEMICAL) NAME	BRAND (TRADE) NAME	DOSAGE FORMS AND STRENGTHS
Rifampin	RIFADIN	Capsules: 150, 300 mg
	RIMACTANE	Capsules: 300 mg

DRUG PROFILE

Rifampin is an antibiotic, which both kills and prevents the growth of new bacteria. For the treatment of tuberculosis, it is usually given in combination with another antituberculosis medicine. Rifampin may also be prescribed for a person who is a carrier of meningitis bacteria, even if that person does not have any symptoms of disease, to prevent the spread of meningitis. It is not used for the treatment of meningitis.

BEFORE USING THIS DRUG

Let your doctor know *IF*

You have ever had allergic reactions or other problems with ■ rifampin.

You have ever had any of the following medical problems: ■ alcoholism ■ liver disease.

You are taking any of the following medicines: ■ other medicines for tuberculosis ■ acetaminophen ■ anticoagulants (blood thinners) ■ corticosteroids ■ medicine for diabetes ■ theophylline or related medicine (medicine for asthma) ■ medicine for abnormal heart rhythms ■ medicine for cancer ■ thyroid hormone ■ digitalis (heart medicine) ■ medicine for seizures ■ estrogens or progestins (female hormones) ■ medicine for fungal infections ■ cyclosporine ■ probenecid (medicine for gout) ■ dapsone (medicine for leprosy) ■ beta-blockers (medicine for chest pain or high blood pressure).

SPECIAL RESTRICTIONS WHILE TAKING THIS DRUG

FOOD AND DRUG INTERACTIONS

Other Drugs	Do not take this drug within six hours of the time you take aminosalicylate (another medicine for tuberculosis).
Foods and Beverages	Take this drug on an empty stomach, at least one hour before or two hours after meals.
Alcohol	Avoid alcohol while taking this medicine.

No special restrictions on smoking.

DAILY LIVING

Examinations or Tests	It is important for you to keep all appointments with your doctor, even if you feel well, so that your progress can be checked. Periodic blood tests may be required.
Other Precautions	It is normal for this drug to cause your urine, stool, saliva, sputum, sweat, and tears to turn reddish-orange or reddish-brown. Since discoloration of the tears may permanently stain soft contact lenses, it is best to avoid wearing soft lenses while you are on this drug. You may continue to wear hard contact lenses.
Helpful Hints	If this medicine upsets your stomach, ask your doctor if you can take it with food.
	If you are unable to swallow capsules, you may open the capsules and mix the contents with applesauce or jelly; you might also ask your pharmacist to make up a liquid preparation for you.

No special restrictions on driving, exertion and exercise, sun exposure, or exposure to excessive heat or cold.

POSSIBLE SIDE EFFECTS

Although this list of adverse effects may seem somewhat intimidating, keep in mind that some are quite rare. Of course, should these or any other problems arise while you are on medication, it is always a good idea to consult your doctor.

IF YOU DEVELOP	WHAT TO DO
difficulty in breathing ■ wheezing ■ flulike symptoms (cough, fever, body aches) ■ dizziness ■ tiredness or weakness ■ headache ■ bloody or cloudy urine ■ decreased urination ■ yellowing of eyes or skin ■ bleeding or bruising ■ sore throat ■ nausea or vomiting ■ loss of appetite	**Urgent: Stop taking the drug and get in touch with your doctor immediately.**
reddish-orange or reddish-brown discoloration of urine, stool, saliva, sputum, sweat, or tears ■ stomach cramps ■ diarrhea ■ sore mouth or tongue ■ skin redness, rash, or itching ■ drowsiness ■ blurred vision or other visual disturbances	If symptoms are disturbing or persist, let your doctor know.

STORAGE INSTRUCTIONS

Store in a cool, dark place (not in a bathroom medicine cabinet). If your medicine is in a liquid form, it should be kept in the refrigerator, but make sure that it does not freeze. If the color, appearance, or taste of the medicine changes or if the expiration date has passed, discard it immediately. If you are uncertain whether your medicine is all right, consult your pharmacist or doctor.

STOPPING OR INTERRUPTING THERAPY

Rifampin should be taken without interruption for the full length of time prescribed by your doctor (sometimes as long as a year or two), even if you begin to feel better. This will ensure that the tuberculosis clears up completely. If, after two or three weeks, your symptoms either do not improve or worsen, contact your doctor. Be careful not to miss any doses because an irregular dosing schedule may lead to more frequent and serious side effects. If you do miss a dose, take it as soon as possible. If it is almost time for your next dose, skip the missed dose and resume your regular schedule. Do not take two doses at the same time.

SPECIAL CONSIDERATIONS FOR THOSE OVER SIXTY-FIVE

None.

Chapter 10
Disorders of the Skin

SKIN PROBLEMS AND AGING

Skin is much more than just the package we come in. It is, in fact, the body's largest organ, playing key roles in temperature regulation, immunity, and blood circulation.

Like other organs, the skin may be subject to various disorders. Unfortunately, skin problems tend to multiply with age; in one study, two-thirds of people older than seventy had at least one skin problem requiring a doctor's attention.

WHY SKIN CHANGES

Among the normal changes that the skin may undergo over the years are the following:

• Gradually, less sweat and protective oil are secreted by the glands, causing the skin to dry out. The chief result can be itchiness. (One welcome result of reduced sweating, however, is diminished body odor.)

• The inner, structural layer of the skin, the dermis, which contains collagen and elastic fibers, gradually becomes thinner and more fragile. This causes a loss of elasticity and paves the way for wrinkles. (Some doctors prescribe an acne medicine, tretinoin, to decrease skin wrinkling. This agent is described on pages 811–814.)

The loss of elasticity also undermines the support for the small blood vessels that feed the skin. Results can include blue "lakes" of dilated veins (especially around the face, lips, and ears); spider-shaped clusters of vessels on the face, neck, or hands (telangiectasia); and a tendency to bruise.

• The skin becomes more permeable, allowing substances that can irritate or cause allergic reactions to penetrate more readily.

• Changes in the skin's pigmentation can occur with age. "Lentigos," flat brown patches typically found on the face and hands, are a common problem. Such spots are very sensitive to sunlight, which makes them darker.

• Exposure to sunlight contributes to many of the skin changes that are often attributed to aging. The ultraviolet rays that strike the skin over an entire lifetime are cumulative and cause changes in the cell makeup in the outer layer of the skin. Degenerative changes also occur in the connective tissue fibers of the skin and cause deep wrinkling, sagging of the skin, nodular elastosis (yellow bumps in the skin), actinic keratosis (scaling, red patches on the skin), and a variety of skin cancers. These photo-aging changes are most marked in light-complexioned, easily sunburned individuals who have spent long periods in the sun during their life.

• Hair growth may also change with aging, resulting in a loss of hair on the scalp. Applying a drug called minoxidil (which, interestingly enough, is a blood pressure–lowering medicine) to the scalp may stimulate new hair growth, though this drug is not a panacea for baldness. Minoxidil, when it works, slows down and reverses the balding process in approximately 20–30% of balding men or women who apply this preparation twice a day. It works only on the crown of the head and not in those individuals with a receding hairline. A patient must use minoxidil a minimum of six months and up to twelve months to determine if he or she will be one of 20–30% of the individuals who may benefit from this treatment. If the treatment is successful then use of the preparation must continue permanently. Discontinuation of minoxidil will result in resumption of the balding process. You might want to talk with your doctor about the drug's benefits and risks.

ITCHING

By far the most common symptom that can develop in the skin is itching, or pruritus. It's an unwelcome feature of many of the skin conditions described in the medical guides in this chapter. It can also be a by-product of diseases affecting other parts of the body, including kidney disease, liver disease, and cancer. Itching, however, may simply result from the drying that occurs as skin ages.

Once itching begins, a number of things can make it worse, including exposure of the skin to dry air, contact with irritating or prickly surfaces such as wool, and excessive washing with soap. In addition, anything that dilates the blood vessels, including coffee and alcohol, can increase the blood flow to an itching region and intensify the sensation. Giving in to the impulse to scratch irritates the skin further and leads to more itching; excessive scratching can also open the way to infection.

The first defense against itching—and scratching—is to keep the skin from drying out in the first place. Especially in the winter months, with cold dry air outdoors and hot dry air indoors, make use of moisturizing cream or lotion. At night, turn down the heat and use a humidifier or put pans of water on the radiator.

When you bathe, use a mild soap, such as Dove or Neutrogena or a skin cleanser such as Cetaphil. If itchiness develops, don't use soap at all. Bath oils can help moisturize the skin, but at the price of making the tub slippery. Better to do your moisturizing after bathing, by applying such products as Eucerin Creme or Lotion, Keri Lotion, or Neutrogena Emulsion to help lock in moisture.

If dry skin leads to itching, your doctor may prescribe an antihistamine (see the drug charts on pages 815–821) or crotamiton cream or lotion (see the drug chart on page 821). Cool compresses can help soothe a region that has become inflamed from scratching. White petrolatum or hydrogenated vegetable oil with menthol may also help soothe the skin. Avoid creams and sprays containing such anesthetics as benzocaine because they can set the stage for allergic skin reactions.

Let your doctor know if itching continues to be a problem, especially if discoloration or skin eruptions occur. Your doctor may want to reevaluate whether there could be a hidden cause that needs attention.

STASIS DERMATITIS

One skin condition that occurs mainly in older people is stasis dermatitis, or eczema on the legs. Symptoms include red, itchy, raised patches on the legs that may ooze fluid and become crusty. People with stasis dermatitis may have other conditions related to poor blood flow in the legs, such as varicose veins or phlebitis (painful inflammation of a leg vein).

If you have circulation problems in your legs, try to avoid sitting or standing too long in any one position. When you sit or lie down, keep your legs elevated above the level of your hips. Your doctor may advise you to wear support hose, elastic bandages, or pressure stockings to help keep blood from collecting in your legs.

Stasis dermatitis is not a condition you should handle on your own. Your doctor will probably recommend that you use a steroid cream to control the inflammation (see the drug chart on pages 822–827). Another medicine that may be prescribed is a topical antibiotic, especially if the skin is broken in the affected area (see pages 827–829).

AVOIDING SKIN PROBLEMS

The most important thing you can do to avoid skin damage is to stay out of the sun. When you do spend time outdoors, use a highly protective sunscreen lotion with an SPF (Sun Protection Factor) of at least 15.

Also, avoid prolonged soaking and contact with soaps and detergents. Wear gloves and long sleeves when engaged in hobbies or other activities that could expose you to irritating chemicals. If you need to use an adhesive bandage, coat the skin with one of the new "liquid bandages" first, or ask your pharmacist about bandages with mild adhesive; the stronger adhesives can damage the top layer of skin.

Caution: Some drugs in this section may affect pregnancy or fetal development. Check with your doctor if this concerns you.

CONDITION: **MISCELLANEOUS SKIN CHANGES**

CATEGORY: **VITAMIN A DERIVATIVES**

GENERIC (CHEMICAL) NAME	BRAND (TRADE) NAME	DOSAGE FORMS AND STRENGTHS
Tretinoin	RETIN-A	Cream: 0.025%, 0.05%, 0.1% Gel: 0.025%, 0.01% Liquid: 0.05%

DRUG PROFILE

Tretinoin, a derivative of vitamin A, is applied to the skin to treat acne. Some doctors also prescribe tretinoin to decrease skin wrinkling. Tretinoin causes a mild peeling of the skin and this may be the mechanism by which it reduces wrinkling and removal of some pigmented aging spots. Use as a dewrinkling agent has not yet been approved by the Food and Drug Administration.

BEFORE USING THIS DRUG

Let your doctor know *IF*

You have ever had allergic reactions or other problems with ■ tretinoin ■ vitamin A–like preparations.

You have ever had any of the following medical problems: ■ eczema ■ sunburn.

You are using any of the following medicines: ■ any other skin medicines ■ any preparation containing a peeling agent (such as benzoyl peroxide, resorcinol, salicylic acid, or sulfur) ■ abrasive soaps or cleansers.

SPECIAL RESTRICTIONS WHILE TAKING THIS DRUG

FOOD AND DRUG INTERACTIONS

Other Drugs	To avoid skin irritation, do not apply any of the following types of products on the same areas you are applying tretinoin unless directed by your doctor: other topical medicines including those for acne, abrasive soaps or cleansers, alcohol-containing preparations, preparations containing peeling agents (such as benzoyl peroxide, resorcinol, salicylic acid, or sulfur), soaps or cosmetics that dry the skin, or medicated cosmetics.

No special restrictions on foods and beverages, alcohol use, or smoking.

DAILY LIVING

Sun Exposure	Skin areas being treated with tretinoin may be more prone to sunburn. Avoid exposure of affected areas to sunlight, including sunlamps. If you must be exposed to the sun, wear protective clothing or apply sunscreen to exposed skin surfaces before going outdoors. Let your doctor know if you should accidentally develop a sunburn.
Excessive Cold	Your skin may become more sensitive to wind and cold temperature while you are using this medicine. It's a good idea to wear protective clothing; let your doctor know if your skin does become windburned or irritated.
Examinations or Tests	It is important for you to keep all appointments with your doctor so your progress can be checked.

Other Precautions

Follow your doctor's instructions and read the patient information brochure carefully. Overuse can cause skin irritation.

Your condition may seem to get worse during the first two or three weeks of treatment. Do not stop using this medicine unless your skin becomes severely irritated or your condition worsens and you've checked with your doctor. Definite improvements may not be seen for three to six weeks, and possibly not for up to four to six months.

Be careful not to get this medicine in your eyes or mouth, around your nose, or on any mucous membranes or open wounds.

You may experience a mild stinging sensation or feeling of warmth after application of this medicine.

Helpful Hints

Wash your skin with a mild soap or skin cleanser and warm water, then pat dry. Allow twenty to thirty minutes before applying this medicine to make sure your skin has dried completely. Do not wash your face more than two or three times a day. Avoid using shaving lotions, astringents, and perfume, since these products tend to irritate treated skin. Nonmedicated cosmetics may be used.

If you are using the cream or gel form, put on enough medicine to cover the affected areas and then rub it in gently. Formation of dry flakes while applying the gel indicates that you are using too much. If you are using the solution, apply enough medicine with your fingertips, a gauze pad, or a cotton swab to cover the affected areas. If your skin becomes irritated from this medicine, try using a little less or stop applying it for a day or two until the irritation subsides.

Cosmetics may be used, but the area to be treated should be thoroughly cleaned before the medication is applied.

Wash your hands thoroughly after applying tretinoin.

No special restrictions on driving, exertion and exercise, or exposure to excessive heat.

POSSIBLE SIDE EFFECTS

Although this list of adverse effects may seem somewhat intimidating, keep in mind that some are quite rare. Of course, should these or any other problems arise while you are on medication, it is always a good idea to consult your doctor.

IF YOU DEVELOP	WHAT TO DO
severe burning (from sun) or skin redness ■ swelling ■ blisters ■ crusting, darkening, or lightening of treated areas	**May be serious** Check with your doctor as soon as possible.
feeling of warmth in treated areas ■ skin peeling ■ mild stinging	If symptoms are disturbing or persist, let your doctor know.

STORAGE INSTRUCTIONS

Store in a cool, dark place (not in a bathroom medicine cabinet). If your medicine is in a liquid form, make sure that it does not freeze.

STOPPING OR INTERRUPTING THERAPY

If you miss a dose of this medicine, skip the missed dose and resume your regular schedule.

SPECIAL CONSIDERATIONS FOR THOSE OVER SIXTY-FIVE

None.

CONDITION: **ITCHING**

CATEGORY: **ANTIHISTAMINES**

GENERIC (CHEMICAL) NAME	BRAND (TRADE) NAME	DOSAGE FORMS AND STRENGTHS
Astemizole	HISMANAL	Tablets: 10 mg
Diphenhydramine hydrochloride	BENADRYL	Capsules: 25, 50 mg Elixir: 12.5 mg per tsp
Hydroxyzine	ATARAX VISTARIL	Syrup: 10 mg per tsp Tablets: 10, 25, 50, 100 mg Capsules: 25, 50, 100 mg Suspension: 25 mg per tsp
Terfenadine	SELDANE	Tablets: 60 mg

DRUG PROFILE

When you are exposed to a substance to which you are allergic, a chemical called histamine is released into the bloodstream and produces the itchy, watery eyes; runny nose; and rashes that are typical of an allergic reaction. Antihistamines work by blocking the action of histamine. They are used to treat allergies as well as to relieve the symptoms of a cold.

The antihistamines listed above are some of those most commonly used. For complete information on these drugs, see pages 753–763.

CONDITION: **ITCHING**

CATEGORY: **ANTIHISTAMINES**

GENERIC (CHEMICAL) NAME	BRAND (TRADE) NAME	DOSAGE FORMS AND STRENGTHS
Trimeprazine tartrate	TEMARIL	Controlled-release capsules: 5 mg Syrup: 2.5 mg per tsp Tablets: 2.5 mg

DRUG PROFILE

Trimeprazine is an antihistamine (see chapter 9, Disorders of the Respiratory System) that is used to relieve the itching associated with hives, rashes, and other skin conditions. When you are exposed to a substance to which you are allergic, a chemical called histamine is released into the bloodstream and produces the symptoms, including itching, watery eyes, runny nose, and rashes that are typical of an allergic reaction. Antihistamines work by blocking the action of histamines.

BEFORE USING THIS DRUG

Let your doctor know *IF*

You have ever had allergic reactions or other problems with ■ trimeprazine ■ other antihistamines ■ phenothiazines (tranquilizers or medicine for nausea).

You have ever had any of the following medical problems: ■ asthma or other lung disease ■ respiratory infections, such as pneumonia ■ heart or blood vessel disease ■ high blood pressure ■ intestinal or urinary blockage ■ other urinary problems ■ enlarged prostate ■ liver disease ■ breast cancer ■ ulcers ■ glaucoma ■ seizures ■ kidney disease ■ overactive thyroid ■ mental illness.

You are taking any of the following medicines: ■ other antihistamines ■ aspirin or aspirinlike medicine ■ medicine for cancer ■ medicine for asthma ■ antibiotics ■ barbiturates ■ muscle relaxants ■ sleep medicines ■ narcotics or other prescription pain-killers ■ tranquilizers ■ medicine for nausea and vomiting ■ medicine for depression ■ diuretics (water pills) ■ medicine for high blood pressure ■ medicine to dilate the blood vessels ■ medicine for seizures ■ antacids ■ appetite suppressants ■ medicine for Parkinson's disease ■ beta-blockers (eg, propranolol, atenolol, metoprolol, etc.) ■ medicine for hay fever, coughs, or colds ■ vitamin C ■ cimetidine (medicine for ulcers) ■ Antabuse (used in the treatment of alcoholism) ■ digoxin or digitalis (heart medicines).

SPECIAL RESTRICTIONS WHILE TAKING THIS DRUG

FOOD AND DRUG INTERACTIONS

Other Drugs	Do not take any other drugs, including over-the-counter (OTC) drugs, before checking with your doctor. This drug increases the effects of other drugs that depress the central nervous system, such as other antihistamines; medicine for hay fever, allergies, or colds; sleep medicines; tranquilizers; narcotics or other prescription pain-killers; muscle relaxants; and medicine for seizures. Antihistamines may mask ringing in the ears caused by aspirin. Let your doctor know if you are taking aspirin or aspirinlike drugs.
Alcohol	This drug increases the effect of alcohol, a central nervous system depressant. Avoid alcohol unless your doctor has approved its use.

No special restrictions on foods and beverages or smoking.

DAILY LIVING

Driving	This drug may cause dizziness, drowsiness, weakness, loss of alertness, or blurred vision. Be careful when driving, operating household appliances, or doing any other tasks that require alertness until you know how this drug affects you.

Exertion and Exercise	This drug may cause you to sweat less than normally. Sweating is your body's natural way of cooling down, and not sweating enough can be dangerous. Use caution not to become overheated when you exercise or exert yourself.
Sun Exposure	When this drug is used for a long time, discoloration of the skin may occur, especially in those areas exposed to the sun. It is a good idea to avoid prolonged sun exposure and to apply a sunscreen to exposed skin surfaces before going outdoors.
Excessive Heat	See "Exertion and Exercise"; use caution during hot weather, since overexertion may result in heat stroke. Avoid extremely hot baths or saunas.
Excessive Cold	This drug may disturb your body's ability to regulate its temperature; use care during very cold weather and make sure all exposed parts are well covered. Also, do not swim in extremely cold water.
Examinations or Tests	If you are taking this drug on a long-term basis (several months), it is important for you to keep all appointments with your doctor so that your progress can be checked.
Other Precautions	Tell any doctor or dentist you consult that you are taking this medicine, especially if you will be undergoing any type of surgery. If you are going to be tested for allergies, tell the doctor in charge that you are taking this drug, since it affects the results of allergy tests.

If you are going to have an X-ray examination of the nervous system that requires an injection into the spinal cord, be sure to tell your doctor that you are taking this drug. Because this drug increases the chances of seizures during such a procedure, it will need to be discontinued a short time before and after the examination.

Helpful Hints	If this drug upsets your stomach, taking it with milk, meals, a snack, or water should help.
	If your mouth or throat feels dry, chewing sugarless gum or sucking ice chips or sugarless hard candy will help.
	Antihistamines sometimes cause insomnia, which can be avoided by taking your last dose several hours before bedtime; check with your doctor about the best dosage schedule for you.
	You may feel dizzy, light-headed, or faint when starting out on this type of drug. This should disappear in a few weeks or so. Getting up slowly from a reclining or sitting position should help.

POSSIBLE SIDE EFFECTS

Although this list of adverse effects may seem somewhat intimidating, keep in mind that some are quite rare. Of course, should these or any other problems arise while you are on medication, it is always a good idea to consult your doctor.

IF YOU DEVELOP

WHAT TO DO

seizures ■ unsteadiness or clumsiness ■ severe drowsiness ■ fainting ■ flushing ■ hallucinations ■ difficulty in breathing ■ dilated pupils ■ sleeplessness ■ confusion ■ difficulty in speech ■ difficulty in swallowing ■ nervousness or restlessness ■ irritability ■ excitement or other mood changes ■ muscle weakness or severe muscle stiffness ■ tremors ■ tightness in chest ■ irregular or fast heartbeat ■ increased sweating ■ incontinence ■ swelling in throat ■ shuffling walk ■ jerky movements of head and face

Urgent Get in touch with your doctor immediately.

fever ■ flulike symptoms (cough, fever, or body aches) ■ sore throat ■ bleeding or bruising ■ tiredness ■ blurred vision or other visual disturbances ■ swelling of hands or feet ■ pain or difficulty in urination ■ rigidity ■ posture changes ■ yellowing of eyes or skin ■ slow, monotonous speech ■ increased skin sensitivity to sunlight ■ nausea or vomiting ■ ringing in the ears ■ nightmares ■ rash ■ upset stomach ■ stomach pain

May be serious Check with your doctor as soon as possible.

drowsiness ■ dizziness or light-headedness ■ decreased alertness ■ loss of appetite ■ headache ■ "high" feeling ■ dry mouth, nose, or throat ■ increased appetite ■ weight gain ■ diarrhea ■ constipation ■ diminished sexual desire ■ difficulty in ejaculating ■ stuffy nose ■ thickened phlegm ■ decreased sweating ■ anxiety ■ depression ■ breast pain or swelling ■ mouth sores ■ redness or whiteness inside the mouth ■ cracking of lips and corners of mouth ■ tongue changes ■ loosening of teeth

If symptoms are disturbing or persist, let your doctor know.

STORAGE INSTRUCTIONS

Store in a cool, dark place (not in a bathroom medicine cabinet). If your medicine is in a liquid form, make sure that it does not freeze.

STOPPING OR INTERRUPTING THERAPY

If you miss a dose of this medicine, take it as soon as possible. If it is almost time for your next dose, skip the missed dose and resume your regular schedule. Do not take two doses at the same time.

SPECIAL CONSIDERATIONS FOR THOSE OVER SIXTY-FIVE

Older people taking trimeprazine may be more prone to develop confusion, pain or difficulty in urination, dizziness, drowsiness, fainting, or dry mouth. Nightmares, restlessness, and irritability are also more apt to occur in those over sixty-five. Thus, doctors may start people over sixty-five on a lower dose.

CONDITION: **ITCHING**

CATEGORY: **OTHER DRUGS FOR ITCHING**

GENERIC (CHEMICAL) NAME	BRAND (TRADE) NAME	DOSAGE FORMS AND STRENGTHS
Crotamiton	EURAX	Cream: 10% Lotion: 10%

DRUG PROFILE

Crotamiton is used to treat scabies infestations of the skin. This medicine cures, but does not prevent, scabies. Crotamiton is also sometimes used to relieve severe itching.

For complete information on this drug, see pages 858–860.

CONDITION: **STASIS DERMATITIS, RASH, AND INFLAMMATION**

CATEGORY: **TOPICAL CORTICOSTEROIDS**

GENERIC (CHEMICAL) NAME	BRAND (TRADE) NAME	DOSAGE FORMS AND STRENGTHS
Alclometasone	ACLOVATE	Cream: 0.05% Ointment: 0.05%
Amcinonide	CYCLOCORT	Cream: 0.1% Lotion: 0.1% Ointment: 0.1%
Betamethasone dipropionate	DIPROLENE AF DIPROLENE DIPROSONE	Cream: 0.05% Cream: 0.05% Lotion: 0.05% Ointment: 0.05% Cream: 0.05% Lotion: 0.05% Ointment: 0.05% Spray: 0.1%
Betamethasone valerate	VALISONE	Cream: 0.01%, 0.1% Lotion: 0.1% Ointment: 0.1%
Clocortolone pivalate	CLODERM	Cream: 0.1%
Desonide	DESOWEN TRIDESILON	Cream: 0.05% Ointment: 0.05% Cream: 0.05% Ointment: 0.05%
Desoximetasone	TOPICORT	Cream: 0.25%

		Gel: 0.05%
	TOPICORT LP	Ointment: 0.25%
		Cream: 0.05%
Dexamethasone	DECADERM	Gel: 0.1%
	AEROSEB-DEX	Spray: 0.01%
	DECASPRAY	Spray: 0.04%
Diflorasone diacetate	FLORONE	Cream: 0.05%
		Ointment: 0.05%
Fluocinolone acetonide	SYNALAR	Cream: 0.01%, 0.025%
		Ointment: 0.025%
		Solution: 0.01%
	SYNALAR-HP	Cream: 0.2%
	SYNEMOL	Cream: 0.025%
Fluocinonide	LIDEX	Cream: 0.05%
		Gel: 0.05%
		Ointment: 0.05%
		Solution: 0.05%
	LIDEX-E	Cream: 0.05%
	VASODERM E	Cream: 0.05%
Flurandrenolide	CORDRAN	Lotion: 0.05%
		Ointment: 0.025%, 0.05%
	CORDRAN SP	Cream: 0.025%, 0.05%
Halcinonide	HALOG	Cream: 0.025%, 0.1%
		Ointment: 0.1%
		Solution: 0.1%
	HALOG-E	Cream: 0.1%
Hydrocortisone	AEROSEB-HC	Spray: 0.5%
	CORT-DOME	Cream: 0.25%, 0.5%, 1%
		Lotion: 0.25%, 0.5%, 1%

	HYTONE	Cream: 0.5%, 1%, 2.5% Lotion: 1%, 2.5% Ointment: 1%, 2.5%
Hydrocortisone acetate	Many brands available	Cream: 0.5%, 1% Ointment: 0.5%, 1%, 2.5% Lotion: 0.5%
Hydrocortisone valerate	WESTCORT	Cream: 0.2% Ointment: 0.2%
Mometasone	ELOCON	Cream 0.1% Lotion: 0.1% Ointment: 0.1%
Polymyxin B sulfate, bacitracin zinc, neomycin sulfate, and hydrocortisone	CORTISPORIN Ointment	Ointment: 5,000 units polymyxin B sulfate, 400 units bacitracin zinc, 5 mg neomycin sulfate, and 10 mg hydrocortisone per g
Polymyxin B sulfate, neomycin sulfate, and hydrocortisone acetate	CORTISPORIN Cream	Cream: 10,000 units polymyxin B sulfate, 5 mg neomycin sulfate, and 5 mg hydrocorti- sone acetate per g
Triamcinolone acetonide	KENALOG ARISTOCORT ARISTOCORT A	Spray Cream: 0.025%, 0.1%, 0.5% Ointment: 0.025%, 0.1%, 0.5% Cream: 0.025%, 0.1%, 0.5% Ointment: 0.1%, 0.5% Cream: 0.025%, 0.1%, 0.5% Ointment: 0.1%, 0.5%

Many brands of topical hydrocortisone are sold over the counter as well.

DRUG PROFILE

Topical corticosteroids are applied directly to the skin to help alleviate the pain, itching, and swelling of rashes and various other skin conditions. They work by blocking the inflammatory response of the skin to irritations, infections, and allergic reactions.

BEFORE USING THIS DRUG

Let your doctor know *IF*

You have ever had allergic reactions or other problems with ■ any corticosteroids ■ any antibiotics.

You have ever had any of the following medical problems: ■ any other skin problems on the area being treated ■ circulation problems ■ current viral or skin infection, such as chickenpox or herpes ■ tuberculosis ■ perforated ear drum, if the drug is being used to treat an external ear infection.

SPECIAL RESTRICTIONS WHILE TAKING THIS DRUG

FOOD AND DRUG INTERACTIONS

No special restrictions on other drugs, foods and beverages, alcohol use, or smoking.

DAILY LIVING

Examinations or Tests	If you are using this drug for a prolonged period of time, it is important for you to keep all appointments with your doctor so that your progress can be checked.
Other Precautions	Use this drug exactly as instructed by your doctor. Do not use it for longer than prescribed or for any other condition than the one for which it has been prescribed.
	Do not cover the treated area of skin with bandages or other material unless your doctor tells you to do so. If you have been instructed to make a dressing,

follow directions carefully. Use only the less potent steroids (desonide, hydrocortisone, and hydrocortisone valerate) on your face or in body folds (eg, under your arms) for long periods of time (greater than four weeks). Use of the more potent steroids for long periods may cause skin atrophy, stretch marks, acne-like eruptions and dilated, small blood vessels (telangiectasis) on the face.

Skin reactions are more likely to occur with long-term therapy with topical corticosteroids or if you are using a dressing. Occasionally, skin reactions may occur after therapy has been stopped; let your doctor know if this occurs. Some topical corticosteroids may cause a mild, brief tingling sensation on the area to which they are applied.

No special restrictions on driving, exertion and exercise, sun exposure, or exposure to excessive heat or cold.

POSSIBLE SIDE EFFECTS

Although this list of adverse effects may seem somewhat intimidating, keep in mind that some are quite rare. Of course, should these or any other problems arise while you are on medication, it is always a good idea to consult your doctor.

IF YOU DEVELOP	WHAT TO DO
Signs of further irritation or infection: itching, redness, swelling, blisters, peeling, pain, or any symptoms not present before using the drug	**May be serious** Check with your doctor as soon as possible.
With combination drugs only: hearing problems	
hair growth ■ bruising ■ purplish lines on skin, especially on face, armpits, and groin ■ acne or other facial eruptions ■ whitening of skin ■ inflammation of hair follicles ■ unusual roundness of face	If symptoms are disturbing or persist, let your doctor know.

STORAGE INSTRUCTIONS

Store in a cool, dark place (not in a bathroom medicine cabinet).

STOPPING OR INTERRUPTING THERAPY

If you are using this medicine on a regular schedule and you miss a dose, apply it as soon as possible. If it is almost time for your next dose, skip the missed dose and resume your regular schedule.

SPECIAL CONSIDERATIONS FOR THOSE OVER SIXTY-FIVE

Steroids may cause thinning of the skin, which may be a particular problem for older people whose skin has already grown thinner with age. Doctors may recommend that people over sixty-five apply this medicine less frequently.

CONDITION: **BACTERIAL INFECTIONS**

CATEGORY: **TOPICAL ANTIBIOTICS**

GENERIC (CHEMICAL) NAME	BRAND (TRADE) NAME	DOSAGE FORMS AND STRENGTHS
Gentamicin sulfate	GARAMYCIN	Cream: 0.1% Ointment: 0.1%
Mupirocin	BACTROBAN	Ointment: 2%
Polymyxin B sulfate and bacitracin zinc	POLYSPORIN	Ointment: 10,000 units polymyxin B sulfate and 500 units of bacitracin zinc per g

Combination products composed of bacitracin, polymyxin B sulfate, and neomycin are available without prescription.

DRUG PROFILE

These topical antibiotics interfere with the basic life processes of the bacteria, eventually causing the bacteria's death. Mupirocin is used to treat special cases of impetigo.

BEFORE USING THIS DRUG

Let your doctor know *IF*

You have ever had allergic reactions or other problems with ■ gentamicin ■ polymyxin B sulfate ■ bacitracin zinc ■ aminoglycoside antibiotics ■ mupirocin ■ preservatives.

You are taking any of the following medicines: ■ other antibiotics.

SPECIAL RESTRICTIONS WHILE TAKING THIS DRUG

FOOD AND DRUG INTERACTIONS

No special restrictions on other drugs, foods and beverages, alcohol use, or smoking.

DAILY LIVING

Other Precautions	If your skin problem becomes worse or does not improve after a week, check with your doctor.
Helpful Hints	Apply the cream or ointment exactly as instructed by your doctor, using a sterile gauze pad to cover the dressing if indicated. Be careful to avoid contaminating the infected area.

No special restrictions on driving, exertion and exercise, sun exposure, or exposure to excessive heat or cold.

POSSIBLE SIDE EFFECTS

Although this list of adverse effects may seem somewhat intimidating, keep in mind other problems arise while you are on medication, it is always a good idea to consult your doctor.

IF YOU DEVELOP	WHAT TO DO
With preparations containing bacitracin zinc only: rash ■ swelling of lips and face ■ increased sweating ■ tightness in chest ■ extreme dizziness ■ fainting ■ difficulty in breathing	**Urgent** Get in touch with your doctor immediately.
With preparations containing mupirocin only: nausea itching, redness, swelling, or other signs of skin irritation that you didn't have before you used the drug	**May be serious** Check with your doctor as soon as possible.

STORAGE INSTRUCTIONS

Store in a cool, dark place (not in a bathroom medicine cabinet).

STOPPING OR INTERRUPTING THERAPY

This medicine should be used without interruption for the full time prescribed by your doctor, even if your symptoms improve or disappear. If you are using this medicine on a regular schedule and you miss a dose, apply it as soon as possible. If it is almost time for your next dose, skip the missed dose and resume your regular schedule.

SPECIAL CONSIDERATIONS FOR THOSE OVER SIXTY-FIVE

None.

CONDITION: **BALDNESS**

CATEGORY: **HAIR GROWTH STIMULANT**

GENERIC (CHEMICAL) NAME	BRAND (TRADE) NAME	DOSAGE FORMS AND STRENGTHS
Minoxidil	ROGAINE	Solution: 2%

DRUG PROFILE

Minoxidil is applied directly to the scalp to encourage hair growth. Exactly how this medicine works is not known.

BEFORE USING THIS DRUG

Let your doctor know *IF*

You have ever had allergic reactions or other problems with ■ minoxidil.

You have ever had any of the following medical problems: ■ skin problems ■ heart disease ■ high blood pressure.

You are taking any of the following medicines: ■ medicine for high blood pressure ■ medicines for anxiety ■ nitrates (medicine for angina) ■ antidepressants.

SPECIAL RESTRICTIONS WHILE TAKING THIS DRUG

FOOD AND DRUG INTERACTIONS

Other Drugs	Do not use any other topical medicine on the scalp while you are using minoxidil.

No special restrictions on foods and beverages, alcohol use, or smoking.

DAILY LIVING

Examinations or Tests	It is important for you to keep all appointments with your doctor so that your progress and any side effects can be checked.
Other Precautions	Keep this medicine away from your face. If you accidentally get the solution in your eyes, nose, or mouth, rinse the area thoroughly with cool tap water.
	Follow your doctor's instructions carefully concerning how much of this medicine to use and how often to apply it. Do not use topical minoxidil on any other part of the body, as using too much may increase your chance of developing side effects.
	For morning application: Shampoo and dry hair and scalp thoroughly before applying minoxidil.
	For bedtime application: Apply minoxidil at least 30 minutes before retiring; this will minimize the amount of solution that will rub off on the pillowcase.
	Wash hands thoroughly after each application.

No special restrictions on driving, exertion and exercise, sun exposure, or exposure to excessive heat or cold.

POSSIBLE SIDE EFFECTS

Although this list of adverse effects may seem somewhat intimidating, keep in mind that some are quite rare. Of course, should these or any other problems arise while you are on medication, it is always a good idea to consult your doctor.

IF YOU DEVELOP	WHAT TO DO
itching or burning of scalp ■ rash ■ swelling of face ■ hives ■ chest pain ■ back pain ■ weight gain ■ dizziness, light-headedness, or faintness ■ fast or irregular heartbeat	**May be serious** Check with your doctor as soon as possible.
increased hair loss ■ visual disturbances ■ dry, flaky, or red scalp ■ sexual problems	If symptoms are disturbing or persist, let your doctor know.

STORAGE INSTRUCTIONS

Store in a cool, dark place (not in a bathroom medicine cabinet), and make sure that it does not freeze.

STOPPING OR INTERRUPTING THERAPY

If you miss a dose of this medicine, apply it as soon as possible. If it is almost time for your next dose, skip the missed dose and resume your regular schedule.

SPECIAL CONSIDERATIONS FOR THOSE OVER SIXTY-FIVE

None.

SKIN INFECTIONS AND INFESTATIONS

Of all the uncomfortable and unsightly ailments the skin is heir to, few are more annoying than the rashes and lesions caused by fungi, yeasts, and mites. Although poor hygiene is commonly blamed for these infections and infestations, the real cause is contact with someone or something that harbors an organism capable of growing on or living in human skin. Parasites and fungi may spread more rapidly when people are crowded together, but unsanitary conditions are certainly *not* prerequisites for contracting any of these organisms.

With a few notable exceptions—such as tinea capitis, a fungal infection of the scalp that mostly affects children—these problems occur with similar frequency in all age groups. The only skin infection that is particularly common in older people is shingles, or herpes zoster.

SHINGLES

Unlike other infections mentioned in this guide, shingles is caused by a virus—the varicella-zoster virus, which also causes chickenpox. The varicella virus is one of the herpes viruses, which have the unique ability to lie dormant in the body after an initial infection and become reactivated months or even years later.

Scientists believe that varicella viruses stay in certain nerve cells after causing chickenpox and may not cause further problems for long periods of time. Sometimes, however, these dormant viruses become active, inflaming the nerve and causing an outbreak of shingles. No one knows precisely what reactivates the virus, but certain factors such as weakened immunity, trauma to the skin, and spinal surgery often precipitate outbreaks. Two-thirds of shingles cases occur in people over fifty.

Shingles usually begins with pain and itching along the course of the nerve in which the virus has become reactivated. The pain may be constant or intermittent, and it is sometimes accompanied by headache and fever. Several days later, a band of tiny, closely grouped blisters erupts on one side of the body. Seven to ten days after they appear, the blisters dry out and form scablike crusts, which remain on the skin for two or three weeks. The pain of shingles sometimes persists for months or years (this is called post-herpetic neuralgia) after the crusts have fallen off.

Until recently, treatment of shingles was limited to pain relief in the form of analgesics, cool compresses, and calamine lotion. While these measures may still be helpful, the current mainstay of treatment is an antiviral drug called acyclovir. (See the drug chart on pages 863–866.) This drug, which may shorten the shingles outbreak, may be given by mouth or intravenously. Treatment usually begins at the first sign of an outbreak and continues until all the lesions have dried. Beginning treatment as early as possible may hasten healing. Some physicians may also give patients over 50 years of age a short course of prednisone since this may decrease the intensity and the occurrence of postherpetic neuralgia.

If you have a shingles outbreak on your face, particularly extending from the side of your nose to your forehead, your doctor may advise hospitalization and intravenous treatment with acyclovir. Shingles in this area can affect the eye, causing serious complications.

FUNGAL INFECTIONS

Fungal infections, which are also called ringworm because of the circular, ridged lesions they produce, are caused by organisms called dermatophytes. People can be infected by a number of different dermatophyte species on different parts of the body.

Tinea Corporis This condition is a fungal infection occurring on any part of the body besides the hands, feet, scalp, beard, or groin. People with such illnesses as leukemia and diabetes run the greatest risk of developing this infection. The rash consists of reddened, itchy, round splotches that may be covered with tiny blisters or bumps. Occasionally, if the rash has been scratched, a bacterial infection may occur, causing more inflammation and leaking of pus or other fluid. Tinea corporis sometimes clears up on its own, though doctors usually advise use of antifungal ointment or lotion. Severe cases are treated with an oral antifungal drug, such as griseofulvin

or ketoconazole, which must be taken for four to six weeks. (See the drug charts on pages 843–846 and 849–852.) Doctors will also treat any secondary bacterial infection with antibiotics, such as erythromycin. (See the drug chart on pages 866–867.) The rash may clear more quickly if the skin is kept cool and dry.

Tinea Pedis This condition, also known as athlete's foot, is the most common fungal infection of the skin. Typically, it causes a dry, scaly rash on the feet, starting between the toes and spreading to the soles. Often, tiny blisters that itch, sting, and drain appear, causing inflammation. Some outbreaks of athlete's foot are brief and self-limiting; others—particularly the dry, scaly kind—can last for years despite treatment.

Several over-the-counter and prescription drugs are available for treating athlete's foot. Antifungal creams, including clotrimazole, haloprogin, and miconazole (see the drug charts on pages 838–840, 847–849, and 853–855), may be helpful, but in severe cases, doctors often prescribe oral griseofulvin. If you have athlete's foot, keep your feet dry, your toes separated with lamb's wool, and wear well-ventilated shoes and absorbent socks to promote healing.

Tinea Cruris This condition, or jock itch, a fungal infection of the groin, affects men much more often than women. Like athlete's foot, it is frequently caused by a fungus that thrives in warm, moist environments. The rash usually begins in the fold between the buttocks or in the area between the thigh and groin and spreads to cover the upper inner thigh. In men, the skin of the scrotum is almost never affected, which is one of the signs doctors use to distinguish jock itch from other skin infections.

Many doctors recommend treating jock itch with cool compresses, an antifungal cream, and dusting powder to soothe the itching. Avoiding tightly fitting clothing and wet bathing suits will also help the rash heal. Active, painful infections may require treatment with oral griseofulvin for four to five weeks.

Onychomycosis   Fungi and other organisms sometimes take hold in the finger- and toenails, causing an infection called onychomycosis. This infection, which causes the nails to become discolored and crumbly, is often difficult to treat, and recurrences are common. It occurs most often in nails that are already fragile because of injury or because of a generalized illness such as a circulatory disorder. Some doctors treat onychomycosis by removing the diseased nail and prescribing griseofulvin for five to six months if fingernails are involved, or at least eighteen months for infected toenails. Older people whose toenails are affected may be advised to forgo drug treatment in favor of a regimen of foot care that will minimize any discomfort.

YEAST INFECTIONS

Candida albicans, a yeast that normally lives in the mouth, gastrointestinal tract, and vagina, sometimes causes a moist, red, itchy rash to develop on the body, particularly in areas where skin surfaces rub together— between the buttocks, beneath the breasts, or in the armpits and groin. Candidal infections can also be involved in paronychia, a condition in which there is redness and swelling with pain around the base of the fingernails. This is particularly common in individuals whose hands are continually wet (eg, food handlers whose hands are frequently in water). Also, a secondary candidal infection may occur due to perlèche—a redness, irritation, and fissuring at the corners of the mouth. This is often the result of saliva accumulating at the corners of the mouth due to poor fitting dentures and the deep skin furrows that occur in this area with age. *Candida albicans* may also cause oral and vaginal infections. Obese people and people with diabetes are especially prone to getting yeast infections.

Yeast infections begin with tiny bumps and blisters that break, drain, and become inflamed. A bacterial infection may also occur.

It is important to keep your skin dry and cool if you have a yeast infection, exposing the affected areas to air and dusting them with powder several times during the day. An oral drug called ketoconazole may be prescribed (see the drug chart on pages 849–852), and clotrimazole (see the drug chart on pages 838–840) applied topically may also be helpful.

LICE AND SCABIES

Three types of lice infest the human. Two set up housekeeping in the hair, while the other lives in the seams of clothing.

Head and body lice are grayish-white bugs that feed on human blood, inject saliva into the skin, and lay seven to ten eggs a day. They are transmitted through hats, combs, and brushes, or, in the case of body lice, clothing and bedding. Bites from these lice produce itchy bumps that the infested person often scratches furiously, paving the way for secondary bacterial infection.

Pubic lice, sometimes called crabs because of their round shape and long, slender front legs, operate in much the same manner as head lice. They are usually transmitted through sexual contact but can be passed on clothing or towels. Bites from these bugs produce blue-gray bumps that are also intensely itchy.

Treatment for both kinds of lice involves application of either lindane cream, lotion, or shampoo or a nonprescription medicine containing pyrethrins (A-200 pyrinate, RID, etc). Permethrin (NIX) is a nonprescription treatment for head lice. (See the drug charts on pages 858–863.) Cloth-ing and bedding must be laundered and, in the case of pubic lice, sex partners must also be treated. Additionally, it may be necessary to take an antibiotic, such as erythromycin (see the drug chart on pages 866–867), if a secondary bacterial infection has developed.

Scabies are tiny mites that lay eggs under the skin, most often in the area of the wrists and between the fingers of the hand, though the waist, genitalia, elbows, and feet may also be affected. They are usually transmitted through close personal contact or picked up from clothing or bedding.

Scabies mites produce curved ridges and red, itching bumps. The itching is so severe, especially at night, that most infested people scratch enough to cause a secondary infection.

Lindane and crotamiton are the agents used to treat scabies. Treatment begins with a bath, followed by application of one of the lotions to all skin below the neck. If a bath is used, allow the skin to dry before applying the cream or lotion. If one member of your family has scabies, your entire household should be treated.

WOUNDS

Any kind of wound—a cut, puncture, burn, abrasion, scratch, or bite—can become infected with bacteria if it is not properly cleaned or if your immune system is weakened. Wash all skin wounds with an antibacterial soap and water and dab them with a disinfectant. For most wounds, this should be sufficient protection against infection. Any bite (animal or human) and all puncture wounds, however, should be cleaned with special care in a doctor's office. After a bite or puncture wound, it is also necessary to get a tetanus booster if you haven't been immunized against tetanus in the past five years.

OUTLOOK

As annoying and unsightly as skin infections and infestations are, they are also highly treatable, both by medical means and other measures. In some cases, such as for shingles, treatment options are expanding, making it even easier to rid yourself of the infection and pain.

CONDITION: **FUNGAL INFECTIONS**
CATEGORY: **ANTIFUNGAL DRUGS**

GENERIC (CHEMICAL) NAME	BRAND (TRADE) NAME	DOSAGE FORMS AND STRENGTHS
Clotrimazole	LOTRIMIN, LOTRIMIN AF	Cream: 1%
		Solution: 1%
	LOTRIMIN	Lotion: 1%
	MYCELEX, MYCELEX OTC	Cream: 1%
		Solution: 1%
	MYCELEX	Lozenges: 10 mg

DRUG PROFILE

Clotrimazole is used to treat fungal and candidal infections. It is given in lozenge (troche) form for the treatment of thrush (white mouth). For skin problems, it can be applied topically as a cream, lotion, or solution. This drug works by altering the permeability of the membrane of the fungal cell so that the fungus loses essential nutrients.

BEFORE USING THIS DRUG

Let your doctor know *IF*

You have ever had allergic reactions or other problems with ■ clotrimazole.

For clotrimazole lozenges:

You have ever had the following medical problem: ■ liver disease.

SPECIAL RESTRICTIONS WHILE TAKING THIS DRUG

FOOD AND DRUG INTERACTIONS

No special restrictions on other drugs, foods and beverages, alcohol use, or smoking.

DAILY LIVING

Examinations or Tests	It is important for you to keep all appointments with your doctor so that your progress can be checked. Periodic blood tests or stool samples may be required.
Other Precautions	Tell your doctor if your mouth symptoms do not improve within a week, if your skin problems do not improve within four weeks, or if any problem worsens. Keep the topical forms of this medicine away from your eyes.
Helpful Hints	Allow the lozenges to dissolve slowly and completely in your mouth (this may take fifteen to thirty minutes). Continue to swallow your saliva during this time. Do not chew the lozenges or swallow them whole. When using the cream, lotion, or solution form, apply enough to cover both the affected and surrounding skin areas and rub it in gently. Do not cover it with anything else, unless your doctor tells you to. Make sure to keep the affected areas clean and dry, as this will help them heal as well as prevent reinfection.

No special restrictions on driving, exertion and exercise, sun exposure, or exposure to excessive heat or cold.

POSSIBLE SIDE EFFECTS

Although this list of adverse effects may seem somewhat intimidating, keep in mind that some are quite rare. Of course, should these or any other problems arise while you are on medication, it is always a good idea to consult your doctor.

IF YOU DEVELOP	WHAT TO DO
blisters ■ skin redness ■ itching ■ burning or stinging sensation ■ peeling ■ hives ■ irritation ■ any other skin problem not present before taking this drug	**May be serious** Check with your doctor as soon as possible.
nausea or vomiting ■ stomach cramps ■ diarrhea	If symptoms are disturbing or persist, let your doctor know.

STORAGE INSTRUCTIONS

Store in a cool, dark place (not in a bathroom medicine cabinet). If your medicine is in a liquid form, make sure that it does not freeze.

STOPPING OR INTERRUPTING THERAPY

Use this medicine for the full length of time prescribed by your doctor even if your symptoms begin to improve. This will ensure that the infection clears up completely and that your symptoms do not return. If you miss a dose of this medicine, take it as soon as possible. If it is almost time for your next dose, skip the missed dose and resume your regular schedule. Do not take two doses at the same time.

SPECIAL CONSIDERATIONS FOR THOSE OVER SIXTY-FIVE

None.

CONDITION: **FUNGAL INFECTIONS**

CATEGORY: **ANTIFUNGAL DRUGS**

GENERIC (CHEMICAL) NAME	BRAND (TRADE) NAME	DOSAGE FORMS AND STRENGTHS
Fluconazole	DIFLUCAN	Tablets: 50, 100, 200 mg

DRUG PROFILE

Fluconazole is used to treat various types of fungal and yeast infections.

BEFORE USING THIS DRUG

Let your doctor know *IF*

You have ever had allergic problems with ■ fluconazole ■ ketoconazole ■ miconazole ■ clotrimazole.

You have had any of the following medical problems: ■ liver disease ■ kidney disease ■ organ transplant ■ AIDS ■ tuberculosis ■ diabetes mellitus ■ cancer ■ seizures.

You are taking any of the following medicines: ■ phenytoin or valproic acid (medicine for seizures) ■ cyclosporine (medicine for organ transplantation) ■ rifampin or isoniazid (medicine for tuberculosis) ■ cimetidine (medicine for ulcers) ■ anticoagulants (blood thinners) ■ thiazide diuretics ■ medicine for diabetes mellitus ■ medicine for cancer.

SPECIAL RESTRICTIONS WHILE TAKING THIS DRUG

FOOD AND DRUG INTERACTIONS

Alcohol	Drinking alcohol while taking this medicine may increase liver problems. Avoid alcohol or minimize intake while you are taking this medicine.

No special restrictions on other drugs, foods and beverages, or smoking.

DAILY LIVING

Examinations and Tests	It is important for you to keep all appointments with your doctor so that your progress can be checked. Periodic blood, urine, and stool cultures may be required.
Other Precautions	It may take several weeks or even months to eradicate the fungus. If your symptoms do not improve within several weeks or if they worsen, check with your doctor. If you have cancer or other medical problems that increase your likelihood of developing a fungal infection and your doctor has prescribed this drug for preventive reasons, be especially careful to follow dosage instructions exactly.

No special restrictions on exertion and exercise or exposure to excessive heat or cold.

POSSIBLE SIDE EFFECTS

Although this list of adverse effects may seem somewhat intimidating, keep in mind that some are quite rare. Of course, should these or any other problems arise while you are on medication, it is always a good idea to consult your doctor.

IF YOU DEVELOP	WHAT TO DO
difficulty in breathing ■ yellowing of skin and eyes ■ red, blistering, peeling skin ■ severe stomach pain ■ dark urine ■ nausea ■ vomiting ■ diarrhea	**Urgent** Get in touch with your doctor immediately.
rash	**May be serious** Check with your doctor immediately.

bloating, abdominal pain ■ headache	If symptoms are disturbing or persist let your doctor know.

STORAGE INSTRUCTIONS

Store in a cool, dark place (not in a bathroom medicine cabinet).

STOPPING OR INTERRUPTING THERAPY

Use this medicine for the full length of time prescribed by your doctor, even if your symptoms begin to improve. This will ensure that the infection clears up completely and that your symptoms do not return. If you miss a dose of this medicine, take it as soon as possible. If it is almost time for your next dose, skip the missed dose and then resume your normal schedule at your next scheduled time.

SPECIAL CONSIDERATIONS FOR THOSE OVER SIXTY-FIVE

None.

CONDITION: **FUNGAL INFECTIONS**

CATEGORY: **ANTIFUNGAL DRUGS**

GENERIC (CHEMICAL) NAME	BRAND (TRADE) NAME	DOSAGE FORMS AND STRENGTHS
Griseofulvin	FULVICIN P/G	Tablets: 125, 165, 250, 330 mg
	FULVICIN-U/F	Tablets: 250, 500 mg
	GRIFULVIN V	Suspension: 125 mg per tsp
		Tablets: 250, 500 mg
	GRISACTIN	Capsules: 125, 250 mg
		Tablets: 500 mg
	GRISACTIN ULTRA	Tablets: 125, 250, 330 mg
	GRIS-PEG	Tablets: 125, 250 mg

DRUG PROFILE

Griseofulvin is a medicine taken by mouth to treat fungal infections of the skin, hair, and nails. This drug works by destroying a part of the fungus cell essential for cell division. Your doctor may prescribe a topical antifungal agent to use along with this medicine.

BEFORE USING THIS DRUG

Let your doctor know *IF*

You have ever had allergic reactions or other problems with ■ griseofulvin ■ penicillin ■ penicillamine (medicine for arthritis).

You have ever had any of the following medical problems: ■ liver disease ■ systemic lupus erythematosus ■ porphyria.

You are taking any of the following medicines: ■ anticoagulants (blood thinners) ■ barbiturates ■ tranquilizers ■ primidone or other medicine for seizures ■ oral contraceptives.

SPECIAL RESTRICTIONS WHILE TAKING THIS DRUG

FOOD AND DRUG INTERACTIONS

Alcohol	Griseofulvin may increase the effects of alcohol and if taken with alcohol may cause flushing and increased heart rate. Check with your doctor or avoid alcohol while taking this medicine.

No special restrictions on other drugs, foods and beverages, or smoking.

DAILY LIVING

Sun Exposure	You may become more sensitive to sunlight while you are taking this medicine. Limit your exposure to bright sunlight or sunlamps until you know how you will react, especially if you normally burn easily. If you have a severe reaction, check with your doctor.
Examinations or Tests	It is important for you to keep all appointments with your doctor so that your progress can be checked. Periodic blood tests may be required.
Other Precautions	It may take several weeks or even months to eradicate the fungus completely, especially if the nails are affected.
Helpful Hints	Make sure to keep the affected areas clean and dry, as this will help them heal, as well as prevent reinfection. Taking this medicine with or after meals, especially fatty ones, will help its absorption by the stomach and reduce your chance of upset stomach. Check with your doctor if you are on a low-fat diet.

No special restrictions on driving, exertion and exercise, or exposure to excessive heat or cold.

POSSIBLE SIDE EFFECTS

Although this list of adverse effects may seem somewhat intimidating, keep in mind that some are quite rare. Of course, should these or any other problems arise while you are on medication, it is always a good idea to consult your doctor.

IF YOU DEVELOP	WHAT TO DO
rash, hives, or itching	**Urgent** Get in touch with your doctor immediately.
confusion ■ behavior changes ■ numbness in hands or feet ■ soreness or irritation of mouth or tongue ■ white patches inside mouth ■ fever ■ sore throat	**May be serious** Check with your doctor as soon as possible.
headache ■ fatigue ■ dizziness ■ sleeplessness ■ nausea or vomiting ■ increased thirst ■ diarrhea ■ upset stomach ■ increased skin sensitivity to sunlight ■ gas ■ hearing problems	If symptoms are disturbing or persist, let your doctor know.

STORAGE INSTRUCTIONS

Store in a cool, dark place (not in a bathroom medicine cabinet). If your medicine is in a liquid form, make sure that it does not freeze.

STOPPING OR INTERRUPTING THERAPY

Use this medicine for the full length of time prescribed by your doctor, even if your symptoms begin to improve. This will ensure that the infection clears up completely and that your symptoms do not return. If you miss a dose of this medicine, take it as soon as possible. If it is almost time for your next dose, skip the missed dose and resume your regular schedule. Do not take two doses at the same time.

SPECIAL CONSIDERATIONS FOR THOSE OVER SIXTY-FIVE

None.

CONDITION: **FUNGAL INFECTIONS**
CATEGORY: **ANTIFUNGAL DRUGS**

GENERIC (CHEMICAL) NAME	BRAND (TRADE) NAME	DOSAGE FORMS AND STRENGTHS
Haloprogin	HALOTEX	Cream: 1% Solution: 1%

DRUG PROFILE

Haloprogin is used to treat fungal infections of the skin. It may be used in combination with other medicines if your skin problem is also caused by bacteria or fungi not susceptible to haloprogin. Haloprogin probably works by causing a sloughing off of the skin in which the fungus lives.

BEFORE USING THIS DRUG

Let your doctor know *IF*

You have ever had allergic reactions or other problems with ■ haloprogin.

SPECIAL RESTRICTIONS WHILE TAKING THIS DRUG

FOOD AND DRUG INTERACTIONS

No special restrictions on other drugs, foods and beverages, alcohol use, or smoking.

DAILY LIVING

Examinations or Tests	It is important for you to keep all appointments with your doctor so that your progress can be checked.
Other Precautions	It may take several weeks or even months to eradicate the fungus. If your symptoms do not improve within four weeks or if they worsen, check with your doctor.
	Be careful not to get this medicine in your eyes.
	You may feel a mild stinging sensation after applying the solution form of this medicine.
Helpful Hints	Make sure you apply enough of this medicine to cover the affected area, and rub it in gently. Do not cover the area with anything else unless instructed to do so by your doctor.
	Make sure to keep the affected areas clean and dry, since this will help them heal as well as prevent reinfection.

No special restrictions on driving, exertion and exercise, sun exposure, or exposure to excessive heat or cold.

POSSIBLE SIDE EFFECTS

Although this list of adverse effects may seem somewhat intimidating, keep in mind that some are quite rare. Of course, should these or any other problems arise while you are on medication, it is always a good idea to consult your doctor.

IF YOU DEVELOP

irritation ■ burning sensation ■ blisters ■ itching
■ worsening of skin condition ■ redness

WHAT TO DO

May be serious Check with your doctor as soon as possible.

STORAGE INSTRUCTIONS

Store in a cool, dark place (not in a bathroom medicine cabinet). If your medicine is in a liquid form, make sure that it does not freeze.

STOPPING OR INTERRUPTING THERAPY

Use this medicine for the full length of time prescribed by your doctor, even if your symptoms begin to improve. This will ensure that the infection clears up completely and that your symptoms do not return. If you miss a dose of this medicine, apply it as soon as possible. If it is almost time for your next dose, skip the missed dose and resume your regular schedule.

SPECIAL CONSIDERATIONS FOR THOSE OVER SIXTY-FIVE

None.

CONDITION: **FUNGAL INFECTIONS**
CATEGORY: **ANTIFUNGAL DRUGS**

GENERIC (CHEMICAL) NAME	BRAND (TRADE) NAME	DOSAGE FORMS AND STRENGTHS
Ketoconazole	NIZORAL	Cream: 2% Suspension: 100 mg per tsp Tablets: 200 mg Shampoo: 2%

DRUG PROFILE

Ketoconazole is used to treat various types of fungal infections. It is usually used in combination with other antifungal medicines. This medicine works by interfering with basic life processes of the fungus cells.

BEFORE USING THIS DRUG

Let your doctor know *IF*

You have ever had allergic reactions or other problems with ■ ketoconazole.

You have ever had any of the following medical problems:

For tablets: ■ achlorhydria (lack of stomach acid) ■ alcoholism ■ liver disease.

You are taking any of the following medicines:

For tablets: ■ acetaminophen ■ oral anticoagulants (blood thinners) ■ medicine for cancer ■ cyclosporine ■ medicine for diabetes ■ rifampin or isoniazid (medicines for tuberculosis) ■ sulfonamides (sulfa drugs) ■ medicine for ulcers (cimetidine, ranitidine, famotidine, etc.) ■ antacids ■ medicine for stomach spasms ■ phenytoin (medicine for seizures) ■ tranquilizers.

SPECIAL RESTRICTIONS WHILE TAKING THIS DRUG

FOOD AND DRUG INTERACTIONS

Alcohol	Drinking alcohol while you are taking this medicine may cause liver problems. Avoid alcohol while you are taking this medicine.

No special restrictions on other drugs, foods and beverages, or smoking.

DAILY LIVING

Driving	This drug may cause drowsiness, light-headedness, dizziness, and loss of alertness and coordination. Be careful when driving, operating household appliances, or doing any other tasks that require alertness until you know how this drug affects you.
Sun Exposure	You may experience increased eye sensitivity to light while taking this drug. Wearing sunglasses if you're exposed to the sun should relieve any discomfort.
Examinations or Tests	It is important for you to keep all appointments with your doctor so that your progress can be checked. Periodic blood, urine, and stool cultures may be required.
Other Precautions	It may take several weeks or even months to eradicate the fungus. If your symptoms do not improve within a few weeks or if they worsen, check with your doctor. If you have cancer or other medical problems that increase your likelihood of developing a fungal infection and your doctor has prescribed this drug for preventive reasons, be especially careful to follow dosage instructions exactly. Be careful not to get this medicine in your eyes.
Helpful Hints	If this medicine upsets your stomach, taking it with a meal or snacks should help. Make sure to keep the affected areas clean and dry, since this will help them heal as well as prevent reinfection.

No special restrictions on exertion and exercise or exposure to excessive heat or cold.

POSSIBLE SIDE EFFECTS

Although this list of adverse effects may seem somewhat intimidating, keep in mind that some are quite rare. Of course, should these or any other problems arise while you are on medication, it is always a good idea to consult your doctor.

IF YOU DEVELOP	WHAT TO DO
dark or red urine ■ pale stools ■ stomach pain ■ yellowing of eyes or skin ■ extreme tiredness or weakness ■ difficulty in breathing	**Urgent** Get in touch with your doctor immediately.
fever and chills ■ joint pain ■ ringing in ears ■ male breast enlargement and tenderness	**May be serious** Check with your doctor as soon as possible.
loss of appetite ■ nausea or vomiting ■ gas ■ diarrhea ■ itching ■ rash or hives ■ drowsiness ■ dizziness ■ male impotence ■ constipation ■ headache ■ nervousness ■ sleeplessness ■ vivid dreams ■ tingling or burning sensations ■ increased eye sensitivity to light	If symptoms are disturbing or persist, let your doctor know.

STORAGE INSTRUCTIONS

Store in a cool, dark place (not in a bathroom medicine cabinet).

STOPPING OR INTERRUPTING THERAPY

Use this medicine for the full length of time prescribed by your doctor, even if your symptoms begin to improve. This will ensure that the infection clears up completely and that your symptoms do not return. If you miss a dose of this medicine, take it as soon as possible. If it is almost time for your next dose, take the missed dose and wait ten to twelve hours before taking your next dose. Then resume your normal schedule.

SPECIAL CONSIDERATIONS FOR THOSE OVER SIXTY-FIVE

None.

CONDITION: **FUNGAL INFECTIONS**

CATEGORY: **ANTIFUNGAL DRUGS**

GENERIC (CHEMICAL) NAME	BRAND (TRADE) NAME	DOSAGE FORMS AND STRENGTHS
Miconazole	MONISTAT-DERM	Cream: 2% Lotion: 2%

DRUG PROFILE

Miconazole is used to treat fungal infections. This drug works by affecting the membrane and certain enzymes in the fungus cells, which results in destruction of the fungus.

BEFORE USING THIS DRUG

Let your doctor know *IF*

You have ever had allergic reactions or other problems with ■ miconazole.

SPECIAL RESTRICTIONS WHILE TAKING THIS DRUG

FOOD AND DRUG INTERACTIONS

No special restrictions on other drugs, foods and beverages, alcohol use, or smoking.

DAILY LIVING

Examinations or Tests	It is important for you to keep all appointments with your doctor so that your progress can be checked.

Other Precautions

It may take several weeks or even months to eradicate the fungus. If your symptoms do not improve within four weeks or if they worsen, check with your doctor.

Keep this medicine away from your eyes.

Helpful Hints

Make sure you apply enough of this drug to cover the affected area, and rub it in gently. Do not cover it with anything else unless instructed to do so by your doctor.

It is best to use the lotion, not cream, for areas between folds of skin (eg, between buttocks, in groin) and rub it in well.

No special restrictions on driving, exertion and exercise, sun exposure, or exposure to excessive heat or cold.

POSSIBLE SIDE EFFECTS

Although this list of adverse effects may seem somewhat intimidating, keep in mind that some are quite rare. Of course, should these or any other problems arise while you are on medication, it is always a good idea to consult your doctor.

IF YOU DEVELOP

irritation ■ burning sensation ■ rash

WHAT TO DO

May be serious Check with your doctor as soon as possible.

STORAGE INSTRUCTIONS

Store in a cool, dark place (not in a bathroom medicine cabinet), and make sure that it does not freeze.

STOPPING OR INTERRUPTING THERAPY

Use this medicine for the full length of time prescribed by your doctor, even if your symptoms begin to improve. This will ensure that the infection clears up completely and that your symptoms do not return. If you miss a dose of this medicine, apply it as soon as possible and resume your regular schedule. If it is almost time for your next dose, skip the missed dose and resume your regular schedule.

SPECIAL CONSIDERATIONS FOR THOSE OVER SIXTY-FIVE

None.

CONDITION: **FUNGAL INFECTIONS**

CATEGORY: **ANTIFUNGAL DRUGS**

GENERIC (CHEMICAL) NAME	BRAND (TRADE) NAME	DOSAGE FORMS AND STRENGTHS
Naftifine hydrochloride	NAFTIN	Cream: 1% Gel: 1%

DRUG PROFILE

Naftifine is used to treat fungal infections.

BEFORE USING THIS DRUG

Let your doctor know *IF*

You have ever had allergic reactions or other problems with ■ naftifine.

SPECIAL RESTRICTIONS WHILE TAKING THIS DRUG

FOOD AND DRUG INTERACTIONS

DAILY LIVING

Examinations or Tests	It is important for you to keep all appointments with your doctor so that your progress can be checked.
Other Precautions	It may take several weeks or even months to eradicate the fungus. If your symptoms do not improve within four weeks or if they worsen, check with your doctor. Keep this medicine away from your eyes, nose, and mouth.
Helpful Hints	Make sure you apply enough of this drug to cover the affected area, and rub it in gently. Do not cover it with anything else unless instructed to do so by your doctor.

No special restrictions on driving, exertion and exercise, sun exposure, or exposure to excessive heat or cold.

POSSIBLE SIDE EFFECTS

Although this list of adverse effects may seem somewhat intimidating, keep in mind that some are quite rare. Of course, should these or any other problems arise while you are on medication, it is always a good idea to consult your doctor.

IF YOU DEVELOP

irritation ■ burning or stinging ■ dryness ■ redness ■ itching ■ skin tenderness

WHAT TO DO

May be serious Discontinue use and check with your doctor as soon as possible.

STORAGE INSTRUCTIONS

Store in a cool, dark place (not in a bathroom medicine cabinet), and make sure that it does not freeze.

STOPPING OR INTERRUPTING THERAPY

Use this medicine for the full length of time prescribed by your doctor, even if your symptoms begin to improve. This will ensure that the infection clears up completely and that your symptoms do not return. If you miss a dose of this medicine, apply it as soon as possible and resume your regular schedule. If it is almost time for your next dose, skip the missed dose and resume your regular schedule.

SPECIAL CONSIDERATIONS FOR THOSE OVER SIXTY-FIVE

None.

CONDITION: **SCABIES**

CATEGORY: **SCABICIDES AND PEDICULICIDES**

GENERIC (CHEMICAL) NAME	BRAND (TRADE) NAME	DOSAGE FORMS AND STRENGTHS
Crotamiton	EURAX	Cream: 10% Lotion: 10%

DRUG PROFILE

Crotamiton is used to treat scabies infestations of the skin. This medicine cures, but does not prevent scabies. Crotamiton is also sometimes used to relieve severe itching.

BEFORE USING THIS DRUG

Let your doctor know *IF*

You have ever had allergic reactions or other problems with ■ crotamiton ■ other skin medicines.

You have ever had the following medical problem: ■ skin that is severely inflamed or has open sores.

SPECIAL RESTRICTIONS WHILE TAKING THIS DRUG

FOOD AND DRUG INTERACTIONS

No special restrictions on other drugs, foods and beverages, alcohol use, or smoking.

DAILY LIVING

Other Precautions
: Since this drug may cause irritation, avoid getting any in your mouth or eyes or in any open scratches, cuts, or sores. Follow your doctor's instructions carefully concerning how much crotamiton to use and how often and for how long to apply it.

Helpful Hints
: If you have just taken a bath or shower, make sure your skin is cool and dry before applying this drug.

Wash all of your recently worn clothing and used bed linens and towels in very hot water or dry-clean them in order to prevent reinfestation of yourself or infestation of other people.

No special restrictions on driving, exertion and exercise, sun exposure, or exposure to excessive heat or cold.

POSSIBLE SIDE EFFECTS

Although this list of adverse effects may seem somewhat intimidating, keep in mind that some are quite rare. Of course, should these or any other problems arise while you are on medication, it is always a good idea to consult your doctor.

IF YOU DEVELOP

burning sensation in the mouth ■ nausea or vomiting ■ stomach pain

WHAT TO DO

Urgent Get in touch with your doctor immediately.

rash or irritation that you didn't have before using this medicine	**May be serious** Check with your doctor as soon as possible.

STORAGE INSTRUCTIONS

Store in a cool, dark place (not in a bathroom medicine cabinet), and make sure that it does not freeze.

STOPPING OR INTERRUPTING THERAPY

One treatment (two applications) is usually enough to get rid of lice or scabies. Your doctor will advise you to reapply this medicine only if he or she sees evidence of continued infestation.

SPECIAL CONSIDERATIONS FOR THOSE OVER SIXTY-FIVE

None.

CONDITION: **SCABIES AND LICE**

CATEGORY: **SCABICIDES AND PEDICULOCIDES**

GENERIC (CHEMICAL) NAME	BRAND (TRADE) NAME	DOSAGE FORMS AND STRENGTHS
Lindane	KWELL	Cream: 1% Lotion: 1% Shampoo: 1%

DRUG PROFILE

Lindane cream or lotion is used to treat scabies and lice infestations of the skin. Lindane shampoo is used to treat lice infestation. This medicine cures, but does not prevent, scabies and lice.

BEFORE USING THIS DRUG

Let your doctor know *IF*

You have ever had allergic reactions or other problems with ■ lindane.

You have ever had the following medical problem: ■ seizures.

You are using any of the following medicines: ■ any other skin preparation, including creams, lotions, ointments, or oils.

SPECIAL INSTRUCTIONS WHILE TAKING THIS DRUG

FOOD AND DRUG INTERACTIONS

Other Drugs	Other skin preparations such as oils, creams, or lotions may increase the absorption of lindane through your skin, which may be harmful; check with your doctor before using any of these products while using lindane.

No special restrictions on foods and beverages, alcohol use, or smoking.

DAILY LIVING

Other Precautions	Since lindane is poisonous if ingested, avoid getting any in your mouth or eyes or in any open scratches, cuts, or sores. If applying lindane to another person, wear plastic or rubber gloves.
	Follow your doctor's instructions carefully concerning how much lindane to use and how often and for how long to apply it.
	Do not use lindane shampoo in the shower or bath, and do not use it for routine hair cleansing.

Helpful Hints	If you have just taken a bath or shower, make sure your skin is cool and dry before applying lindane cream or lotion.
	Wash all of your recently worn clothing and used bed linens and towels in very hot water or dry-clean them in order to prevent reinfestation of yourself or infestation of other people.

No special restrictions on driving, exertion and exercise, sun exposure, or exposure to excessive heat or cold.

POSSIBLE SIDE EFFECTS

Although this list of adverse effects may seem somewhat intimidating, keep in mind that some are quite rare. Of course, should these or any other problems arise while you are on medication, it is always a good idea to consult your doctor.

IF YOU DEVELOP	WHAT TO DO
clumsiness or unsteadiness ■ seizures ■ muscle cramps ■ nervousness or restlessness ■ irritability ■ fast heartbeat ■ vomiting	**Urgent** Get in touch with your doctor immediately.
rash or irritation that you didn't have before using this medicine	**May be serious** Check with your doctor as soon as possible.
itching for several weeks after you stop using this medicine	If symptoms are disturbing or persist, let your doctor know.

STORAGE INSTRUCTIONS

Store in a cool, dark place (not in a bathroom medicine cabinet) and make sure that it does not freeze.

STOPPING OR INTERRUPTING THERAPY

Only one application of this medicine is usually required for cure. Do not repeat the treatment unless directed to by your doctor.

SPECIAL CONSIDERATIONS FOR THOSE OVER SIXTY-FIVE

None.

CONDITION: **VIRAL INFECTIONS**

CATEGORY: **ANTIVIRAL DRUGS**

GENERIC (CHEMICAL) NAME	BRAND (TRADE) NAME	DOSAGE FORMS AND STRENGTHS
Acyclovir	ZOVIRAX	Capsules: 200 mg Tablets: 800 mg Ointment: 5% Suspension: 200 mg per 5 ml

DRUG PROFILE

Acyclovir is used to treat infections of the external genitalia or skin caused by the herpes simplex virus. This medicine interferes with the ability of the virus to multiply within infected cells. Both the ointment and capsule forms of acyclovir may reduce pain, speed up the healing of sores, and prevent new blisters from forming during the first flare-up of infection. However, only the capsule form is effective for preventing recurrent flare-ups. Oral acyclovir is also used for the treatment of infection with the herpes zoster virus, more commonly known as shingles.

BEFORE USING THIS DRUG

Let your doctor know *IF*

You have ever had allergic reactions or other problems with ■ acyclovir.

You have ever had the following medical problem:

With oral acyclovir only: ■ kidney disease.

You are taking the following medicine:

With oral acyclovir only: ■ probenecid (medicine for gout).

SPECIAL INSTRUCTIONS WHILE TAKING THIS DRUG

FOOD AND DRUG INTERACTIONS

No special restrictions on other drugs, foods and beverages, alcohol use, or smoking.

DAILY LIVING

Driving	The oral form of this drug may cause drowsiness, light-headedness, dizziness, and loss of alertness and coordination. Be careful when driving, operating household appliances, or doing any other tasks that require alertness until you know how this drug affects you.
Examinations or Tests	If you are a woman who has genital herpes, your doctor may recommend that you have a Pap smear at least annually to test for cervical cancer.
Other Precautions	If your herpes infection does not begin to improve after you have been taking this medicine for a few days, check with your doctor. Your doctor may caution you to refrain from sexual relations during a flare-up of genital herpes.

Helpful Hints	This medicine works best if you use it as soon as you notice such herpes symptoms as pain, burning, or blistering.
	When applying the ointment, wear a rubber glove or finger sheath to avoid spreading the infection from one area to another.

No special restrictions on sun exposure or exposure to excessive heat or cold.

POSSIBLE SIDE EFFECTS

Although this list of adverse effects may seem somewhat intimidating, keep in mind that some are quite rare. Of course, should these or any other problems arise while you are on medication, it is always a good idea to consult your doctor.

IF YOU DEVELOP	WHAT TO DO
rash	**May be serious** Get in touch with your doctor as soon as possible.
headache ■ diarrhea ■ nausea ■ vomiting ■ dizziness ■ joint pain ■ acne ■ loss of appetite ■ sleep disturbances ■ tiredness ■ sore throat ■ constipation *With ointment only:* mild pain, burning, or stinging ■ itching	If symptoms are disturbing or persist, let your doctor know.

STORAGE INSTRUCTIONS

Store in a cool, dark place (not in a bathroom medicine cabinet). Do not let the ointment freeze.

STOPPING OR INTERRUPTING THERAPY

Use this medicine for the full length of time prescribed by your doctor, even if your symptoms begin to improve. This will ensure that the infection clears up completely and that your symptoms do not return. If you do miss a dose, take it as soon as possible. If it is almost time for your next dose, skip the missed dose and resume your regular schedule. Do not take this medicine more often or for a longer period of time than your doctor has advised.

SPECIAL CONSIDERATIONS FOR THOSE OVER SIXTY-FIVE

None.

CONDITION: **BACTERIAL INFECTIONS**

CATEGORY: **ANTIBIOTICS (ERYTHROMYCINS)**

GENERIC (CHEMICAL) NAME	BRAND (TRADE) NAME	DOSAGE FORMS AND STRENGTHS
Erythromycin	ERY-TAB	Tablets: 250, 333, 500 mg
	ERYC	Capsules: 250 mg
	E-MYCIN	Tablets: 250, 333 mg
	PCE	Tablets: 333, 500 mg
Erythromycin estolate	ILOSONE	Capsules: 250 mg Chewable tablets: 125, 250 mg Drops: 100 mg per ml Suspension: 125, 250 mg per tsp Tablets: 500 mg
Erythromycin ethylsuccinate	E.E.S.	Chewable tablets: 200 mg Drops: 100 mg per 2.5 ml

		Suspension: 200, 400 mg per tsp
		Suspension granules: 200 mg per tsp
		Tablets: 400 mg
	WYAMYCIN E	Suspension: 200, 400 mg per tsp

Erythromycin stearate	ERYTHROCIN Stearate	Tablets: 250, 500 mg
	WYAMYCIN S	Tablets: 250, 500 mg

This type of drug is available under other brand names as well.

DRUG PROFILE

Erythromycins are antibiotics that are used to treat a variety of bacterial infections, including such respiratory tract infections as bronchitis and pneumonia. These drugs suppress the growth of the bacteria and keep them from multiplying by blocking the bacteria's ability to manufacture protein.

For complete information on these drugs, see pages 710–713.

CONDITION: **BACTERIAL INFECTIONS**

CATEGORY: **ANTIBIOTICS (PENICILLINS)**

GENERIC (CHEMICAL) NAME	BRAND (TRADE) NAME	DOSAGE FORMS AND STRENGTHS
Amoxicillin	AMOXIL	Capsules: 250, 500 mg
		Chewable tablets: 125, 250 mg
		Suspension: 125, 250 mg per tsp
	LAROTID	Capsules: 250, 500 mg
		Suspension: 125, 250 mg per tsp

	POLYMOX	Capsules: 250, 500 mg Suspension: 125, 250 mg per tsp
	TRIMOX	Capsules: 250, 500 mg Suspension: 125, 250 mg per tsp
Ampicillin	AMCILL	Capsules: 250, 500 mg Suspension 125, 250 mg per tsp
	OMNIPEN	Capsules: 250, 500 mg Suspension: 125, 250 mg per tsp
	POLYCILLIN	Capsules: 250, 500 mg Suspension: 125, 250, 500 mg per tsp
	TOTACILLIN	Capsules: 250, 500 mg Suspension: 125, 250 mg per tsp

Bacampicillin
  hydrochloride
	SPECTROBID	Suspension: 125
		  mg per tsp
		Tablets: 400 mg

Carbenicillin indanyl sodium	GEOCILLIN	Tablets: 382 mg
Cloxacillin sodium	TEGOPEN	Capsules: 250, 500 mg Solution: 125 mg per tsp
Cyclacillin	CYCLAPEN-W	Suspension: 125, 250 mg per tsp Tablets: 250, 500 mg

Nafcillin sodium	UNIPEN	Capsules: 250 mg Solution: 250 mg per tsp Tablets: 500 mg
Oxacillin sodium	PROSTAPHLIN	Capsules: 250, 500 mg Solution: 250 mg per tsp
Penicillin G potassium	PENTIDS	Tablets: 125, 250, 500 mg Solution: 250 mg per tsp
Penicillin V potassium	LEDERCILLIN VK	Solution: 125, 250 mg per tsp Tablets: 250, 500 mg
	PEN•VEE•K	Solution: 125, 250 mg per tsp Tablets: 250, 500 mg
	V-CILLIN K	Solution: 125, 250 mg per tsp Tablets: 125, 250, 500 mg

This type of drug is available under other brand names as well.

DRUG PROFILE

Penicillins are antibiotics that are used to treat a wide variety of bacterial infections, including infections of the ear, nose, and throat and such respiratory tract infections as bronchitis and pneumonia. Penicillins suppress the growth of bacteria by interfering with the bacteria's ability to form new protective cell walls.

For complete information on these drugs, see pages 714–718.

CONDITION: **BACTERIAL INFECTIONS**

CATEGORY: **ANTIBIOTICS (TETRACYCLINES)**

GENERIC (CHEMICAL) NAME	BRAND (TRADE) NAME	DOSAGE FORMS AND STRENGTHS
Tetracycline hydrochloride	ACHROMYCIN V	Capsules: 250, 500 mg Suspension: 125 mg per tsp
	PANMYCIN	Capsules: 250 mg
	ROBITET	Capsules: 250, 500 mg
	SUMYCIN	Capsules: 250, 500 mg Syrup: 125 mg per tsp Tablets: 250, 500 mg

DRUG PROFILE

Tetracyclines are antibiotics that are used to treat a wide variety of bacterial infections, including skin eruptions and bronchitis and pneumonia. These antibiotics suppress the growth of bacteria by interfering with their manufacture of protein.

For complete information on this drug, see pages 706–710.

BENIGN AND MALIGNANT TUMORS OF THE SKIN

Older people often develop skin growths, particularly if they have blond or red hair and light skin and have spent a lot of time outdoors in the sun. While some of these growths are harmless, others may be precursors of serious skin cancers. Therefore, it is important that you see your doctor about any unusual growth or localized change in the texture or color of your skin. If a suspicious-looking growth does turn out to be malignant, early treatment can usually bring about a complete cure.

Some of the signs of skin malignancy are : 1) growths that are unusually asymmetric; 2) growths that bleed and may break apart easily; 3) the presence of an ulcer or an area that does not heal (if a sore does not heal in two to four weeks a physician should be consulted); 4) growths that have irregular, black, blue, red, or even white discolorations; 5) spots that grow rapidly (may be a skin cancer, but many cancers of the skin grow slowly); 6) any mole that evolves suddenly, and especially if it itches, develops brown, black, and blue colors, or bleeds. Any such growth may be cancerous; it should be seen immediately by a physician.

EPIDERMAL CYSTS

One type of benign growth that often frightens people because it appears as a solid lump is the relatively common epidermoid cyst. These cysts, which are caused by the growth of superficial skin cells in deeper layers of the skin, are most often found on the face, neck, chest, or upper back. Usually, the cyst causes no unusual sensation, but if it gets infected from friction or scratching, it may become red and tender. Doctors usually remove an epidermoid cyst either by excising, or cutting away, the entire cyst or by opening it and scraping out all the walls of the cyst.

SEBORRHEIC KERATOSES

These benign growths are the most common tumors among older people. When they first appear, they are sharply defined yellow or brown spots with either smooth or warty surfaces. People usually get a crop of seborrheic keratoses rather than just one, and they are usually located on the chest, back, or abdomen. Over time, these early seborrheic keratoses enlarge and thicken.

These small, benign tumors can easily be burned off electrically or frozen off with liquid nitrogen in your doctor's office. Your doctor may choose, in some cases, to take a biopsy of a growth that resembles a seborrheic keratosis to make sure it is not a malignant skin growth.

SENILE SEBACEOUS HYPERPLASIA

This yellowish, rough-surfaced growth is also more common among older people than among other age groups. It is caused by a malformation of the oil-producing glands in the skin, and usually appears on the face, particularly the forehead and nose. These growths can be removed with electrosurgery.

ACTINIC KERATOSES AND SQUAMOUS CELL CARCINOMA

Older men and women who work in the sun often develop actinic keratoses; these are small bumps of reddish, brown, or gray color on the face, lower lip, or the backs of the hands—areas that are seldom covered and thus receive the most ultraviolet radiation. It's extremely important to treat actinic keratoses right away, since there is the potential for them to develop into squamous cell carcinoma. The growths can be removed by scraping, chemical burning, or electrosurgery; if they are particularly large, surgical excision may be necessary. Occasionally, if a large area of skin is involved, doctors treat actinic keratoses with an ointment containing the anticancer drug 5-fluorouracil (see the drug chart on pages 875–877), which is rubbed onto the skin for at least thirty days.

The average age of onset of squamous cell carcinoma—a condition caused by skin exposure—is sixty. People who work with compounds containing arsenic are also prone to this cancer.

Squamous cell carcinomas appear in the same areas of skin as do actinic keratoses. Tumors that do not begin as actinic keratoses start out as firm, irregular bumps that may slowly or rapidly enlarge and develop crusty, fragile, and readily bleeding centers that eventually turn into deep open sores. The lower lip is a common place for aggressive squamous cell cancers to develop; on the lip, they appear as an ulcerating crusted lump. Squamous cell cancers can also occur on both male and female genitalia. Use of drugs such as prednisone or cyclosporine (which suppress the body's immune system, as must be done for organ transplantation) has resulted in increased squamous cell cancers in these immunosuppressed patients. The appearance of any new skin spot in such patients should be carefully followed by their physician to be sure squamous cell cancers are identified early and removed.

If unchecked, any squamous cell carcinoma can invade deeply and spread to cover a large area of skin. To prevent this progression, prompt treatment of precancerous actinic keratoses and early tumors is essential. Small squamous cell lesions that have not invaded deeply can be effectively scraped and burned off. More serious lesions require surgical removal. Occasionally, older people who may not be able to tolerate surgery receive radiation therapy for this form of cancer.

BASAL CELL CARCINOMA

This skin cancer, which is the most common malignancy in white people, is caused by a proliferation of cells from the skin's surface. The same conditions that predispose people to squamous cell carcinoma—exposure to sun and certain chemicals or radiation—also increase the risk of basal cell carcinoma. Fortunately, however, basal cell carcinoma progresses more slowly than squamous cell carcinoma, and 95 percent of cases can be cured.

Several types of basal cell carcinoma have been identified. The most common variety, called noduloulcerative, usually appears on the face; the tumor begins as a small bump, or node, that eventually develops an indented center and ulcerates. In another type, superficial basal cell carcinoma, the lesions are round rough spots with slightly elevated borders. This form of skin cancer is usually a chronic condition developing after long-term exposure to arsenical compounds. Sclerosing basal cell carcinoma, which most often affects the head and neck, is a yellowish-white lesion with no distinct border. It enlarges slowly but, on occasion, invades deeper tissues. Another type of basal cell cancer is the pigmented basal cell cancer that appears as a dark brown to blue bump or lump.

All types of basal cell lesions can be removed by burning or surgical excision. Some tumors are treated with 5-fluorouracil ointment as well (see the drug chart on pages 875–877).

MALIGNANT MELANOMA

This type of cancer has a reputation for being particularly lethal but is actually highly curable—if it is discovered early and treated promptly. There is a 100 percent cure rate for malignant melanomas removed at their earliest stage, before they invade below the outermost layer of the skin. Even when a malignant melanoma invades the first layer of the dermis, the cure rate is 90 percent. Still, of all skin cancer, this is the most serious and most likely to spread to other parts of the body.

Many scientists believe that malignant melanoma, which develops in the pigment-producing cells of the skin, is caused by sun exposure. Some evidence indicates that being in the sun intermittently and getting burned increases the risk for malignant melanoma more than does long-term sun exposure. For unknown reasons, women are more likely to be cured of this disease than are men.

It is estimated that anywhere from 20 percent to 85 percent of malignant melanomas have their origins in already existing moles, which are also called nevi. Typically, a malignant melanoma grows wider on the skin surface for a long period—perhaps as long as ten years—before it invades the deeper skin. It starts as a brown or black spot that is barely raised above the skin's surface. The initial spot may have an irregular border and, as it spreads, its hue may vary from red to blue to black. At the time of invasion, the lesion becomes raised into a lump or node.

Another, less common, type of malignant melanoma, called lentigo maligna melanoma, affects older people primarily. It develops from a benign lesion called a melanotic freckle of Hutchinson—an irregularly shaped brown splotch, usually on the face. Thirty percent to 50 percent of these lesions eventually change to malignant melanoma, a transformation heralded by a roughening of the surface and a darkening of the pigment.

Two other types of malignant melanoma, nodular and acral lentiginous melanoma, are particularly difficult to treat. The nodular type never goes through the typical early growth phase on the skin's surface; instead, it begins as an invasive node. Acral malignant melanoma is difficult to spot because it often occurs on the palms of the hands or soles of the feet, where the skin is thicker and changes are hard to identify. Hence, it is often not detected until it has become invasive.

Patients with highly pigmented, easily sunburned skin with many pigmented moles, and especially patients with a family history of melanoma, should examine their skin every two months for the presence of pigmented spots and for the ABCDs of a melanoma. This would help early recognition of a melanoma. Hand and wall mirrors may be used to examine skin in hard to see areas like the soles of the feet, genitalia, back, and scalp.

A simple mnemonic to use is the following ABCDs of melanoma recognition:

A. *Asymmetry*—of the lesion, ie, half of the lesion is unlike the other half.

B. *Border*—the borders of the melanomas are highly irregular and scalloped and indistinct in some areas.

C. *Color*—great variations in color are seen in melanomas, ie, browns, blues, blacks, reds, and white.

D. *Diameter*—any pigmented spot that grows to a diameter greater than a pencil eraser should be suspected of being a melanoma.

The mainstay of treatment for all types of malignant melanoma is surgical excision of the tumor. The doctor will examine the excised tumor microscopically to determine how far the disease has progressed; sometimes, if the lesion is particularly thick, the doctor will also take biopsies of nearby lymph nodes to see whether they have been affected. If the disease has spread to other parts of the body, radiation therapy and chemotherapy may be recommended (see the drug charts on pages 875–879).

OUTLOOK

Although many growths on the skin are harmless, all skin tumors should receive immediate medical attention because of the possibility of malignancy. Fortunately, skin cancer is generally curable, but chances are best if detection is early and treatment prompt.

Caution: Some drugs in this section may affect pregnancy or fetal development. Check with your doctor if this concerns you.

CONDITION: **SKIN CANCER**

CATEGORY: **DRUGS FOR ACTINIC KERATOSES AND SKIN CANCER**

GENERIC (CHEMICAL) NAME	BRAND (TRADE) NAME	DOSAGE FORMS AND STRENGTHS
5-Fluorouracil	EFUDEX	Cream: 5%
		Solution: 2%, 5%
	FLUOROPLEX	Cream: 1%
		Solution: 1%

DRUG PROFILE

5-Fluorouracil is used to treat precancerous or cancerous skin conditions. This drug interferes with the manufacture of DNA, which is necessary for the growth and multiplication of cells.

BEFORE USING THIS DRUG

Let your doctor know *IF*

You have ever had allergic reactions or other problems with ■ 5-fluorouracil.

You have ever had the following medical problem: ■ other skin problems.

SPECIAL RESTRICTIONS WHILE TAKING THIS DRUG

FOOD AND DRUG INTERACTIONS

No special restrictions on other drugs, foods and beverages, alcohol use, or smoking.

DAILY LIVING

Sun Exposure	Avoid excessive sun exposure; your skin may become more sensitive to sunlight while you are on this drug and for one to two months after you stop using it. In addition, too much sun may increase the effect of this drug. It is a good idea to apply a sunscreen to exposed skin surfaces before going outdoors.
Examinations or Tests	It is important for you to keep all appointments with your doctor so that your progress can be checked.
Other Precautions	Follow your doctor's instructions carefully concerning how much, how often, and for how long you should use this medicine. The treated skin may become red and sore and peel or scale for several weeks, even after you stop using the medicine. Once the skin heals, the area may remain pink and smooth for another month or two. If the area being treated becomes very uncomfortable, check with your doctor, but do not stop using fluorouracil unless your doctor tells you to.
Helpful Hints	When applying the medicine, use a cotton-tipped applicator or your fingertips to cover the entire affected area with a thin layer. A gauze dressing may be placed over the medicine.
	If you apply this medicine with your fingertips, wash your hands thoroughly afterwards.
	If you are using this medicine on your face, be careful not to get any in your eyes, nose, or mouth.

No special restrictions on driving, exertion and exercise, or exposure to excessive heat or cold.

POSSIBLE SIDE EFFECTS

Although this list of adverse effects may seem somewhat intimidating, keep in mind that some are quite rare. Of course, should these or any other problems arise while you are on medication, it is always a good idea to consult your doctor.

IF YOU DEVELOP	WHAT TO DO
redness and swelling of normal skin	**Urgent** Get in touch with your doctor immediately.
sleeplessness ■ irritability	**May be serious** Check with your doctor as soon as possible.
burning sensation following application ■ rash, scaling, or oozing ■ soreness or tenderness ■ itching ■ increased skin sensitivity to sunlight ■ skin darkening ■ scarring ■ watery eyes ■ sores inside mouth	If symptoms are disturbing or persist, let your doctor know.

STORAGE INSTRUCTIONS

Store in a cool, dark place (not in a bathroom medicine cabinet). If your medicine is in a liquid form, make sure that it does not freeze.

STOPPING OR INTERRUPTING THERAPY

If you miss a dose of this medicine, apply it as soon as possible. If more than a few hours have passed, skip the missed dose and resume your regular schedule. Check with your doctor if you miss more than one dose.

SPECIAL CONSIDERATIONS FOR THOSE OVER SIXTY-FIVE

None.

CONDITION: **SKIN CANCER**

CATEGORY: **CHEMOTHERAPEUTIC AGENTS**

GENERIC (CHEMICAL) NAME	BRAND (TRADE) NAME	DOSAGE FORMS AND STRENGTHS
Cyclophosphamide	CYTOXAN	Tablets: 25, 50 mg

DRUG PROFILE

Cyclophosphamide is used to treat many types of cancer, including leukemia, cancers of the lymph nodes (including Hodgkin's disease), and cancers of the retina, skin, nervous system, ovaries, and breast. This drug slows or stops the spread of cancer, keeping the cancer cells from multiplying.

For complete information on this drug, see pages 1059–1063.

CONDITION: **SKIN CANCER**

CATEGORY: **CHEMOTHERAPEUTIC AGENTS**

GENERIC (CHEMICAL) NAME	BRAND (TRADE) NAME	DOSAGE FORMS AND STRENGTHS
Methotrexate		Tablets: 2.5 mg

DRUG PROFILE

Methotrexate is used to treat certain types of leukemia, cancer of the lymph nodes, cancer of the breast, and certain cancers of the head, neck, skin, and lung. This drug is also sometimes used to treat rheumatoid arthritis and severe cases of psoriasis—a skin disorder. Methotrexate slows and halts the growth and spread of cancer cells by interfering with one of the steps in cell growth.

For complete information on this drug, see pages 1072–1076.

SKIN ALLERGIES AND IRRITATIONS

A number of conditions can develop in the skin as the body responds to allergy-triggering substances and other materials, both man-made and natural. These skin disorders are considered forms of dermatitis, a catchall term meaning "inflammation of the skin." Itchiness, sometimes intense, occurs in all of them. Some also produce reddened, blistery regions that can ooze fluid and become scaly. The treatments for these conditions vary somewhat but are drawn from the same basic groups of medicines.

CONTACT DERMATITIS

If you've ever had poison ivy dermatitis, you've had firsthand experience with the skin disorder known as contact dermatitis—inflammation resulting from skin contact with an offending substance. Depending on the substance involved, contact dermatitis can involve an allergic reaction (as with poison ivy) or a direct irritation. Symptoms can range from redness and hardening of the skin to severe eczema (another term for dermatitis). In older people, the allergic reaction may take longer to occur (up to 24–48 hours) than in younger individuals.

Common sources of allergic contact dermatitis include plant products, cosmetics, metals, and dyes. Various household chemicals, as well as those used in hobbies, can bring about irritant contact dermatitis. The allergic form generally requires at least one prior exposure to the substance to cause the immune system to become sensitized. Subsequent encounters then produce the rash, which may appear in minutes or be delayed for many hours. Contact dermatitis can occur anywhere on the body, though it tends to spare the scalp.

Contact dermatitis usually first breaks out at the site of contact and then may spread. Sometimes the source is obvious—for example, when a rash breaks out just where a new piece of jewelry has touched the skin. Other times, though, identifying the source will require some detective work by you and your doctor. Your doctor may recommend having a specialist perform a "patch test," in which a variety of common allergens are applied to a small area of your skin. A rash indicates an allergic reaction.

The severity of contact dermatitis depends in part on how easily the substance can penetrate the skin. Skin that is broken or damaged from frequent contact with soap can be easier to penetrate, as can skin that has grown thinner with age. Contact dermatitis also tends to be worse in winter because of the effects of cold, dry air. With this and all other forms of dermatitis, scratching leads to more itching and can increase the risk of infection.

HAND ECZEMA

This condition is simply contact dermatitis of the hands. It has sometimes been called housewives' dermatitis, but anyone whose hands come in frequent contact with detergents, shampoos, bleaches, cleansers, and other chemicals is a potential candidate.

Hand eczema usually involves direct skin irritation, though a contact allergy is also possible. It can range in severity from redness and roughness to blistering, crusting, and cracking. It usually clears up in a few days if contact is discontinued. However, severe inflammation, especially if accompanied by infection, should be treated by a doctor.

Sensible hand care is the best protection against hand eczema. Whenever possible, wear cotton-lined rubber gloves with additional soft cotton gloves underneath during exposure to an irritating substance. If your hands are frequently immersed in water, be sure to keep a moisturizing lotion nearby, and use it frequently. Superfatted soaps and other cleaning products designed to cut down on the loss of natural skin oils may also help.

ATOPIC DERMATITIS

This intensely itchy form of dermatitis tends to run in families that also have a high incidence of hay fever and allergic asthma. It usually develops in infancy or early childhood, flares up and dies down a number of times over the years, and may disappear for good by the teens or twenties. In some cases, however, it persists throughout life.

A vicious cycle of scratching leading to more itching is common in atopic dermatitis. Strong emotions, extreme temperatures, and contact with scratchy materials can readily reignite the inflammation.

HIVES

Slightly raised, pink wheals with well-defined borders are the hallmark of this condition, also called urticaria. The itchy wheals can appear and disappear within hours, often to be replaced by new wheals elsewhere. Hives generally last for a day or two, though chronic cases can continue for many weeks.

The most common cause of hives is a food allergy. Shellfish, nuts, strawberries, chocolate, and some food additives are common triggers. Some chemicals and drugs, including aspirin and certain opiates and antibiotics, can also produce this skin condition. In some people, physical pressure, a simple scratch, or exposure to cold may lead to hives. Emotional stress can worsen an existing case of hives or can even actually trigger a case.

Hives themselves are usually annoying but harmless. However, in a more severe form of hives called angioedema, swelling develops not just in the top layer of skin but also in the inner layer, or dermis. Sometimes, the swelling becomes severe enough to threaten breathing, requiring immediate medical attention.

DRUG-TRIGGERED
SKIN REACTIONS

Medicines, most often antibiotics, can produce hives and other kinds of rashes. The rash may appear within minutes to hours after the drug has been started or may take about a week to develop.

Sometimes, if a person's immune system is sensitized to a drug, a subsequent exposure can trigger a life-threatening condition known as anaphylactic shock. But if you and your doctor keep close track of any drug allergies you have, the problem can generally be avoided by substituting another medicine.

Sunlight can sometimes set off a rash in people who are on certain medicines. Your doctor may recommend that you stay out of the sun as much as possible while using the drug; an effective sunscreen on the face, hands, and other exposed areas can also help.

TREATMENT

For all the conditions described in this guide, the smartest treatment plan is to steer clear of whatever it is that's causing the problem. But that may not always be possible, either because you don't know what's affecting your skin or because there's no avoiding it.

The two main types of medicine used in treating these conditions are topical steroids (see the drug chart on pages 883–886) and antihistamines (see the drug chart on pages 886–887).

Topical steroids help relieve redness, itching, and swelling, whatever their cause. Antihistamines counter the effects of histamine (a chemical in your body involved in allergic reactions) and are the drugs of choice in treating hives. Your doctor may also prescribe an antihistamine for contact and atopic dermatitis, especially when an allergy is clearly involved.

Antibiotics are sometimes necessary to prevent or reverse infection in situations in which the skin is broken. Erythromycin or dicloxacillin is often used for this purpose. (See the drug chart on pages 887–888.) In cases of severe hives, angioedema, or anaphylaxis, an injection of epinephrine may be necessary as part of emergency treatment.

OUTLOOK

Steering clear of poison ivy, while a good idea, is only one approach available to you in dealing with skin allergies and irritations. The medicines used to treat these conditions are quite effective in relieving the inflammation, itchiness, and other typical symptoms. As researchers sharpen their techniques for identifying the offending substances and learn more about the underlying processes, even better treatment methods are likely to evolve.

Caution. Some drugs in this section may affect pregnancy or fetal development. Check with your doctor if this concerns you.

CONDITION: **ALLERGIC SKIN REACTIONS**

CATEGORY: **TOPICAL CORTICOSTEROIDS**

GENERIC (CHEMICAL) NAME	BRAND (TRADE) NAME	DOSAGE FORMS AND STRENGTHS
Alclometasone	ACLOVATE	Cream: 0.05% Ointment: 0.05%
Amcinonide	CYCLOCORT	Cream: 0.1% Lotion: 0.1% Ointment: 0.1%
Betamethasone dipropionate	DIPROLENE	Cream: 0.05% Lotion: 0.05%
	DIPROLENE AF	Cream: 0.05% Ointment: 0.05%
	DIPROSONE	Cream: 0.05% Lotion: 0.05% Ointment: 0.05% Spray: 0.1%
Betamethasone valerate	VALISONE	Cream: 0.01%, 0.1% Lotion: 0.1% Ointment: 0.1%
Clocortolone pivalate	CLODERM	Cream: 0.1%
Desonide	DESOWEN	Cream: 0.05% Ointment: 0.05%
	TRIDESILON	Cream: 0.05% Ointment: 0.05%

Desoximetasone	TOPICORT	Cream: 0.25% Gel: 0.05% Ointment: 0.25%
	TOPICORT LP	Cream: 0.05%
Dexamethasone	DECADERM AEROSEB-DEX DECASPRAY	Gel: 0.1% Spray: 0.01% Spray: 0.04%
Diflorasone diacetate	FLORONE	Cream: 0.05% Ointment: 0.05%
Fluocinolone acetonide	SYNALAR	Cream: 0.01%, 0.025% Ointment: 0.025% Solution: 0.01%
	SYNALAR-HP SYNEMOL	Cream: 0.2% Cream: 0.025%
Fluocinonide	LIDEX	Cream: 0.05% Gel: 0.05% Ointment: 0.05% Solution: 0.05%
	LIDEX-E VASODERM E	Cream: 0.05% Cream: 0.05%
Flurandrenolide	CORDRAN	Lotion: 0.05% Ointment: 0.025%, 0.05%
	CORDRAN SP	Cream: 0.025%, 0.05%
Halcinonide	HALOG	Cream: 0.025%, 0.1% Ointment: 0.1% Solution: 0.1%
	HALOG-E	Cream: 0.1%

Hydrocortisone	AEROSEB-HC	Spray: 0.5%
	CORT-DOME	Cream: 0.25%, 0.5%, 1% Lotion: 0.25%, 0.5%, 1%
	HYTONE	Cream: 0.5%, 1%, 2.5% Lotion: 1%, 2.5% Ointment: 1%, 2.5%
Hydrocortisone acetate	Many brands available	Cream: 0.5%, 1% Ointment: 0.5%, 1%, 2.5% Lotion: 0.5%
Hydrocortisone valerate	WESTCORT	Cream: 0.2% Ointment: 0.2%
Mometasone	ELOCON	Cream: 0.1% Lotion: 0.1% Ointment: 0.1%
Polymyxin B sulfate, bacitracin zinc, neomycin sulfate, and hydrocortisone	CORTISPORIN Ointment	Ointment: 5,000 units polymyxin B sulfate, 400 units bacitracin zinc, 5 mg neomycin sulfate, and 10 mg hydrocortisone per g
Polymyxin B sulfate, neomycin sulfate, and hydrocortisone acetate	CORTISPORIN Cream	Cream: 10,000 units polymyxin B sulfate, 5 mg neomycin sulfate, and 5 mg hydrocortisone acetate per g
Triamcinolone acetonide	KENALOG	Spray Cream: 0.025%, 0.1%, 0.5% Ointment: 0.025%, 0.1%, 0.5%
	ARISTOCORT	Cream: 0.025%, 0.1%, 0.5% Ointment: 0.1%, 0.5%
	ARISTOCORT A	Cream: 0.025%, 0.1%, 0.5% Ointment: 0.1%, 0.5%

Many brands of topical hydrocortisone are sold over the counter as well.

DRUG PROFILE

Topical corticosteroids are applied directly to the skin to help alleviate the pain, itching, and swelling of rashes and various other skin conditions. They work by blocking the inflammatory response of the skin to irritations, infections, and allergic reactions.

For complete information on these drugs, see pages 822–827.

CONDITION: **ALLERGIC SKIN REACTIONS**

CATEGORY: **ANTIHISTAMINES**

GENERIC (CHEMICAL) NAME	BRAND (TRADE) NAME	DOSAGE FORMS AND STRENGTHS
Astemizole	HISMANAL	Tablets: 10 mg
Diphenhydramine hydrochloride	BENADRYL	Capsules: 25, 50 mg Elixir: 12.5 mg per tsp
Hydroxyzine hydrochloride	ATARAX	Syrup: 10 mg per tsp Tablets: 10, 25, 50, 100 mg
Hydroxyzine pamoate	VISTARIL	Capsules: 25, 50, 100 mg Suspension: 25 mg per tsp
Terfenadine	SELDANE	Tablets: 60 mg

DRUG PROFILE

When you are exposed to a substance to which you are allergic, a chemical called histamine is released into the bloodstream and produces the itchy, watery eyes; runny nose; and rashes that are typical of an allergic reaction. Antihistamines work by blocking the action of histamine. They are used to treat allergies as well as to relieve the symptoms of a cold.

For complete information on these drugs, see pages 753–763.

CONDITION: **ALLERGIC SKIN REACTIONS**

CATEGORY: **ANTIHISTAMINES**

GENERIC (CHEMICAL) NAME	BRAND (TRADE) NAME	DOSAGE FORMS AND STRENGTHS
Trimeprazine tartrate	TEMARIL	Controlled-release capsules: 5 mg Syrup: 2.5 mg per tsp Tablets: 2.5 mg

DRUG PROFILE

Trimeprazine is an antihistamine (see chapter 9, Disorders of the Respiratory System) that is used to relieve the itching associated with hives, rashes, and other skin conditions. When you are exposed to a substance to which you are allergic, a chemical called histamine is released into the bloodstream and produces the symptoms, including itching, that are typical of an allergic reaction. Antihistamines work by blocking the action of histamines.

For complete information on this drug, see pages 816–821.

CONDITION: **ALLERGIC SKIN REACTIONS**

CATEGORY: **ANTIBIOTICS (ERYTHROMYCINS)**

GENERIC (CHEMICAL) NAME	BRAND (TRADE) NAME	DOSAGE FORMS AND STRENGTHS
Erythromycin	E-MYCIN	Tablets: 250, 333 mg
	ERYC	Capsules: 250 mg
	ERY-TAB	Tablets: 250, 333, 500 mg
	PCE	Tablets: 333, 500 mg

Erythromycin estolate	ILOSONE	Capsules: 250 mg
		Chewable tablets: 125,
		   250 mg
		Drops: 100 mg per ml
		Suspension: 125, 250 mg
		   per tsp
		Tablets: 500 mg

Erythromycin
   ethylsuccinate
	E.E.S.	Chewable tablets: 200 mg
		Drops: 100 mg per 2.5 ml
		Suspension: 200, 400 mg
		   per tsp
		Suspension granules: 200 mg
		   per tsp
		Tablets: 400 mg

	WYAMYCIN E	Suspension: 200, 400 mg per tsp
Erythromycin Stearate	ERYTHROCIN Stearate WYAMYCIN S	Tablets: 250, 500 mg Tablets: 250, 500 mg

This type of drug is available under other brand names as well.

DRUG PROFILE

Erythromycins are antibiotics that are used to treat a variety of bacterial infections, including such respiratory tract infections as bronchitis and pneumonia. These drugs suppress the growth of the bacteria and keep them from multiplying by blocking the bacteria's ability to manufacture protein.

For complete information on these drugs, see pages 710–713.

PSORIASIS, ROSACEA, AND SEBORRHEIC DERMATITIS

The skin conditions known as psoriasis, rosacea, and seborrheic dermatitis are all irritating nuisances of unknown cause. Cures for them have also proven elusive—but these disorders can often be controlled, and you can look and feel as well as ever.

PSORIASIS

Psoriasis, a skin condition that affects one out of fifty people in the United States, can occur for the first time at any age. You may suspect you have it if you notice a raised, sometimes itchy, red patch of skin with silvery scales. These so-called plaques most often appear on the elbows, knees, and scalp but can affect the skin of any portion of the body. Because blood supply to the skin diminishes with age, plaques don't become as inflamed in older people as in younger ones. Some people with psoriasis also have fingernails that are pitted or discolored.

Psoriasis is not contagious (passed from person to person), but it may run in families. At least three out of ten people with psoriasis report a family history of the problem. Despite this genetic aspect, some researchers believe that psoriasis doesn't show itself until set off by some triggering factor. The culprits might include psychological stress, infection, injury to the skin, or vaccination.

It's not hard for a doctor to tell, by looking at the plaques, that the problem is psoriasis. But to confirm the diagnosis, your doctor may stroke this thickened patch of skin with a wooden spatula to dislodge the silvery-white scales that are a sure sign of this annoying disorder.

Many people find that sunlight helps relieve psoriasis. Some doctors prescribe PUVA therapy, a light treatment that uses long-wave ultraviolet light in combination with a drug called methoxsalen.

Steroid creams have been found to be effective in controlling psoriasis (see the drug chart on pages 891–894). Another product, anthralin, may also be used to treat psoriasis of the skin and scalp (see the drug chart on pages 894–896); methotrexate (see the drug chart on page 904) may be prescribed for the most severe cases. However, because psoriasis often recurs, these remedies generally must be usedrepeatedly.

ROSACEA

Rosacea, formerly known as acne rosacea, has some similarities to the form of acne so embarrassing to adolescents—notably, pimples and oiliness of the skin. But rosacea, which is most common in people over thirty-five, also causes the skin to flush and most often occurs in the middle of the face (mid-forehead, chin, and nose). In fact, a severe form of rosacea that affects men results in enlargement of the nose. Additionally, more than half the people who have rosacea have accompanying eye problems, such as conjunctivitis.

Some researchers had thought that an abnormality of the intestinal tract caused the disease, while others blamed alcohol, spicy foods, stress, or vitamin deficiencies. Recent research shows no evidence that any of these cause rosacea. However, some doctors suggest that people with rosacea avoid spicy foods, caffeine, alcohol, hot drinks, and exposure to extreme heat or cold, since those factors lead to flushing.

A few people will have only one attack of rosacea and then aren't troubled again. But in most cases the condition will get increasingly worse if it's not properly treated. Such antibiotics as tetracycline or minocycline may help improve this harmless but unsightly skin disorder (see the drug chart on page 909). Usually these drugs are taken in high doses for two or three months and then continued in lower doses for another six weeks. This treatment prevents recurrences in about one out of three people. If the condition does recur, low doses of antibiotics are continued. If tetracycline or minocycline doesn't prove effective in your case, your doctor may switch you to a drug called metronidazole. (For more information on this drug, see the chart on page 910).

SEBORRHEIC DERMATITIS

Seborrheic dermatitis is not a single disorder but actually refers to a variety of skin conditions. These range from simple dandruff to dandruff accompanied by inflammation of the scalp to greasy, scaling patches on the chest and eyebrows, behind the ears, and around the nose. Those areas have high concentrations of sebaceous glands, which coat the surface of the skin with an oily substance called sebum. Contrary to popular belief, seborrheic dermatitis does *not* cause baldness, nor is it contagious. This skin condition is quite common in older men and postmenopausal women.

Seborrheic dermatitis cannot be cured but can be treated effectively. If you have dandruff, shampoo with a product that contains zinc, selenium, or tar every other day until the dandruff is under control (see the drug charts on pages 897–899 and 904–909); to *keep* it under control, continue to use those shampoos once or twice a week. Hydrocortisone cream can successfully control seborrheic dermatitis on the face or body. (See the drug chart on pages 891–894 for descriptions of appropriate medicines.) In some patients, the antiyeast cream, ketoconazole (see pages 907–908), has been effective in seborrheic dermatitis.

Caution: Some drugs in this section may affect pregnancy or fetal development. Check with your doctor if this concerns you.

CONDITION: **PSORIASIS**

CATEGORY: **TOPICAL CORTICOSTEROIDS**

GENERIC (CHEMICAL) NAME	BRAND (TRADE) NAME	DOSAGE FORMS AND STRENGTHS
Alclometasone	ACLOVATE	Cream: 0.05% Ointment: 0.05%
Amcinonide	CYCLOCORT	Cream: 0.1% Lotion: 0.1% Ointment: 0.1%
Betamethasone dipropionate	DIPROLENE	Cream: 0.05% Lotion: 0.05% Ointment: 0.05%
	DIPROSONE	Cream: 0.05% Lotion: 0.05% Ointment: 0.05% Spray: 0.1%
Betamethasone valerate	VALISONE	Cream: 0.01%, 0.1% Lotion: 0.1% Ointment: 0.1%
Clocortolone pivalate	CLODERM	Cream: 0.1%
Desonide	DESOWEN	Cream: 0.05% Ointment: 0.05%
	TRIDESILON	Cream: 0.05% Ointment: 0.05%

Desoximetasone	TOPICORT	Cream: 0.25% Gel: 0.05% Ointment: 0.25%
	TOPICORT LP	Cream: 0.05%
Dexamethasone	AEROSEB-DEX	Spray: 0.01%
Diflorasone diacetate	FLORONE	Cream: 0.05% Ointment: 0.05%
Fluocinolone acetonide	SYNALAR	Cream: 0.025%, 0.01% Ointment: 0.025% Solution: 0.01%
	SYNALAR-HP	Cream: 0.2%
	SYNEMOL	Cream: 0.025%
Fluocinonide	LIDEX	Cream: 0.05% Gel: 0.05% Ointment: 0.05% Solution: 0.05%
	LIDEX-E	Cream: 0.05%
	VASODERM E	Cream: 0.05%
Flurandrenolide	CORDRAN	Lotion: 0.05% Ointment: 0.025%, 0.05%
	CORDRAN SP	Cream: 0.025%, 0.05%
Halcinonide	HALOG	Cream: 0.025%, 0.1% Ointment: 0.1% Solution: 0.1%
	HALOG-E	Cream: 0.1%

Hydrocortisone	AEROSEB-HC	Spray: 0.5%
	CORT-DOME	Cream: 0.25%, 0.5%, 1%
		Lotion: 0.25%, 0.5%, 1%
	HYTONE	Cream: 0.5%, 1%, 2.5%
		Lotion: 1%, 2.5%
		Ointment: 1%, 2.5%
Hydrocortisone acetate	Many brands available	Ointment: 1%, 2.5%
Hydrocortisone valerate	WESTCORT	Cream: 0.2%
		Ointment: 0.2%
Mometasone	ELOCON	Cream: 0.1%
		Lotion: 0.1%
		Ointment: 0.1%
Polymyxin B sulfate, bacitracin zinc, neomycin sulfate, and hydrocortisone	CORTISPORIN Ointment	Ointment: 5,000 units polymyxin B sulfate, 400 units bacitracin zinc, 5 mg neomycin sulfate, and 10 mg hydrocortisone per g
Polymyxin B sulfate, neomycin sulfate, and hydrocortisone acetate	CORTISPORIN Cream	Cream: 10,000 units polymyxin B sulfate, 5 mg neomycin sulfate, and 5 mg hydrocortisone acetate per g
Triamcinolone acetonide	ARISTOCORT	Cream: 0.025%, 0.1%, 0.5%
		Ointment: 0.1%, 0.5%
	ARISTOCORT A	Cream: 0.025%, 0.1%, 0.5%
		Ointment: 0.1%, 0.5%

Many brands of topical hydrocortisone are sold over the counter as well.

DRUG PROFILE

Topical corticosteroids are applied directly to the skin to help alleviate the pain, itching, and swelling of rashes and various other skin conditions. They work by blocking the inflammatory response of the skin to irritations, infections, and allergic reactions.

For complete information on these drugs, see pages 822–827.

CONDITION: **PSORIASIS**

CATEGORY: **KERATOLYTIC DRUGS**

GENERIC (CHEMICAL) NAME	BRAND (TRADE) NAME	DOSAGE FORMS AND STRENGTHS
Anthralin	ANTHRA-DERM	Ointment: 0.1%, 0.25%, 0.5%, 1%
	DRITHOCREME	Cream: 0.1%, 0.25%, 0.5%, 1%
	DRITHO-SCALP	Cream: 0.25%, 0.5%

DRUG PROFILE

Anthralin is used to treat psoriasis of the skin and scalp. It works by inhibiting the growth of skin cells in the areas to which it is applied.

BEFORE USING THIS DRUG

Let your doctor know *IF*

You have ever had allergic reactions or other problems with ■ anthralin.

You have ever had the following medical problem: ■ kidney disease.

You are taking any of the following medicines: ■ other medicine for psoriasis (especially coal tar preparations or methoxsalen).

SPECIAL RESTRICTIONS WHILE TAKING THIS DRUG

FOOD AND DRUG INTERACTIONS

No special restrictions on other drugs, foods and beverages, alcohol use, or smoking.

DAILY LIVING

Precautions	Avoid getting this medicine in your mouth, your eyes, or the inside of your nose or in any open scratches, cuts, or sores.
	Follow your doctor's instructions carefully concerning how much of this medicine to use and how often and for how long to apply it. This medicine can stain your skin and hair, though the stain will fade after you stop using it. It can also stain your clothing and bed linens.
Helpful Hints	Since this medicine can irritate normal skin, surround the affected areas with a ring of petroleum jelly before applying it. Remove any medicine accidentally applied to normal skin.
	Always wash your hands after applying this medicine, or wear plastic gloves. To remove it from your bathtub or shower, wash it off first with hot water and then with a household cleanser.

No special restrictions on driving, exertion and exercise, sun exposure, or exposure to excessive heat or cold.

POSSIBLE SIDE EFFECTS

IF YOU DEVELOP

rash or irritation that you didn't have before using this medicine

WHAT TO DO

May be serious Check with your doctor as soon as possible.

STORAGE INSTRUCTIONS

Store in a cool, dark place (not in a bathroom medicine cabinet) and make sure that it does not freeze.

STOPPING OR INTERRUPTING THERAPY

If you miss a dose of this medicine, apply it as soon as possible. If it is almost time for your next dose, skip the missed dose and resume your regular schedule.

SPECIAL CONSIDERATIONS FOR THOSE OVER SIXTY-FIVE

None.

CONDITION: **ECZEMA, PSORIASIS, SEBORRHEA, AND DANDRUFF**

CATEGORY: **KERATOLYTIC DRUGS (COAL TAR PREPARATIONS)**

GENERIC (CHEMICAL) NAME	BRAND (TRADE) NAME	DOSAGE FORMS AND STRENGTHS
Coal tar	FOTOTAR	Cream: 2%
		Stick: 5%
	ZETAR EMULSION	Lotion: 30%

Numerous coal tar preparations are also available over the counter in a variety of brand names, dosage forms, and strengths.

DRUG PROFILE

Coal tar products are used for relief of the itching, irritation, and skin flaking seen in such conditions as eczema, psoriasis, seborrhea, and dandruff.

BEFORE USING THIS DRUG

Let your doctor know *IF*

You have ever had allergic reactions or other problems with ■ coal tar.

You have ever had any of the following medical problems: ■ sensitivity to sunlight ■ systemic lupus erythematosus ■ skin cancer.

You are taking any of the following medicines: ■ other medicine for psoriasis, especially methoxsalen and anthralin ■ tetracycline (antibiotic) ■ tretinoin (medicine for acne) ■ trioxsalen (medicine for vitiligo, in which skin color is lost).

SPECIAL RESTRICTIONS WHILE TAKING THIS DRUG

FOOD AND DRUG INTERACTIONS

No special restrictions on other drugs, foods and beverages, alcohol use, or smoking.

DAILY LIVING

Sun Exposure	Avoid sun exposure of any skin area treated with this medicine for twenty-four hours following application unless your doctor tells you otherwise. Use clothing, sunscreens, or sunblocks for protection. Before sun exposure, remove the medicine from your skin. If you have psoriasis, your doctor may recommend sunlight or ultraviolet light treatment in combination with this medicine.
Other Precautions	Avoid getting this medicine in your eyes; in any open scratches, cuts, or sores; or in the anogenital area. Follow your doctor's instructions carefully concerning how much of this medicine to use and how often and for how long to apply it. If your problem continues or worsens, check with your doctor. This medicine can stain your skin and hair, though the stain will fade after you stop using it. It can also stain your clothing and bed linens.
Helpful Hints	If your skin becomes dry, apply an emollient (a moisturizer) to the treated area one hour after application of this medicine.

No special restrictions on driving, exertion and exercise, or exposure to excessive heat or cold.

POSSIBLE SIDE EFFECTS

Although this list of adverse effects may seem intimidating, keep in mind that some are quite rare. Of course, should these or any other problems arise while you are on medication, it is always a good idea to consult your doctor.

IF YOU DEVELOP	WHAT TO DO
rash or irritation that you didn't have before using this medicine	**May be serious** Check with your doctor as soon as possible.
mild stinging upon application of this medicine	If symptoms are disturbing or persist, let your doctor know.

STORAGE INSTRUCTIONS

Store in a cool, dark place (not in a bathroom medicine cabinet). If your medicine is in a liquid form, make sure that it does not freeze.

STOPPING OR INTERRUPTING THERAPY

If you miss a dose of this medicine, apply it as soon as possible. If it is almost time for your next dose, skip the missed dose and resume your regular schedule.

SPECIAL CONSIDERATIONS FOR THOSE OVER SIXTY-FIVE

None.

CONDITION: **PSORIASIS**

CATEGORY: **ANTIPSORIATIC DRUGS**

GENERIC (CHEMICAL) NAME	BRAND (TRADE) NAME	DOSAGE FORMS AND STRENGTHS
Etretinate	TEGISON	Capsules: 10, 25 mg

DRUG PROFILE

Etretinate is used to treat severe cases of psoriasis, when other therapy has not been effective. It controls epithelial (skin) cell growth.

BEFORE USING THIS DRUG

Let your doctor know *IF*

You have ever had allergic reactions or other problems with ■ etretinate ■ isotretinoin ■ tretinoin ■ vitamin A–containing medicine.

You have ever had any of the following medical problems: ■ diabetes (or family history of diabetes) ■ high cholesterol (or family history of high cholesterol) ■ high triglyceride levels ■ liver disease (or family history of liver disease) ■ heart or blood vessel disease (or family history of heart or blood vessel disease) ■ obesity ■ alcoholism.

You are taking any of the following medicines: ■ isotretinoin (medicine for acne) ■ tretinoin (medicine for acne and facial peeling) ■ methotrexate (used to treat certain kinds of cancer and severe psoriasis) ■ tetracyclines ■ vitamin A or any medicine containing vitamin A ■ alcohol-containing preparations (perfumes, aftershaves, toners) ■ topical medicine or soaps for acne including drying or abrasive agents ■ cosmetics to dry up or cover blemishes.

SPECIAL RESTRICTIONS WHILE TAKING THIS DRUG

FOOD AND DRUG INTERACTIONS

Other Drugs	Do not take vitamin A or any supplements containing vitamin A, as they may increase side effects of etretinate therapy.
Foods and Beverages	It is best to take this medicine with a glass of milk or a fatty snack or meal. Otherwise, you should reduce your intake of high-fat foods, as etretinate tends to increase blood cholesterol.

Alcohol	Reduce your ingestion of alcohol while you are taking this drug, as alcohol increases blood cholesterol (see above).

No special restrictions on smoking.

DAILY LIVING

Driving	This drug may cause vision problems, including decreased night vision. Be careful when driving, operating household appliances, or doing any other tasks that require alertness until you know how this drug affects you.
Sun Exposure	Avoid excessive sun exposure; your skin may become more sensitive to sunlight while you are on this drug. It is a good idea to apply a sunscreen to exposed skin surfaces before going outdoors.
Examinations or Tests	It is important for you to keep all appointments with your doctor so that your progress can be checked. Blood tests, X rays, or eye examinations may be required.
Other Precautions	Etretinate must not be taken by women who can or who intend to become pregnant. This drug may cause severe birth defects if taken during pregnancy. Women who have the potential of getting pregnant should have a negative pregnancy test and be on an effective contraceptive for at least one month before receiving this medicine and for an extended period after stopping etretinate. Do not give this drug to anyone else.

If you have diabetes, be aware that this medicine may raise blood-sugar levels. If you notice any change when testing sugar levels in your blood or urine, let your doctor know.

Tell any doctor or dentist you consult that you are taking this medicine, especially if you will be undergoing blood tests.

Because etretinate can remain in the blood for some time, you should not donate blood to a blood bank while you are taking etretinate and for two or three months after you stop therapy.

Helpful HInts

If your mouth or throat feels dry, chewing sugarless gum or sucking ice chips or sugarless hard candy will help. Also, since etretinate may make you more prone to cavities, gum disease, and mouth infections, be sure to see your dentist regularly.

Your eyes may become dry and if you wear contact lenses, you may experience trouble with them. If this becomes a problem, your doctor may suggest the use of eye lubricants, such as artificial tears.

During the first month of therapy, your psoriasis may worsen; you should see improvement by the second or third month. If your symptoms become severe, contact your doctor.

No special restrictions on exertion and exercise or exposure to excessive heat or cold.

POSSIBLE SIDE EFFECTS

Although this list of adverse effects may seem somewhat intimidating, keep in mind that some are quite rare. Of course, should these or any other problems arise while you are on medication, it is always a good idea to consult your doctor.

IF YOU DEVELOP	WHAT TO DO
flulike symptoms ■ severe headache ■ blurred or double vision or other vision problems ■ severe nausea or vomiting ■ difficulty breathing ■ dark-colored urine ■ yellowing of eyes or skin ■ swelling of face, hands, or lower legs	**Urgent** Get in touch with your doctor immediately.
bleeding or bruising ■ muscle cramps or rigidity ■ pain or stiffness in bones or joints ■ stomach pain ■ burning, irritated, or itching eyes ■ dry eyes, tearing, or other eye problems ■ earache or ear discharge ■ hearing problems ■ depression ■ anxiety ■ memory problems ■ mood changes ■ confusion ■ bleeding or swollen gums	**May be serious** Check with your doctor as soon as possible.
headache ■ dizziness ■ dry mouth ■ sore tongue ■ fever ■ nausea ■ increased or decreased appetite ■ increased skin sensitivity to sunlight ■ sensitivity to contact lenses ■ bleeding fingertips, palms, or soles ■ redness or soreness around fingernails or loosened fingernails ■ cold or clammy skin ■ blisters, warts, or other skin problems ■ dry nose ■ nosebleed ■ tiredness ■ increased thirst ■ hair loss	If symptoms are disturbing or persist, let your doctor know.

STORAGE INSTRUCTIONS

Store in a cool, dark place (not in a bathroom medicine cabinet).

STOPPING OR INTERRUPTING THERAPY

Take this medicine exactly as instructed by your doctor. If you miss a dose, take it as soon as possible with milk or a fatty snack. If it is almost time for your next dose, skip the missed dose and resume your regular schedule. Do not take two doses at the same time.

SPECIAL CONSIDERATIONS FOR THOSE OVER SIXTY-FIVE

None.

CONDITION: **PSORIASIS**

CATEGORY: **ANTIPSORIATIC DRUGS**

GENERIC (CHEMICAL) NAME	BRAND (TRADE) NAME	DOSAGE FORMS AND STRENGTHS
Methotrexate		Tablets: 2.5 mg

DRUG PROFILE

Methotrexate is used to treat certain types of leukemia, cancer of the lymph nodes, cancer of the breast, and certain cancers of the head, neck, skin, and lung. This drug is also sometimes used to treat rheumatoid arthritis and severe cases of psoriasis—a skin disorder. Methotrexate slows and halts the growth and spread of cancer cells by interfering with one of the steps in cell growth.

For complete information on this drug, see pages 1072–1076.

CONDITION: **DANDRUFF AND SEBORRHEA**

CATEGORY: **ANTISEBORRHEIC DRUGS**

GENERIC (CHEMICAL) NAME	BRAND (TRADE) NAME	DOSAGE FORMS AND STRENGTHS
Selenium sulfide	SELSUN	Lotion: 2.5%
	EXSEL	Lotion: 2.5%
	SELSUN BLUE	Shampoo

DRUG PROFILE

Selenium sulfide is used to control dandruff and seborrhea of the scalp. It is also sometimes used to treat certain fungal infections of the skin.

BEFORE USING THIS DRUG

Let your doctor know *IF*

You have ever had allergic reactions or other problems with ■ selenium sulfide.

SPECIAL RESTRICTIONS WHILE TAKING THIS DRUG

FOOD AND DRUG INTERACTIONS

No special restrictions on other drugs, foods and beverages, alcohol use, or smoking.

DAILY LIVING

Other Precautions	Avoid getting this medicine in your eyes or in any open scratches, cuts, or sores.
	Remove all jewelry before using selenium sulfide lotion to avoid possible damage.
Helpful Hints	Rinse your hair thoroughly after applying this medicine to minimize the chance of hair discoloration.

No special restrictions on driving, exertion and exercise, sun exposure, or exposure to excessive heat or cold.

POSSIBLE SIDE EFFECTS

Although this list of adverse effects may seem intimidating, keep in mind that some are quite rare. Of course, should these or any other problems arise while you are on medication, it is always a good idea to consult your doctor.

IF YOU DEVELOP	WHAT TO DO
irritation or rash that you didn't have before using this medicine	**May be serious** Check with your doctor as soon as possible.
dryness or oiliness of the hair or scalp ■ hair loss	If symptoms are disturbing or persist, let your doctor know.

STORAGE INSTRUCTIONS

Keep this medicine in a tight container in a cool, dark place (not in a bathroom medicine cabinet), and make sure that it does not freeze.

STOPPING OR INTERRUPTING THERAPY

Although dandruff usually responds well to selenium sulfide products, the problem tends to recur once treatment is stopped. It is best to continue to use this medicine on a regular, relatively infrequent basis (once every one to four weeks) as needed.

SPECIAL CONSIDERATIONS FOR THOSE OVER SIXTY-FIVE

None.

CONDITION: **DANDRUFF AND SEBORRHEA**

CATEGORY: **ANTISEBORRHEIC DRUGS**

GENERIC (CHEMICAL) NAME	BRAND (TRADE) NAME	DOSAGE FORMS AND STRENGTHS
Ketoconazole	NIZORAL	Shampoo: 2%

DRUG PROFILE

Ketoconazole is used to treat fungal infections. In tablet form it is used to treat systemic fungal infections. The cream is used to treat fungal infections of the skin. The shampoo is used to treat dandruff that is associated with fungal infections of the scalp.

For complete information on this drug, see pages 849–852 (in the section of this chapter on Skin Infections and Infestations).

BEFORE USING THIS DRUG

Let your doctor know *IF*

You have ever had allergic reactions or other problems with ■ ketoconazole.

SPECIAL RESTRICTIONS WHILE TAKING THIS DRUG

FOOD AND DRUG INTERACTIONS

No special restrictions on other drugs, foods and beverages, alcohol use, or smoking.

DAILY LIVING

Other Precautions	Avoid getting this medicine in your eyes.

Helpful Hints	This shampoo may interfere with hair permanent waving.

No special restrictions on driving, exertion and exercise, sun exposure, or exposure to excessive heat or cold.

POSSIBLE SIDE EFFECTS

IF YOU DEVELOP	WHAT TO DO
irritation or rash that you did not have before using this medicine ■ scalp pimples or blisters	**May be serious** Check with your doctor as soon as possible.
oiliness or dryness of the hair and scalp ■ itching ■ change in hair texture	If symptoms are disturbing or persist, let your doctor know.

STORAGE INSTRUCTIONS

Store at room temperature and protect from direct sunlight or freezing.

STOPPING OR INTERRUPTING THERAPY

Ketaconazole shampoo is generally used twice a week for four weeks with at least three days between each use. Intermittent use is often prescribed to maintain dandruff control.

SPECIAL CONSIDERATIONS FOR THOSE OVER SIXTY-FIVE

None.

CONDITION: **ROSACEA**

CATEGORY: **ANTIBIOTICS FOR SKIN DISORDERS (TETRACYCLINES)**

GENERIC (CHEMICAL) NAME	BRAND (TRADE) NAME	DOSAGE FORMS AND STRENGTHS
Tetracycline hydrochloride	ACHROMYCIN V	Capsules: 250, 500 mg Suspension: 125 mg per tsp
	PANMYCIN	Capsules: 250 mg
	ROBITET	Capsules: 250, 500 mg
	SUMYCIN	Capsules: 250, 500 mg Syrup: 125 mg per tsp Tablets: 250, 500 mg
Minocycline	MINOCIN	Capsules: 50, 100 mg Suspension: 50 mg per tsp

DRUG PROFILE

Tetracyclines are antibiotics that are used to treat a wide variety of bacterial infections, including skin eruptions and bronchitis and pneumonia. These antibiotics suppress the growth of bacteria by interfering with their manufacture of protein.

For complete information on these drugs, see pages 706–710.

CONDITION: **ROSACEA**

CATEGORY: **ANTIBIOTICS FOR SKIN DISORDERS**

GENERIC (CHEMICAL) NAME	BRAND (TRADE) NAME	DOSAGE FORMS AND STRENGTHS
Metronidazole	FLAGYL METROGEL	Tablets: 250, 500 mg Gel: 0.75%

DRUG PROFILE

Metronidazole is an antibiotic that is used to treat trichomoniasis (a vaginal infection) as well as a wide variety of systemic infections including dysentery and infections of the respiratory tract, skin, bones and joints, and stomach.

For complete information on this drug, see pages 971–974.

BEDSORES

Decubitus ulcers, better known as bedsores, are open wounds that can develop when someone lies or sits in the same position for a long time. Most often, they affect people who are bedridden because of a long-term illness or a major disability. But bedsores are more than an unsightly accompaniment to a long stay in bed. These ulcers may become infected, and if they're not treated properly, the infected area may expand.

CAUSES

Bedsores don't occur randomly on different parts of the body. Instead, they tend to develop in certain ulcer sites that vary with the person's position. When someone who is bedridden lies on his or her back, the body's weight presses most heavily at the shoulders, elbows, base of the spine, buttocks, and heels. Lying on one's side produces different pressure points —at the outside of the ankle and the thigh. Being confined to a wheelchair means still different areas of pressure— on the rim of the pelvic bones and in the lower part of the buttocks.

These areas of pressure are prime targets for bedsores. What happens is that the body weight, pressing down day after day, squeezes the small blood vessels that nourish the skin. The vessels can actually be compressed to the point at which the blood can't continue to flow; the skin, deprived of its blood supply, begins to die, and an ulcer forms. This process can happen to anyone confined to bed or a wheelchair, but people who have a chronic vascular disease are particularly vulnerable.

DIAGNOSIS

The first sign of a bedsore is a red or purple blotch on the skin over one of the pressure points. It may be painful and feel hot. If the pressure is relieved, the skin will return to normal within a few weeks. Otherwise, the bedsore will get worse. The skin will crack, and blisters will form. Bacteria then usually invade the site, doing further damage as the hole in the skin widens and deepens, opening a channel that can go all the way down to the bone.

PREVENTION AND TREATMENT

Confinement to bed does not necessarily produce bedsores. They may be avoided if the person's position is changed frequently, his or her skin kept clean and dry, and the bedsheets kept absolutely smooth so that wrinkles won't irritate the skin. At the very first sign of a bedsore, you should ask your doctor what to do, since healing is much easier to accomplish before the skin begins to break and blister.

If your doctor is concerned about the possibility of infection—or if bacteria have already invaded the wound—you may be given a prescription for a medicine you can apply right to the affected area. Such topical medicines are described in the drug chart on page 912. In cases where bedsores are neglected and penetrate far below the skin, surgery may be necessary to remove the damaged area and close the opening.

CONDITION: **BEDSORES**

CATEGORY: **TOPICAL ANTIBIOTICS**

GENERIC (CHEMICAL) NAME	BRAND (TRADE) NAME	DOSAGE FORMS AND STRENGTHS
Gentamicin sulfate	GARAMYCIN	Cream: 0.1% Ointment: 0.1%
Polymyxin B sulfate and bacitracin zinc	POLYSPORIN	Ointment: 10,000 units polymyxin B sulfate and 500 units of bacitracin zinc, per gram
Silver sulfadiazine	SILVADENE	Cream: 1%

Combination products composed of bacitracin, polymyxin B sulfate, and neomycin are available without prescription.

DRUG PROFILE

Gentamicin works by interfering with the bacteria's ability to manufacture protein. Polymyxin B alters the membrane of the bacterial cell so that the bacteria lose essential nutrients. Bacitracin interferes with the bacteria's ability to form new protective cell walls.

For complete information on these drugs, see pages 827–829.

Chapter 11
Disorders of the
Genitourinary Tract

URINARY TRACT INFECTION

Infections are among the most common problems of the urinary tract, especially in older people. The organs that may be affected are the kidneys, the bladder, the urethra (the tube that carries urine out of the bladder), and, in men, the prostate gland.

It's possible to have a urinary tract infection and have no symptoms at all. But more commonly, the problem is signaled by one or more of the following problems: a burning sensation when urinating; an urgent need to urinate frequently; blood in the urine; pain in the lower abdomen, groin, or back; and fever. A headache and loss of appetite may also accompany this condition.

CAUSES

The most common cause of urinary tract infections is a bacterium called *Escherichia coli (E. coli* for short), though other bacteria as well as fungi may be involved. *E. coli* normally resides in the colon, but it can migrate to, and multiply in, the urinary tract.

Older people may be especially prone to bacterial invasion of the urinary tract for several reasons. In the first place, the body's immune system, which fights off infection, may not be as efficient as it once was. Therefore, bacteria can multiply more easily.

Physical changes in the urinary tract may also set the stage for infection. In older men, the prostate gland sometimes enlarges and squeezes the urethra; urine therefore pools in the bladder and becomes a breeding ground for bacteria. A loss of bladder muscle strength that leaves women unable to empty their bladders completely can have a similar effect. Although women do not have a prostate gland, the urethra is shorter and closes less tightly, thereby making the bladder more vulnerable to bacteria from the outside. Atrophic vaginitis (see page 960) may add to discomfort.

Other sources of infection may include surgical procedures or urinary catheters, which can irritate the urinary tract and even introduce bacteria into the body. Lurking behind some urinary tract infections is a kidney stone or other blockage to the flow of urine.

DIAGNOSIS

Infections of different areas of the urinary tract have different names: pyelonephritis if the infection is in the kidneys; cystitis if it is in the bladder; urethritis, in the urethra; and prostatitis, in the prostate.

Whatever you call it, a urinary tract infection can make you quite uncomfortable and definitely warrants medical attention. Your doctor will probably want to examine a urine specimen under the microscope to determine precisely what is bothering you and to devise an appropriate treatment plan.

You may be asked simply to produce a specimen by urinating as you ordinarily would. Or the doctor may tell you to cleanse yourself thoroughly, empty your bladder partially, and then release the remaining urine into a specimen bottle. Men may have to use three specimen bottles so that the doctor can do different tests for cystitis, prostatitis, and urethritis.

TREATMENT

Antibiotics are usually quite effective in clearing up urinary tract infections within a week to ten days, though your doctor may prescribe the medicine for two weeks to be certain that the bacteria are all gone. For more information on these drugs, refer to the drug charts on pages 916–940.

Sometimes symptoms return within about two to four weeks of the end of therapy. This happens because the infecting organism was not completely eradicated. Or a new infection may occur caused by a different organism; this usually happens within six months of the original infection. If these relapses or reinfections occur frequently, your doctor may do further tests or prescribe the antibiotic for a longer period of time.

Most doctors choose not to prescribe medicine for older people who have urinary tract infections without any symptoms, since the potential side effects of the medicine outweigh the benefits of treatment in this case. However, if the infection is a symptom of another problem such as a kidney stone or obstruction, that condition will have to be addressed.

OUTLOOK

Urinary tract infections are highly treatable, especially those involving the bladder and urethra. When treatment is started at an early stage, continued for the proper length of time, and resumed or changed appropriately if a relapse occurs, these infections pose no serious threat to health.

Caution: Some drugs in this section may affect pregnancy or fetal development. Check with your doctor if this concerns you.

CONDITION: **URINARY TRACT INFECTIONS**

CATEGORY: **URINARY ANTI-INFECTIVES**

GENERIC (CHEMICAL) NAME	BRAND (TRADE) NAME	DOSAGE FORMS AND STRENGTHS
Sulfamethoxazole and phenazopyridine hydrochloride	AZO GANTANOL	Tablets: 500 mg sulfamethoxazole and 100 mg phenazopyridine hydrochloride
Sulfisoxazole	GANTRISIN	Tablets: 500 mg Suspension: 500 mg per tsp
Sulfisoxazole and phenazopyridine hydrochloride	AZO GANTRISIN	Tablets: 500 mg sulfisoxazole and 50 mg phenazopyridine hydrochloride

DRUG PROFILE

Sulfamethoxazole and sulfisoxazole are "sulfa" antibiotics, which suppress the growth of bacteria. They are used to treat infections of the urinary tract. Phenazopyridine relieves such symptoms of urinary tract infections as pain, burning, and irritation.

BEFORE USING THIS DRUG

Let your doctor know *IF*

You have ever had allergic reactions or other problems with ■ sulfonamides (sulfa drugs) ■ thiazide diuretics (water pills) ■ medicine for diabetes.

You have ever had any of the following medical problems: ■ glucose-6-phosphate dehydrogenase (G-6-PD) deficiency ■ porphyria ■ kidney disease ■ liver disease ■ blood disease ■ asthma or severe allergies.

You are taking any of the following medicines: ■ other sulfa drugs ■ any oral medicine containing para-aminobenzoic acid (PABA) ■ phenytoin (medicine for seizures) ■ digoxin or digitalis (heart medicines) ■ sulfinpyrazone (medicine for gout) ■ aspirin, aspirinlike medicine, or other medicine for pain and inflammation ■ methotrexate (medicine for cancer and severe psoriasis) ■ anticoagulants (blood thinners) ■ medicine for diabetes ■ tricyclic antidepressants ■ methenamine (other medicine for urinary tract infections) ■ barbiturates.

SPECIAL RESTRICTIONS WHILE TAKING THIS DRUG

FOOD AND DRUG INTERACTIONS

No special restrictions on other drugs, foods and beverages, alcohol use, or smoking.

DAILY LIVING

Sun Exposure	Your skin may become more sensitive to sunlight and more likely to develop a sunburn while you are taking this drug. It is a good idea to avoid too much sun and to apply a sunscreen to exposed skin surfaces before going outdoors.
Examinations or Tests	It is important for you to keep all appointments with your doctor so that your progress can be checked. Blood or urine tests may be required.
Other Precautions	Tell any doctor or dentist you consult that you are taking this medicine, especially if you will be undergoing any type of surgery or diagnostic testing. Phenazopyridine-containing medicine causes the urine to turn a reddish-orange color. This effect will disappear when you stop taking it. Clothing and other fabric may also be stained.

If you have diabetes, be aware that this drug may affect urine-sugar and ketone tests. Check with your doctor to see whether you should use a different type of test.

If your symptoms do not improve within a few days or if they worsen, check with your doctor.

Helpful Hints

For maximum benefit, take this drug on an empty stomach (one hour before or two hours after meals).

Be sure to drink four to six extra glasses of water a day while taking this drug.

No special restrictions on driving, exertion and exercise, or exposure to excessive heat or cold.

POSSIBLE SIDE EFFECTS

Although this list of adverse effects may seem somewhat intimidating, keep in mind that some are quite rare. Of course, should these or any other problems arise while you are on medication, it is always a good idea to consult your doctor.

IF YOU DEVELOP

seizures ■ bluish tinge to skin ■ rash ■ difficulty in breathing

Symptoms of hypoglycemia: "hot" feeling, increased sweating, dizziness, unsteadiness, tremors, weakness, blurred vision, hunger, headache, tingling in lips, slurred speech

WHAT TO DO

Urgent Get in touch with your doctor immediately.

numbness, tingling, or pain in hands or feet
■ paleness ■ sore throat or fever ■ bleeding or bruising ■ hives, itching, or other skin problems ■ severe
headache ■ mouth sores ■ red, itching eyes with
runny nose ■ swelling around eyes or neck ■ swelling
of the tip of the penis ■ joint pain ■ yellowing of eyes
or skin ■ stomach pain ■ blood in urine ■ decreased
or increased urination ■ pain or burning sensation in
urination ■ low back pain ■ clumsiness ■ depression
■ confusion ■ hallucinations ■ behavior changes
■ tiredness or weakness ■ swelling of tongue or vocal cords ■ ringing or buzzing sound in ears or other
hearing problems

With Azo Gantrisin and Gantrisin only: vomiting, with
blood or vomit that looks like coffee grounds ■ bloody
or black, tarry stools ■ flushing ■ irregular or fast
heartbeat ■ fainting ■ spasms ■ chest pain ■ muscle
pain ■ swelling of hands or feet ■ swelling around
ears

May be serious Check with
your doctor as soon as
possible.

upset stomach ■ nausea or vomiting ■ increased skin
sensitivity to sunlight ■ headache ■ dizziness
■ drowsiness ■ restlessness ■ sleeplessness ■ loss
of appetite ■ diarrhea ■ gas ■ skin color changes
■ anxiety

If symptoms are disturbing
or persist, let your doctor
know.

STORAGE INSTRUCTIONS

Store in a cool, dark place (not in a bathroom medicine cabinet).

STOPPING OR INTERRUPTING THERAPY

This medicine should be taken without interruption for the full length of time
prescribed by your doctor, even if you begin to feel better. If you do miss a dose,
take it as soon as possible. If it is almost time for your next dose, skip the missed
dose and resume your regular schedule. Do not take two doses at the same time.

SPECIAL CONSIDERATIONS FOR THOSE OVER SIXTY-FIVE

Because sulfa drugs are excreted through the kidneys and kidney function commonly decreases with age, doctors may start people over sixty-five on a lower dosage of this drug.

CONDITION: **URINARY TRACT INFECTIONS**

CATEGORY: **URINARY ANTI-INFECTIVES**

GENERIC (CHEMICAL) NAME	BRAND (TRADE) NAME	DOSAGE FORMS AND STRENGTHS
Nalidixic acid	NegGRAM	Suspension: 250 mg per tsp Tablets: 250, 500, 1000 mg

DRUG PROFILE

Nalidixic acid is used to treat bacterial infections of the urinary tract. This antibiotic drug interferes with the growth of bacteria.

BEFORE USING THIS DRUG

Let your doctor know *IF*

You have ever had allergic reactions or other problems with ■ nalidixic acid ■ oxolinic acid (another urinary antibiotic).

You have ever had any of the following medical problems: ■ seizures ■ cerebral atherosclerosis ■ asthma or other lung disease ■ kidney disease ■ liver disease.

You are taking any of the following medicines: ■ anticoagulants (blood thinners) ■ antacids ■ nitrofurantoin (another urinary antibiotic).

SPECIAL RESTRICTIONS WHILE TAKING THIS DRUG

FOOD AND DRUG INTERACTIONS

Other Drugs	If you are taking an antacid, take it two hours before or after a dose of this medicine.

No special restrictions on foods and beverages, alcohol use, or smoking.

DAILY LIVING

Sun Exposure	This drug may make your skin become more sensitive to sunlight, causing redness and blisters after sun exposure. It is a good idea to avoid prolonged sun exposure and to apply a sunscreen to exposed skin surfaces before going outdoors.
Examinations or Tests	It is important for you to keep all appointments with your doctor so that your progress can be checked. If you are on long-term therapy, periodic blood or urine tests may be required.
Other Precautions	If you have diabetes, be aware that this drug may affect urine-sugar tests. Check with your doctor before increasing your diabetes medicine or altering your diet. If your symptoms do not improve within two days or if they worsen, check with your doctor.
Helpful Hints	For maximum benefit, take this medicine one hour before meals. However, if this medicine upsets your stomach, ask your doctor if you can take it with food or milk.

No special restrictions on driving, exertion and exercise, or exposure to excessive heat or cold.

POSSIBLE SIDE EFFECTS

Although this list of adverse effects may seem somewhat intimidating, keep in mind that some are quite rare. Of course, should these or any other problems arise while you are on medication, it is always a good idea to consult your doctor.

IF YOU DEVELOP	WHAT TO DO
seizures ■ difficulty in breathing ■ personality changes ■ severe drowsiness ■ severe or continuing nausea or vomiting	**Urgent** Get in touch with your doctor immediately.
blurred or double vision ■ trouble focusing ■ change in color vision ■ increased skin sensitivity to sunlight ■ severe stomach pain ■ sore throat or fever ■ chills ■ bleeding or bruising ■ dark urine ■ yellowing of eyes or skin ■ extreme tiredness or weakness ■ fainting ■ muscle ache ■ joint stiffness ■ excitement ■ confusion ■ depression ■ change in hearing, smell, taste, or touch ■ eye pain or burning ■ jerky eye movements	**May be serious** Check with your doctor as soon as possible.
diarrhea ■ stomach pain ■ nausea or vomiting ■ rash, hives, or itching ■ dizziness ■ drowsiness ■ headache ■ general ill feeling ■ sleeplessness	If symptoms are disturbing or persist, let your doctor know.

STORAGE INSTRUCTIONS

Store in a cool, dark place (not in a bathroom medicine cabinet). If your medicine is in a liquid form, make sure that it does not freeze.

STOPPING OR INTERRUPTING THERAPY

This medicine should be taken without interruption for the full length of time prescribed by your doctor, even if you begin to feel better. If you do miss a dose, take it as soon as possible. If it is almost time for your next dose and you take three or more doses per day, either space the missed dose and the following dose two to four hours apart or double the following dose.

SPECIAL CONSIDERATIONS FOR THOSE OVER SIXTY-FIVE

Patients over sixty-five may be more sensitive to this medicine and be more prone to the possible side effects of mental changes or seizures, especially if the prescribed dose is exceeded. Your doctor may want to check your progress carefully.

CONDITION: **URINARY TRACT INFECTIONS**
CATEGORY: **URINARY ANTI-INFECTIVES**

GENERIC (CHEMICAL) NAME	BRAND (TRADE) NAME	DOSAGE FORMS AND STRENGTHS
Trimethoprim	PROLOPRIM	Tablets: 100, 200 mg
	TRIMPEX	Tablets: 100 mg

DRUG PROFILE

Trimethoprim is used to treat bacterial infections of the urinary tract. This antibiotic suppresses the growth of bacteria.

BEFORE USING THIS DRUG

Let your doctor know *IF*

You have ever had allergic reactions or other problems with ■ trimethoprim.

You have ever had any of the following medical problems: ■ kidney disease ■ liver disease ■ anemia ■ gout ■ malaria.

You are taking any of the following medicines: ■ phenytoin (medicine for seizures) ■ anticoagulants (blood thinners) ■ folic acid ■ medicine for diabetes ■ methotrexate (medicine for cancer and severe psoriasis) ■ thiazide diuretics (water pills) ■ medicine for arthritis.

SPECIAL RESTRICTIONS WHILE TAKING THIS DRUG

FOOD AND DRUG INTERACTIONS

No special restrictions on other drugs, foods and beverages, alcohol use, or smoking.

DAILY LIVING

Examinations or Tests	It is important for you to keep all appointments with your doctor so that your progress can be checked.
Other Precautions	If your symptoms do not improve within a few days or if they should worsen, check with your doctor.
Helpful Hints	If this medicine upsets your stomach, taking it with milk, meals, or snacks should help.

No special restrictions on driving, exertion and exercise, sun exposure, or exposure to excessive heat or cold.

POSSIBLE SIDE EFFECTS

Although this list of adverse effects may seem somewhat intimidating, keep in mind that some are quite rare. Of course, should these or any other problems arise while you are on medication, it is always a good idea to consult your doctor.

IF YOU DEVELOP	WHAT TO DO
severe or continuing nausea or vomiting ■ headache ■ dizziness ■ difficulty in breathing	**Urgent** Get in touch with your doctor immediately.
sore throat ■ fever ■ pale skin ■ extreme tiredness ■ bluish nails, lips, or skin ■ bleeding or bruising	**May be serious** Check with your doctor as soon as possible.

rash, itching, or other skin problems ■ nausea or vomiting ■ upset stomach ■ tongue inflammation ■ taste changes ■ diarrhea ■ loss of appetite ■ stomach cramps ■ sore mouth

If symptoms are disturbing or persist, let your doctor know.

STORAGE INSTRUCTIONS

Store in a cool, dark place (not in a bathroom medicine cabinet).

STOPPING OR INTERRUPTING THERAPY

This medicine should be taken without interruption for the full length of time prescribed by your doctor, even if you begin to feel better. If you miss a dose, take it as soon as possible. If it is almost time for your next dose, space the missed dose and following dose ten to twelve hours apart. Then return to your regular schedule.

SPECIAL CONSIDERATIONS FOR THOSE OVER SIXTY-FIVE

None.

CONDITION: **URINARY TRACT INFECTIONS**
CATEGORY: **URINARY ANTI-INFECTIVES**

GENERIC (CHEMICAL) NAME	BRAND (TRADE) NAME	DOSAGE FORMS AND STRENGTHS
Trimethoprim and sulfamethoxazole	BACTRIM	Suspension: 40 mg trimethoprim and 200 mg sulfamethoxazole per tsp Tablets: 80 mg trimethoprim and 400 mg sulfamethoxazole
	BACTRIM DS	Tablets: 160 mg trimethoprim and 800 mg sulfamethoxazole
	SEPTRA	Suspension: 40 mg trimethoprim and 200 mg sulfamethoxazole per tsp Tablets: 80 mg trimethoprim and 400 mg sulfamethoxazole
	SEPTRA DS	Tablets: 160 mg trimethoprim and 800 mg sulfamethoxazole

DRUG PROFILE

This combination drug is used to treat bacterial infections, including those that affect the urinary tract. The antibiotics trimethoprim and sulfamethoxazole work together to suppress the growth of bacteria. It is also used to treat travelers' diarrhea.

BEFORE USING THIS DRUG

Let your doctor know *IF*

You have ever had allergic reactions or other problems with ■ trimethoprim ■ sulfamethoxazole ■ other sulfonamides (sulfa drugs) ■ thiazide diuretics (water pills) ■ medicine for diabetes.

You have ever had any of the following medical problems: ■ glucose-6-phosphate dehydrogenase (G-6-PD) deficiency ■ folate deficiency ■ anemia ■ porphyria ■ kidney disease ■ liver disease ■ blood disease ■ asthma or other lung disease.

You are taking any of the following medicines: ■ sulfonamides (sulfa drugs) or other urinary antibiotics ■ anticoagulants (blood thinners) ■ medicine for seizures ■ methotrexate (medicine for cancer, severe psoriasis, or severe rheumatoid arthritis) ■ medicine for diabetes ■ aspirin, aspirinlike medicine, or other medicine for pain and inflammation ■ sulfinpyrazone (medicine for gout) ■ folic acid.

SPECIAL RESTRICTIONS WHILE TAKING THIS DRUG

FOOD AND DRUG INTERACTIONS

Foods and Beverages	Because this medicine can cause folic acid deficiency, be sure to eat a well-balanced diet including plenty of B vitamins.

No special restrictions on other drugs, alcohol use, or smoking.

DAILY LIVING

Sun Exposure	Your skin may become more sensitive to sunlight and more likely to develop a sunburn while you are taking this drug. It is a good idea to avoid too much sun and to apply a sunscreen to exposed skin surfaces before going outdoors.

Examinations or Tests	It is important for you to keep all appointments with your doctor so that your progress can be checked. Periodic urine tests may be required.
Other Precautions	If you have diabetes, be aware that this drug may affect urine-sugar and ketone tests. Check with your doctor to see whether you should use a different type of test.
	If your symptoms do not improve within a few days or if they worsen, check with your doctor.
Helpful Hints	If this medicine upsets your stomach, taking it with milk, meals, or snacks should help.
	Be sure to drink four to six glasses of water a day while taking this medicine so that your body can easily eliminate the waste products of the medicine.

No special restrictions on driving, exertion and exercise, or exposure to excessive heat or cold.

POSSIBLE SIDE EFFECTS

Although this list of adverse effects may seem somewhat intimidating, keep in mind that some are quite rare. Of course, should these or any other problems arise while you are on medication, it is always a good idea to consult your doctor.

IF YOU DEVELOP	**WHAT TO DO**
difficulty in breathing ■ sore throat or fever ■ chills ■ extreme tiredness ■ bleeding or bruising ■ joint pain ■ blood in urine if not present earlier ■ dramatically increased or decreased urination ■ swelling in neck ■ severe diarrhea	**Urgent: Stop taking this drug and get in touch with your doctor immediately.**
rash, hives, or other skin problems ■ very pale skin ■ swelling around eyes ■ red, itching eyes ■ tiredness ■ nervousness ■ muscle weakness ■ clumsiness ■ ringing or buzzing sound in ears ■ depression ■ hallucinations ■ yellowing of eyes or skin ■ change in urine or stool color ■ numbness, tingling, or pain in hands or feet ■ bluish nails, lips, or skin ■ low back pain	**May be serious** Check with your doctor as soon as possible.
headache ■ diarrhea ■ dizziness ■ nausea or vomiting ■ stomach pain ■ increased skin sensitivity to sunlight ■ tongue inflammation ■ mouth sores ■ sleeplessness	If symptoms are disturbing or persist, let your doctor know.

STORAGE INSTRUCTIONS

Store in a cool, dark place (not in a bathroom medicine cabinet). If your medicine is in a liquid form, make sure that it does not freeze.

STOPPING OR INTERRUPTING THERAPY

This medicine should be taken without interruption for the full length of time prescribed by your doctor, even if you begin to feel better. If you do miss a dose, space the missed dose between the time you should have taken it and your next scheduled dose or simply double the next scheduled dose and resume your regular schedule.

SPECIAL CONSIDERATIONS FOR THOSE OVER SIXTY-FIVE

Because this medicine is excreted through the kidneys and kidney function commonly decreases with age, doctors may start people over sixty-five on a lower dosage of this medicine.

CONDITION: **URINARY TRACT INFECTIONS**

CATEGORY: **URINARY ANTI-INFECTIVES**

GENERIC (CHEMICAL) NAME	BRAND (TRADE) NAME	DOSAGE FORMS AND STRENGTHS
Methenamine hippurate	HIPREX	Tablets: 1 g
	UREX	Tablets: 1 g
Methenamine mandelate	MANDELAMINE	Granules: 1 g Suspension: 250, 500 mg per tsp Tablets: 0.5, 1 g
Methenamine, methylene blue, phenyl salicylate, benzoic acid, atropine sulfate, and hyoscyamine	URISED	Tablets: 40.8 mg methenamine, 5.4 mg methylene blue, 18.1 mg phenyl salicylate, 4.5 mg benzoic acid, 0.03 mg atropine sulfate, and 0.03 mg hyoscyamine

DRUG PROFILE

Methenamine is used to prevent urinary tract infections from recurring. It is converted into an antibacterial drug in the acidic environment of the urinary tract.

BEFORE USING THIS DRUG

Let your doctor know *IF*

You have ever had allergic reactions or other problems with ■ methenamine ■ tartrazine (FD&C Yellow Dye No. 5) (contained in Hiprex tablets).

You have ever had any of the following medical problems: ■ liver disease ■ kidney disease.

With Urised only: ■ heart disease ■ difficulty in urination ■ enlarged prostate ■ glaucoma ■ fecal (stool) impaction or severe constipation.

You are taking any of the following medicines: ■ sulfonamides (sulfa drugs) ■ diuretics (water pills) ■ medicine to make the urine less acidic ■ baking soda ■ any medicine containing potassium citrate, sodium acetate, sodium citrate, or sodium lactate ■ antacids.

With Urised only: ■ medicine for stomach cramps or pain ■ amantadine, benztropine, or trihexyphenidyl (medicine for Parkinson's disease) ■ antihistamines ■ haloperidol (tranquilizer) ■ phenothiazines (tranquilizers and medicine for nausea) ■ medicine for depression.

SPECIAL RESTRICTIONS WHILE TAKING THIS DRUG

FOOD AND DRUG INTERACTIONS

Other Drugs	Do not take any other drugs, including over-the-counter (OTC) drugs, before checking with your doctor. OTC antacids and allergy or cold medicines may interfere with the action of these drugs.
Foods and Beverages	These drugs are most effective when the urine is very acidic. Foods and beverages that make the urine more acidic include cranberry juice, plums, prunes, and protein-rich foods. Avoid foods and beverages that make the urine alkaline, such as most fruits, especially citrus fruits and juices, milk, cheese, and other dairy products.

No special restrictions on alcohol use or smoking.

DAILY LIVING

Driving	Urised may cause blurred vision or loss of alertness. Be careful when driving, operating household appliances, or doing any other tasks that require alertness until you know how this drug affects you.

Exertion and Exercise	Urised may cause you to sweat less than normally. Sweating is your body's natural way of cooling down, and not sweating enough can be dangerous. Use caution not to become overheated when you exercise or exert yourself.
Excessive Heat	See above; use caution during hot weather, as overexertion may result in heat stroke. Avoid extremely hot baths and saunas.
Examinations or Tests	It is important for you to keep all appointments with your doctor so that your progress can be checked. Periodic blood or urine tests may be required. Your doctor will probably instruct you to test the acidity of your urine with urine acid test paper once a day; follow directions exactly.
Other Precautions	If your symptoms do not improve within a few days or if they should worsen, check with your doctor. If you are taking Urised, be aware that your urine and stools may be discolored to a blue or blue-green because of the methylene blue component (a dye) in the drug.
Helpful Hints	Taking this medicine after meals and at bedtime may help reduce the chance of upset stomach. Swallow tablets whole, without crushing or chewing. Dissolve the granules in two to four ounces of water and stir well before drinking. If your mouth or throat feels dry, chewing sugarless gum or sucking ice chips or sugarless hard candy will help.

No special restrictions on sun exposure or exposure to excessive cold.

POSSIBLE SIDE EFFECTS

Although this list of adverse effects may seem somewhat intimidating, keep in mind that some are quite rare. Of course, should these or any other problems arise while you are on medication, it is always a good idea to consult your doctor.

IF YOU DEVELOP	WHAT TO DO
fever ■ difficulty in breathing *With Urised only:* irregular or fast heartbeat ■ dizziness ■ blurred vision ■ hot, dry, flushed skin ■ decreased or difficult urination ■ red or painful eyes	**Urgent** Get in touch with your doctor immediately.
blood in urine ■ lower back pain ■ pain in urination ■ urinary frequency ■ dry mouth ■ swelling of face, feet, or hands ■ muscle cramps ■ ringing or buzzing sound in ears	**May be serious** Check with your doctor as soon as possible.
nausea or vomiting ■ rash, hives, or itching ■ diarrhea ■ stomach cramps ■ loss of appetite ■ mouth sores	If symptoms are disturbing or persist, let your doctor know.

STORAGE INSTRUCTIONS

Store in a cool, dark place (not in a bathroom medicine cabinet). If your medicine is in a liquid form, make sure that it does not freeze.

STOPPING OR INTERRUPTING THERAPY

This medicine should be taken without interruption for the full length of time prescribed by your doctor, even if you begin to feel better. If you do miss a dose, take it as soon as possible. If it is almost time for your next dose and you take two doses a day, space the missed dose and following dose five to six hours apart; if you take three or more doses a day, space the missed dose and the following dose two to four hours apart, or simply double the following dose. Then resume your regular schedule.

SPECIAL CONSIDERATIONS FOR THOSE OVER SIXTY-FIVE

Doctors may start people over sixty-five on a lower-than-usual adult dosage. Older people may be more prone to the side effects of Urised and doctors may wish to check them frequently while they are taking this drug.

CONDITION: **URINARY TRACT INFECTIONS**

CATEGORY: **URINARY ANTI-INFECTIVES**

GENERIC (CHEMICAL) NAME	BRAND (TRADE) NAME	DOSAGE FORMS AND STRENGTHS
Ciprofloxacin hydrochloride	CIPRO	Tablets: 250, 500, 750 mg
Ofloxacin	FLOXIN	Tablets: 200, 300, 400 mg
Norfloxacin	NOROXIN	Tablets: 400 mg

DRUG PROFILE

Ciprofloxacin, ofloxacin, and norfloxacin are antibiotics that are used to treat infections of the urinary tract. These drugs keep bacteria from multiplying by interfering with the action of the bacteria's genetic material. Ciprofloxacin and ofloxacin are also used to treat other bacterial infections.

BEFORE USING THIS DRUG

Let your doctor know *IF*

You have ever had allergic reactions or other problems with ■ ciprofloxacin ■ ofloxacin ■ norfloxacin ■ nalidixic acid.

You have ever had any of the following medical problems: ■ kidney disease ■ liver disease ■ seizures.

You are taking any of the following medicines: ■ antacids ■ probenecid (medicine for gout) ■ nitrofurantoin (medicine for urinary tract infection) ■ chloramphenicol ■ theophylline ■ sucralfate (medicine for ulcers).

SPECIAL RESTRICTIONS WHILE TAKING THIS DRUG

FOOD AND DRUG INTERACTIONS

Other Drugs	Antacids containing calcium or magnesium interfere with the absorption of this drug. Allow two hours between the time you take this medicine and the time you take this kind of antacid.
Food and Beverages	Food interferes with the absorption of norfloxacin and ofloxacin. These medicines should be taken one hour before or two hours after a meal with a glass of water. Ciprofloxacin may be taken without regard to meals.

No special restrictions on alcohol use or smoking.

DAILY LIVING

Driving	These medicines may cause drowsiness, light-headedness, or vision disturbances. Be careful when driving, operating household appliances, or doing any other tasks that require alertness until you know how this drug affects you.
Sun Exposure	You may develop a sensitivity to light, especially sunlight, while taking this medicine. Therefore, it is a good idea to avoid too much sun while you are taking this medicine. If you feel a tingling or burning sensation on your hands, feet, or nose or any other unusual reaction after being exposed to the sun, let your doctor know right away. If necessary, dark glasses may be worn to protect your eyes.

Examinations or Tests	It is important for you to keep all appointments with your doctor, even if you feel well, so that your progress can be checked. Urine tests may be required.
Other Precautions	Tell any doctor or dentist you consult that you are taking this drug.
Helpful Hints	Take norfloxacin and ofloxacin with a full glass of water and on an empty stomach, that is, one hour before or two hours after a meal. Make sure you drink plenty of water—several glasses a day in addition to your regular liquid intake—in order to avoid urinary side effects.
	If your mouth or throat feels dry, chewing sugarless gum or sucking ice chips or sugarless hard candy will help.

No special restrictions on exertion and exercise or exposure to excessive heat or cold.

POSSIBLE SIDE EFFECTS

Although this list of adverse effects may seem somewhat intimidating, keep in mind that some are quite rare. Of course, should these or any other problems arise while you are on medication, it is always a good idea to consult your doctor.

IF YOU DEVELOP

■ seizures ■ swelling of eyes, face, neck, lips, hands ■ difficulty swallowing ■ trouble breathing ■ shortness of breath ■ confusion ■ mood or behavior changes

WHAT TO DO

Urgent: Stop taking this drug and get in touch with your doctor immediately.

dizziness ■ light-headedness ■ headache ■ depression ■ blurred vision or other vision problems ■ increased sensitivity to light ■ increased skin sensitivity to sunlight ■ lower back pain ■ blood in urine, or pain while urinating ■ upset stomach	**May be serious** Check with your doctor as soon as possible.
heartburn ■ nausea or vomiting ■ loss of appetite ■ indigestion ■ stomach pain ■ diarrhea ■ constipation ■ gas ■ drowsiness ■ rash, itching, or redness ■ pain or stiffness in joints or tendons ■ sleeplessness ■ tiredness ■ fever	If symptoms are disturbing or persist, let your doctor know.

STORAGE INSTRUCTIONS

Store in a cool, dark place (not in a bathroom medicine cabinet).

STOPPING OR INTERRUPTING THERAPY

Take this drug without interruption for the full length of time prescribed by your doctor, even if you begin to feel better. This will ensure that the infection clears up completely and that your symptoms do not return. If you miss a dose, take it as soon as possible. If it is almost time for your next dose, skip the missed dose and resume your regular schedule. Do not take two doses at the same time.

SPECIAL CONSIDERATIONS FOR THOSE OVER SIXTY-FIVE

Because this drug is excreted by the kidney and some elderly patients may have decreased kidney function, doctors may start certain older patients at a lower dosage of this drug.

CONDITION: **URINARY TRACT INFECTIONS**

CATEGORY: **URINARY ANTI-INFECTIVES**

GENERIC (CHEMICAL) NAME	BRAND (TRADE) NAME	DOSAGE FORMS AND STRENGTHS
Nitrofurantoin	MACRODANTIN	Capsules: 25, 50, 100 mg

DRUG PROFILE

Nitrofurantoin is used to treat infections of the urinary tract. It is also sometimes prescribed as a single dose before bedtime to prevent recurrent urinary tract infections. This drug is thought to work by interfering with bacterial enzymes.

BEFORE USING THIS DRUG

Let your doctor know *IF*

You have ever had allergic reactions or other problems with ■ nitrofurantoin ■ furazolidone.

You have ever had any of the following medical problems: ■ kidney disease ■ lack of urination or excessive urination ■ anemia ■ diabetes ■ mineral deficiency ■ vitamin B deficiency ■ lung disease ■ nerve damage ■ glucose-6-phosphate dehydrogenase (G-6-PD) deficiency.

You are taking any of the following medicines: ■ other antibiotics ■ probenecid or sulfinpyrazone (medicine for gout) ■ magnesium trisilicate-containing antacids ■ medicine for seizures.

SPECIAL RESTRICTIONS WHILE TAKING THIS DRUG

FOOD AND DRUG INTERACTIONS

No special restrictions on other drugs, foods and beverages, alcohol use, or smoking.

DAILY LIVING

Examinations or Tests	It is important for you to keep all appointments with your doctor so that your progress can be checked. Periodic blood and urine tests may be required.
Other Precautions	Tell any doctor or dentist you consult that you are taking this medicine, especially if you will be undergoing any type of surgery.
	This medicine may cause the urine to turn a rusty or brownish color. This effect will disappear when you stop taking it.
	If you have diabetes, be aware that this drug may affect urine-sugar tests. Check with your doctor to see whether you should use a different type of test.
	If symptoms do not improve within a few days or if they worsen, check with your doctor.
Helpful Hints	For maximum benefit, and to lessen the chance of stomach upset, take this drug with milk or food.

No special restrictions on sun exposure, exertion and exercise, driving or exposure to excessive heat or cold.

POSSIBLE SIDE EFFECTS

Although this list of adverse effects may seem somewhat intimidating, keep in mind that some are quite rare. Of course, should these or any other problems arise while you are on medication, it is always a good idea to consult your doctor.

IF YOU DEVELOP	WHAT TO DO
shortness of breath ■ difficulty in breathing ■ general ill feeling ■ fever ■ chills ■ cough ■ chest pain ■ headache ■ tiredness or weakness ■ numbness, tingling, or burning of face or mouth ■ yellowing of eyes or skin ■ skin rashes ■ drowsiness ■ paleness	**Urgent: Stop taking this drug and get in touch with your doctor immediately.**
itching ■ rash ■ abdominal or stomach pain ■ upset stomach ■ nausea or vomiting ■ loss of appetite ■ diarrhea ■ headache ■ dizziness	If symptoms are disturbing or persist, let your doctor know.

STORAGE INSTRUCTIONS

Store in a cool, dark place (not in a bathroom medicine cabinet).

STOPPING OR INTERRUPTING THERAPY

This medicine should be taken without interruption for the full length of time prescribed by your doctor, even if you begin to feel better. If you miss a dose of this medicine, take it as soon as possible. If it is almost time for your next dose, space the missed dose and your next scheduled dose two to four hours apart or simply double the next dose and resume your regular schedule. If you are taking this drug to *prevent* urinary tract infections and you miss a dose, take it as soon as possible. If it is almost time for your next dose, take the missed dose and wait ten to twelve hours before taking your next dose. Then resume your regular schedule.

SPECIAL CONSIDERATIONS FOR THOSE OVER SIXTY-FIVE

None.

CONDITION: **URINARY TRACT INFECTIONS**

CATEGORY: **URINARY ANALGESICS**

GENERIC (CHEMICAL) NAME	BRAND (TRADE) NAME	DOSAGE FORMS AND STRENGTHS
Phenazopyridine hydrochloride	PYRIDIUM	Tablets: 100, 200 mg
Phenazopyridine hydrochloride, hyoscyamine hydrobromide, and butabarbital	PYRIDIUM PLUS	Tablets: 150 mg phenazopyridine hydrochloride, 0.3 mg hyoscyamine hydrobromide, and 15 mg butabarbital

DRUG PROFILE

Phenazopyridine is prescribed to relieve symptoms of urinary tract infections such as pain, burning, irritation, and frequency and urgency of urination.

BEFORE USING THIS DRUG

Let your doctor know *IF*

You have ever had allergic reactions or other problems with ■ phenazopyridine ■ hyoscyamine ■ butabarbital.

You have ever had any of the following medical problems: ■ hepatitis ■ kidney disease ■ glucose-6-phosphate dehydrogenase (G-6-PD) deficiency.

With Pyridium Plus only: ■ glaucoma ■ porphyria ■ difficult urination ■ enlarged prostate.

You are taking any of the following medicines:

With Pyridium Plus only: ■ anticoagulants (blood thinners) ■ amantadine, benztropine, or trihexyphenidyl (medicine for Parkinson's disease) ■ antihistamines ■ medicine for hay fever, coughs, or colds ■ narcotics or other prescription pain-killers ■ sleep medicines ■ tranquilizers ■ medicine for seizures ■ medicine for stomach cramps ■ antacids ■ medicine for diarrhea ■ corticosteroids ■ digoxin or digitalis (heart medicines) ■ griseofulvin (medicine for fungal infections) ■ tetracyclines ■ medicine for depression.

SPECIAL RESTRICTIONS WHILE TAKING THIS DRUG

FOOD AND DRUG INTERACTIONS

Other Drugs	Do not take any other drug, including over-the-counter (OTC) drugs, before checking with your doctor—especially if you are taking Pyridium Plus. Pyridium Plus increases the effects of drugs that depress the central nervous system, such as antihistamines; medicine for hay fever, allergies, or colds; sleep medicines; tranquilizers; narcotics or other prescription pain-killers; muscle relaxants; and medicine for seizures.
Alcohol	Pyridium Plus increases the effects of alcohol, a central nervous system depressant. Avoid alcohol if you are taking Pyridium Plus unless your doctor has approved its use.

No special restrictions on foods and beverages or smoking.

DAILY LIVING

Driving	Pyridium Plus may cause blurred vision, dizziness, or drowsiness. If you are taking Pyridium Plus, be careful when driving, operating household appliances, or doing any other tasks that require alertness until you know how this drug affects you.

Exertion and Exercise	Pyridium Plus may cause you to sweat less than normally. Sweating is your body's natural way of cooling down, and not sweating enough can be dangerous. Use caution not to become overheated when you exercise or exert yourself.
Excessive Heat	See above; use caution during hot weather, as overexertion may result in heat stroke. Avoid extremely hot baths and saunas.
Other Precautions	These drugs cause the urine to turn a reddish-orange color. This effect will disappear when you stop taking the drug. These drugs may also stain clothing; wipe carefully.
	If your symptoms do not improve within a few days or if they worsen, check with your doctor.
	If you have diabetes, be aware that this drug may affect urine-sugar and ketone tests. Check with your doctor to see whether you should use a different type of test.
	Especially for Pyridium Plus: Do not take this drug more often or for a longer period of time than directed by your doctor, since it may become habit-forming.
Helpful Hints	If this medicine upsets your stomach, taking it with or immediately after meals should help.

No special restrictions on sun exposure or exposure to excessive cold.

POSSIBLE SIDE EFFECTS

Although this list of adverse effects may seem somewhat intimidating, keep in mind that some are quite rare. Of course, should these or any other problems arise while you are on medication, it is always a good idea to consult your doctor.

IF YOU DEVELOP	WHAT TO DO
pain in urination ■ bluish tinge to skin *With Pyridium Plus only:* difficulty in breathing ■ fast heartbeat ■ hot, dry, flushed skin ■ dry mouth ■ delirium ■ fever ■ seizures ■ extreme drowsiness ■ red or painful eyes	**Urgent** Get in touch with your doctor immediately.
extreme tiredness ■ skin color changes ■ yellowing of eyes or skin ■ hives ■ rash *With Pyridium Plus only:* blurred vision ■ nausea or vomiting ■ decreased urination	**May be serious** Check with your doctor as soon as possible.
headache ■ dizziness ■ upset stomach *With Pyridium Plus only:* drowsiness ■ confusion	If symptoms are disturbing or persist, let your doctor know.

STORAGE INSTRUCTIONS

Store in a cool, dark place (not in a bathroom medicine cabinet).

STOPPING OR INTERRUPTING THERAPY

If you miss a dose, take it as soon as possible. If it is almost time for your next dose, skip the missed dose and resume your regular schedule. Do not take two doses at the same time.

SPECIAL CONSIDERATIONS FOR THOSE OVER SIXTY-FIVE

Older people may be more prone to the side effects of Pyridium Plus. Doctors may wish to check people over sixty-five frequently.

URINARY INCONTINENCE

Urinary incontinence—a loss of urinary control—is a problem that occurs more frequently with aging, but is neither normal nor a part of normal aging. Incontinence can range from the discomfort of slight losses of urine to the distress and disability of severe, frequent wetting.

Most people don't realize that many cases of incontinence can be cured and that the majority of cases can be treated and controlled. Incontinence is not a disease. Rather, it is a symptom of an underlying problem, such as a neurologic disorder, or the result of using certain medicines. Because the underlying problem may occasionally be serious, medical evaluation should be sought in all cases. The three major types of incontinence are discussed below.

STRESS INCONTINENCE

The leakage of urine during activities that put pressure on the bladder, such as coughing or laughing, is called stress incontinence. In women, it may be caused by changes in the anatomy resulting from childbirth or brought on by surgery or by inflammation of the urethra—the canal through which urine flows to the outside. Inflammation may be triggered by infection or by lowered levels of the female hormone estrogen, associated with menopause. Men rarely develop stress incontinence, and when they do, it's usually as a result of surgery. Stress incontinence may be complicated by urge incontinence (see the following).

OVERACTIVE BLADDER

Overactive bladder means that the muscular layer lining the bladder is hyperactive, causing the bladder to contract in spasms. This leads to frequent urination, and excessive urination at night. Some causes of this type of incontinence are Parkinson's disease, cancer, infection, cerebrovascular disease, and Alzheimer's disease. If you have an overactive bladder, you may also experience urge incontinence. Urge incontinencerefers to the inability to reach the toilet in time. It may accompany an enlarged prostate gland in men. Urge incontinence can also be due to such physical conditions as arthritis or muscle weakness, or such emotional problems as depression and anger (which can be expressed either consciously or unconsciously as incontinence). But it can also occur in otherwise healthy older people. The best approach is to deal with any underlying difficulty, while at the same time making it easy for you to get to the toilet promptly. If you are physically incapacitated, a bedside commode should help. Medications may also be helpful.

OVERFLOW INCONTINENCE

In this type of incontinence, small amounts of urine leak frequently from a constantly filled bladder. In men, this is often caused by an enlarged prostate gland, which prevents emptying of the bladder. Some people with diabetes experience overflow incontinence because the bladder cannot contract normally. The use of drugs that relax the bladder may also produce this problem.

DIAGNOSIS

People who have trouble controlling their urination should see a doctor for a complete medical examination. This examination will include a history so the doctor can find out what circumstances, such as coughing or laughing, cause leakage; whether you are able to stop urine flow; and other relevant information, such as medicines you use. Your doctor may ask you to develop an incontinence chart to record the timing of your symptoms. A physical exam will focus on the urinary, reproductive, and neurologic systems. Laboratory tests may also be conducted. Your doctor may then refer you to a specialist in diseases of the urinary tract, for further tests.

TREATMENT

Various medicines are available for the treatment of urinary incontinence. Although they must be taken under close medical supervision, they cause remarkable improvement in most people. These remedies are described in the drug charts on pages 947–956.

Certain behavioral conditioning techniques, such as bladder retraining, have proven useful in people with urinary incontinence. These techniques help the person sense bladder filling and delay urination until a toilet is available. If the problem is the result of an enlarged prostate, however, surgical correction may be necessary.

For stress incontinence, some doctors recommend that women perform pelvic floor exercises (Kegel exercises) to strengthen the muscles that help close the bladder outlet. This involves the repeated tightening and then relaxation of these sphincter muscles. Yet another approach to this type of incontinence involves the use of vaginal appliances, such as pessaries and tampons, to raise the urethra. This relieves the problem in some women. If these simple methods fail, surgical correction may be recommended.

Catheterization—inserting a flexible, slender tube into the urethra and collecting the urine in a container—is another treatment alternative. It is generally not done continuously, but intermittently, to reduce the likelihood of urinary infection. In men, the collecting device is sometimes worn externally, over the genitalia, and connected to a drainage bag.

Specially designed absorbent underwear is available, as are layered sheets that will make the person more comfortable. Diapers, however, should be used only as a last resort. This approach to the problem may be convenient, but it is generally both emotionally and physically damaging.

OUTLOOK

Many people who are incontinent shy away from socializing and try to hide their problem from friends and family. But this condition *can* be managed, and often totally cured. Once the problem is confronted and medical help sought, modern treatment approaches can ease the discomfort, the inconvenience, and the embarrassment and allow you to live normally.

CONDITION: **URINARY RETENTION**

CATEGORY: **URINARY TRACT STIMULANTS**

GENERIC (CHEMICAL) NAME	BRAND (TRADE) NAME	DOSAGE FORMS AND STRENGTHS
Bethanechol chloride	DUVOID	Tablets: 10, 25, 50 mg
	URECHOLINE	Tablets: 5, 10, 25, 50 mg

DRUG PROFILE

Bethanechol is used to treat urinary retention, that is, difficulty in urinating or in emptying the bladder completely. This drug, which belongs to a class of drugs known as parasympathomimetic agents, stimulates the bladder and relaxes the muscles that control the flow of urine.

BEFORE USING THIS DRUG

Let your doctor know *IF*

You have ever had allergic reactions or other problems with ■ bethanechol.

You have ever had any of the following medical problems: ■ asthma or other lung disease ■ seizures ■ heart or blood vessel disease ■ high or low blood pressure ■ digestive or urinary tract blockage ■ slow heartbeat ■ spastic disease of the digestive tract ■ ulcers ■ overactive thyroid ■ Parkinson's disease or other nerve disorders ■ recent bladder or intestinal surgery ■ enlarged prostate.

You are taking any of the following medicines: ■ medicine for myasthenia gravis ■ mecamylamine (medicine for high blood pressure) ■ medicine for abnormal heart rhythms ■ medicine for Parkinson's disease ■ medicine for asthma ■ medicine for irritable bowel syndrome or spastic colon ■ narcotics or other prescription pain-killers.

SPECIAL RESTRICTIONS WHILE TAKING THIS DRUG

FOOD AND DRUG INTERACTIONS

No special restrictions on other drugs, foods and beverages, alcohol use, or smoking.

DAILY LIVING

Driving	This medicine may cause blurred vision or dizziness. Be careful when driving, operating household appliances, or doing any other tasks that require alertness until you know how this drug affects you.
Other Precautions	Tell any doctor or dentist you consult that you are taking this medicine, especially if you will be undergoing any type of surgery.
Helpful Hints	Dizziness or light-headedness may occur, especially when getting up from a reclining or sitting position. Getting up slowly may help this. To reduce the chance of nausea or vomiting, take this medicine on an empty stomach—one hour before or two hours after meals.

No special restrictions on exertion and exercise, sun exposure, or exposure to excessive heat or cold.

POSSIBLE SIDE EFFECTS

Although this list of adverse effects may seem somewhat intimidating, keep in mind that some are quite rare. Of course, should these or any other problems arise while you are on medication, it is always a good idea to consult your doctor.

IF YOU DEVELOP	WHAT TO DO
severe dizziness ■ fainting ■ irregular or fast heartbeat ■ bloody diarrhea ■ cold, clammy skin ■ difficulty in breathing ■ tightness in chest ■ convulsions	**Urgent** Get in touch with your doctor immediately.
fever ■ difficulty controlling bowel movements ■ blurred vision ■ irritability	**May be serious** Check with your doctor as soon as possible.
diarrhea ■ stomach pain or cramps ■ dizziness ■ headache ■ nausea or vomiting ■ belching ■ flushing or warm skin ■ increased sweating ■ increased salivation ■ tearing ■ urinary urgency ■ increased bowel sounds ■ general ill feeling	If symptoms are disturbing or persist, let your doctor know.

STORAGE INSTRUCTIONS

Store in a cool, dark place (not in a bathroom medicine cabinet).

STOPPING OR INTERRUPTING THERAPY

If you miss a dose of this medicine, take it as soon as possible. If it is more than two hours since the scheduled time of the missed dose, skip it and resume your regular schedule. Do not take two doses at the same time.

SPECIAL CONSIDERATIONS FOR THOSE OVER SIXTY-FIVE

None.

CONDITION: **URINARY INCONTINENCE**

CATEGORY: **ANTISPASMODICS**

GENERIC (CHEMICAL) NAME	BRAND (TRADE) NAME	DOSAGE FORMS AND STRENGTHS
Oxybutynin chloride	DITROPAN	Syrup: 5 mg per tsp Tablets: 5 mg

DRUG PROFILE

Oxybutynin is used to relieve urinary conditions caused by bladder spasms. This drug increases the capacity of the bladder to hold urine, helps control bladder spasms, and delays the desire to urinate.

BEFORE USING THIS DRUG

Let your doctor know *IF*

You have ever had allergic reactions or other problems with ■ oxybutynin.

You have ever had any of the following medical problems: ■ stomach or intestinal problems, including colitis ■ enlarged prostate ■ digestive or urinary tract blockage ■ difficulty in urination ■ recent diarrhea ■ hiatal hernia ■ heart disease ■ abnormal heart rhythms ■ kidney disease ■ liver disease ■ myasthenia gravis ■ overactive thyroid ■ fast heartbeat ■ nerve disorders ■ glaucoma.

You are taking any of the following medicines: ■ any other urinary antibiotics ■ cimetidine (medicine for ulcers) ■ digoxin or digitalis (heart medicines) ■ medicine for Parkinson's disease ■ thiazide diuretics (water pills) ■ tranquilizers ■ medicine for nausea or vomiting ■ medicine for abnormal heart rhythms ■ medicine for depression ■ antihistamines ■ beta-blockers (eg, propranolol, atenolol, metoprolol).

SPECIAL RESTRICTIONS WHILE TAKING THIS DRUG

FOOD AND DRUG INTERACTIONS

Other Drugs	Do not take any other drugs, including over-the-counter (OTC) drugs, before checking with your doctor. This drug increases the effects of drugs that depress the central nervous system, such as antihistamines; medicine for hay fever, allergies, or colds; sleep medicines; tranquilizers; narcotics or other prescription pain-killers; muscle relaxants; and medicines for seizures.
Alcohol	The combination of this drug with alcohol may increase such side effects as drowsiness or dizziness. Avoid alcohol unless your doctor has approved its use.

No special restrictions on foods and beverages or smoking.

DAILY LIVING

Driving	This drug may cause blurred vision or loss of alertness. Be careful when driving, operating household appliances, or doing any other tasks that require alertness until you know how this drug affects you.
Exertion and Exercise	This drug may cause you to sweat less than normally. Sweating is your body's natural way of cooling down, and not sweating enough can be dangerous. Use caution not to become overheated when you exercise or exert yourself.
Excessive Heat	See above; use caution during hot weather, since overexertion may result in heat stroke. Avoid extremely hot baths and saunas.

Other Precautions	This drug may cause your eyes to become more sensitive to light. Wearing tinted glasses should help ease any discomfort.
Helpful Hints	If your mouth or throat feels dry, chewing sugarless gum or sucking ice chips or sugarless hard candy will help.

No special restrictions on sun exposure or exposure to excessive cold.

POSSIBLE SIDE EFFECTS

Although this list of adverse effects may seem somewhat intimidating, keep in mind that some are quite rare. Of course, should these or any other problems arise while you are on medication, it is always a good idea to consult your doctor.

IF YOU DEVELOP	WHAT TO DO
fever ■ very fast heartbeat ■ agitation ■ excitement ■ restlessness ■ irritation ■ behavior changes ■ flushing ■ loss of balance ■ confusion ■ drowsiness ■ hallucinations ■ difficulty in breathing ■ convulsions ■ eye pain	**Urgent** Get in touch with your doctor immediately.
rash or hives ■ difficulty in urination ■ dizziness ■ sleeplessness	**May be serious** Check with your doctor as soon as possible.
constipation ■ decreased sweating ■ drowsiness ■ dry mouth or throat ■ blurred vision ■ changes in pupil size ■ increased eye sensitivity to light ■ nausea or vomiting ■ impotence ■ bloating	If symptoms are disturbing or persist, let your doctor know.

STORAGE INSTRUCTIONS

Store in a cool, dark place (not in a bathroom medicine cabinet). If your medicine is in a liquid form, make sure that it does not freeze.

STOPPING OR INTERRUPTING THERAPY

If you miss a dose, take it as soon as possible. If it is almost time for your next dose, skip the missed dose and resume your regular schedule. Do not take two doses at the same time.

SPECIAL CONSIDERATIONS FOR THOSE OVER SIXTY-FIVE

Older people may be more prone to the side effects of this drug. Doctors may wish to check people over sixty-five frequently.

CONDITION: URINARY INCONTINENCE

CATEGORY: ANTISPASMODICS

GENERIC (CHEMICAL) NAME	BRAND (TRADE) NAME	DOSAGE FORMS AND STRENGTHS
Flavoxate hydrochloride	URISPAS	Tablets: 100 mg

DRUG PROFILE

Flavoxate is used to relieve symptoms associated with urinary tract infections such as painful urination, urinary urgency or frequency, urination during the night, bladder pain, and inability to retain urine. This drug acts directly on the muscles of the bladder to stop spasms and increase capacity (the amount of urine the bladder can hold). A urinary antibiotic is occasionally prescribed along with this drug.

BEFORE USING THIS DRUG

Let your doctor know *IF*

You have ever had allergic reactions or other problems with ■ flavoxate.

You have ever had any of the following medical problems: ■ stomach or intestinal problems ■ urinary tract blockage ■ glaucoma ■ enlarged prostate.

You are taking any of the following medicines: ■ digoxin or digitalis (heart medicines) ■ tranquilizers ■ medicine for nausea or vomiting ■ medicine for abnormal heart rhythms ■ medicine for depression ■ antihistamines.

SPECIAL RESTRICTIONS WHILE TAKING THIS DRUG

FOOD AND DRUG INTERACTIONS

Other Drugs	Do not take any other drugs, including over-the-counter (OTC) drugs, before checking with your doctor. This drug increases the effects of drugs that depress the central nervous system, such as antihistamines; medicines for hay fever, allergies, or colds; sleep medicines; tranquilizers; narcotics or other prescription pain-killers; muscle relaxants; and medicine for seizures, and may cause you to become drowsy or dizzy.
Alcohol	This drug increases the effect of alcohol, a central nervous system depressant. Avoid alcohol unless your doctor has approved its use.

No special restrictions on foods and beverages or smoking.

DAILY LIVING

Driving	This drug may cause blurred vision, drowsiness, or dizziness. Be careful when driving, operating household appliances, or doing any other tasks that require alertness until you know how this drug affects you.
Exertion and Exercise	This drug may cause you to sweat less than normally. Sweating is your body's natural way of cooling down, and not sweating enough can be dangerous. Use caution not to become overheated when you exercise or exert yourself.

Excessive Heat	See above; use caution during hot weather, since overexertion may result in heat stroke. Avoid extremely hot baths and saunas.
Examinations or Tests	It is important for you to keep all appointments with your doctor so that your progress can be checked.
Other Precautions	This drug may cause your eyes to become more sensitive to light. Wearing tinted glasses should help ease any discomfort.
Helpful Hints	If your mouth or throat feels dry, chewing sugarless gum or sucking ice chips or sugarless hard candy will help. If this medicine upsets your stomach, taking it with milk, meals, or snacks should help.

No special restrictions on sun exposure or exposure to excessive cold.

POSSIBLE SIDE EFFECTS

Although this list of adverse effects may seem somewhat intimidating, keep in mind that some are quite rare. Of course, should these or any other problems arise while you are on medication, it is always a good idea to consult your doctor.

IF YOU DEVELOP	WHAT TO DO
confusion ■ irregular or fast heartbeat	**Urgent** Get in touch with your doctor immediately.
eye pain ■ rash or hives ■ sore throat ■ fever ■ pain in urination ■ inability to concentrate	**May be serious** Check with your doctor as soon as possible.

drowsiness ■ dry mouth or throat ■ blurred vision or other visual disturbances ■ constipation ■ dizziness ■ headache ■ nausea or vomiting ■ nervousness ■ stomach pain ■ difficulty in urination ■ decreased sweating

If symptoms are disturbing or persist, let your doctor know.

STORAGE INSTRUCTIONS

Store in a cool, dark place (not in a bathroom medicine cabinet).

STOPPING OR INTERRUPTING THERAPY

If you miss a dose, take it as soon as possible. If it is almost time for your next dose, skip the missed dose and resume your regular schedule. Do not take two doses at the same time.

SPECIAL CONSIDERATIONS FOR THOSE OVER SIXTY-FIVE

Older people may be more prone to such side effects of this drug as confusion. Doctors may want to check people over sixty-five frequently.

KIDNEY STONES

Although some people save their kidney stones as souvenirs of surgery weathered well, most would prefer to forget the surgery and the stones, as well as the accompanying pain. Kidney stones are actually crystallized deposits of substances—usually calcium phosphate, calcium oxalate, or uric acid—that are normally found in solution in our urine.

In some fortunate people, the crystal deposits may be as small as a grain of sand or piece of gravel and cause little discomfort (other than the urge to urinate more frequently) as they make their way through the urinary tract. Larger stones, some of which may have staghornlike branches, are another story, however. These stones can cause excruciating pain as they pass into the ureter, the duct that transports urine from the kidney to the bladder. Sometimes, the pain is accompanied by inflammation, infection, and fever as well as the appearance of blood in the urine.

CAUSES

Most commonly, stones form because the concentration of calcium or uric acid (or some other offending substance) becomes too high for it to remain dissolved in the urine (just as a heaping spoonful of sugar may refuse to dissolve completely in a cup of tea). As a result, the calcium or uric acid crystallizes out of solution, and the crystals band together to form stones.

Sometimes, the problem can be traced to excess intake of calcium in dairy foods, calcium supplements, or calcium-containing antacids; a diet high in oxalate-containing foods, like rhubarb and spinach; or overuse of vitamin D supplements. Almost never, however, are they caused by ingestion of the normally recommended daily requirement for calcium (800–1,200 mg) and vitamin D (400–600 International Units). Other conditions that may lead to the buildup of calcium stones include prolonged immobilization; overactivity of the parathyroid glands, which sit beside the thyroid; and certain kidney problems. An infection or blockage of the urinary tract is sometimes at the root of stone formation. People who are troubled by gout, a disorder caused by too much uric acid, may develop uric acid stones. Heredity is also often to blame for kidney stones, as this problem tends to run in families.

DIAGNOSIS

To confirm the diagnosis of kidney stones, doctors usually take X rays of the kidney, ureter, and bladder. A urine sample is also important, to see whether and how the chemical composition, acidity, or bacterial flora of the urine may be contributing to the problem. If you've already passed a kidney stone, your doctor will probably want to analyze its makeup for clues to why you formed the stone.

TREATMENT

Surgery to remove kidney stones is no longer done routinely. It's usually reserved for people whose stones are extremely large, become infected, or are blocking the urinary tract. Surgery will help relieve the acute pain, but stones will continue to form unless the underlying cause is discovered and treated.

A new therapy for people with kidney stones is called extracorporeal shock wave lithotripsy. This is a nonsurgical procedure in which the stones are broken up by shock waves conveyed through a bath of water.

The one treatment prescribed for everyone with kidney stones—regardless of cause—is water. Drinking at least two quarts a day can help prevent new stones from forming and can even help dissolve some types of stones and wash them out of your system.

Other steps may include dietary changes that depend on the chemical makeup of your kidney stones. For example, doctors generally recommend that people who are prone to form calcium stones follow a diet that is low in calcium and vitamin D. Similarly, people with calcium oxalate stones may be told to watch their intake of oxalate-containing foods, such as tea, chocolate, rhubarb, and spinach. People with uric acid stones may be told to make their urine less acidic by taking sodium bicarbonate or drinking a citrate solution.

Specific medicines may also be prescribed—the diuretic hydrochlorothiazide for some people with calcium stones and allopurinol for those who recurrently form uric acid stones. For more information on these drugs, see the drug charts on page 959.

OUTLOOK

Many people stop taking their medicine and become lax in other parts of their treatment program as soon as their symptoms improve. But treatment must be continued for three to five years. It's considered successful if during that time no new stones are formed, old stones either disappear or stay the same size, pain and infection subside, and kidney function does not deteriorate because of urinary tract blockage. Kidney stones, left untreated, *can* lead to serious problems. But carefully supervised therapy continued for the appropriate length of time can prevent unnecessary surgery and disability.

CONDITION: **KIDNEY STONES**

CATEGORY: **URIC ACID REDUCERS**

GENERIC (CHEMICAL) NAME	BRAND (TRADE) NAME	DOSAGE FORMS AND STRENGTHS
Allopurinol	LOPURIN	Tablets: 100, 300 mg
	ZYLOPRIM	Tablets: 100, 300 mg

DRUG PROFILE

Allopurinol is used in conditions such as gout and kidney stones caused by an excess amount of uric acid in the body. This drug blocks xanthine oxidase, an enzyme necessary for the production of uric acid; it may be used in combination with other drugs.

For complete information on this drug, see pages 546–549.

CONDITION: **KIDNEY STONES**

CATEGORY: **THIAZIDE DIURETICS**

GENERIC (CHEMICAL) NAME	BRAND (TRADE) NAME	DOSAGE FORMS AND STRENGTHS
Hydrochlorothiazide	ESIDRIX	Tablets: 25, 50, 100 mg
	HydroDIURIL	Tablets: 25, 50, 100 mg
	ORETIC	Tablets: 25, 50 mg

DRUG PROFILE

Thiazide and thiazide-type diuretics are often used to help control high blood pressure. They are also used in the treatment of kidney stones because they decrease the amount of calcium eliminated through urination.

For complete information on this drug, see pages 23–28.

VAGINITIS

Atrophic vaginitis is one of the symptomatic conditions that follow menopause as the ovaries gradually produce less of the female hormone estrogen. The decrease in estrogen production leads to a slowdown in the normal process by which the lining of the vagina sheds old cells and renews itself. In time, the lining of the vagina becomes thin, loses its elasticity and can no longer produce enough natural lubrication. In that fragile state, the vagina may become particularly prone to irritation, injury, and infection.

Whether these changes cause troublesome symptoms varies from woman to woman. Some women may experience itching, burning, and pain, particularly after sexual intercourse. Others may notice a watery or blood-stained discharge or find that they have an unusually frequent and urgent need to urinate. Some actually develop urinary incontinence, the unexpected and unwanted loss of urine.

DIAGNOSIS

To confirm that your discomfort is caused by atrophic vaginitis, your doctor will perform an internal examination and take a Pap smear and cultures, with the goal of ruling out such other problems as an infection or an abnormal growth.

TREATMENT

Fortunately, the irksome symptoms of atrophic vaginitis, as well as other disturbing menopausal symptoms such as hot flashes, can be relieved by taking oral estrogen tablets or by wearing a skin patch that releases estrogen through the skin into the bloodstream. (See the chart on page 961.) Or, your doctor may prescribe estrogen cream to be applied to the vagina. Estrogen cream helps restore the normal thickness, strength, and lubrication of the lining of the vagina.

Estrogen creams are not for everyone. Although only limited amounts of estrogen cream are absorbed by the body, these products may still pose hazards for women who have had blood clots or breast cancer.

Because of the increased fragility of the vagina, it is especially important to treat vaginal fungal infections in women past menopause. (For information on the drugs used to treat these infections, see the charts on pages 966–974.) Let your doctor know if you develop itching, burning, or irritation or a white discharge from the vagina.

OUTLOOK

Daily application of an estrogen cream should clear up the discomfort within one to three weeks. Many experts advise that a woman use the cream daily for three weeks a month, followed by a one-week vacation from estrogen. Others recommend only one or two applications of estrogen cream a week to maintain the improvement. For more information on estrogen cream see the chart on pages 962–966.

CONDITION: **ATROPHIC VAGINITIS**
CATEGORY: **ESTROGENS**

GENERIC (CHEMICAL) NAME	BRAND (TRADE) NAME	DOSAGE FORMS AND STRENGTHS
Conjugated estrogens	PREMARIN	Tablets: 0.3, 0.625, 0.9, 1.25, and 2.5 mg
Chlorotrianisene	TACE	Capsules: 12, 25, 72 mg
Diethylstilbestrol		Tablets: 1, 5 mg
Estradiol	ESTRACE ESTRADERM	Tablets: 1, 2 mg Skin patch: 0.05, 0.1 mg per 24 hours
Estropipate	OGEN	Tablets: 0.625, 1.25, 2.5, 5 mg
Ethinyl estradiol	ESTINYL	Tablets: 0.02, 0.05, 0.5 mg
Quinestrol	ESTROVIS	Tablets: 100 mcg

DRUG PROFILE

Estrogens (female hormones) are used to help treat the bone loss that occurs in women after menopause or after surgical removal of the uterus and/or ovaries, when the body no longer produces natural estrogens. These drugs are also used in other medical conditions such as breast or prostate cancer as well as for atrophic vaginitis (dryness of the vagina) and other symptoms of menopause. Estrogens are usually administered in a cycle: three weeks on therapy and one week off therapy. You may be given a low dose of progesterone along with estrogens, which will help counteract some of estrogen's side effects.

For complete information on these drugs, see pages 560–565.

CONDITION: **ATROPHIC VAGINITIS**

CATEGORY: **TOPICAL ESTROGENS**

GENERIC (CHEMICAL) NAME	BRAND (TRADE) NAME	DOSAGE FORMS AND STRENGTHS
Conjugated estrogens	PREMARIN	Cream: 0.0625%
Dienestrol	ORTHO DIENESTROL CREAM	Cream: 0.01%
Estradiol	ESTRACE	Cream: 0.01%
Estropipate	OGEN VAGINAL CREAM	Cream: 0.15%

DRUG PROFILE

Topical estrogens are prescribed for atrophic vaginitis (vaginal dryness) or kraurosis vulvae (dry, sore, or itching vulvae), conditions that sometimes occur after menopause or after surgical removal of the uterus and/or ovaries, when the body no longer produces natural estrogen. These uncomfortable changes can be treated by direct application of estrogens in a cream. Although these medicines are applied topically, some drug is absorbed into the bloodstream and may cause side effects similar to those caused by estrogens taken orally.

BEFORE USING THIS DRUG

Let your doctor know *IF*

You have ever had allergic reactions or other problems with ■ estrogens.

With Ortho Dienestrol Cream and Ogen Vaginal Cream only: ■ tartrazine (FD&C Yellow Dye No. 5) ■ aspirin.

You have ever had any of the following medical problems: ■ asthma ■ circulation disorders or blood clots ■ breast lumps or breast cancer ■ any other kind of cancer ■ diabetes ■ seizures ■ gallbladder disease or gallstones ■ heart disease, including heart attacks ■ high blood pressure or a family history of high blood pressure ■ high blood-calcium levels ■ jaundice ■ kidney disease ■ liver disease ■ depression ■ migraine headaches ■ stroke ■ high cholesterol or a family history of high cholesterol.

You smoke.

You are taking any of the following medicines: ■ medicine for seizures ■ barbiturates ■ rifampin (antibiotic) ■ tricyclic antidepressants ■ vitamin C ■ anticoagulants (blood thinners).

SPECIAL RESTRICTIONS WHILE TAKING THIS DRUG

FOOD AND DRUG INTERACTIONS

Smoking	Smoking increases the chance of developing serious side effects such as thromboembolism, heart attack, and stroke with estrogen therapy. If you smoke, try to stop or at least cut down.

No special restrictions on other drugs, foods and beverages, or alcohol use.

DAILY LIVING

Sun Exposure

You may find that you sunburn more easily or that you develop brown, splotchy spots on your skin after exposure to the sun while taking estrogens. Try to minimize sun exposure, and apply a sunscreen to all exposed skin surfaces before going outdoors.

Examinations or Tests

It is important for you to keep all appointments with your doctor so that your progress can be checked. You will probably need periodic gynecologic examinations, including Pap smears and mammograms. Periodic blood pressure or blood and urine tests may be required while you are on estrogen therapy.

Other Precautions

Tell any doctor or dentist you consult that you are on estrogen therapy, especially if you will be undergoing any type of surgery or any kind of diagnostic testing.

If you wear contact lenses, you may find your eyes becoming sensitive to them during estrogen therapy. If this happens, discuss with your eye doctor whether it may be necessary for you to wear eyeglasses while you are on estrogen.

Estrogen therapy has been associated with a number of serious side effects. Long-term use of estrogens in women after menopause increases the possibility of developing endometrial cancer. Your doctor may be able to tailor your dosage schedule to minimize such a risk. If your uterus has been surgically removed (hysterectomy), there is no chance of your developing endometrial cancer. On the other hand, the risk of developing many other conditions, such as high cholesterol, heart attack, or ovarian cancer may be diminished. It is best to consult with your doctor when weighing these risks.

No special restrictions on driving, exertion and exercise, or exposure to excessive heat or cold.

POSSIBLE SIDE EFFECTS

Although this list of adverse effects may seem somewhat intimidating, keep in mind that some are quite rare. Of course, should these or any other problems arise while you are on medication, it is always a good idea to consult your doctor.

IF YOU DEVELOP	WHAT TO DO
Possible signs of a blood clot: sharp pain or heavy feeling in chest; sharp pains in groin or legs (especially the calves); weakness or numbness in arms or legs; severe and sudden headache, sometimes with vomiting; visual disturbances; difficulty in speech; sudden dizziness or faintness; unexplained cough	**Urgent: Stop taking this drug and get in touch with your doctor immediately.**
pain, swelling, or tenderness in stomach or side ■ vaginal bleeding ■ vaginal discharge ■ breast lumps ■ discharge from nipples ■ depression ■ uncontrollable jerky movements ■ yellowing of eyes or skin ■ bleeding ■ fever ■ joint pain ■ rash	**May be serious** Check with your doctor as soon as possible.
nausea or vomiting ■ increase or decrease in appetite ■ weight gain or loss ■ tenderness and swelling of breasts ■ stomach cramps ■ bloating ■ diarrhea ■ headaches, including migraine headaches ■ dizziness ■ change in sex drive ■ hair growth or loss ■ intolerance to contact lenses or other eye problems ■ increased skin sensitivity to sunlight, including development of brown, splotchy patches ■ reddened skin or other skin problems	If symptoms are disturbing or persist, let your doctor know.

STORAGE INSTRUCTIONS

Store in a cool, dry place (not in a bathroom medicine cabinet). If your medicine is in a cream form, make sure it does not freeze.

STOPPING OR INTERRUPTING THERAPY

If you miss a dose of this medicine, apply it as soon as possible. If you do not remember until the following day, skip the missed dose and resume your regular schedule. Do not apply two doses at the same time.

SPECIAL CONSIDERATIONS FOR THOSE OVER SIXTY-FIVE

None.

CONDITION: **VAGINAL INFECTIONS**

CATEGORY: **TOPICAL VAGINAL ANTIFUNGAL AGENTS**

GENERIC (CHEMICAL) NAME	BRAND (TRADE) NAME	DOSAGE FORMS AND STRENGTHS
Sulfanilamide	VAGITROL	Vaginal cream: 15%
	AVC	Vaginal cream: 15% sulfanilamide
		Vaginal suppositories: 1.05 g sulfanilamide

DRUG PROFILE

These sulfonamides (sulfa drugs) are applied directly in the vagina to treat fungal infections of the vagina (yeast infections).

BEFORE USING THIS DRUG

Let your doctor know *IF*

You have ever had allergic reactions or other problems with ■ sulfonamides (sulfa drugs) ■ furosemide or thiazide diuretics ■ oral medicine for diabetes ■ oral medicine for glaucoma ■ dapsone or sulfoxone (antibiotics).

With AVC only: ■ tartrazine (FD&C Yellow Dye No. 5) (contained in suppository).

SPECIAL RESTRICTIONS WHILE TAKING THIS DRUG

FOOD AND DRUG INTERACTIONS

No special restrictions on other drugs, foods and beverages, alcohol use, or smoking.

DAILY LIVING

Other Precautions	These drugs usually come with patient instructions, which you should read carefully before use. Unless your doctor instructs you otherwise, this medicine should be applied at bedtime.
	Ask your doctor about intercourse or douching while on treatment.
Helpful Hints	A sanitary pad may be used to protect your clothing from vaginal discharge. To keep fungal infections from recurring, wear panties and pantyhose with crotches made of cotton rather than of synthetics (such as nylon).
	If you have been storing the suppository form of this medicine in a warm place, it may be too soft to use. Put it in the refrigerator for half an hour or run cold water over the wrapped suppository before use.

No special restrictions on driving, exertion and exercise, sun exposure, or exposure to excessive heat or cold.

POSSIBLE SIDE EFFECTS

IF YOU DEVELOP	WHAT TO DO
increased discomfort ■ burning sensation ■ rash ■ sore throat ■ fever ■ increased urination	**Urgent** Get in touch with your doctor immediately.

STORAGE INSTRUCTIONS

Store in a cool place (not in a bathroom medicine cabinet). Keep from freezing.

STOPPING OR INTERRUPTING THERAPY

This medicine should be taken for the full length of time prescribed by your doctor, even if you begin to feel better. This will ensure that the infection clears up completely and that your symptoms don't return. If you miss a dose, simply resume your regular schedule the following day. Do not apply two doses at the same time.

SPECIAL CONSIDERATIONS FOR THOSE OVER SIXTY-FIVE

None.

CONDITION: **VAGINAL INFECTIONS**

CATEGORY: **TOPICAL VAGINAL ANTIFUNGAL AGENTS**

GENERIC (CHEMICAL) NAME	BRAND (TRADE) NAME	DOSAGE FORMS AND STRENGTHS
Butoconazole	FEMSTAT	Vaginal cream: 2%
Clotrimazole*	GYNE-LOTRIMIN	Vaginal cream: 1% Vaginal tablets: 100, 500 mg
	MYCELEX-G	Vaginal cream: 1% Vaginal tablets: 100, 500 mg

*Some strengths of clotrimazole and miconazole are available without a prescription (OTC).

Miconazole nitrate*	MONISTAT 3	Vaginal suppositories: 200 mg
	MONISTAT 7	Vaginal cream: 2%
		Vaginal suppositories: 100 mg
Nystatin	MYCOSTATIN	Vaginal tablets: 100,000 units
Terconazole	TERAZOL 7	Vaginal cream: 0.4%
	TERAZOL 3	Vaginal suppositories: 80 mg
Tioconazole	VAGISTAT	Vaginal ointment: 6.5%

*Some strengths of clotrimazole and miconazole are available without a prescription (OTC).

DRUG PROFILE

These antifungal drugs are applied directly in the vagina to treat fungal infections of the vagina (yeast infections).

BEFORE USING THIS DRUG

Let your doctor know *IF*

You have ever had allergic reactions or other problems with ■ clotrimazole ■ miconazole ■ nystatin ■ terconazole ■ butoconazole.

SPECIAL RESTRICTIONS WHILE TAKING THIS DRUG

FOOD AND DRUG INTERACTIONS

No special restrictions on other drugs, foods and beverages, alcohol use, or smoking.

DAILY LIVING

Other Precautions

These drugs usually come with patient instructions, which you should read carefully before use. Unless your doctor instructs you otherwise, this medicine should be applied at bedtime.

Ask your doctor about intercourse or douching while on treatment.

Helpful Hints

A sanitary pad may be used to protect your clothing from vaginal discharge.

To keep fungal infections from recurring, wear panties and pantyhose with crotches made of cotton rather than of synthetics (such as nylon).

If you have been storing the suppository form of this medicine in a warm place, it may be too soft to use. Put it in the refrigerator for half an hour or run cold water over the wrapped suppository before use.

No special restrictions on driving, exertion and exercise, sun exposure, or exposure to excessive heat or cold.

POSSIBLE SIDE EFFECTS

Although this list of adverse effects may seem somewhat intimidating, keep in mind that some are quite rare. Of course, should these or any other problems arise while you are on medication, it is always a good idea to consult your doctor.

IF YOU DEVELOP

vaginal burning, itching, redness, or irritation that was not present before use of the medicine ■ rash or hives

WHAT TO DO

Urgent Get in touch with your doctor immediately.

headache ■ pelvic cramps

With clotrimazole only: increased urination ■ bladder irritation ■ bloating

With terconazole only: fever ■ chills ■ general pain

May be serious Check with your doctor as soon as possible.

STORAGE INSTRUCTIONS

Store in a cool, dry place (not in a bathroom medicine cabinet). Keep from freezing.

STOPPING OR INTERRUPTING THERAPY

This medicine should be used for the full length of time prescribed by your doctor, even if you begin to feel better. This will ensure that the infection clears up completely and that your symptoms don't return. If you miss a dose, simply resume your regular schedule the following day. Do not apply two doses at the same time.

SPECIAL CONSIDERATIONS FOR THOSE OVER SIXTY-FIVE

None.

CONDITION: **VAGINAL INFECTIONS**

CATEGORY: **ANTI-TRICHOMONAL DRUGS**

GENERIC (CHEMICAL) NAME	BRAND (TRADE) NAME	DOSAGE FORMS AND STRENGTHS
Metronidazole	FLAGYL	Tablets: 250, 500 mg

DRUG PROFILE

Metronidazole is an antibiotic that is used to treat bacterial and trichomonal vaginitis as well as a wide variety of systemic infections including dysentery and infections of the respiratory tract, skin, bones and joints, and stomach.

BEFORE USING THIS DRUG

Let your doctor know *IF*

You have ever had allergic reactions or other problems with ■ metronidazole.

You have ever had any of the following medical problems: ■ blood disease ■ seizures ■ severe liver disease ■ alcoholism.

You are taking any of the following medicines: ■ anticoagulants (blood thinners) ■ Antabuse (used in the treatment of alcoholism) ■ barbiturates ■ phenytoin (medicine for seizures) ■ cimetidine (medicine for ulcers) ■ lithium.

SPECIAL RESTRICTIONS WHILE TAKING THIS DRUG

FOOD AND DRUG INTERACTIONS

Alcohol	Do not drink alcohol while taking this drug and for at least one day before and following the end of therapy. The combination may result in nausea or vomiting, stomach pains, and flushing.

No special restrictions on other drugs, foods and beverages, or smoking.

DAILY LIVING

Examinations or Tests	It is important for you to keep all appointments with your doctor so that your condition can be reevaluated after therapy. Blood tests may be required before and after therapy with this drug.
Other Precautions	If you are being treated for trichomonal infection, your sexual partner should see a doctor, as he may be infected and need treatment as well. Also, it may be necessary to use a condom for a while to prevent both of you from reinfecting each other.
	If your symptoms do not improve within a few days or if they worsen, check with your doctor.

Let your doctor know if you develop itching, burning, soreness, or general irritation in the genital area; a white vaginal discharge; or a white coating on the inside of your mouth.

Helpful Hints	If this medicine causes upset stomach, taking it with milk, meals, or snacks should help.

No special restrictions on driving, exertion and exercise, sun exposure, or exposure to excessive heat or cold.

POSSIBLE SIDE EFFECTS

Although this list of adverse effects may seem somewhat intimidating, keep in mind that some are quite rare. Of course, should these or any other problems arise while you are on medication, it is always a good idea to consult your doctor.

IF YOU DEVELOP

WHAT TO DO

numbness, tingling, pain, or weakness in hands or feet ■ seizures

Urgent Get in touch with your doctor immediately.

clumsiness or unsteadiness ■ rash or hives ■ sore throat ■ fever ■ confusion ■ irritability ■ weakness ■ depression ■ sleeplessness ■ flushing ■ dryness of the vagina or vulva ■ painful intercourse ■ decreased sex drive ■ pain in urination ■ urinary frequency ■ bladder irritation ■ feeling of pressure in the pelvic area

May be serious Check with your doctor as soon as possible.

unpleasant taste in mouth ■ nausea or vomiting ■ diarrhea ■ loss of appetite ■ stomach cramps ■ constipation ■ dry mouth ■ mouth sores ■ furry or inflamed tongue ■ dizziness ■ headache ■ stuffy nose ■ dark urine

If symptoms are disturbing or persist, let your doctor know.

STORAGE INSTRUCTIONS

Store in a cool, dark place (not in a bathroom medicine cabinet).

STOPPING OR INTERRUPTING THERAPY

This medicine should be taken for the full length of time prescribed by your doctor, even if you begin to feel better. This will ensure that the infection clears up completely and that your symptoms don't return. If you miss a dose, take it as soon as possible. If it is almost time for your next dose, skip the missed dose and resume your regular schedule.

SPECIAL CONSIDERATIONS FOR THOSE OVER SIXTY-FIVE

In older people, metabolism of metronidazole may be altered. Doctors may want to monitor and check the blood level of metronidazole to make sure patients are receiving the correct dosage.

Chapter 12
Disorders of the Eye

GLAUCOMA

You may have noticed that you don't see quite as clearly as you used to. The world sometimes has a fuzzy look to it, and your eyes sometimes give you an aching feeling. These may be symptoms of glaucoma, an eye disorder that occurs when too much fluid is trapped inside the eye, causing a buildup of pressure. If glaucoma is not controlled by surgical techniques or drugs described in this section, it can lead to blindness. Glaucoma is, in fact, a major cause of blindness in the United States.

Present in more than two million people in the United States, glaucoma is most common in men and women over sixty-five, affecting three out of every one hundred people in this age group. Glaucoma tends to run in families, so don't be surprised if a relative of yours had it before you did. This eye condition is also particularly prevalent in people with diabetes.

CAUSES

Your eyes are constantly manufacturing a fluid called aqueous humor, which flows around the lens and through the pupil. In a normal eye, it then drains away through tiny canals in the front of the eye. But in an eye that is affected by glaucoma, that drainage system is blocked. More aqueous humor is continuously produced, but the fluid can't leave the eye. This creates pressure within the eye—pressure that can damage the retina and the optic nerve.

DIAGNOSIS

There are two basic types of glaucoma, each with its own set of symptoms. One type is known as acute angle-closure (or narrow-angle) glaucoma. In this variation, the drainage path is tightly closed, and the pressure from the trapped aqueous humor becomes very high. The results are intense pain, redness of the affected eye, and blurring (halos around lights) or loss of vision. If the pressure from an acute attack is not treated, it can lead to blindness in one to five days.

In the other type, called open-angle (or chronic) glaucoma, the person has virtually no symptoms except for a slow, progressive peripheral vision loss when tested for it. This condition is often referred to as the "sneak thief of sight," since vision is irreversibly lost without the person being aware of even having the disease until it is too late. Over time, permanent damage to the retina and optic nerve occurs. Treatment can keep the condition from becoming worse but cannot restore any loss of vision that has already occurred. Because of this, patients should have their intraocular pressures measured yearly by an ophthalmologist if they have a family history of glaucoma, have diabetes, or are known to have even mildly elevated eye pressure. Otherwise, the eye pressure should be measured every two years. During most routine eye exams by an ophthalmologist, a pressure check is done with an instrument placed on the cornea for a few seconds. This procedure lets the doctor know if the pressure in your eye is too high. The doctor can also look at the drainage pathways in the front of your eye and at the optic nerve and retina to check for any glaucomalike changes.

TREATMENT

Should you experience the symptoms of acute glaucoma described above, go immediately to a doctor or a hospital emergency room, where you will be given eyedrops or other medicine to bring the pressure down. In addition, an eye surgeon might make a tiny opening in your iris to allow the fluid to drain out. This procedure can save your vision. The operation can now be done with the intense light of a laser beam rather than with sharp surgical instruments. The surgeon may recommend a similar operation on the other eye to prevent a second acute attack. (After one attack, the other eye is at an increased risk for a similar attack.)

If you are diagnosed as having glaucoma, and your doctor feels that drug treatment is appropriate, you may be prescribed pills or eyedrops to use at home. Some of the more commonly prescribed medicines used to control glaucoma are listed on pages 978–993.

OUTLOOK

Glaucoma can lead to blindness—whether or not you are aware of its symptoms. However, recognition of its presence can allow treatment to prevent irreversible vision loss. If you see your doctor for regular eye checkups and get medical attention as soon as you experience any symptoms of glaucoma, it's likely that the disease process can be halted before significant or total loss of vision occurs.

CONDITION: **GLAUCOMA**

CATEGORY: **TOPICAL BETA-BLOCKERS**

GENERIC (CHEMICAL) NAME	BRAND (TRADE) NAME	DOSAGE FORMS AND STRENGTHS
Betaxolol hydrochloride	BETOPTIC	Solution: 0.5%
Levobunolol hydrochloride	BETAGAN	Solution: 0.25%, 0.5%
Metipranolol hydrochloride	OPTIPRANOLOL	Solution: 0.3%
Timolol maleate	TIMOPTIC	Solution: 0.25%, 0.5%

DRUG PROFILE

The topical beta-blockers are prescribed, either alone or in combination with other medicine, to treat glaucoma. They are believed to work by lessening the production of aqueous fluid and thereby reducing increased pressure in the eye.

BEFORE USING THIS DRUG

Let your doctor know *IF*

You have ever had allergic reactions or other problems with ■ any beta-blocker.

You have ever had any of the following medical problems: ■ asthma or other lung disease ■ slow heartbeat ■ diabetes ■ any heart or blood vessel disease ■ overactive thyroid ■ myasthenia gravis.

You are taking any of the following medicines: ■ other medicine for glaucoma ■ other beta-blockers ■ medicine for high blood pressure ■ calcium blockers (eg, diltiazem, nifedipine, verapamil) ■ medicine for asthma or other lung disease ■ medicine for hay fever, allergies, or colds ■ tranquilizers ■ digoxin or digitalis (heart medicines) ■ medicine for diabetes.

SPECIAL RESTRICTIONS WHILE TAKING THIS DRUG

FOOD AND DRUG INTERACTIONS

Other Drugs	It is especially important to let your doctor know if you are taking the blood pressure–lowering drug reserpine or medicines called calcium blockers, since the use of these drugs with a beta-blocker may cause low blood pressure, slow heartbeat, or dizziness.

No special restrictions on foods and beverages, alcohol use, or smoking.

DAILY LIVING

Driving	Do not drive until you know how this drug will affect you, since it may cause blurring of vision. If your vision remains clear, you may drive, but with caution. Also be careful when operating household appliances or doing any other tasks that require clear vision until you know how this drug affects you.
Exertion and Exercise	Be careful when you exert yourself or exercise since you may become more tired than usual.
Examinations or Tests	It is important for you to keep all appointments with your doctor so that your eye pressure can be checked and your eyes can be examined for any adverse effects from this drug.
Other Precautions	Tell any doctor or dentist you consult that you are taking this medicine, especially if you will be undergoing any type of surgery. If you have diabetes, be aware that this medicine may mask the signs of low blood sugar, such as changes in pulse rate or increased blood pressure.

Your eyes may become especially sensitive to light. Wearing tinted glasses should help ease any discomfort.

Helpful Hints	Wash your hands thoroughly before and after each use. After dropping the solution into your eye, apply pressure to the inner corner of your eye with the middle finger for one to two minutes to prevent the medicine from draining into your nose and throat. To prevent contamination, avoid touching the dropper tip to the eye, eyelid, or any other surface, and keep the container tightly closed when not in use.

No special restrictions on sun exposure or exposure to excessive heat or cold.

POSSIBLE SIDE EFFECTS

Although this list of adverse effects may seem somewhat intimidating, keep in mind that some are quite rare. Of course, should these or any other problems arise while you are on medication, it is always a good idea to consult your doctor.

IF YOU DEVELOP	WHAT TO DO
irregular or slow heartbeat ■ dizziness, weakness, light-headedness, or fainting ■ difficulty in breathing ■ confusion ■ headache ■ nausea ■ rash or hives	**Urgent** Get in touch with your doctor immediately.
eye irritation ■ blurred or double vision ■ drooping of the upper eyelids ■ depression ■ lack of coordination ■ lethargy ■ numbness or tingling of fingers, hands, or feet	**May be serious** Check with your doctor as soon as possible.
temporary burning or stinging in eye ■ tearing ■ increased eye sensitivity to light ■ insomnia ■ upset stomach	If symptoms are disturbing or persist, let your doctor know.

STORAGE INSTRUCTIONS

Store in a cool, dry place, away from direct sun light.

STOPPING OR INTERRUPTING THERAPY

If you miss a dose and you are taking this medicine more than once a day, apply it as soon as possible and resume your regular schedule. If you miss a dose and you are taking this medicine once a day, apply the missed dose as soon as possible. If you do not remember until the following day, skip the missed dose and resume your regular schedule.

SPECIAL CONSIDERATIONS FOR THOSE OVER SIXTY-FIVE

Older people may be more susceptible to the side effects of this drug. Doctors may want to start people over sixty-five on a lower dosage.

CONDITION: **GLAUCOMA**

CATEGORY: **CARBONIC ANHYDRASE INHIBITORS**

GENERIC (CHEMICAL) NAME	BRAND (TRADE) NAME	DOSAGE FORMS AND STRENGTHS
Acetazolamide	DIAMOX	Controlled-release capsules: 500 mg Tablets: 125, 250 mg
Dichlorphenamide	DARANIDE	Tablets: 50 mg
Methazolamide	NEPTAZANE	Tablets: 25, 50 mg

DRUG PROFILE

These drugs are used as supplemental therapy for glaucoma, along with topical medicines that are applied directly to the eye. They decrease the formation of aqueous humor (the fluid inside the front of the eyeball), thereby reducing the increased pressure inside the eye that is the hallmark of glaucoma. This type of drug has a slight diuretic effect as well; that is, it helps your body rid itself of excess water through increased urination.

BEFORE USING THIS DRUG

Let your doctor know *IF*

You have ever had allergic reactions or other problems with ■ acetazolamide ■ dichlorphenamide ■ methazolamide ■ sulfonamides (sulfa drugs).

You have ever had any of the following medical problems: ■ emphysema or other lung disease ■ potassium or sodium deficiency ■ Addison's disease ■ kidney disease, including kidney stones ■ liver disease ■ diabetes ■ leukemia ■ anemia.

You are taking any of the following medicines: ■ corticosteroids or corticotropin (ACTH) ■ medicine for diabetes ■ digoxin or digitalis (heart medicines) ■ aspirin or aspirinlike medicine ■ methenamine (medicine to prevent urinary tract infections) ■ phenobarbital ■ lithium ■ diuretics (water pills) ■ amphetamines ■ procainamide or quinidine (medicine for abnormal heart rhythms) ■ tricyclic antidepressants ■ primidone or phenytoin (medicine for seizures) ■ medicine for stomach spasms or cramps.

SPECIAL RESTRICTIONS WHILE TAKING THIS DRUG

FOOD AND DRUG INTERACTIONS

Foods and Beverages	This medicine may decrease potassium levels in your blood. Your doctor may give you special instructions about eating foods or drinking beverages that have a high potassium content (such as bananas and citrus fruit juices), taking a potassium supplement, or using salt substitutes.

No special restrictions on other drugs, alcohol use, or smoking.

DAILY LIVING

Driving	This drug may cause drowsiness. Use caution when driving, operating household appliances, or doing any other tasks that require alertness until you know how this drug affects you.
Examinations or Tests	It is important for you to keep all appointments with your doctor so that your progress can be checked.
Other Precautions	If you have diabetes, be aware that this medicine may raise blood-sugar levels. If you notice any change when testing sugar levels in your blood or urine, let your doctor know.

Helpful Hints

When first starting on this medicine, you may feel tired or depressed and will probably experience both greater volume and frequency of urination. Until your individual pattern of urination has been established with this medicine, it may be wise to time carefully any activity that will put you out of convenient reach of a bathroom, such as bus or car travel. In addition, taking this medicine at bedtime may interfere with sleep; you should discuss your dosage schedule with your doctor.

Check with your doctor if you become ill with flulike symptoms, such as cough, fever, or body aches; lose your appetite; vomit; or have diarrhea. This may cause you to lose a great deal of fluid, making it important not to take the diuretic for one or more doses.

If this medicine upsets your stomach, taking it with meals, milk, or snacks should help.

No special restrictions on exertion and exercise, sun exposure, or exposure to excessive heat or cold.

POSSIBLE SIDE EFFECTS

Although this list of adverse effects may seem somewhat intimidating, keep in mind that some are quite rare. Of course, should these or any other problems arise while you are on medication, it is always a good idea to consult your doctor.

IF YOU DEVELOP

irregular heartbeat ■ tiredness or weakness ■ confusion ■ seizures ■ shortness of breath ■ difficulty in breathing ■ bluish skin ■ bloody or black, tarry stools ■ vomiting, with blood ■ pain in urination ■ blood in urine ■ lower back pain ■ red rash ■ slow blood clotting

WHAT TO DO

Urgent: Stop using this drug and get in touch with your doctor immediately.

weak pulse ■ depression ■ nausea or vomiting ■ dry mouth ■ increased thirst ■ drowsiness ■ headache ■ irritability ■ nervousness ■ excitement ■ dizziness ■ clumsiness ■ tremors ■ increased or decreased urination ■ dark urine ■ rash, hives, or itching ■ sore throat or fever ■ bleeding or bruising ■ yellowing of eyes or skin ■ pale stools ■ muscle paralysis ■ hearing disturbances, ringing in the ears ■ taste alterations

May be serious Stop using this drug and check with your doctor as soon as possible.

loss of appetite ■ diarrhea ■ weight loss ■ changes in taste or smell ■ constipation ■ bloating ■ general ill feeling ■ increased skin sensitivity to sunlight ■ numbness or tingling in hands, feet, lips, tongue, or anus ■ development or worsening of nearsighted-ness ■ upset stomach

If symptoms are disturbing or persist, let your doctor know.

STORAGE INSTRUCTIONS

Store in a cool, dry place, away from direct sunlight.

STOPPING OR INTERRUPTING THERAPY

If you miss a dose, take it as soon as possible. If it is almost time for your next dose, skip the missed dose and resume your regular schedule. Do not take two doses at the same time.

SPECIAL CONSIDERATIONS FOR THOSE OVER SIXTY-FIVE

None.

CONDITION: **GLAUCOMA**

CATEGORY: **MIOTICS**

GENERIC (CHEMICAL) NAME	BRAND (TRADE) NAME	DOSAGE FORMS AND STRENGTHS
Carbachol	ISOPTO CARBACHOL	Solution: 0.75%, 1.5%, 2.25%, 3%
Demecarium bromide	HUMORSOL	Solution: 0.125%, 0.25%
Echothiophate iodide	PHOSPHOLINE IODIDE	Solution: 0.03%, 0.06%, 0.125%, 0.25%
Isoflurophate	FLOROPRYL	Ointment: 0.025%
Pilocarpine hydrochloride	ADSORBOCARPINE	Solution: 1%, 2%, 4%
	AKARPINE	Solution: 1%, 2%, 3%, 4%
	ALMOCARPINE	Solution: 1%, 2%, 4%
	ISOPTO CARPINE	Solution: 0.25%, 0.5%, 1%, 2%, 3%, 4%, 5%, 6%, 8%, 10%
	OCUSERT	Eye insert medication-release system: 20, 40 μg per hour
	PILOCAR	Solution: 0.5%, 1%, 2%, 3%, 4%, 6%
	PILOPINE HS	Gel: 4%
Pilocarpine nitrate	P.V. CARPINE	Solution: 1%, 2%, 4%

DRUG PROFILE

Miotics are a family of drugs that constrict the pupil and are thought to place tension on the drainage canals at the front of the eye, allowing the fluid to flow out more easily and thereby reducing pressure in the eye.

BEFORE USING THIS DRUG

Let your doctor know *IF*

You have ever had allergic reactions or other problems with ■ carbachol ■ echothiophate iodide ■ pilocarpine ■ preservatives.

You have ever had any of the following medical problems: ■ any injury to or inflammation of the eye ■ asthma ■ heart disease, including recent heart attack ■ ulcers or other problems of the digestive tract ■ urinary tract blockage ■ slow heartbeat ■ low or high blood pressure ■ Parkinson's disease ■ nervous disorders ■ overactive thyroid ■ seizures.

You are using any other eye medications or being treated for myasthenia gravis.

For Phospholine Iodide only: You are often exposed to organophosphate-type pesticides (ie, if you are a professional gardener or farmer or if you work at a plant that manufactures such pesticides).

SPECIAL RESTRICTIONS WHILE TAKING THIS DRUG

FOOD AND DRUG INTERACTIONS

Other Drugs	If you are being treated for myasthenia gravis with drugs, your doctor may need to adjust your dosage of these agents while you are on antiglaucoma therapy.

No special restrictions on foods and beverages, alcohol use, or smoking.

DAILY LIVING

Driving	Do not drive until you know how this drug will affect you, since it may cause blurring of vision. If your vision remains clear, you may drive, but with caution. Also be careful when operating household appliances or doing any other tasks that require clear vision until you know how this drug affects you.
Other Precautions	Tell any doctor or dentist you consult that you are using this medicine, especially if you will be undergoing any type of surgery. Adverse effects usually disappear within a few days of beginning regular use. If your eye feels painful, try taking aspirin. If side effects fail to subside or if your eye remains irritated, let your doctor know.
Helpful Hints	*If you are using eyedrops:* If you wear soft contact lenses, it is a good idea to remove them before using drops. After dropping the solution into your eye, apply pressure to the inner corner of your eye with your middle finger for one to two minutes to keep the medicine from draining into your nose and throat. Remove any excess solution from around the eyes with a tissue. Wash your hands thoroughly before and after use of this medicine. To prevent contamination, avoid touching the dropper tip to the eye, eyelid, or any other surface and keep the bottle tightly closed when not in use.
	If you are using the eye insert system: Be sure to wash your hands thoroughly before and after inserting the system. You may experience temporary blurred and dim vision after insertion; these effects can be reduced by inserting the system at bedtime. Any discomfort should improve after one to six weeks of therapy.

No special restrictions on exertion and exercise, sun exposure, or exposure to excessive heat or cold.

POSSIBLE SIDE EFFECTS

Although this list of adverse effects may seem somewhat intimidating, keep in mind that some are quite rare. Of course, should these or any other problems arise while you are on medication, it is always a good idea to consult your doctor.

IF YOU DEVELOP

nausea or vomiting ■ diarrhea ■ tremors or weakness ■ stomach pain or cramps ■ increased salivation ■ excessive sweating ■ dizziness ■ tingling sensations ■ slow heartbeat ■ wheezing ■ difficulty in breathing ■ tightness in chest ■ fainting ■ excitement ■ depression ■ clumsiness ■ seizures ■ urinary frequency or incontinence ■ flushing ■ paleness ■ bluish skin ■ flashing lights or floating spots in your field of vision ■ curtain of darkness over part of your vision

WHAT TO DO

Urgent: Stop using this drug and get in touch with your doctor immediately.

pain, stinging, or burning in eye ■ blurred or dim vision or other visual disturbances ■ redness or irritation of eyes or edge of eyelids ■ watery eyes ■ twitching of eyelids ■ headache ■ browache ■ increased eye sensitivity to light ■ poor vision in dim light

If symptoms are disturbing or persist, let your doctor know.

STORAGE INSTRUCTIONS

Store in a cool, dry place, away from direct sunlight, and make sure that it does not freeze.

STOPPING OR INTERRUPTING THERAPY

Take this medicine exactly as prescribed by your doctor. If you miss a dose and you are taking this medicine more than once a day, apply it as soon as possible and resume your regular schedule. If you miss a dose and you take this medicine once a day, apply the missed dose as soon as possible. If you do not remember until the following day, skip the missed dose and resume your regular schedule. If you take this medicine every other day and miss a day, apply the missed dose on the day you remember and skip the following day. If you are using the eye insert system, follow the instructions in the package circular.

SPECIAL CONSIDERATIONS FOR THOSE OVER SIXTY-FIVE

Some older people, especially those with cataracts, will be unable to tolerate miotics; if this is the case, doctors will prescribe another antiglaucoma medicine.

CONDITION: **GLAUCOMA**

CATEGORY: **EPINEPHRINE PREPARATIONS**

GENERIC (CHEMICAL) NAME	BRAND (TRADE) NAME	DOSAGE FORMS AND STRENGTHS
Dipivefrin hydrochloride	PROPINE	Solution: 0.01%
Epinephrine hydrochloride	EPIFRIN GLAUCON	Solution: 0.25%, 0.5%, 1%, 2% Solution: 1%, 2%
Epinephrine bitartrate	EPITRATE	Solution: 2%
Epinephrine borate	EPINAL EPPY/N	Solution: 0.5%, 1% Solution: 0.5%, 1%, 2%

DRUG PROFILE

These epinephrine preparations are mydriatics—drugs that dilate the pupil—and are used to treat glaucoma. Epinephrine and dipivefrin, which is converted into epinephrine in the eye, are thought to reduce increased pressure in the eye by lessening the production of aqueous fluid and increasing aqueous fluid outflow. Your doctor may prescribe this type of drug to be used either alone or in combination with another medicine.

BEFORE USING THIS DRUG

Let your doctor know *IF*

You have ever had allergic reactions or other problems with ■ epinephrine ■ preservatives.

You have ever had any of the following medical problems: ■ past attack of narrow-angle glaucoma ■ other eye disease ■ cataract surgery ■ heart disease, including abnormal heart rhythm ■ blood vessel disease ■ high blood pressure ■ overactive thyroid.

You are taking any of the following medicines: ■ digoxin or digitalis (heart medicines) ■ medicine for depression.

SPECIAL RESTRICTIONS WHILE TAKING THIS DRUG

FOOD AND DRUG INTERACTIONS

Other Drugs	There is a greater risk of developing irregular heartbeat when this drug is used with heart medicine (digoxin or digitalis) or tricyclic antidepressants.
Foods and Beverages	The caffeine in cocoa, chocolate, coffee, tea, and cola drinks may add to the effects of this drug and result in palpitations.

No special restrictions on alcohol use or smoking.

DAILY LIVING

Driving

Do not drive until you know how this drug will affect you, since it may cause blurring of vision. If your vision remains clear, you may drive, but with caution. Also, be careful when operating appliances or doing any other tasks that require alertness until you know how this drug affects you.

Examinations or Tests

It is important for you to keep all appointments with your doctor so that your eye pressure can be checked and your eyes can be examined for any adverse effects from this drug.

Other Precautions

Tell any doctor or dentist you consult that you are on this kind of therapy, especially if you will be undergoing any type of surgery.

If your eye symptoms do not improve or if they worsen, stop using this drug and check with your doctor.

You should not wear soft contact lenses while instilling this drug.

Your eyes may become especially sensitive to light; wearing tinted glasses should help ease any discomfort.

Helpful Hints

Wash your hands thoroughly before and after each use. After dropping the solution into your eye, apply pressure to the inner corner of your eye with the middle finger for one to two minutes to prevent the medicine from draining into your nose and throat. To prevent contamination, avoid touching the dropper tip to the eye, eyelid, or any other surface and keep the container tightly closed when not in use. Although epinephrine usually causes discomfort when it is first instilled, your eye should begin to feel better in a few minutes. Also, if you experience headache or brow-ache, these symptoms may improve with continued treatment.

No special restrictions on exertion and exercise or exposure to excessive heat or cold.

POSSIBLE SIDE EFFECTS

Although this list of adverse effects may seem somewhat intimidating, keep in mind that some are quite rare. Of course, should these or any other problems arise while you are on medication, it is always a good idea to consult your doctor.

IF YOU DEVELOP	WHAT TO DO
irregular, pounding, or fast heartbeat ■ severe pain in the back of the head ■ faintness ■ excessive sweating ■ tremors ■ paleness ■ difficulty in breathing ■ bluish skin ■ chest pain ■ black spots floating across your field of vision	**Urgent: Stop using this drug and get in touch with your doctor immediately.**
aching or pain in brow or head ■ aching, pain, stinging, burning, irritation, or watering of the eyes ■ eyelid irritations ■ temporary blurred vision ■ increased eye sensitivity to light ■ difficulty seeing at night	If symptoms are disturbing or persist, let your doctor know.

STORAGE INSTRUCTIONS

Store in a cool, dry place, away from direct sunlight.

STOPPING OR INTERRUPTING THERAPY

If you miss a dose of this medicine, apply it as soon as possible. If it is almost time for your next dose, skip the missed dose and resume your regular schedule.

SPECIAL CONSIDERATIONS FOR THOSE OVER SIXTY-FIVE

None.

CONJUNCTIVITIS

Conjunctivitis, popularly called red-eye or pink-eye, is an inflammation of the membrane that covers the eyeball and lines the eyelid. Most of the white of the eye appears red, a color change caused by the dilation of blood vessels in the eye. This condition differs from bloodshot eyes, in which tiny red veins are visible in the whites of the eyes. (The problem, in that case, is usually only lack of sleep or localized eye irritation, from smoke, for example.)

The redness of conjunctivitis may be present in either one eye or in both. Often, the eyes feel itchy and there may be mild discomfort, but usually no pain. Another sign of conjunctivitis is a discharge from the eyes. You may first notice this as a crust on your eyelashes when you wake up in the morning.

CAUSES

Conjunctivitis may be caused by bacterial infections, fungal infections, allergies such as hay fever, or viruses. It can also be brought on by such ailments as arthritis or certain strains of herpes.

DIAGNOSIS

Your doctor may take a smear from your eye to test for bacteria and examine the cells. Your pattern of symptoms will also provide a clue to the diagnosis. Bacterial conjunctivitis often begins with a discharge of pus from the eye; viral conjunctivitis is likely to be accompanied by a watery discharge and by a painful sensitivity to light, called photophobia; allergic conjunctivitis commonly causes severe itching and accompanying swollen lids.

TREATMENT

To treat conjunctivitis, most doctors prescribe eyedrops or an ointment (see the drug charts pages 996–1034). If the source of the problem is a bacterial infection, the drugs will often bring relief in one to three days. But even when the symptoms have disappeared, you should continue to use the antibiotic for as long as the doctor has directed to prevent a relapse. Viral conjunctivitis doesn't respond to antibiotics and takes longer to heal, perhaps one to two weeks (which is the life cycle of the virus). Although antibiotics will not help viral conjunctivitis, the doctor may prescribe them to prevent a secondary infection by bacteria.

Conjunctivitis can be extremely contagious, so when red-eye first appears, you should take some simple precautions to prevent spreading it to a family member. Avoid touching the affected eye; wash your hands frequently; and do not share towels, washcloths, or pillowcases. Launder these linens after each use, if possible. Contact lenses and eye makeup can make conjunctivitis worse—stop using them until the doctor says the infection has cleared. Be sure to sterilize contact lenses carefully before using them again.

OUTLOOK

Symptoms affecting your eyes should be checked by a doctor, but if you're told that conjunctivitis is the cause, you have little to worry about. If you follow the medical advice your doctor gives you, and the practical advice outlined above, both you and your family should be none the worse for your bout with red-eye.

CONDITION: **INFLAMMATION**

CATEGORY: **OPHTHALMIC CORTICOSTEROIDS**

GENERIC (CHEMICAL) NAME	BRAND (TRADE) NAME	DOSAGE FORMS AND STRENGTHS
Dexamethasone	AK-DEX	Ointment: 0.05% Solution: 0.1%
	DECADRON Phosphate	Ointment: 0.05% Solution: 0.1%
	MAXIDEX	Ointment: 0.05% Suspension: 0.1%
Fluorometholone	FML	Ointment: 0.1% Suspension: 0.1%
	FML Forte	Suspension: 0.25%
Medrysone	HMS	Suspension: 1%
Prednisolone	AK-TATE	Suspension: 1%
	ECONOPRED	Suspension: 0.125%
	ECONOPRED Plus	Suspension: 1%
	INFLAMASE	Solution: 0.125%
	INFLAMASE Forte	Solution: 1%
	PRED Forte	Suspension: 1%
	PRED Mild	Suspension: 0.12%

DRUG PROFILE

These topical drugs are used to reduce the inflammation and other discomfort associated with such eye conditions as allergies, certain types of conjunctivitis, and uveitis (inflammation of the iris and neighboring parts of the eye).

BEFORE USING THIS DRUG

Let your doctor know *IF*

You have ever had allergic reactions or other problems with ■ corticosteroids ■ sulfites ■ other preservatives.

You have ever had any of the following medical problems: ■ glaucoma ■ cataracts ■ tuberculosis of the eye ■ eye injury ■ any type of eye infection ■ herpes simplex keratitis ■ diabetes (or family history of diabetes) ■ recent chickenpox or other viral disease ■ fungal infections ■ rheumatoid arthritis.

SPECIAL RESTRICTIONS WHILE TAKING THIS DRUG

FOOD AND DRUG INTERACTIONS

No special restrictions on other drugs, foods and beverages, alcohol use, or smoking.

DAILY LIVING

Driving	Do not drive until you know how this drug will affect you, since it may cause blurring of vision. If your vision remains clear, you may drive, but with caution. Also be careful when operating household appliances or doing any other tasks that require clear vision until you know how this drug affects you.
Examinations or Tests	Prolonged therapy with ophthalmic corticosteroids may lead to glaucoma or cataracts. It is important for you to keep all appointments with your doctor—particularly if you are on long-term therapy with this drug—so that your eye pressure can be checked and your eyes can be examined for any adverse effects from this drug.

Other Precautions

If your eye symptoms do not improve or if they worsen, check with your doctor. Also, if you develop any signs of infection not present when you first started using this drug, let your doctor know.

The ointment should not be applied while wearing contact lenses.

The use of these drugs slows wound healing, which may be important if you have surgery done in or around the eyes. Let your doctor know that you are taking this drug, if you are undergoing this kind of surgery.

Helpful Hints

To use: After washing your hands thoroughly, pull the lower eyelid down to form a pouch; drop in the solution or squeeze about a one-third-inch strip of ointment into the pouch. Keep your eyes closed for one to two minutes. You may experience a temporary burning or stinging sensation or blurred vision after use of the ointment.

To prevent contamination, avoid touching either the dropper or tube tip to the eye, eyelid, or any other surface and keep the container tightly closed when not in use. Wipe off the tip of the tube of ointment with a clean tissue before replacing the cap.

No special restrictions on exertion and exercise, sun exposure, or exposure to excessive heat or cold.

POSSIBLE SIDE EFFECTS

Although this list of adverse effects may seem somewhat intimidating, keep in mind that some are quite rare. Of course, should these or any other problems arise while you are on medication, it is always a good idea to consult your doctor.

IF YOU DEVELOP	WHAT TO DO
sudden eye pain ■ loss of vision	**Urgent: Stop using this drug and get in touch with your doctor immediately.**
blurred vision or other visual disturbances ■ drooping or swelling of eyelids ■ eye pain ■ increased redness of the eyes ■ dilated pupils ■ headache ■ tearing ■ painful rash ■ increased sensitivity to light ■ sensation of a foreign body in the eye ■ any sign of eye infection not present before beginning use of this drug	**May be serious** Stop using this drug and check with your doctor as soon as possible.
stinging and burning of the eye	If symptoms are disturbing or persist, let your doctor know.

STORAGE INSTRUCTIONS

Store in a cool, dry place, away from direct sunlight.

STOPPING OR INTERRUPTING THERAPY

If you miss a dose, apply it as soon as possible. If it is almost time for your next dose, skip the missed dose and resume your regular schedule.

SPECIAL CONSIDERATIONS FOR THOSE OVER SIXTY-FIVE

None.

CONDITION: **BACTERIAL INFECTIONS**

CATEGORY: **OPHTHALMIC ANTI-INFECTIVES (AMINOGLYCOSIDES)**

GENERIC (CHEMICAL) NAME	BRAND (TRADE) NAME	DOSAGE FORMS AND STRENGTHS
Gentamicin	GARAMYCIN	Ointment: 0.3% Solution: 0.3%
	GENOPTIC	Ointment: 0.3% Solution: 0.3%
	GENTACIDIN	Ointment: 0.3% Solution: 0.3%
	GENT-AK	Ointment: 0.3% Solution: 0.3%
Neomycin sulfate, polymyxin B sulfate, gramicidin	AK-SPORE	Solution: neomycin sulfate equivalent to 1.75 mg of neomycin, 10,000 units of polymyxin B sulfate, and 0.025 mg gramicidin per ml
	NEOSPORIN	Solution: neomycin sulfate equivalent to 1.75 mg of neomycin, 10,000 units of polymyxin B sulfate, and 0.025 mg gramicidin per ml
Tobramycin	TOBREX	Ointment: 0.3% Solution: 0.3%

DRUG PROFILE

These antibiotics are applied directly to the eye to treat infections caused by bacteria. They work by interfering with the manufacture of protein inside the bacterial organism.

BEFORE USING THIS DRUG

Let your doctor know *IF*

You have ever had allergic reactions or other problems with ■ gentamicin ■ tobramycin ■ any other aminoglycoside antibiotic, including amikacin, kanamycin, neomycin, netilmicin, or streptomycin ■ preservatives.

You are taking any of the following medicines: ■ other eye preparations.

SPECIAL RESTRICTIONS WHILE TAKING THIS DRUG

FOOD AND DRUG INTERACTIONS

No special restrictions on other drugs, foods and beverages, alcohol use, or smoking.

DAILY LIVING

Driving	Do not drive until you know how this drug will affect you, since the ointment form of this medication may cause blurring of vision. If your vision remains clear, you may drive, but with caution. Also be careful when operating household appliances or doing any other tasks that require clear vision until you know how this drug affects you.
Examinations or Tests	It is important for you to keep all appointments with your doctor so that your progress can be checked.
Other Precautions	If your eye symptoms do not improve or if they worsen, check with your doctor. Also, if you develop any signs of eye infection not present when you first started using this drug, let your doctor know.
Helpful Hints	*To use:* After washing your hands thoroughly, pull the lower lid down to form a pouch; drop in the solution or squeeze about a one-third-inch strip of ointment

into the pouch. Keep your eyes closed for one to two minutes. You may experience a temporary burning or stinging sensation or blurred vision after use of the ointment.

To prevent contamination, avoid touching either the dropper or tube tip to the eye, eyelid, or any other surface, and keep the container tightly closed when not in use. Wipe off the tip of the tube of ointment or cream with a clean tissue before replacing the cap.

No special restrictions on exertion and exercise, sun exposure, or exposure to excessive heat or cold.

POSSIBLE SIDE EFFECTS

Although this list of adverse effects may seem somewhat intimidating, keep in mind that some are quite rare. Of course, should these or any other problems arise while you are on medication, it is always a good idea to consult your doctor.

IF YOU DEVELOP	WHAT TO DO
eye irritation ■ itching of eyes ■ swelling of eyelids ■ red eyes ■ watering of the eyes ■ any sign of eye infection not present before beginning use of this drug	**May be serious** Stop taking this drug and check with your doctor as soon as possible.
stinging and burning of the eye	If symptoms are disturbing or persist, let your doctor know.

STORAGE INSTRUCTIONS

Store in a cool, dry place, away from direct sunlight, and make sure that it does not freeze.

STOPPING OR INTERRUPTING THERAPY

If you miss a dose, apply it as soon as possible. If it is almost time for your next dose, however, skip the missed dose and resume your regular schedule.

SPECIAL CONSIDERATIONS FOR THOSE OVER SIXTY-FIVE

None.

CONDITION: **BACTERIAL INFECTIONS**

CATEGORY: **OPHTHALMIC ANTI-INFECTIVES (ERYTHROMYCIN)**

GENERIC (CHEMICAL) NAME	BRAND (TRADE) NAME	DOSAGE FORMS AND STRENGTHS
Erythromycin	AK-MYCIN	Ointment: 0.5%
	ILOTYCIN	Ointment: 0.5%

DRUG PROFILE

This type of antibiotic is applied directly to the eye to treat infections caused by bacteria. It suppresses the growth of bacteria by interfering with the manufacture of protein inside the bacterial organism.

BEFORE USING THIS DRUG

Let your doctor know *IF*

You have ever had allergic reactions or other problems with ■ any form of erythromycin ■ preservatives.

You are taking any of the following medicines: ■ other eye preparations.

SPECIAL RESTRICTIONS WHILE TAKING THIS DRUG

FOOD AND DRUG INTERACTIONS

No special restrictions on other drugs, foods and beverages, alcohol use, or smoking.

DAILY LIVING

Driving	Do not drive until you know how this drug will affect you, since the ointment form of this medication may cause blurring of vision. If your vision remains clear, you may drive, but with caution. Also be careful when operating household appliances or doing any other tasks that require clear vision until you know how this drug affects you.
Examinations or Tests	It is important for you to keep all appointments with your doctor so that your progress can be checked.
Other Precautions	If your eye symptoms do not improve or if they worsen, check with your doctor. Also, if you develop any signs of eye infection not present when you first started using this drug, let your doctor know.
Helpful Hints	*To use:* Pull the lower eyelid down to form a pouch; squeeze about a one-third-inch strip of ointment into the pouch. Keep your eyes closed for one to two minutes. You may experience a temporary burning or stinging sensation or blurred vision after use of this ointment.
	To prevent contamination, avoid touching the tube tip to the eye, eyelid, or any other surface, and keep the container tightly closed when not in use. Wipe off the tip of the tube with a clean tissue before replacing the cap.

No special restrictions on exertion and exercise, sun exposure, or exposure to excessive heat or cold.

POSSIBLE SIDE EFFECTS

Although this list of adverse effects may seem somewhat intimidating, keep in mind that some are quite rare. Of course, should these or any other problems arise while you are on medication, it is always a good idea to consult your doctor.

IF YOU DEVELOP	WHAT TO DO
eye irritation ■ itching of eyes ■ swelling of eyelids ■ red eyes ■ watering of the eyes ■ any sign of eye infection not present before beginning use of this drug	**May be serious** Stop using this drug and check with your doctor as soon as possible.
stinging or burning of eyes	If symptoms are disturbing or persist, let your doctor know.

STORAGE INSTRUCTIONS

Store in a cool, dry place, away from direct sunlight.

STOPPING OR INTERRUPTING THERAPY

If you miss a dose, apply it as soon as possible. If it is almost time for your next dose, skip the missed dose and resume your regular schedule.

SPECIAL CONSIDERATIONS FOR THOSE OVER SIXTY-FIVE

None.

CONDITION: **BACTERIAL INFECTIONS**

CATEGORY: **OPHTHALMIC ANTI-INFECTIVES (SULFONAMIDES)**

GENERIC (CHEMICAL) NAME	BRAND (TRADE) NAME	DOSAGE FORMS AND STRENGTHS
Sulfacetamide sodium	AK-SULF	Ointment: 10%
		Solution: 10%, 15%, 30%
	BLEPH-10	Ointment: 10%
		Solution: 10%
	CETAMIDE	Ointment: 10%
	ISOPTO CETAMIDE	Solution: 15%
	Sodium SULAMYD	Ointment: 10%
		Solution: 10%, 30%
	SULF-10	Solution: 10%
	SULTEN-10	Solution: 10%
Sulfacetamide sodium and phenylephrine hydrochloride	VASOSULF	Solution: 15% sulfacetamide sodium and 0.125% phenylephrine
Sulfisoxazole	GANTRISIN	Ointment: 4%
		Solution: 4%

DRUG PROFILE

Ophthalmic sulfonamides (sulfa drugs) are used to treat bacterial infections of the eye such as conjunctivitis and ulcers of the cornea. These antibiotics suppress the growth of bacteria by interfering with the manufacture of folic acid. Phenylephrine, a decongestant drug, relieves redness, watering, and itching by constricting the blood vessels in the eye.

These drugs are sometimes used in combination with other ophthalmic preparations or with oral sulfonamide therapy.

BEFORE USING THIS DRUG

Let your doctor know *IF*

You have ever had allergic reactions or other problems with ■ any sulfonamides (sulfa drugs) ■ furosemide or thiazide diuretics (water pills) ■ oral medicine for diabetes ■ oral medicine for glaucoma ■ sulfites or other preservatives.

You are taking any of the following medicines: ■ other eye preparations.

SPECIAL RESTRICTIONS WHILE TAKING THIS DRUG

FOOD AND DRUG INTERACTIONS

No special restrictions on other drugs, foods and beverages, alcohol use, or smoking.

DAILY LIVING

Driving	Do not drive until you know how this drug will affect you, since the ointment form of this medication may cause blurring of vision. If your vision remains clear, you may drive, but with caution. Also be careful when operating household appliances or doing any other tasks that require clear vision until you know how this drug affects you.
Examinations or Tests	It is important for you to keep all appointments with your doctor so that your progress can be checked.
Other Precautions	If your eye symptoms do not improve or if they worsen, stop using this drug and check with your doctor. Also, if you develop any signs of eye infection not present when you first started using this drug or if you start to have a pus-filled discharge from the eye, let your doctor know. Tell any doctor you consult that you are using this drug, if you will be undergoing eye surgery.

Helpful Hints

To use: After washing your hands thoroughly, pull the lower eyelid down to form a pouch; drop in the solution or squeeze about a half-inch to one-inch strip of ointment into the pouch. Keep your eyes closed for one to two minutes. You may experience a temporary burning or stinging sensation or blurred vision after use of the ointment.

To prevent contamination, avoid touching either the dropper or tube tip to the eye, eyelid, or any other surface, and keep the container tightly closed when not in use. Wipe off the tip of the tube of ointment with a clean tissue before replacing the cap.

No special restrictions on exertion and exercise, sun exposure, or exposure to excessive heat or cold.

POSSIBLE SIDE EFFECTS

Although this list of adverse effects may seem somewhat intimidating, keep in mind that some are quite rare. Of course, should these or any other problems arise while you are on medication, it is always a good idea to consult your doctor.

IF YOU DEVELOP	WHAT TO DO
redness, hives, peeling, scaling, or blisters	**Urgent: Stop using this drug and get in touch with your doctor immediately.**
eye irritation ■ itching of eyes ■ swelling of eyelids ■ red eyes ■ watering of the eyes ■ any sign of eye infection not present before beginning use of this drug	**May be serious** Stop using this drug and check with your doctor as soon as possible.
stinging and burning of the eyes ■ headache ■ browache ■ blurred vision ■ increased eye sensitivity to light	If symptoms are disturbing or persist, let your doctor know.

STORAGE INSTRUCTIONS

Store in a cool, dry place, away from direct sunlight.

STOPPING OR INTERRUPTING THERAPY

If you miss a dose, apply it as soon as possible. If it is almost time for your next dose, skip the missed dose and resume your regular schedule.

SPECIAL CONSIDERATIONS FOR THOSE OVER SIXTY-FIVE

None.

CONDITION: **BACTERIAL INFECTIONS**

CATEGORY: **OPHTHALMIC ANTI-INFECTIVES (TETRACYCLINES)**

GENERIC (CHEMICAL) NAME	BRAND (TRADE) NAME	DOSAGE FORMS AND STRENGTHS
Chlortetracycline	AUREOMYCIN	Ointment: 1%
Tetracycline hydrochloride	ACHROMYCIN	Ointment: 1% Suspension: 1%

DRUG PROFILE

Ophthalmic tetracyclines are used to treat various types of bacterial infections of the eye. These antibiotics suppress the growth of bacteria by interfering with the manufacture of protein inside the bacterial organism. If you are being treated for trachoma, your doctor will probably prescribe an oral antibiotic along with the ophthalmic tetracycline.

BEFORE USING THIS DRUG

Let your doctor know *IF*

You are taking any of the following medicines: ■ other eye preparations.

SPECIAL RESTRICTIONS WHILE TAKING THIS DRUG

FOOD AND DRUG INTERACTIONS

No special restrictions on other drugs, foods and beverages, alcohol use, or smoking.

DAILY LIVING

Driving	Do not drive until you know how this drug will affect you, since the ointment form of this medication may cause blurring of vision. If your vision remains clear, you may drive, but with caution. Also be careful when operating household appliances or doing any other tasks that require clear vision until you know how this drug affects you.
Examinations or Tests	It is important for you to keep all appointments with your doctor so that your progress can be checked. If your eye symptoms do not improve or if they worsen, stop taking this drug and check with your doctor. Also, if you develop any signs of eye infection not present when you first started using this drug, let your doctor know.
Helpful Hints	*To use:* After washing your hands thoroughly, pull the lower lid down to form a pouch; drop in the solution or squeeze about a one-third-inch strip of ointment into the pouch. Keep your eyes closed for one to two minutes. You may experience a temporary burning or stinging sensation or blurred vision after use of the ointment.

To prevent contamination, avoid touching either the dropper or tube tip to the eye, eyelid, or any other surface, and keep the container tightly closed when not in use. Wipe off the tip of the tube of ointment with a clean tissue before replacing the cap.

No special restrictions on exertion and exercise, sun exposure, or exposure to excessive heat or cold.

POSSIBLE SIDE EFFECTS

Although this list of adverse effects may seem somewhat intimidating, keep in mind that some are quite rare. Of course, should these or any other problems arise while you are on medication, it is always a good idea to consult your doctor.

IF YOU DEVELOP	WHAT TO DO
eye irritation ■ itching of eyes ■ swelling of the eye-lids ■ red eyes ■ watering of the eyes ■ any sign of eye infection not present before beginning use of this drug ■ sensation of a foreign body in the eye	**May be serious** Stop using this drug and check with your doctor as soon as possible.
stinging and burning of the eyes	If symptoms are disturbing or persist, let your doctor know.

STORAGE INSTRUCTIONS

Store in a cool, dry place, away from direct sunlight.

STOPPING OR INTERRUPTING THERAPY

If you miss a dose, apply it as soon as possible. If it is almost time for your next dose, skip the missed dose and resume your regular schedule.

SPECIAL CONSIDERATIONS FOR THOSE OVER SIXTY-FIVE

None.

CONDITION: **BACTERIAL INFECTIONS**

CATEGORY: **OPHTHALMIC ANTI-INFECTIVES (BACITRACIN AND BACITRACIN COMBINATIONS)**

GENERIC (CHEMICAL) NAME	BRAND (TRADE) NAME	DOSAGE FORMS AND STRENGTHS
Bacitracin	BACIGUENT	Ointment: 500 units per g
Bacitracin, neomycin sulfate, and polymyxin B sulfate	MYCITRACIN	Ointment: 500 units bacitracin, 10,000 units polymyxin B sulfate, and neomycin sulfate equivalent to 3.5 mg of neomycin
Bacitracin zinc and polymyxin B sulfate	AK-POLY-BAC	Ointment: 500 units bacitracin zinc and 10,000 units polymyxin B sulfate per g
	POLYSPORIN	Ointment: 500 units bacitracin zinc and 10,000 units polymyxin B sulfate per g
Bacitracin zinc, polymyxin B sulfate, and neomycin sulfate	NEOSPORIN	Ointment: 400 units bacitracin zinc, 10,000 units polymyxin B sulfate, and neomycin sulfate equivalent to 3.5 mg of neomycin per g
	AK-SPORE	Ointment: 400 units bacitracin zinc, 10,000 units polymyxin B sulfate, and neomycin sulfate equivalent to 3.5 mg of neomycin

DRUG PROFILE

Bacitracin and bacitracin combinations are used for short-term treatment of bacterial infections of the eye. These antibiotics suppress the growth of bacteria by interfering with the manufacture of protein inside the bacterial organism.

BEFORE USING THIS DRUG

Let your doctor know *IF*

You have ever had allergic reactions or other problems with ■ bacitracin ■ neomycin ■ polymyxin.

With products containing neomycin only: ■ aminoglycoside antibiotics including amikacin, gentamicin, kanamycin, tobramycin, or streptomycin.

You are taking any of the following medicines: ■ other eye preparations.

SPECIAL RESTRICTIONS WHILE TAKING THIS DRUG

FOOD AND DRUG INTERACTIONS

No special restrictions on other drugs, foods and beverages, alcohol use, or smoking.

DAILY LIVING

Driving	Do not drive until you know how this drug will affect you, since the ointment form of this medication may cause blurring of vision. If your vision remains clear, you may drive, but with caution. Also be careful when operating household appliances or doing any other tasks that require clear vision until you know how this drug affects you.
Examinations or Tests	It is important for you to keep all appointments with your doctor so that your progress can be checked.

Other Precautions	If your eye symptoms do not improve or if they worsen, check with your doctor. Also, if you develop any signs of eye infection not present when you first started using this drug, let your doctor know.
Helpful Hints	*To use:* After washing your hands thoroughly, pull the lower eyelid down to form a pouch; squeeze about a one-third-inch strip of ointment into the pouch. Keep your eyes closed for one to two minutes. You may experience a temporary burning or stinging sensation or blurred vision after use of the ointment. To prevent contamination, avoid touching the tube tip to the eye, eyelid, or any other surface, and keep the container tightly closed when not in use. Wipe off the tip of the tube with a clean tissue before replacing the cap.

No special restrictions on exertion and exercise, sun exposure, or exposure to excessive heat or cold.

POSSIBLE SIDE EFFECTS

Although this list of adverse effects may seem somewhat intimidating, keep in mind that some are quite rare. Of course, should these or any other problems arise while you are on medication, it is always a good idea to consult your doctor.

IF YOU DEVELOP	WHAT TO DO
difficulty in breathing ■ fainting ■ tightness in chest ■ swelling of lips and face	**Urgent: Stop using this drug and get in touch with your doctor immediately.**
itching of eyes ■ increased sweating ■ inflammation of the eye ■ any sign of eye infection not present before beginning use of this drug ■ rash	**May be serious** Check with your doctor as soon as possible.

STORAGE INSTRUCTIONS

Store in a cool, dry place, away from direct sunlight.

STOPPING OR INTERRUPTING THERAPY

If you miss a dose, apply it as soon as possible. If it is almost time for your next dose, skip the missed dose and resume your regular schedule.

SPECIAL CONSIDERATIONS FOR THOSE OVER SIXTY-FIVE

None.

CONDITION: BACTERIAL INFECTIONS
**CATEGORY: OPHTHALMIC ANTI-INFECTIVES
(CHLORAMPHENICOL)**

GENERIC (CHEMICAL) NAME	BRAND (TRADE) NAME	DOSAGE FORMS AND STRENGTHS
Chloramphenicol	AK-CHLOR	Ointment: 1% Solution: 0.5%
	CHLOROMYCETIN	Ointment: 1% Powder: to be mixed with sterile distilled water to make 0.16% to 0.5% solution
	CHLOROPTIC	Ointment: 1% Solution: 0.5%
	OPHTHOCHLOR	Solution: 0.5%

DRUG PROFILE

Chloramphenicol is used for short-term treatment of bacterial infections of the eye. This drug suppresses the growth of bacteria by interfering with the manufacture of protein inside the bacterial organism. Your doctor may prescribe an oral antibiotic for you to take as well.

BEFORE USING THIS DRUG

Let your doctor know *IF*

You have ever had allergic reactions or other problems with ■ chloramphenicol ■ sulfites or other preservatives.

SPECIAL RESTRICTIONS WHILE TAKING THIS DRUG

FOOD AND DRUG INTERACTIONS

No special restrictions on other drugs, foods and beverages, alcohol use, or smoking.

DAILY LIVING

Driving	Do not drive until you know how this drug will affect you, since the ointment form of this medication may cause blurring of vision. If your vision remains clear, you may drive, but with caution. Also be careful when operating household appliances or doing any other tasks that require clear vision until you know how this drug affects you.
Examinations or Tests	It is important for you to keep all appointments with your doctor so that your progress can be checked.
Other Precautions	If your eye symptoms do not improve or if they worsen, check with your doctor. Also, if you develop any signs of eye infection not present when you first started using this drug, stop using it and let your doctor know.
Helpful Hints	*To use:* After washing your hands thoroughly, pull the lower lid down to form a pouch; drop in the solution or squeeze about a one-third-inch strip of ointment into the pouch. Keep your eyes closed for one to two

minutes. You may experience a temporary burning or stinging sensation or blurred vision after use of the ointment.

To prevent contamination, avoid touching either the dropper or tube tip to the eye, eyelid, or any other surface, and keep the container tightly closed when not in use. Wipe off the tip of the tube with a clean tissue before replacing the cap.

No special restrictions on exertion and exercise, sun exposure, or exposure to excessive heat or cold.

POSSIBLE SIDE EFFECTS

Although this list of adverse effects may seem somewhat intimidating, keep in mind that some are quite rare. Of course, should these or any other problems arise while you are on medication, it is always a good idea to consult your doctor.

IF YOU DEVELOP	WHAT TO DO
shortness of breath ■ swelling of lips or face ■ fever, chills, or sore throat ■ tiredness ■ paleness ■ delayed blood clotting	**Urgent: Stop using this drug and get in touch with your doctor immediately.**
inflammation, itching, stinging, or burning of the eyes ■ hives, rash, blisters, or changes in skin color ■ any sign of eye infection not present before beginning use of this drug	**May be serious** Check with your doctor as soon as possible.

STORAGE INSTRUCTIONS

Store in a cool, dry place, away from direct sunlight. If your medicine is in a liquid form, make sure that it does not freeze.

STOPPING OR INTERRUPTING THERAPY

If you miss a dose, apply it as soon as possible. If it is almost time for your next dose, skip the missed dose and resume your regular schedule.

SPECIAL CONSIDERATIONS FOR THOSE OVER SIXTY-FIVE

None.

CONDITION: **BACTERIAL INFECTIONS**

CATEGORY: **OPHTHALMIC ANTI-INFECTIVES (TRIMETHOPRIM AND POLYMYXIN)**

GENERIC (CHEMICAL) NAME	BRAND (TRADE) NAME	DOSAGE FORMS AND STRENGTHS
Trimethoprim and polymyxin B sulfate	POLYTRIM	Solution: Trimethoprim 1 mg per ml and polymyxin sulfate 10,000 units per ml

DRUG PROFILE

The combination of trimethoprim and polymyxin B sulfate is used to treat bacterial infections of the eye. These antibiotics suppress the growth of bacteria.

BEFORE USING THIS DRUG

Let your doctor know *IF*

You have ever had allergic reactions or other problems with ■ trimethoprim ■ polymyxin.

You are using any of the following medicines: ■ other eye preparations.

SPECIAL RESTRICTIONS WHILE TAKING THIS DRUG

FOOD AND DRUG INTERACTIONS

No special restrictions on other drugs, foods and beverages, alcohol use, or smoking.

DAILY LIVING

Other Precautions:	If your eye symptoms do not improve or if they worsen, check with your doctor. Also, if you develop any signs of eye infection not present when you first started using this drug, stop using it and let your doctor know.
Helpful Hints	To use: After washing your hands thoroughly, pull the lower lid down to form a pouch: drop the solution into the pouch. Keep your eyes closed for one or two minutes. You may experience a temporary burning, stinging, itching, or redness when the drops are instilled. To prevent contamination, avoid touching the dropper to the eye, eyelid, or any other surface, and keep the container tightly closed when not in use.

No special restrictions on exertion and exercise, sun exposure or exposure to excessive heat or cold.

POSSIBLE SIDE EFFECTS

Although this list of adverse effects may seem intimidating, keep in mind that some are quite rare. Of course, should these or any other problems arise while you are on medication, it is always a good idea to consult your doctor.

IF YOU DEVELOP	WHAT TO DO
any sign of eye infection not present before beginning use of this drug ■ inflammation or redness of the eye ■ itching of the eyes ■ rash ■ eye pain ■ swelling of the eyelids	**May be serious** Stop using this drug and check with your doctor as soon as possible
stinging and burning of the eyes ■ tearing	If symptoms are disturbing or persist, let your doctor know.

STORAGE INSTRUCTIONS

Store in a cool, dry place, away from direct sunlight.

STOPPING OR INTERRUPTING THERAPY

If you miss a dose, apply as soon as possible. If it is almost time for your next dose, skip the missed dose and resume your regular schedule.

SPECIAL CONSIDERATIONS FOR THOSE OVER SIXTY-FIVE

None.

CONDITION: **VIRAL INFECTIONS**

CATEGORY: **OPHTHALMIC ANTI-INFECTIVES (ANTIVIRAL AGENTS)**

GENERIC (CHEMICAL) NAME	BRAND (TRADE) NAME	DOSAGE FORMS AND STRENGTHS
Idoxuridine	HERPLEX	Solution: 0.1%
	STOXIL	Ointment: 0.5%
		Solution: 0.1%
Trifluridine	VIROPTIC	Solution: 1%
Vidarabine	VIRA-A	Ointment: 3%

DRUG PROFILE

These drugs are used for short-term treatment of eye infections caused by the virus herpes simplex. They work by preventing the virus from multiplying.

BEFORE USING THIS DRUG

Let your doctor know *IF*

You have ever had allergic reactions or other problems with ■ idoxuridine ■ trifluridine ■ vidarabine.

SPECIAL RESTRICTIONS WHILE TAKING THIS DRUG

FOOD AND DRUG INTERACTIONS

No special restrictions on other drugs, foods and beverages, alcohol use, or smoking.

DAILY LIVING

Driving	Do not drive until you know how this drug will affect you, since the ointment form of this medication may cause blurring of vision. If your vision remains clear, you may drive, but with caution. Also be careful when operating household appliances or doing any other tasks that require clear vision until you know how this drug affects you.
Examinations or Tests	It is important for you to keep all appointments with your doctor so that your progress can be checked.
Other Precautions	If your eye remains irritated, let your doctor know. Do not use this drug for longer than three weeks unless directed by your ophthalmologist.
Helpful Hints	*To use:* After washing your hands thoroughly, pull the lower eyelid down to form a pouch; drop in the solution or squeeze about a half-inch strip of ointment into the pouch (refer to the package instructions for the exact amount). Keep your eyes closed for one to two minutes. You may experience a temporary burning or stinging sensation or blurred vision after use of the ointment.
	To prevent contamination, avoid touching either the dropper or tube tip to the eye, eyelid, or any other surface, and keep the container tightly closed when not in use. Wipe off the tip of the tube with a clean tissue before replacing the cap.

No special restrictions on exertion and exercise, sun exposure, or exposure to excessive heat or cold.

POSSIBLE SIDE EFFECTS

Although this list of adverse effects may seem somewhat intimidating, keep in mind that some are quite rare. Of course, should these or any other problems arise while you are on medication, it is always a good idea to consult your doctor.

IF YOU DEVELOP	WHAT TO DO
eye pain or irritation ■ any signs of eye infection not present before beginning use of this drug ■ blurred vision ■ increased sensitivity to light	**May be serious** Stop using this drug and check with your doctor as soon as possible.
burning or stinging of the eyes ■ swelling of eyelids ■ dry eyes ■ redness in or around eyes *With vidarabine only:* tearing ■ sensation of a foreign body in the eye	If symptoms are disturbing or persist, let your doctor know.

STORAGE INSTRUCTIONS

Store this medicine in the refrigerator, but make sure that it does not freeze.

STOPPING OR INTERRUPTING THERAPY

If you miss a dose, apply it as soon as possible. If it is almost time for your next dose, skip the missed dose and resume your regular schedule.

SPECIAL CONSIDERATIONS FOR THOSE OVER SIXTY-FIVE

None.

CONDITION: **INFLAMMATION AND INFECTION**

CATEGORY: **OPHTHALMIC CORTICOSTEROID—
ANTI-INFECTIVE COMBINATIONS**

GENERIC (CHEMICAL) NAME	BRAND (TRADE) NAME	DOSAGE FORMS AND STRENGTHS
Dexamethasone, neomycin sulfate, and polymyxin B sulfate	AK-TROL	Ointment: 0.1% dexamethasone, 0.5% neomycin sulfate, and 10,000 units polymyxin B sulfate per g Suspension: 0.1% dexamethasone, 0.5% neomycin sulfate, and 10,000 units polymyxin B sulfate per ml
	DEXACIDIN	Ointment: 0.1% dexamethasone, 0.5% neomycin sulfate, and 10,000 units polymyxin B sulfate per g Suspension: 0.1% dexamethasone, 0.5% neomycin sulfate, and 10,000 units polymyxin B sulfate per ml
	MAXITROL	Ointment: 0.1% dexamethasone, 0.5% neomycin sulfate, and 10,000 units polymyxin B sulfate per g Suspension: 0.1% dexamethasone, 0.5% neomycin sulfate, and 10,000 units polymyxin B sulfate per ml
Dexamethasone and neomycin sulfate	NeoDECADRON	Ointment: 0.05% dexamethasone and 0.5% neomycin sulfate per g Solution: 0.1% dexamethasone and 0.5% neomycin sulfate per ml

Dexamethasone and tobramycin	TOBRADEX	Ointment: 0.1% dexamethasone and 0.3% tobramycin Suspension: 0.1% dexamethasone and 0.3% tobramycin
Hydrocortisone, bacitracin zinc, polymyxin B sulfate, and neomycin sulfate	CORTISPORIN	Ointment: 1% hydrocortisone, 400 units bacitracin zinc, 10,000 units polymyxin B sulfate, and 0.5% neomycin sulfate per g
Hydrocortisone acetate, polymyxin B sulfate, and chloramphenicol	OPHTHOCORT	Ointment: 0.5% hydrocortisone acetate, 10,000 units polymyxin B sulfate, and 1% chloramphenicol
Hydrocortisone, polymyxin B sulfate, and neomycin sulfate	CORTISPORIN	Suspension: 1% hydrocortisone, 10,000 units polymyxin B sulfate, and 0.5% neomycin sulfate per ml
	AK-SPORE HC	Suspension: 1% hydrocortisone, 10,000 units polymyxin B sulfate, and 0.5% neomycin sulfate per ml
Prednisolone and gentamicin	PRED G	Suspension: 1.0% prednisolone and 0.3% gentamicin
Prednisolone acetate, polymyxin B sulfate, and neomycin sulfate	POLY-PRED	Suspension: 0.5% prednisolone acetate, 10,000 units polymyxin B sulfate, and 0.5% neomycin sulfate per ml

Prednisolone acetate and sulfacetamide sodium	AK-CIDE	Ointment: 0.5% prednisolone acetate and 10% sulfacetamide sodium per g
		Suspension: 0.5% prednisolone acetate and 10% sulfacetamide sodium per ml
	BLEPHAMIDE	Ointment: 0.2% prednisolone acetate and 10% sulfacetamide sodium per g
		Suspension: 0.2% prednisolone acetate and 10% sulfacetamide sodium per ml
	CETAPRED	Ointment: 0.25% prednisolone acetate and 10% sulfacetamide sodium per g
	ISOPTO CETAPRED	Suspension: 0.25% prednisolone acetate and 10% sulfaacetamide sodium per ml
	VASOCIDIN	Ointment: 0.5% prednisolone acetate and 10% sulfacetamide sodium per g

DRUG PROFILE

These combination drugs are prescribed to treat eye infections, injuries, and other inflammatory conditions. The antibiotic component suppresses the growth of bacteria, while the corticosteroid reduces inflammation and discomfort.

BEFORE USING THIS DRUG

Let your doctor know *IF*

You have ever had allergic reactions or other problems with ■ corticosteroids ■ sulfites or other preservatives ■ neomycin sulfate ■ polymyxin B sulfate.

With sulfacetamide combinations only: ■ any sulfonamides (sulfa drugs) ■ furosemide or thiazide diuretics (water pills) ■ oral medicine for diabetes ■ oral medicine for glaucoma.

You have ever had any of the following medical problems: ■ any type of eye infection ■ glaucoma ■ cataracts ■ tuberculosis of the eye ■ herpes simplex keratitis ■ recent eye injury (including foreign object in the eye) ■ diabetes (or family history of diabetes) ■ recent chickenpox or other viral diseases.

You are taking any of the following medicines: ■ other eye preparations.

SPECIAL RESTRICTIONS WHILE TAKING THIS DRUG

FOOD AND DRUG INTERACTIONS

No special restrictions on other drugs, foods and beverages, alcohol use, or smoking.

DAILY LIVING

Driving	Do not drive until you know how this drug will affect you, since the ointment form of this medication may cause blurring of vision. If your vision remains clear, you may drive, but with caution. Also be careful when operating household appliances or doing any other tasks that require clear vision until you know how this drug affects you.
Examinations or Tests	It is important for you to keep all appointments with your doctor—particularly if you are on long-term therapy with this drug—so that your eye pressure can be checked and your eyes can be examined for any adverse effects from this drug.
Other Precautions	If your eye symptoms do not improve or if they worsen, check with your doctor. Also, if you develop any signs of eye infection not present when you first started using this drug, let your doctor know. If you will be undergoing eye surgery, let your doctor know that you have been using any of these medicines.

Helpful Hints

To use: After washing your hands thoroughly, pull the lower eyelid down to form a pouch; drop in the solution or squeeze about a one-third-inch strip of ointment into the pouch. Keep your eyes closed for one to two minutes. You may experience a temporary burning or stinging sensation or blurred vision after use of an ointment.

To prevent contamination, avoid touching either the dropper or tube tip to the eye, eyelid, or any other surface, and keep the container tightly closed when not in use. Wipe off the tip of the tube with a clean tissue before replacing the cap.

No special restrictions on exertion and exercise, sun exposure, or exposure to excessive heat or cold.

POSSIBLE SIDE EFFECTS

Although this list of adverse effects may seem somewhat intimidating, keep in mind that some are quite rare. Of course, should these or any other problems arise while you are on medication, it is always a good idea to consult your doctor.

IF YOU DEVELOP	WHAT TO DO
severe eye pain ■ blurred vision	**Urgent: Stop using this drug and get in touch with your doctor immediately.**
blurred vision, seeing halos around lights, or other visual disturbances ■ drooping eyelids ■ eye pain or irritation ■ dilated pupils ■ headache or browache ■ herpes ■ itching of the eyelids ■ eye redness or itching ■ any sign of eye infection not present before beginning use of this drug	**May be serious** Stop using this drug and check with your doctor as soon as possible.

burning or stinging of the eyes ■ increased eye sensitivity to light

If symptoms are disturbing or persist, let your doctor know.

STORAGE INSTRUCTIONS

Store in a cool, dry place, away from direct sunlight, and make sure that it does not freeze.

STOPPING OR INTERRUPTING THERAPY

If you miss a dose, apply it as soon as possible. If it is almost time for your next dose, skip the missed dose and resume your regular schedule.

SPECIAL CONSIDERATIONS FOR THOSE OVER SIXTY-FIVE

None.

CONDITION: **IRRITATION**

CATEGORY: **OPHTHALMIC DECONGESTANTS**

GENERIC (CHEMICAL) NAME	BRAND (TRADE) NAME	DOSAGE FORMS AND STRENGTHS
Naphazoline hydrochloride	AK-CON	Solution: 0.1%
	ALBALON	Solution: 0.1%
	MURO'S OPCON	Solution: 0.1%
	NAPHCON	Solution: 0.012%
	NAPHCON Forte	Solution: 0.1%
	VASOCON	Solution: 0.1%
Naphazoline hydrochloride and antazoline phosphate	ALBALON-A	Solution: 0.05% naphazoline hydrochloride and 0.5% antazoline phosphate
	VASOCON-A	Solution: 0.05% naphazoline hydrochloride and 0.5% antazoline phosphate
Naphazoline hydrochloride and pheniramine maleate	AK-CON-A	Solution: 0.025% naphazoline hydrochloride and 0.3% pheniramine maleate
	MURO'S OPCON-A	Solution: 0.025% naphazoline hydrochloride and 0.3% pheniramine maleate
	NAPHCON-A	Solution: 0.025% naphazoline hydrochloride and 0.3% pheniramine maleate
Phenylephrine hydrochloride	NEO-SYNEPHRINE	Solution: 2.5%, 10%

Phenylephrine hydrochloride, pyrilamine maleate, and antipyrine	PREFRIN-A	Solution: 0.12% phenylephrine hydrochloride, 0.1% pyrilamine maleate, and 0.1% antipyrine

DRUG PROFILE

These decongestant drugs are prescribed to relieve the redness, watering, and itching of the eyes associated with minor irritations and allergies. They work by constricting the blood vessels in the eye. The antihistamine components prevent the inflammatory response of the eye to allergens.

BEFORE USING THIS DRUG

Let your doctor know *IF*

You have ever had allergic reactions or other problems with ■ any ophthalmic decongestants.

You have ever had any of the following medical problems: ■ glaucoma ■ recent eye infections or a foreign body in the eye ■ diabetes ■ high blood pressure ■ overactive thyroid ■ any disease of the heart or blood vessels.

You are taking any of the following medicines: ■ monoamine oxidase inhibitors (MAOIs) for depression (in the past two weeks).

With phenylephrine only: ■ tricyclic antidepressants ■ beta-blockers (eg, propranolol, atenolol, metoprolol) ■ reserpine, guanethidine, or methyldopa (medicine for high blood pressure).

SPECIAL RESTRICTIONS WHILE TAKING THIS DRUG

FOOD AND DRUG INTERACTIONS

Other Drugs	Do not take any other drugs, including over-the-counter (OTC) drugs, before checking with your doctor. The combination of these drugs and certain other medicines—especially monoamine oxidase inhibitors—can result in a severe and dangerous rise in blood pressure.

No special restrictions on foods and beverages, alcohol use, or smoking.

DAILY LIVING

Sun Exposure	Your eyes may become especially sensitive to sunlight; wearing tinted glasses should help ease any discomfort.
Examinations or Tests	If you are hypertensive, it is important to have your blood pressure checked regularly.
Other Precautions	If your eye symptoms do not improve within forty-eight hours or if they worsen, check with your doctor. Avoid frequent, prolonged use of these drugs, as chronic redness of the eyes may develop.

No special restrictions on driving, exertion and exercise, or exposure to excessive heat or cold.

POSSIBLE SIDE EFFECTS

Although this list of adverse effects may seem somewhat intimidating, keep in mind that some are quite rare. Of course, should these or any other problems arise while you are on medication, it is always a good idea to consult your doctor.

IF YOU DEVELOP	WHAT TO DO
irregular, pounding, or fast heartbeat ■ nervousness ■ nausea ■ dizziness ■ weakness ■ drowsiness ■ faintness ■ tremors ■ increased sweating ■ eye pain ■ headache or browache ■ seeing halos around lights	**Urgent: Stop using this drug and get in touch with your doctor immediately.**
colored spots floating across your field of vision ■ dilated pupils ■ stuffy or runny nose ■ swelling of the eyes ■ worsened eye irritation	**May be serious** Stop using this drug and check with your doctor as soon as possible.
burning or stinging of the eye	If symptoms are disturbing or persist, let your doctor know.

STORAGE INSTRUCTIONS

Store in a cool, dry place, away from direct sunlight.

STOPPING OR INTERRUPTING THERAPY

If you miss a dose, apply it as soon as possible. If it is almost time for your next dose, skip the missed dose and resume your regular schedule. Most of these medicines can be used as needed for eye redness or itching and can be discontinued without adverse effects.

SPECIAL CONSIDERATIONS FOR THOSE OVER SIXTY-FIVE

Older people may be especially susceptible to the effects of these products on the heart and blood vessels. Therefore, it is important that people over sixty-five inform their doctor if they have high blood pressure or a heart condition. In addition, older people may be more prone to the side effect of seeing colored spots floating across the field of vision.

CATARACTS

Clear vision depends on the eye's ability to focus light rays to a point on the retina, a tissue that lines the inside of the back of the eye and relays images to the brain. For light rays to reach the retina at the correct point, they must be bent through two transparent organs—the cornea, which arches like a dome over the iris (the colored part of the eye), and the lens, a pea-shaped organ just behind the iris.

CAUSES

With age, the lens may begin to lose some of its transparency as the result of certain chemical changes in the eye. Cloudy areas, called opacities, may develop. At the same time, the center of the lens—its nucleus—hardens, and the entire lens loses some of its clarity and elasticity. These changes occur in about 80 percent of people over sixty-five, and, for a little less than half of that group, are severe enough to disrupt vision. When a cloudy lens interferes with sight, it is called a cataract.

About two million Americans have cataracts, and, while the condition sometimes affects younger people, 90 percent of cases are age related. Because high blood sugar also has an adverse effect on the lens, diabetics, too, are prone to cataracts. Cataracts are quite unpredictable; for unknown reasons, they progress much more quickly in some people than in others.

DIAGNOSIS

Depending on its exact location in the lens, a cataract may make itself known through a number of different symptoms, some subtle, some greatly annoying. The condition is almost always painless, however, and for many people, the only noticeable change is a gradual deterioration of vision. Some cataract sufferers have said that they seem to be viewing the world through smudged glass.

Cataracts can also cause very distressing double vision. This symptom is the result of a cataract that has some areas that are denser than others. Ironically, another common symptom of cataracts may appear, at first, as an improvement in eyesight—specifically, in near vision, reducing the need for the reading glasses that so many older people rely on. This is due to nuclear sclerosis, which is hardening of the nucleus. This type of cataract, however, may worsen nearsightedness, forcing many people with the condition to change eyeglass or contact lens prescriptions frequently.

Another symptom may be poor vision in bright light, caused by an opacity in the center of the lens's rear surface. This kind of cataract often occurs as a result of long-term use of cortisone, a steroid, to treat disorders such as arthritis and asthma. It may also be due to chronic ocular inflammation, known as uveitis. Finally, an advanced cataract can mute color vision, causing everything to have a yellowish tinge.

TREATMENT

Frequently, when cataracts are first diagnosed, the best course of action is to wait and watch. Your ophthalmologist may be able to reduce the vision problems caused by the cataract with a new prescription for glasses, bifocals, or, rarely, contact lenses. Most of the time, cataract surgery is performed when the person decides it is necessary, although if vision loss is severe enough, the ophthalmologist may recommend an operation. Increased glare may also suggest that earlier surgical intervention be considered.

Certain conditions of the eye make cataract surgery a poor choice for some people. For example, if your retina is already damaged from diabetes, high blood pressure, or a retinal disorder called macular degeneration that is common in older people, your ophthalmologist may not recommend surgery, since the resulting improvement in vision may be minimal.

Three types of cataract surgery are currently performed. The most common type had been intracapsular excision, where the entire lens is removed with a cryoprobe—a pencil probe that freezes itself to the cataract. Most cataract surgeons are now performing extracapsular extractions, however, where parts of the cataract are removed separately, starting with the front part of the capsule surrounding the lens. The back portion of the capsule is purposely left behind. Modern microsurgical techniques have made extracapsular surgery safe and effective. The third type of surgery, phacoemulsification, requires the smallest incision of all—only about one-tenth of an inch. The surgeon again removes the front part of the capsule, and then inserts a titanium needle that vibrates at a rapid rate (ultrasound) to pulverize the nucleus. The remaining cortex is then sucked out, and the back portion of the capsule left behind.

Which type of surgery is best for you depends both on the condition of your eye and on your surgeon's preferred technique. Each type is equally effective, since the end result—removal of the cataract—is always the same. However, the types that do not extract the back part of the capsule (extracapsular extraction and phacoemulsification) allow a wider choice of intraocular implants—quarter-inch plastic lenses that may be inserted during cataract surgery and are designed to help make up for the loss of your natural lens. Therefore, these techniques are preferred by most cataract surgeons.

For the first twenty-four hours after your operation, you'll have to wear a patch and shield over your eye, and you may, for a few days, experience some pain, tearing, and discharge. After that, complete recovery can take from three or four weeks to three months, depending on the type of operation you had and your individual healing characteristics.

During the recovery period, your ophthalmologist may prescribe cortisone drops to clear up inflammation, which may persist for four to six weeks. Any of several brands of cortisone drops, including Pred Forte,

Inflamase, Econopred, and Decadron, may be used. (See the drug chart on page 1038 for more information.) You may also need antibiotic drops, such as Garamycin, Tobrex, Neosporin, or Chloroptic, to help prevent infection for a few weeks after surgery. (The drug charts for these products appear on pages 1039 and 1041.) Also, to control pressure increases within the eye during the first few days after the operation, you might have to use drops such as Timoptic or pills such as Diamox to lower that pressure. (See the drug charts on pages 1042–1043.)

Surgery takes away your cataract, but it also takes away your lens, which, when functioning properly, holds one-third of the eye's refractory power (which is most important for focusing on near objects). To make up for this loss, you will need glasses, a contact lens, or an intraocular implant. Intraocular implants, which are permanent and rarely have to be changed, are particularly popular in people over forty-five. They are not recommended, however, for young people or people with other serious eye problems.

OUTLOOK

Cataract surgery is one of the most successful types of operations, restoring normal, clear vision to about 95 percent of people who undergo it. Advances in microsurgical techniques have led to this high level of success.

CONDITION: **CATARACTS**

CATEGORY: **OPHTHALMIC CORTICOSTEROIDS**

GENERIC (CHEMICAL) NAME	BRAND (TRADE) NAME	DOSAGE FORMS AND STRENGTHS
Dexamethasone	AK-DEX	Ointment: 0.05% Solution: 0.1%
	DECADRON Phosphate	Ointment: 0.05% Solution: 0.1%
	MAXIDEX	Ointment: 0.05% Suspension: 0.1%
Fluorometholone	FML	Ointment: 0.1% Suspension: 0.1%
	FML Forte	Suspension: 0.25%
Medrysone	HMS	Suspension: 1%
Prednisolone	AK-TATE	Suspension: 1%
	ECONOPRED	Suspension: 0.125%
	ECONOPRED Plus	Suspension: 1%
	INFLAMASE	Solution: 0.125%
	INFLAMASE Forte	Solution: 1%
	PRED Forte	Suspension: 1%
	PRED Mild	Suspension: 0.12%

DRUG PROFILE

These topical drugs are used to reduce the inflammation and other discomfort associated with such eye conditions as allergies, certain types of conjunctivitis, burns, and uveitis (inflammation of the iris and neighboring parts of the eye).

For complete information on these drugs, see pages 996–999.

CONDITION: **CATARACTS**

CATEGORY: **OPHTHALMIC ANTI-INFECTIVES
(AMINOGLYCOSIDES)**

GENERIC (CHEMICAL) NAME	BRAND (TRADE) NAME	DOSAGE FORMS AND STRENGTHS
Gentamicin	GARAMYCIN	Ointment: 0.3% Solution: 0.3%
	GENOPTIC	Ointment: 0.3% Solution: 0.3%
	GENTACIDIN	Ointment: 0.3% Solution: 0.3%
	GENT-AK	Ointment: 0.3% Solution: 0.3%
Neomycin sulfate, polymyxin B sulfate, gramicidin	AK-SPORE	Solution: neomycin sulfate equivalent to 1.75 mg neomycin, 10,000 units polymyxin B sulfate, and 0.025 mg gramicidin per ml
	NEOSPORIN	Solution: neomycin sulfate equivalent to 1.75 mg neomycin, 10,000 units polymyxin B sulfate, and 0.025 mg gramicidin per ml
Tobramycin	TOBREX	Ointment: 0.3% Solution: 0.3%

DRUG PROFILE

These antibiotics are applied directly to the eye to treat infections caused by bacteria. They work by interfering with the manufacture of protein inside the bacterial organism.

For complete information on these drugs, see pages 1000–1003.

CONDITION: **CATARACTS**

CATEGORY: **OPHTHALMIC ANTI-INFECTIVES (BACITRACIN AND BACITRACIN COMBINATIONS)**

GENERIC (CHEMICAL) NAME	BRAND (TRADE) NAME	DOSAGE FORMS AND STRENGTHS
Bacitracin	BACIGUENT	Ointment: 500 units per g
Bacitracin, neomycin sulfate, and polymyxin B sulfate	MYCITRACIN	Ointment: 500 units bacitracin, 10,000 units polymyxin B sulfate, and neomycin sulfate equivalent to 3.5 mg of neomycin
Bacitracin zinc and polymyxin B sulfate	AK-POLY-BAC	Ointment: 500 units bacitracin zinc and 10,000 units polymyxin B sulfate per g
	POLYSPORIN	Ointment: 500 units bacitracin zinc and 10,000 units polymyxin B sulfate per g
Bacitracin zinc, polymyxin B sulfate, and neomycin sulfate	NEOSPORIN	Ointment: 400 units bacitracin zinc, 10,000 units polymyxin B sulfate, and neomycin sulfate equivalent to 3.5 mg of neomycin per g
	AK-SPORE	Ointment: 400 units bacitracin zinc, 10,000 units polymyxin B sulfate, and neomycin sulfate equivalent to 3.5 mg of neomycin

DRUG PROFILE

Bacitracin and bacitracin combinations are used for short-term treatment of bacterial infections of the eye. These antibiotics suppress the growth of bacteria by interfering with the manufacture of protein inside the bacterial organism.

For complete information on these drugs, see pages 1012–1015.

CONDITION: **CATARACTS**

CATEGORY: **OPHTHALMIC ANTI-INFECTIVES (CHLORAMPHENICOL)**

GENERIC (CHEMICAL) NAME	BRAND (TRADE) NAME	DOSAGE FORMS AND STRENGTHS
Chloramphenicol	AK-CHLOR	Ointment: 1% Solution: 0.5%
	CHLOROMYCETIN	Ointment: 1% Powder: to be mixed with sterile distilled water to make 0.16% to 0.5% solution
	CHLOROPTIC	Ointment: 1% Solution: 0.5%
	OPHTHOCHLOR	Solution: 0.5%

DRUG PROFILE

Chloramphenicol is used for short-term treatment of bacterial infections of the eye. This drug suppresses the growth of bacteria by interfering with the manufacture of protein inside the bacterial organism.

For complete information on this drug, see pages 1015–1018.

CONDITION: **CATARACTS**

CATEGORY: **TOPICAL BETA-BLOCKERS**

GENERIC (CHEMICAL) NAME	BRAND (TRADE) NAME	DOSAGE FORMS AND STRENGTHS
Betaxolol hydrochloride	BETOPTIC BETOPTIC S	Solution: 0.5% Suspension: 0.25%
Levobunolol hydrochloride	BETAGAN	Solution: 0.25%, 0.5%
Metipranolol hydrochloride	OPTIPRANOLOL	Solution: 0.3%
Timolol maleate	TIMOPTIC	Solution: 0.25%, 0.5%

DRUG PROFILE

The topical beta-blockers are prescribed, either alone or in combination with other medicine, to treat glaucoma. They are believed to work by lessening the production of aqueous fluid and thereby reducing increased pressure in the eye.

For complete information on these drugs, see pages 978–981.

CONDITION: **CATARACTS**

CATEGORY: **CARBONIC ANHYDRASE INHIBITORS**

GENERIC (CHEMICAL) NAME	BRAND (TRADE) NAME	DOSAGE FORMS AND STRENGTHS
Acetazolamide	DIAMOX	Controlled-release capsules: 500 mg Tablets: 125, 250 mg
Dichlorphenamide	DARANIDE	Tablets: 50 mg
Methazolamide	NEPTAZANE	Tablets: 25, 50 mg

DRUG PROFILE

These drugs are used as supplemental therapy for glaucoma, along with topical medicines that are applied directly to the eye. They decrease the formation of aqueous humor (the fluid inside the front of the eyeball), thereby reducing the increased pressure inside the eye that is the hallmark of glaucoma. These drugs have a slight diuretic effect as well; that is, they help your body rid itself of excess water through increased urination.

For complete information on these drugs, see pages 982–985.

Chapter 13
Cancer

CANCER

Cancer is a major threat to health in this country but no longer the inevitable harbinger of death it was once considered. Great progress has been made in the past twenty-five years in both detecting and managing cancer, resulting in improved survival rates associated with some types of the disease.

CAUSES

No one knows exactly how or why a normal cell loses its blueprint for orderly reproduction and starts to multiply abnormally—spreading, invading, and destroying healthy tissue. We do know, however, that certain risk factors, or conditions, may be related to the development of some cancers in some people. For instance, a woman whose mother or sister had breast cancer is considered at greater risk for developing it herself; childless women are at greater risk for cancers of the reproductive system than are women who were younger than thirty-five when they gave birth. But it's important to remember that not everyone at risk does get cancer, and some people get cancer who were not known to be at any special risk.

We also know that the earlier cancer is found, the more likely it is to be cured or put into a stage of remission, in which it disappears for long periods of time. So it's vital for you to be aware of cancer's warning signals and to consult your doctor promptly if you notice any of them.

DIAGNOSIS AND TREATMENT

Cancer can strike anybody at any age, but certain types of cancer are most often found in people over fifty.

Breast Cancer Changes that might signal breast cancer include a lump or thickening; secretion from the nipples; scaling or puckering of the skin around the nipple; and any alterations in the contour of the breast. The most frequently reported symptom is a breast lump, or tumor. In many cases, this is felt first by the woman herself during a monthly breast self-examination. Most breast lumps are *not* malignant; your doctor may be able to reassure you just by feeling it. Or he or she might biopsy it—that is, remove it surgically, or draw out its contents with a syringe, so that it can be carefully analyzed. Your doctor might also send you for a mammogram, or breast X ray. In fact, experts generally recommend that women past fifty have mammograms once a year in order to discover cancers too small to be found by physical examination.

Breast cancer is most often treated by surgical removal of the breast, the portion of breast that contains the tumor, or the tumor alone. In some cases, the lymph nodes under the arm are also removed. For women with early breast cancer, the trend is definitely toward less radical procedures.

If the breast is not removed, radiation is used to kill any cancer cells remaining in the breast and the area around it. If malignancy has spread to the lymph nodes under the arm, chemotherapy with drugs that kill rapidly dividing cells is usually prescribed. See the drug charts on pages 1059–1079 for a further discussion of these agents. (There are also other available medications that are administered by injection in a hospital or a doctor's office.) In older women, hormone therapy aimed at cutting off the supply of estrogen to the cancer is frequently helpful as well. These agents are described in the drug charts on pages 1051–1056.

Endometrial Cancer Abnormal bleeding or discharge is the primary symptom of this type of cancer, which develops in the tissue lining the uterus. This symptom does not always signal cancer, but it should be reported promptly to your doctor. Early detection of endometrial cancer is possible through regular pelvic exams and Pap tests. (In a Pap test, cells normally shed from the uterus and cervix are examined under the microscope.) The diagnosis is confirmed through biopsy. Treatment is usually removal of the uterus (hysterectomy), sometimes preceded by radiation therapy. In some cases, a synthetic hormone, progestin, which resembles the hormone progesterone, is used to shrink the abnormal endometrium. See the drug chart on pages 1054–1056 for more information on this drug.

Ovarian Cancer The most common symptom of ovarian cancer is abnormal swelling of the abdomen, but persistent stomach discomfort and gas may also be experienced. Evaluation

of this condition often includes X rays of the colon, kidneys, and uterus. To check further, the doctor may perform a procedure known as laparoscopy. This involves inserting a lighted instrument through a small cut in the abdomen so the ovaries can be seen and biopsied. The usual treatment for this type of cancer is removal of one or both ovaries, the fallopian tubes, and the uterus. Chemotherapy often follows. Drugs used to slow or stop the spread of ovarian cancer are discussed in the drug charts on pages 1059–1063 and 1076–1079.

Prostate Cancer Malignancy in this little gland located at the base of the bladder can cause urinary problems in men—but so can the noncancerous enlargement of the prostate that almost always occurs with age. The doctor might suspect cancer from the way the prostate feels during a rectal examination but will probably perform a biopsy to confirm the diagnosis. Many prostate cancers are not considered dangerous, and no treatment is administered. But they are followed up by annual examinations. Treatment alternatives include surgery, radiation, and medicines that deprive the tumor of male hormones or introduce female hormones. These drugs are described in the chart on page 1059.

Lung Cancer Lung cancer is the most common cancer in the United States. It is estimated that 70% of all lung cancer is caused by smoking or environmental pollutants. At present there are, unfortunately, no good screening tests for this malignancy since it develops quickly. Usually, it is found by chest X ray during the course of a routine check-up.

Treatment for this condition may require surgical removal of the lung, or a portion of it. If the cancer has spread, then chemotherapy and/or radiation may be useful in some cases. Usually, when chemotherapy is given in this disease, it must be given by intravenous injection.

Since a large portion of lung cancer in the United States is believed to be the result of smoking and environmental pollutants, prevention must be accomplished by educating the public about the causes of this disease and by encouraging people to stop smoking and to improve the air quality of our environment.

Cancer of the Colon Malignancy of the large intestine is the second most common cancer in the United States. It can arise anywhere from the anus to the beginning of the large intestine. In many families, this cancer seems to be inherited. It is known that in people with polyps of the colon, or with ulcerative colitis, there is an increased chance to develop cancer of the colon.

Colon cancer is cured 50% of the time by surgical removal of the diseased portion of the colon. If the cancer is toward the anus, it may be necessary to perform a colostomy (removal of the anus and rectum and creation of an opening in the abdominal wall for the fecal waste to pass). If

the cancerous tissue is discovered early and it is small in size then the rate of cure is very high, greater than 90%. If the cancer is not detected early and it has spread, then intravenous chemotherapy may be required.

Because early detection is so important for a successful cure and the fact that colon cancer is so common, it is recommended that everyone should have several simple tests to ensure early detection of cancer of the colon. Everyone should consider having a colon examination every 1–3 years. Since intestinal bleeding may be a sign of colon cancer, each person should also have his or her stool checked for blood annually. At least three stools should be checked annually for hidden blood by the use of special cards supplied by your doctor. If there is any blood in the stool or there is obvious rectal bleeding, the colon should be examined either by X ray (barium enema), or by direct visualization (colonoscopy). Every person over the age of 50 should have an annual rectal examination since approximately 50% of these cancers can be detected this way. Individuals with a family history of colon cancer or with ulcerative colitis should have their colon examined annually after age 50.

Cancer of the Bladder and Kidney A portion of the bladder and kidney cancers are caused by environmental pollutants that have entered the body and are excreted into the urine. The hallmark sign of bladder and kidney cancer is bleeding into the urine.

Everyone should have their urine checked annually for the presence of blood. If blood in the urine is detected then the bladder and kidney should be examined. The bladder may be visualized by cystoscopy and the kidney may be examined by X ray, intravenous pyelography, ultrasound, or CT scanning.

Chronic Lymphocytic Leukemia

This cancer creates an excess of immature white cells in the blood that crowd out normal blood cells. Normally the disease comes on slowly, without warning signs. After several years, such symptoms as fatigue, bruising or bleeding, and a decreased ability to fight off infection may develop. This form of leukemia is discovered and diagnosed through blood tests and the analysis of bone marrow. Many times this type of leukemia is asymptomatic and does not require treatment, as it may remain dormant for many years. When leukemia causes symptoms, however, chemotherapy is necessary. For more information on the chemotherapeutic agents used to treat leukemia, see the drug charts on pages 1079–1089.

Multiple Myeloma This malignant tumor of the bone marrow, consisting most often of abnormal plasma cells, leads to the destruction of bone. Painful fractures or curving of the spine may be the first apparent symptoms. X rays may show bone loss, and analysis of the bone marrow will confirm the diagnosis. Chemotherapy is used to decrease the number of abnormal cells. Treatment with drugs generally

continues for at least twelve months. The drugs used are described in the drug charts on pages 1076–1079.

Hodgkin's Disease Although this disease is often considered a young person's disease, it is also common among people over sixty-five. Hodgkin's disease begins in the lymphatic system, which produces certain blood cells and body fluids, filters out bacteria, and temporarily traps cancer cells. The earliest symptom is usually a swollen lymph gland, or node, in the neck, armpit, or groin. Intermittent fevers, night sweats, fatigue, and weight loss may also occur. The first step in diagnosing the condition is a biopsy of the lymph node. If Hodgkin's disease is present, laboratory tests are performed and X rays taken to determine whether the cancer has spread. Treatment generally involves radiation and/or chemotherapy. This therapeutic approach has greatly prolonged the lives of people with advanced Hodgkin's disease. See the drug charts on pages 1059–1063 for detailed information on the chemotherapeutic agents used to treat this disease.

OUTLOOK

Although many cancers in older people tend to grow slowly, cancer may be fatal at any age, and timely detection is vital to achieve the best outcome. If therapy is initiated early in the course of the illness, the large array of treatment possibilities now at hand offers a good chance of remission or cure.

Pregnancy Caution: The drugs in this section can cause birth defects or fetal harm if taken during pregnancy. Check with your doctor if you are or intend to become pregnant.

CONDITION: **BREAST CANCER**
CATEGORY: **HORMONES**

GENERIC (CHEMICAL) NAME	BRAND (TRADE) NAME	DOSAGE FORMS AND STRENGTHS
Tamoxifen citrate	NOLVADEX	Tablets: 10 mg

DRUG PROFILE

Tamoxifen, a hormone, is used to treat advanced cases of breast cancer in post-menopausal women. It is also used to delay recurrence of breast cancer when there is no evidence of tumor spread after breast surgery and in post-menopausal women after breast surgery. Tamoxifen suppresses growth of the tumor, possibly by preventing estrogen from affecting certain tissues.

BEFORE USING THIS DRUG

Let your doctor know *IF*

You have ever had allergic reactions or other problems with ■ tamoxifen.

You have ever had any of the following medical problems: ■ cataracts ■ other eye problems ■ blood clotting disease.

You are taking any of the following medicines: ■ anticoagulants (blood thinners).

SPECIAL RESTRICTIONS WHILE TAKING THIS DRUG

FOOD AND DRUG INTERACTIONS

No special restrictions on other drugs, foods and beverages, alcohol use, or smoking.

DAILY LIVING

Examinations or Tests	It is very important for you to keep all appointments with your doctor so that your progress can be monitored and you can be checked for the occurrence of unwanted side effects.
Other Precautions	See the warning regarding usage during pregnancy on page 1050.
Helpful Hints	This drug may make you vomit or feel nauseated. Eat small, frequent meals to avoid an empty stomach, and keep dry crackers or toast by your bed to nibble on before you get out of bed in the morning. Make sure you get plenty of clear liquids such as carbonated beverages, clear soups, gelatin, and ices or sherbet. Tart foods, such as lemons and sour pickles, may help relieve your nausea. If you vomit shortly after taking a dose of this drug, consult your doctor. Nausea and vomiting often decrease with continued use of this drug. However, if you continue to feel nauseated or to vomit, your doctor may be able to prescribe a drug for your symptoms.

No special restrictions on driving, exertion and exercise, sun exposure, or exposure to excessive heat or cold.

POSSIBLE SIDE EFFECTS

Although this list of adverse effects may seem somewhat intimidating, keep in mind that some are quite rare. Of course, should these or any other problems arise while you are on medication, it is always a good idea to consult your doctor.

IF YOU DEVELOP	WHAT TO DO
blurred vision or other visual disturbances ■ weakness or drowsiness ■ shortness of breath ■ pain or swelling in legs ■ increased bone pain	**May be serious** Check with your doctor as soon as possible.
nausea or vomiting ■ loss of appetite ■ weight gain ■ hot flashes ■ headache ■ dizziness ■ light-headedness ■ depression ■ rash or dry skin ■ itching in genital area ■ vaginal bleeding or discharge ■ changes in menstruation	If symptoms are disturbing or persist, let your doctor know.

STORAGE INSTRUCTIONS

Store in a cool, dark place (not in a bathroom medicine cabinet).

STOPPING OR INTERRUPTING THERAPY

Use this medicine exactly as directed by your doctor, because your dosage has been tailored especially to your needs. Frequent side effects of tamoxifen are nausea and vomiting; even if you experience these effects, do not stop taking this medicine without first checking with your doctor. If you miss a dose, skip it and resume your regular schedule, and check with your doctor.

SPECIAL CONSIDERATIONS FOR THOSE OVER SIXTY-FIVE

None.

CONDITION: **BREAST CANCER AND ENDOMETRIAL CANCER**
CATEGORY: **HORMONES**

GENERIC (CHEMICAL) NAME	BRAND (TRADE) NAME	DOSAGE FORMS AND STRENGTHS
Megestrol acetate	MEGACE	Tablets: 20, 40 mg

DRUG PROFILE

Synthetic progestins like megestrol are used to treat advanced cases of cancer of the uterus (endometrial cancer) and of the breast. Synthetic progestins resemble progesterone, one of the two major female sex hormones. It is not known exactly how megestrol works to suppress the growth of tumors.

BEFORE USING THIS DRUG

Let your doctor know *IF*

You have ever had allergic reactions or other problems with ■ megestrol.

You have ever had the following medical problem: ■ thrombophlebitis (inflammation of the veins of the legs).

SPECIAL RESTRICTIONS WHILE TAKING THIS DRUG

FOOD AND DRUG INTERACTIONS

No special restrictions on other drugs, foods and beverages, alcohol use, or smoking.

DAILY LIVING

Examinations or Tests	It is very important for you to keep all appointments with your doctor so that your progress can be monitored and you can be checked for the occurrence of unwanted side effects.
Other Precautions	See the warning regarding usage during pregnancy on page 1050.

No special restrictions on driving, exertion and exercise, sun exposure, or exposure to excessive heat or cold.

POSSIBLE SIDE EFFECTS

Although this list of adverse affects may seem somewhat intimidating, keep in mind that some are quite rare. Of course, should these or any other problems arise while you are on medication, it is always a good idea to consult your doctor.

IF YOU DEVELOP	WHAT TO DO
severe sudden headaches ■ sudden loss of vision or other visual disturbances ■ chest pain	**Urgent** Get in touch with your doctor immediately.
pain, burning, or tingling in fingers, hands, or elbows ■ pain or swelling of legs, especially calves ■ shortness of breath ■ difficulty breathing ■ rash	**May be serious** Check with your doctor as soon as possible.
weight gain ■ swelling of ankles or feet ■ tiredness or weakness ■ depression ■ hair loss ■ hair growth ■ breast tenderness ■ acne ■ nausea ■ increase or decrease in appetite	If symptoms are disturbing or persist, let your doctor know.

STORAGE INSTRUCTIONS

Store in a cool, dark place (not in a bathroom medicine cabinet).

STOPPING OR INTERRUPTING THERAPY

Use this medicine exactly as directed by your doctor, because your dosage has been tailored especially to your needs. Do not stop taking this medicine without first checking with your doctor. If you miss a dose, skip it and resume your regular schedule, and check with your doctor.

SPECIAL CONSIDERATIONS FOR THOSE OVER SIXTY-FIVE

Older people with reduced liver function may be started on lower dosages of this drug.

CONDITION: **PROSTATIC CANCER**

CATEGORY: **ANTIANDROGENS**

GENERIC (CHEMICAL) NAME	BRAND (TRADE) NAME	DOSAGE FORMS AND STRENGTHS
Flutamide	EULEXIN	Capsules: 125 mg

DRUG PROFILE

Flutamide belongs to the drug category called antiandrogens. It blocks the action of testosterone on the body. Giving flutamide with another medicine is one way of treating cancer of the prostate.

BEFORE USING THIS DRUG

Let your doctor know *IF*

You have ever had allergic problems with ■ flutamide.

SPECIAL RESTRICTIONS WHILE TAKING THIS DRUG

FOOD AND DRUG INTERACTIONS

Other Drugs

In the treatment of cancer of the prostate, flutamide is often taken with another medicine. It is very important that the two medicines be used exactly as directed by your doctor.

No special restrictions on foods and beverages, alcohol use, or smoking.

DAILY LIVING

Examinations and Tests

It is important to keep all appointments with your doctor so that your progress can be checked and to also prevent the occurrence of unwanted side effects.

Other Precautions

See the warning regarding usage during pregnancy on page 1050.

Eulexin lowers sperm count and the medicine used along with it causes sterility. If you intend to have children be sure that you have discussed this with your doctor before taking this medicine.

Helpful Hints

If you vomit soon after taking this drug check with your doctor. You will be told whether to take this dose again or wait until the next scheduled dose.

No special restrictions on driving, exertion and exercise, sun exposure, or exposure to excessive heat or cold.

POSSIBLE SIDE EFFECTS

Although this list of adverse effects may seem somewhat intimidating, keep in mind that some are quite rare. Of course, should these or any other problems arise while you are on medication, it is always a good idea to consult your doctor.

IF YOU DEVELOP	WHAT TO DO
yellowing of eyes or skin	**May be serious** Check with your doctor immediately.
hot flashes ■ decrease in sexual desire ■ impotence ■ nausea or vomiting ■ diarrhea ■ sudden sweating ■ loss of appetite ■ numbness or tingling of hands or feet ■ swelling and increased tenderness of breast ■ swelling of feet or lower legs ■ difficulty in urinating ■ rash	If symptoms are disturbing or persist, let your doctor know.

STORAGE INSTRUCTIONS

Store in a cool, dark place (not in a bathroom medicine cabinet).

STOPPING OR INTERRUPTING THEREAPY

Take this medicine exactly as prescribed by your doctor; it may take several weeks before you see an effect. Do not suddenly discontinue taking this medicine. If you miss a dose take it as soon as possible. If it is almost time for your next dose skip the missed dose and resume your regular schedule. Do not take two doses at the same time.

SPECIAL CONSIDERATIONS FOR THOSE OVER SIXTY-FIVE

None.

CONDITION: **BREAST CANCER AND PROSTATIC CANCER**

CATEGORY: **HORMONES**

GENERIC (CHEMICAL) NAME	BRAND (TRADE) NAME	DOSAGE FORMS AND STRENGTHS
Diethylstilbestrol (DES)		Tablets: 1, 5 mg

DRUG PROFILE

Systemic estrogens (female hormones) are used to help treat the bone loss that occurs in women after menopause or after surgical removal of the uterus and/or ovaries, when the body no longer produces natural estrogens. This drug is also used in other medical conditions such as breast cancer or prostate cancer.

For complete information on this drug, see pages 560–565.

CONDITION: **CANCER (VARIOUS TYPES)**

CATEGORY: **CHEMOTHERAPEUTIC AGENTS**

GENERIC (CHEMICAL) NAME	BRAND (TRADE) NAME	DOSAGE FORMS AND STRENGTHS
Cyclophosphamide	CYTOXAN	Tablets: 25, 50 mg

DRUG PROFILE

Cyclophosphamide is used to treat many types of cancer including leukemia, cancers of the lymph nodes (including Hodgkin's disease), and cancers of the retina of the eye, skin, nervous system, ovaries, and breast. This drug slows or stops the spread of cancer, keeping the cancer cells from multiplying.

BEFORE USING THIS DRUG

Let your doctor know *IF*

You have ever had allergic reactions or other problems with ■ cyclophosphamide.

You have ever had any of the following medical problems: ■ kidney disease ■ liver disease ■ chronic or recurrent infectious disease, such as shingles ■ chickenpox or recent exposure to chickenpox ■ gout ■ diabetes ■ deficient immune system.

You are taking any of the following medicines: ■ any other medicine for cancer ■ medicine for gout ■ corticosteroids ■ sleep medicines ■ medicine for seizures ■ barbiturates ■ diuretics (water pills) ■ insulin ■ estrogens or other sex hormones ■ tranquilizers ■ medicine for bacterial, viral, or fungal infections ■ medicine for malaria ■ medicine for depression ■ cough medicine ■ vitamin A ■ anticoagulants (blood thinners) ■ digoxin (heart medicine).

You have previously received radiation therapy.

SPECIAL RESTRICTIONS WHILE TAKING THIS DRUG

FOOD AND DRUG INTERACTIONS

Other Drugs	If you have diabetes and are taking insulin, your dosage may have to be adjusted.
	Allopurinol (medicine for gout) may increase the side effects of cyclophosphamide.
	Do not have any vaccinations during therapy or for several weeks after stopping therapy without first checking with your doctor. Because of your lowered resistance, which may persist for one to two months after you stop taking this drug, you may get the infection that the immunization is meant to prevent.
Foods and Beverages	To help your kidneys eliminate waste products of this drug, it is very important to drink seven to twelve glasses of water or other fluid every day.

No special restrictions on alcohol use or smoking.

DAILY LIVING

Examinations or Tests	It is very important for you to keep all appointments with your doctor so that your progress can be monitored and the occurrence of unwanted side effects can be checked. Periodic blood tests may be required.
Other Precautions	See the warning regarding usage during pregnancy on page 1050.
	This medicine temporarily makes you more susceptible to infections. While taking this medicine, avoid being with people suffering from colds and other infectious diseases. Call your doctor if you develop a fever.
	Tell any doctor you consult that you are taking this drug, especially if you will be undergoing any type of skin test.
Helpful Hints	This drug may make you vomit or feel nauseated. Eat small, frequent meals to avoid an empty stomach, and keep dry crackers or toast by your bed to nibble on before you get out of bed in the morning. Make sure you get plenty of clear liquids such as carbonated beverages, clear soups, gelatin, and ices or sherbet. Tart foods, such as lemons and sour pickles, may help relieve your nausea. If you vomit shortly after taking a dose of this drug, consult your doctor. Nausea and vomiting often decrease with continued use of this drug. However, if you continue to feel nauseated, your doctor may be able to prescribe a drug for your symptoms.

No special restrictions on driving, exertion and exercise, sun exposure, or exposure to excessive heat or cold.

POSSIBLE SIDE EFFECTS

Although this list of adverse effects may seem somewhat intimidating, keep in mind that some are quite rare. Of course, should these or any other problems arise while you are on medication, it is always a good idea to consult your doctor.

IF YOU DEVELOP	WHAT TO DO
blood in urine ■ pain in urination or other urinary problems ■ fever, chills, or sore throat ■ fast heartbeat ■ difficulty in breathing ■ cough ■ swelling of feet or legs ■ weight gain ■ side, stomach, or joint pain ■ unusual bleeding or bruising *After you STOP taking this medicine:* blood in urine	**Urgent** Get in touch with your doctor immediately.
dizziness ■ confusion ■ nervousness ■ headache ■ diarrhea ■ red or white spots in mouth ■ yellowing of eyes or skin ■ swelling of face ■ slow healing of wounds	**May be serious** Check with your doctor as soon as possible.
loss of appetite ■ nausea or vomiting ■ tiredness or weakness ■ hair loss ■ darkening of the fingernails ■ changes in skin color ■ rash	If symptoms are disturbing or persist, let your doctor know.

STORAGE INSTRUCTIONS

Store in a cool, dark place (not in a bathroom medicine cabinet).

STOPPING OR INTERRUPTING THERAPY

Use this medicine exactly as directed by your doctor, because your dosage has been tailored especially to your needs. Do not stop taking this medicine without first checking with your doctor. If you miss a dose, skip it and resume your regular schedule, and check with your doctor.

SPECIAL CONSIDERATIONS FOR THOSE OVER SIXTY-FIVE

Since kidney function can decrease with age, it is especially important for older people to drink enough water and other fluids to help their kidneys get rid of waste products of this drug. Older people who are especially prone to anemia and especially susceptible to infectious diseases may need frequent medical checkups while on this drug.

CONDITION: **CANCER (VARIOUS TYPES)**

CATEGORY: **CHEMOTHERAPEUTIC AGENTS**

GENERIC (CHEMICAL) NAME	BRAND (TRADE) NAME	DOSAGE FORMS AND STRENGTHS
Chlorambucil	LEUKERAN	Tablets: 2 mg

DRUG PROFILE

Chlorambucil is used to treat chronic lymphatic leukemia and cancers of the lymph nodes (including Hodgkin's disease). This drug slows the growth and spread of cancer cells by interfering with the cell's genetic machinery.

BEFORE USING THIS DRUG

Let your doctor know *IF*

You have ever had allergic reactions or other problems with ■ chlorambucil ■ mephalan.

You have ever had any of the following medical problems: ■ kidney stones ■ chickenpox or recent exposure to chickenpox ■ gout ■ chronic or recurrent infectious diseases, including shingles ■ anemia or other blood disease ■ cancer.

You are taking any of the following medicines: ■ other medicine for cancer ■ medicine for gout ■ corticosteroids ■ medicine for fungal, bacterial, or viral infections ■ medicine for overactive thyroid ■ medicine to prevent rejection of an organ transplant ■ any type of vaccine.

You have previously received radiation therapy or medicine for cancer.

SPECIAL RESTRICTIONS WHILE TAKING THIS DRUG

FOOD AND DRUG INTERACTIONS

Other Drugs	To treat cancer, chlorambucil is sometimes given along with other chemotherapeutic agents. If your doctor has prescribed such combination therapy, be sure to take each medicine at the exact time specified. Your doctor or pharmacist can help you work out a dosing schedule. Do not mix medicines.
	To help your body eliminate uric acid, a metabolic waste product of chlorambucil therapy, your doctor may suggest that you take allopurinol, a medicine that helps the body excrete uric acid.
	Do not have any vaccinations during therapy or for several weeks after stopping therapy without first checking with your doctor. Because of your lowered resistance, which may persist for one to two months after you stop taking this drug, you may get the infection that the immunization is meant to prevent. In addition, you should avoid exposure to individuals who have recently taken oral polio vaccine; if you cannot avoid contact with such persons, consider wearing a mask that will protect your mouth and nose.
Foods and Beverages	To help your kidneys eliminate waste products of this drug, it is very important to drink seven to twelve glasses of water or other fluids every day.

No special restrictions on alcohol use or smoking.

DAILY LIVING

Examinations and Tests	Because this medicine is such a powerful drug and affects many different parts of the body, your doctor will perform a number of tests before and during therapy. It is very important for you to keep all appointments with your doctor so that your progress can be checked.
Other Precautions	See the warning regarding usage during pregnancy on page 1050.

Chlorambucil may cause depression of blood-forming tissues, which leads to easy bleeding and bruising, and increased susceptibility to infections. Therefore, it is important for you to avoid injuries, including small cuts. Check with your doctor before having any dental work done. Instead of brushing, flossing, and using toothpicks, your doctor or dentist may suggest other ways to keep your teeth and gums clean that will minimize the chances of bleeding. Be extra careful when shaving (if you use a safety razor) or when trimming your finger and toe nails. While taking this medicine, avoid being with people who are suffering from colds and other infectious diseases. Make sure not to touch your eyes or the inside of your nose unless you have just washed your hands.

Call your doctor immediately if you develop chills or a fever. |
| Helpful Hints | This drug may make you vomit or feel nauseated. Eat small, frequent meals to avoid an empty stomach, and keep dry crackers or toast by your bed to nibble on before you get out of bed in the morning. Make sure you get plenty of clear liquids such as carbonated beverages, clear soups, gelatin, and ices or sherbet. Tart foods, such as lemons and sour pickles, may help relieve your nausea. If you vomit shortly after taking a dose of this drug, consult your doctor. Nausea and vomiting often decrease with continued use of this drug. However, if you continue |

to feel nauseated, your doctor may be able to pre-scribe a drug for your symptoms.

Even if you feel ill, DO NOT STOP TAKING THIS DRUG without checking with your doctor.

Exertion and Exercise

Discuss with your doctor which kinds of physical ex-ercises are safe for you to undertake, since this drug may make you more susceptible to bleeding from bumps and bruises.

No special restrictions on driving, sun exposure, or exposure to excessive heat or cold.

POSSIBLE SIDE EFFECTS

Although this list of adverse effects may seem somewhat intimidating, keep in mind that some are quite rare. Of course, should these or any other problems arise while you are on medication, it is always a good idea to consult your doctor.

IF YOU DEVELOP

fever or chills and general feeling of being sick ■ bleeding or bruising ■ sores in mouth or on lips ■ difficulty in walking ■ vomiting ■ stomach pain ■ muscle twitching ■ excitement ■ joint pain ■ lower back or side pain ■ seizures ■ swelling of feet, ankles, or legs ■ rash ■ shortness of breath ■ coughing ■ yellowing of eyes or skin ■ unusual lumps

After you STOP taking this medicine: bleeding or bruising ■ fever or chills ■ shortness of breath ■ coughing

WHAT TO DO

Urgent Get in touch with your doctor immediately.

nausea ■ itching ■ for men, diminished fertility ■ absence of menstruation

If symptoms are disturbing or persist, let your doctor know.

STORAGE INSTRUCTIONS

Store in a cool, dark place (not in a bathroom medicine cabinet).

STOPPING OR INTERRUPTING THERAPY

Use this medicine exactly as directed by your doctor because your dosage has been tailored especially to your needs. Do not stop taking this medicine without first checking with your doctor. If you take chlorambucil once a day and you miss a dose, take the missed dose as soon as you remember and resume your regular schedule; if you do not remember until the following day, take the regular dose for that day only and resume your regular schedule. If you take chlorambucil more than once a day and you miss a dose, take the missed dose as soon as you remember; if it is almost time for your next dose, skip the missed dose and resume your regular schedule. Do not take two doses at the same time.

SPECIAL CONSIDERATIONS FOR THOSE OVER SIXTY-FIVE

None.

CONDITION: CANCER (VARIOUS TYPES)

CATEGORY: CHEMOTHERAPEUTIC AGENTS

GENERIC (CHEMICAL) NAME	BRAND (TRADE) NAME	DOSAGE FORMS AND STRENGTHS
Hydroxyurea	HYDREA	Capsules: 500 mg

DRUG PROFILE

Hydroxyurea is used to treat melanoma, cancer of the ovary, cancer of the cervix, advanced cancer of the prostate, and chronic myelocytic leukemia that does not respond to other therapy. This drug may also be used in combination with radiation therapy to treat cancer of the head and neck. It slows and halts the spread of cancer by interfering with the growth and repair mechanisms of cancer cells.

BEFORE USING THIS DRUG

Let your doctor know *IF*

You have ever had allergic reactions or other problems with ■ hydroxyurea.

You have ever had any of the following medical problems: ■ kidney disease ■ kidney stones ■ anemia or other blood disease ■ chickenpox or recent exposure to chickenpox ■ gout ■ chronic or recurrent infectious diseases, including shingles ■ cancer.

You are taking any of the following medicines: ■ other medicine for cancer ■ medicine for gout ■ medicine for overactive thyroid ■ medicine for bacterial, fungal, or viral infections ■ medicine to prevent rejection of an organ transplant ■ azathioprine ■ any type of vaccine.

You have previously received radiation therapy or medicine for cancer.

SPECIAL RESTRICTIONS WHILE TAKING THIS DRUG

FOOD AND DRUG INTERACTIONS

Other Drugs	To treat cancer, hydroxyurea is sometimes given along with another chemotherapeutic agent. If your doctor has prescribed such combination therapy, be sure to take each medicine at the exact time specified. Do not mix medicines.
	To help your body eliminate uric acid, a metabolic waste product of hydroxyurea therapy, your doctor may suggest that you take allopurinol, a medicine that helps the body excrete uric acid.

Do not have any vaccinations during therapy or for several weeks after stopping therapy without first checking with your doctor. Because of your lowered resistance, which may persist for one to two months after you stop taking this drug, you may get the infection that the immunization is meant to prevent. In addition, you should avoid exposure to individuals who have recently taken oral polio vaccine; if you cannot avoid contact with such persons, consider wearing a mask that will protect your mouth and nose.

Foods and Beverages	To help your kidneys eliminate waste products of this drug, it is very important to drink seven to twelve glasses of water or other fluids every day.

No special restrictions on alcohol use or smoking.

DAILY LIVING

Examinations and Tests	Because this medicine is such a powerful drug and affects many different parts of the body, your doctor will perform a number of tests before and during therapy. It is very important for you to keep all appointments with your doctor so that your progress can be checked.
Other Precautions	See the warning regarding usage during pregnancy on page 1050.

See the warning regarding usage during pregnancy on page 1050.

Hydroxyurea may cause depression of blood-forming tissues, which leads to easy bleeding and bruising, and increased susceptibility to infections. Therefore, it is important for you to avoid injuries, including small cuts. Check with your doctor before having any dental work done. Instead of brushing, flossing, and using toothpicks, your doctor or dentist may suggest other ways to keep your teeth and gums clean that will minimize the chances of bleeding.

Be extra careful when shaving (if you use a safety razor) or when trimming your finger and toe nails. While taking this medicine, avoid being with people who are suffering from colds and other infectious diseases. Make sure not to touch your eyes or the inside of your nose unless you have just washed your hands.

Call your doctor immediately if you develop chills or a fever.

Helpful Hints

If you find the capsules difficult to swallow, you can empty the contents of a capsule into a glass of water and drink the mixture immediately.

This drug may make you vomit or feel nauseated. Eat small, frequent meals to avoid an empty stomach, and keep dry crackers or toast by your bed to nibble on before you get out of bed in the morning. Make sure you get plenty of clear liquids such as carbonated beverages, clear soups, gelatin, and ices or sherbet. Tart foods, such as lemons and sour pickles, may help relieve your nausea. If you vomit shortly after taking a dose of this drug, consult your doctor. Nausea and vomiting often decrease with continued use of this drug. However, if you continue to feel nauseated, your doctor may be able to prescribe a drug for your symptoms.

Driving

This drug may cause drowsiness. Avoid driving until you know how this drug will affect you.

Exertion and Exercise

Discuss with your doctor which kinds of physical exercises are safe for you to undertake, since this drug may make you more susceptible to bleeding from bumps and bruises.

You are taking any of the following medicines: ■ aspirin or aspirinlike medicine ■ vitamins containing folic acid ■ anticoagulants (blood thinners) ■ medicine for infections ■ medicine for seizures ■ medicine for gout ■ nonsteroidal anti-inflammatory drugs, NSAIDs (medicine for arthritis) ■ medicine for malaria.

You have previously received radiation therapy or medicine for cancer.

SPECIAL RESTRICTIONS WHILE TAKING THIS DRUG

FOOD AND DRUG INTERACTIONS

Other Drugs	While you are taking this medicine, it is important to tell your doctor about all other drugs you may be taking.
	Do not have any vaccinations during therapy or for several weeks after stopping therapy without checking with your doctor. Because of your lowered resistance, which may persist for one to two months after you stop taking the drug, you may get the infection that the immunization is meant to prevent.
Foods and Beverages	To help your kidneys eliminate waste products of this drug, it is very important to drink seven to twelve glasses of water or other liquids every day.
Alcohol	Do not drink alcohol while taking this medicine. This combination may be especially damaging to your liver.

No special restrictions on smoking.

DAILY LIVING

Driving	This medicine may cause drowsiness or dizziness. Be careful when driving, operating household appliances, or doing any other tasks that require alertness until you know how this drug affects you.

Sun Exposure	Your skin may become more sensitive to sunlight and more likely to develop a sunburn, and your eyes may become more sensitive to light. It is a good idea to avoid too much sun, wear tinted sunglasses, and apply a sunscreen to exposed skin surfaces before going outdoors.
Examinations or Tests	Because this medicine is such a powerful drug and affects many different parts of the body, your doctor will perform a number of tests before and during therapy. It is very important for you to keep all appointments with your doctor so that your progress can be monitored and the occurrence of unwanted side effects can be checked.
Other Precautions	See the warning regarding usage during pregnancy on page 1050. This medicine temporarily makes you more susceptible to infections. While taking this medicine, avoid being with people who are suffering from colds and other infectious diseases. Call your doctor if you develop a fever.
Helpful Hints	This drug may make you vomit or feel nauseated. Eat small, frequent meals to avoid an empty stomach, and keep dry crackers or toast by your bed to nibble on before you get out of bed in the morning. Make sure you get plenty of clear liquids such as carbonated beverages, clear soups, gelatin, and ices or sherbet. Tart foods, such as lemons and sour pickles, may help relieve your nausea. If you vomit shortly after taking a dose of this drug, consult your doctor. Nausea and vomiting often decrease with continued use of this drug. However, if you continue to vomit or to feel nauseated, your doctor may be able to prescribe a drug for your symptoms.

No special restrictions on exertion and exercise or exposure to excessive heat or cold.

POSSIBLE SIDE EFFECTS

Although this list of adverse effects may seem somewhat intimidating, keep in mind that some are quite rare. Of course, should these or any other problems arise while you are on medication, it is always a good idea to consult your doctor.

IF YOU DEVELOP

diarrhea ■ stomach pain ■ bloody or black, tarry stools ■ vomiting, with blood or vomit that looks like coffee grounds ■ fever, chills, or sore throat ■ bleeding or bruising ■ red spots on skin ■ sores or bleeding around the mouth ■ irritation or bleeding of gums ■ swelling of the tongue or vocal cords ■ shortness of breath ■ dark or bloody urine ■ seizures

WHAT TO DO

Urgent Get in touch with your doctor immediately.

---

nausea or vomiting ■ stomach discomfort ■ cough ■ headache ■ drowsiness ■ blurred vision ■ dizziness ■ swelling of feet, ankles, or legs ■ joint pain ■ decreased urination

After you STOP taking this medicine: blurred vision ■ confusion ■ dizziness ■ drowsiness ■ headache ■ tiredness or weakness

May be serious Check with your doctor as soon as possible.

---

hair loss ■ loss of appetite ■ rash, hives, or itching ■ acne ■ change in skin color ■ increased skin or eye sensitivity to sunlight

If symptoms are disturbing or persist, let your doctor know.

STORAGE INSTRUCTIONS

Store in a cool, dark place (not in a bathroom medicine cabinet).

STOPPING OR INTERRUPTING THERAPY

Use this medicine exactly as directed by your doctor, because your dosage has been tailored especially to your needs. If you miss a dose, skip it and resume your regular schedule, and check with your doctor.

SPECIAL CONSIDERATIONS FOR THOSE OVER SIXTY-FIVE

Since kidney function can decrease with age, it is especially important for older people to drink plenty of water and other fluids to help their kidneys get rid of waste products of this drug. Older people may be especially prone to the side effects of dizziness or drowsiness. Those older people who are especially prone to anemia and especially susceptible to infectious disease may need frequent medical check-ups while on this drug.

CONDITION: **CANCER (VARIOUS TYPES)**

CATEGORY: **CHEMOTHERAPEUTIC AGENTS**

GENERIC (CHEMICAL) NAME	BRAND (TRADE) NAME	DOSAGE FORMS AND STRENGTHS
Melphalan	ALKERAN	Tablets: 2 mg

DRUG PROFILE

Melphalan is used to treat breast cancer, multiple myeloma (bone cancer), and cancer of the ovaries that cannot be operated on. This drug slows and halts the growth and spread of cancer cells.

BEFORE USING THIS DRUG

Let your doctor know *IF*

You have ever had allergic reactions or other problems with ■ melphalan
■ chlorambucil (another medicine for cancer).

You have ever had any of the following medical problems: ■ kidney disease, including kidney stones ■ gout ■ chronic or recurrent infectious diseases, including shingles ■ chickenpox or recent exposure to chickenpox.

You are taking any of the following medicines: ■ any other medicine for cancer ■ medicine for gout.

You have previously received radiation therapy or medicine for cancer.

SPECIAL RESTRICTIONS WHILE TAKING THIS DRUG

FOOD AND DRUG INTERACTIONS

Other Drugs	Do not have any vaccinations during therapy or for several weeks after stopping therapy without checking with your doctor. Because of your lowered resistance, which may persist for one to two months after you stop taking the drug, you may get the infection that the immunization is meant to prevent.
Foods and Beverages	To help your body eliminate waste products of this drug, it is very important to drink seven to twelve glasses of water or other fluids every day.

No special restrictions on alcohol use or smoking.

DAILY LIVING

Examinations or Tests	It is very important for you to keep all appointments with your doctor so that your progress can be monitored and the occurrence of unwanted side effects can be checked. Periodic blood tests may be required.
Other Precautions	See the warning regarding usage during pregnancy on page 1050. This medicine temporarily makes you more susceptible to infections. While taking this medicine, avoid

being with people who are suffering from colds and other infectious diseases. Call your doctor if you develop a fever.

Let any doctor you consult know you are taking this drug, especially if you will be undergoing any type of skin test.

Helpful Hints

This drug may make you vomit or feel nauseated. Eat small, frequent meals to avoid an empty stomach, and keep dry crackers or toast by your bed to nibble on before you get out of bed in the morning. Make sure you get plenty of clear liquids, such as carbonated beverages, clear soups, gelatin, and ices or sherbet. Tart foods, such as lemons and sour pickles, may help relieve your nausea. If you vomit shortly after taking a dose of this drug, consult your doctor. Nausea and vomiting often decrease with continued use of this drug. However, if you continue to feel nauseated or to vomit, your doctor may be able to prescribe a drug for your symptoms.

No special restrictions on driving, exertion and exercise, sun exposure, or exposure to excessive heat or cold.

POSSIBLE SIDE EFFECTS

Although this list of adverse effects may seem somewhat intimidating, keep in mind that some are quite rare. Of course, should these or any other problems arise while you are on medication, it is always a good idea to consult your doctor.

IF YOU DEVELOP

rash, hives, or itching ■ bleeding or bruising ■ fever, chills, or sore throat ■ shortness of breath ■ cough ■ side, stomach, or joint pain ■ swelling of feet, ankles, or legs ■ bloody or black, tarry stools ■ chest pain ■ unusual lumps

WHAT TO DO

Urgent Get in touch with your doctor immediately.

nausea or vomiting	**May be serious** Check with your doctor as soon as possible.
hair loss ■ diarrhea ■ mouth sores ■ absence of menstruation	If symptoms are disturbing or persist, let your doctor know.

STORAGE INSTRUCTIONS

Store in a cool, dark place (not in a bathroom medicine cabinet).

STOPPING OR INTERRUPTING THERAPY

Use this medicine exactly as directed by your doctor, because your dosage has been tailored especially to your needs. Do not stop taking this medicine without first checking with your doctor. If you miss a dose, skip it and resume your regular schedule, and check with your doctor.

SPECIAL CONSIDERATIONS FOR THOSE OVER SIXTY-FIVE

Since kidney function can decrease with age, it is especially important for older people to drink enough water and other fluids to help their kidneys eliminate waste products of this drug. Those older people who are especially prone to anemia and especially susceptible to infectious disease may need frequent medical checkups while on this drug.

CONDITION: **LEUKEMIA**

CATEGORY: **CHEMOTHERAPEUTIC AGENTS**

GENERIC (CHEMICAL) NAME	BRAND (TRADE) NAME	DOSAGE FORMS AND STRENGTHS
Busulfan	MYLERAN	Tablets: 2 mg

DRUG PROFILE

Busulfan is used to treat certain types of leukemia. It works by interfering with the growth of cancer cells—especially in the bone marrow, where many blood cells are manufactured.

BEFORE USING THIS DRUG

Let your doctor know *IF*

You have ever had allergic reactions or other problems with ■ busulfan.

You have ever had any of the following medical problems: ■ kidney disease, including kidney stones ■ chronic or recurrent infectious diseases, such as shingles ■ chickenpox or recent exposure to chickenpox ■ gout ■ asthma or other lung disease ■ anemia.

You are taking the following medicine: ■ medicines for gout.

You have previously received radiation therapy or medicine for cancer.

SPECIAL RESTRICTIONS BEFORE USING THIS DRUG

FOOD AND DRUG INTERACTIONS

Other Drugs	Do not have any vaccinations during therapy or for several weeks after stopping therapy without checking with your doctor. Because of your lowered resistance, which may persist for one to two months after you stop taking the drug, you may get the infection that the immunization is meant to prevent.
Foods and Beverages	To help your body eliminate the waste products of this drug, it is very important to drink seven to twelve glasses of water or other fluids every day.

No special restrictions on alcohol use or smoking.

DAILY LIVING

Examinations or Tests	It is very important for you to keep all appointments with your doctor so that your progress can be monitored and the occurrence of unwanted side effects can be checked. Blood tests may be required before and during therapy.
Other Precautions	See the warning regarding usage during pregnancy on page 1050. This medicine temporarily makes you more susceptible to infections. While taking this medicine, avoid being with people suffering from colds and other infectious diseases. Call your doctor if you develop a fever. Let any doctor you consult know you are taking this drug, especially if you will be undergoing any type of skin test.
Helpful Hints	This drug may make you vomit or feel nauseated. Eat small, frequent meals to avoid an empty stomach, and keep dry crackers or toast by your bed to nibble on before you get out of bed in the morning. Make sure you get plenty of clear liquids such as carbonated beverages, clear soups, gelatin, and ices or sherbet. Tart foods, such as lemons and sour pickles, may help relieve your nausea. If you vomit shortly after taking a dose of this drug, consult your doctor. Nausea and vomiting often decrease with continued use of this drug. However, if you continue to feel nauseated or to vomit, your doctor may be able to prescribe a drug for your symptoms.

No special restrictions on driving, exertion and exercise, sun exposure, or exposure to excessive heat or cold.

POSSIBLE SIDE EFFECTS

Although this list of adverse effects may seem somewhat intimidating, keep in mind that some are quite rare. Of course, should these or any other problems arise while you are on medication, it is always a good idea to consult your doctor.

IF YOU DEVELOP	WHAT TO DO
bleeding or bruising ■ fever, chills, or sore throat ■ shortness of breath or difficulty breathing ■ cough ■ chest congestion ■ side, stomach, or joint pain ■ sores or cracks on lips or in mouth ■ swelling of tongue ■ gout ■ yellowing of eyes or skin	**Urgent** Get in touch with your doctor immediately.
swelling of feet, ankles, or legs ■ confusion ■ rash or hives ■ unusual tiredness or weakness *After you STOP taking this medicine:* bleeding or bruising ■ fever ■ cough ■ shortness of breath	**May be serious** Check with your doctor as soon as possible.
diarrhea ■ nausea or vomiting ■ weight loss ■ loss of appetite ■ drowsiness ■ male breast swelling ■ darkening of skin or other skin changes ■ dry mouth, throat, or nose ■ hair loss ■ decreased sweating ■ absence of menstruation	If symptoms are disturbing or persist, let your doctor know.

STORAGE INSTRUCTIONS

Store in a cool, dark place (not in a bathroom medicine cabinet).

STOPPING OR INTERRUPTING THERAPY

Use this medicine exactly as directed by your doctor, because your dosage has been tailored especially to your needs. Do not stop taking this medicine without first checking with your doctor. If you miss a dose, skip it and resume your regular schedule, and check with your doctor.

SPECIAL CONSIDERATIONS FOR THOSE OVER SIXTY-FIVE

Since kidney function can decrease with age, it is especially important for older people to drink enough water and other fluids to help their kidneys get rid of the waste products of this drug. Those older people who are especially prone to anemia and especially susceptible to infectious disease may need frequent medical checkups while on this drug.

CONDITION: **LEUKEMIA**

CATEGORY: **CHEMOTHERAPEUTIC AGENTS**

GENERIC (CHEMICAL) NAME	BRAND (TRADE) NAME	DOSAGE FORMS AND STRENGTHS
Mercaptopurine	PURINETHOL	Tablets: 50 mg

DRUG PROFILE

Mercaptopurine is used to treat certain forms of leukemia. It halts the growth and spread of cancer cells by interfering with the ability of these cells to manufacture and use DNA, a building block of all life.

BEFORE USING THIS DRUG

Let your doctor know *IF*

You have ever had allergic reactions or other problems with ■ mercaptopurine.

You have ever had any of the following medical problems: ■ kidney disease ■ liver disease ■ chronic or recurrent infectious disease, such as shingles ■ chickenpox or recent exposure to chickenpox ■ gout ■ anemia.

You are taking the following medicine: ■ medicines for gout, especially allopurinol.

You have previously received radiation therapy or medicine for cancer.

SPECIAL RESTRICTIONS WHILE TAKING THIS DRUG

FOOD AND DRUG INTERACTIONS

Other Drugs	Medicine for gout (especially allopurinol) may worsen some side effects of this drug when the drugs are taken together. Check with your doctor if you are taking medicine for gout.
	Do not have any vaccinations during therapy or for several weeks after stopping therapy without checking with your doctor. Because of your lowered resistance, which may persist for one to two months after you stop taking this drug, you may get the infection that the immunization is meant to prevent.
Foods and Beverages	To help your body eliminate the waste products of this drug, it is very important to drink seven to twelve glasses of water or other fluids every day.
	Although you may lose your appetite or feel sick when taking this drug, it is important to follow a nutritious diet.

No special restrictions on alcohol use or smoking.

DAILY LIVING

Examinations or Tests	Because this drug is very powerful and affects many different parts of the body, your doctor will perform a number of tests before and during therapy. It is very important for you to keep all appointments with your doctor so that your progress can be monitored and the occurrence of unwanted side effects can be checked.

Other Precautions	See the warning regarding usage during pregnancy on page 1050.
	This medicine temporarily makes you more susceptible to infections. While taking this medicine, avoid being with people who are suffering from colds or other infectious diseases. Call your doctor if you develop a fever.

No special restrictions on driving, exertion and exercise, sun exposure, or exposure to excessive heat or cold.

POSSIBLE SIDE EFFECTS

Although this list of adverse effects may seem somewhat intimidating, keep in mind that some are quite rare. Of course, should these or any other problems arise while you are on medication, it is always a good idea to consult your doctor.

IF YOU DEVELOP	WHAT TO DO
fever, chills, or sore throat ■ bleeding or bruising ■ side, stomach, or joint pain ■ swelling of feet, ankles, or legs ■ blood in urine ■ decreased urination ■ yellowing of eyes or skin ■ loss of appetite with stomach tenderness	**Urgent** Get in touch with your doctor immediately.
diarrhea ■ darkening of skin ■ rash ■ headache ■ sores on lips or in mouth *After you STOP taking this medicine:* fever, chills, or sore throat ■ bleeding or bruising ■ yellowing of eyes or skin	**May be serious** Check with your doctor as soon as possible.
loss of appetite ■ nausea or vomiting ■ weakness	If symptoms are disturbing or persist, let your doctor know.

STORAGE INSTRUCTIONS

Store in a cool, dark place (not in a bathroom medicine cabinet).

STOPPING OR INTERRUPTING THERAPY

Use this medicine exactly as directed by your doctor, because your dosage has been tailored especially to your needs. Do not stop taking this medicine without first checking with your doctor. If you miss a dose, skip it and resume your regular schedule, and check with your doctor.

SPECIAL CONSIDERATIONS FOR THOSE OVER SIXTY-FIVE

Since kidney function can decrease with age, it is especially important for older people to drink plenty of water and other fluids to help their kidneys get rid of waste products of this drug. Those older patients who are also especially prone to anemia and especially susceptible to infectious disease may need frequent checkups while on this drug.

CONDITION: **LEUKEMIA**

CATEGORY: **CHEMOTHERAPEUTIC AGENTS**

GENERIC (CHEMICAL) NAME	BRAND (TRADE) NAME	DOSAGE FORMS AND STRENGTHS
Thioguanine		Tablets: 40 mg

DRUG PROFILE

Thioguanine is used to treat certain forms of leukemia. It halts the growth and spread of cancer cells by interfering with the ability of these cells to manufacture and use DNA, a building block of all life.

BEFORE USING THIS DRUG

Let your doctor know *IF*

You have ever had allergic reactions or other problems with ■ thioguanine.

You have ever had any of the following medical problems: ■ kidney disease, including kidney stones ■ liver disease ■ current infection ■ chronic or recurrent infectious disease, such as shingles ■ chickenpox or recent exposure to chickenpox ■ gout.

You are taking the following medicine: ■ medicines for gout, especially allopurinol.

You have previously received radiation therapy or medicine for cancer.

SPECIAL RESTRICTIONS WHILE TAKING THIS DRUG

FOOD AND DRUG INTERACTIONS

Other Drugs	Do not have any vaccinations during therapy or for several weeks after stopping therapy without checking with your doctor. Because of your lowered resistance, which may persist for one to two months after you stop taking the drug, you may get the infection that the immunization is meant to prevent.
Foods and Beverages	To help your body eliminate the waste products of this drug, it is very important to drink seven to twelve glasses of water or other fluids every day.

No special restrictions on other drugs, alcohol use, or smoking.

DAILY LIVING

Examinations or Tests	It is very important for you to keep all appointments with your doctor so that your progress can be monitored and the occurrence of unwanted side effects can be checked. Blood tests before and during therapy are usually required.
Other Precautions	See the warning regarding usage during pregnancy on page 1050. This medicine temporarily makes you more susceptible to infections. While taking this medicine, avoid being with people suffering from colds or other infectious diseases. Call your doctor if you develop a fever.
Helpful Hints	This drug may make you vomit or feel nauseated. Eat small, frequent meals to avoid an empty stomach, and keep dry crackers or toast by your bed to nibble on before you get out of bed in the morning. Make sure you get plenty of clear liquids such as carbonated beverages, clear soups, gelatin, and ices or sherbet. Tart foods, such as lemons and sour pickles, may help relieve your nausea. If you vomit shortly after taking a dose of this drug, consult your doctor. Nausea and vomiting usually decrease with continued use of this drug. However, if you continue to feel nauseated or to vomit, your doctor may be able to prescribe a drug for your symptoms.

No special restrictions on driving, exertion and exercise, sun exposure, or exposure to excessive heat or cold.

POSSIBLE SIDE EFFECTS

Although this list of adverse effects may seem somewhat intimidating, keep in mind that some are quite rare. Of course, should these or any other problems arise while you are on medication, it is always a good idea to consult your doctor.

IF YOU DEVELOP	WHAT TO DO
fever, chills, or sore throat ■ bleeding or bruising ■ side, stomach, or joint pain ■ swelling of feet, ankles, or legs ■ yellowing of eyes or skin	**Urgent** Get in touch with your doctor immediately.
diarrhea, sometimes severe ■ nausea or vomiting ■ rash, itching, or skin irritation ■ unsteady walk ■ mouth sores *After you STOP taking this medicine:* fever, chills, or sore throat ■ bleeding or bruising	**May be serious** Check with your doctor as soon as possible.
loss of ability to sense vibrations	If symptoms are disturbing or persist, let your doctor know.

STORAGE INSTRUCTIONS

Store in a cool, dark place (not in a bathroom medicine cabinet).

STOPPING OR INTERRUPTING THERAPY

Use this medicine exactly as directed by your doctor, because your dosage has been tailored especially to your needs. Do not stop taking this medicine without first checking with your doctor. If you miss a dose, skip it and resume your regular schedule, and check with your doctor.

SPECIAL CONSIDERATIONS FOR THOSE OVER SIXTY-FIVE

Since kidney function can decrease with age, it is especially important for older people to drink enough water and other fluids to help their kidneys get rid of the waste products of this drug. Those older patients who are especially prone to anemia and especially susceptible to infectious disease may need frequent checkups while on this drug.

CONDITION: **LEUKEMIA**
CATEGORY: **CORTICOSTEROIDS**

GENERIC (CHEMICAL) NAME	BRAND (TRADE) NAME	DOSAGE FORMS AND STRENGTHS
Prednisone	DELTASONE	Tablets: 2.5, 5, 10, 20, 50 mg

DRUG PROFILE

Oral corticosteroids (also known as steroids) are used to treat a wide variety of inflammatory diseases, such as arthritis, and other rheumatic disorders such as lupus. Prednisone is a corticosteroid that also is used as part of a regimen to treat certain types of leukemia and Hodgkin's disease.

For complete information on this drug, see pages 530–535.

CONDITION: **CANCER**
CATEGORY: **FOLIC ACID—ANTAGONIST ANTIDOTE**

GENERIC (CHEMICAL) NAME	BRAND (TRADE) NAME	DOSAGE FORMS AND STRENGTHS
Leucovorin calcium	WELLCOVORIN	Tablets: 5, 25 mg Oral Solution: 5 mg per tsp

DRUG PROFILE

Leucovorin is used to treat and counteract the harmful effects of certain cancer medications such as methotrexate. It is also used in combination with other cancer drugs to treat colon and rectal cancers. It is sometimes used to treat certain kinds of anemia.

BEFORE USING THIS DRUG

Let your doctor know *IF*

You have ever had allergic reactions or other problems with ■ leucovorin.

You have ever had any of the following medical problems: ■ kidney disease ■ nausea or vomiting caused by current drug therapy or illness ■ anemia or vitamin B_{12} deficiencies.

SPECIAL RESTRICTIONS WHILE TAKING THIS DRUG

FOOD AND DRUG INTERACTIONS

No special restrictions on other drugs, foods and beverages, alcohol use, or smoking.

DAILY LIVING

Examinations or Tests	It is important for you to keep all appointments with your doctor so that your progress can be checked. Periodic blood tests will be required.
Other Precautions	See the warning regarding usage during pregnancy on page 1050.
	If you vomit soon after a dose of this drug, or if you inadvertently miss a dose, contact your doctor immediately for instructions.

No special restrictions on driving, exertion and exercise, sun exposure, or exposure to excessive heat or cold.

POSSIBLE SIDE EFFECTS

Although this list of adverse effects may seem somewhat intimidating, keep in mind that some are quite rare. Of course, should these or any other problems arise while you are on medication, it is always a good idea to consult your doctor.

IF YOU DEVELOP	WHAT TO DO
wheezing ■ rash or hives ■ itching	**Urgent** Get in touch with your doctor immediately.

STORAGE INSTRUCTIONS

Store in a cool, dark place (not in a bathroom medicine cabinet).

STOPPING OR INTERRUPTING THERAPY

This medicine should be taken exactly as prescribed by your doctor. If you miss a dose, contact your doctor immediately for instructions.

SPECIAL CONSIDERATIONS FOR THOSE OVER SIXTY-FIVE

None.

INDICES

INDEX TO THE COLOR IDENTIFICATION GUIDE

Drugs are listed in this index alphabetically by brand (trade) name and dosage strength. Each entry in this index will direct you to the page (A1 through A35) and row (a through e) where the color picture of the particular drug is located. Only tablets and capsules appear in the Color Identification Guide.

INDEX OF DRUGS

Words in all capital letters are brand-name drugs. Bold-face page numbers in this index refer to the chart that summarizes information about the particular drug.

INDEX OF MEDICAL CONDITIONS

Note: Bold-face page numbers in this index refer to descriptions of medical conditions in the text. Following each medical description are the drug charts that summarize information about the drugs prescribed for a particular condition. Page numbers for the drug charts are given in the table of contents at the beginning of this book.

Color Identification Guide

a				
LEVOTHROID 0.2 mg levothyroxine	ZESTRIL 5 mg lisinopril	DIULO 2.5 mg metolazone	CALAN 40 mg verapamil	MELLARIL 15 mg thioridazine	PROLIXIN 1 mg fluphenazine

b				
SYNTHROID 0.2 mg levothyroxine	SYNTHROID 0.112 mg levothyroxine	ISORDIL Oral 5 mg isosorbide dinitrate	MICRONASE 2.5 mg glyburide	ZESTRIL 10 mg lisinopril	ZESTRIL 20 mg lisinopril

c				
LOTENSIN 20 mg benazepril	CELESTONE 0.6 mg betamethasone	ESTINYL 0.05 mg ethinyl estradiol	SER-AP-ES reserpine, hydralazine & hydrochlorothiazide	COUMADIN 1 mg warfarin	PROCARDIA XL 30 mg nifedipine

d				
PARNATE 10 mg tranylcypromine	DIUPRES-250 reserpine & chlorothiazide	PHENERGAN 50 mg promethazine	METAHYDRIN 2 mg trichlormethiazide	LITHOBID 300 mg lithium carbonate	LARODOPA 250 mg levodopa

e				
ORGANIDIN iodinated glycerol	BUTISOL Sodium 100 mg sodium butabarbital	CORDARONE 200 mg amiodarone	PROCARDIA XL 60 mg nifedipine	DIUPRES-500 reserpine & chlorothiazide	ELAVIL 100 mg amitriptyline

Color Identification Guide

a	SEPTRA trimethoprim & sulfamethoxazole	ROBAXISAL methocarbamol & aspirin	RUFEN 400 mg ibuprofen	ETRAFON 2-25 perphenazine & amitriptyline hydrochloride	COMBIPRES 0.1 mg clonidine hydrochloride & chlorthalidone
b	MEDROL 2 mg methylprednisolone	LARODOPA 100 mg levodopa	DEPAKOTE 125 mg divalproex sodium	BUMEX 2 mg bumetanide	CALAN SR 180 mg verapamil
c	ISOPTIN SR 180 mg verapamil	ERY-TAB 250 mg erythromycin	DEPAKOTE 500 mg divalproex sodium	ERY-TAB 500 mg erythromycin	E.E.S. 400 erythromycin ethylsuccinate
d	ERYTHROCIN Stearate 500 mg erythromycin stearate	SEPTRA DS trimethoprim & sulfamethoxazole		CHOLEDYL SA 400 mg oxtriphylline	DIAβETA 2.5 mg glyburide
e	LOPRESSOR 50 mg metoprolol tartrate	TEGRETOL 200 mg carbamazepine	LOPRESSOR HCT 100/25 metoprolol tartrate & hydrochlorothiazide	NAPROSYN 375 mg naproxen	LARODOPA 500 mg levodopa

PROCARDIA XL
90 mg
nifedipine

Color Identification Guide

a					
TRENTAL 400 mg pentoxifylline	CARAFATE 1 g sucralfate		LITHONATE 300 mg lithium carbonate	DARVON 65 mg propoxyphene hydrochloride	
b					
SINEQUAN 75 mg doxepin	SUMYCIN 250 mg tetracycline	DILATRATE-SR 40 mg isosorbide dinitrate	ACTIGALL 300 mg ursodiol	BENADRYL 25 mg diphenhydramine hydrochloride	BENADRYL 50 mg diphenhydramine hydrochloride
c					
SERAX 10 mg oxazepam	MINIPRESS 2 mg prazosin	APRESAZIDE 50/50 hydralazine & hydrochlorothiazide	SUMYCIN 500 mg tetracycline	SINEQUAN 50 mg doxepin	AMOXIL 250 mg amoxicillin
d					
AMOXIL 500 mg amoxicillin	HYDREA 500 mg hydroxyurea	DIFLUCAN 50 mg fluconazole	REGROTON reserpine & chlorthalidone	NAQUA 2 mg trichlormethiazide	TRANXENE T-TAB 15 mg chlorazepate
e					
VASERETIC 10-25 enalapril & hydrochlorothiazide	INDERAL 60 mg propranolol	TENEX 1 mg guanfacine	DIFLUCAN 100 mg fluconazole	DIFLUCAN 200 mg fluconazole	

Color Identification Guide

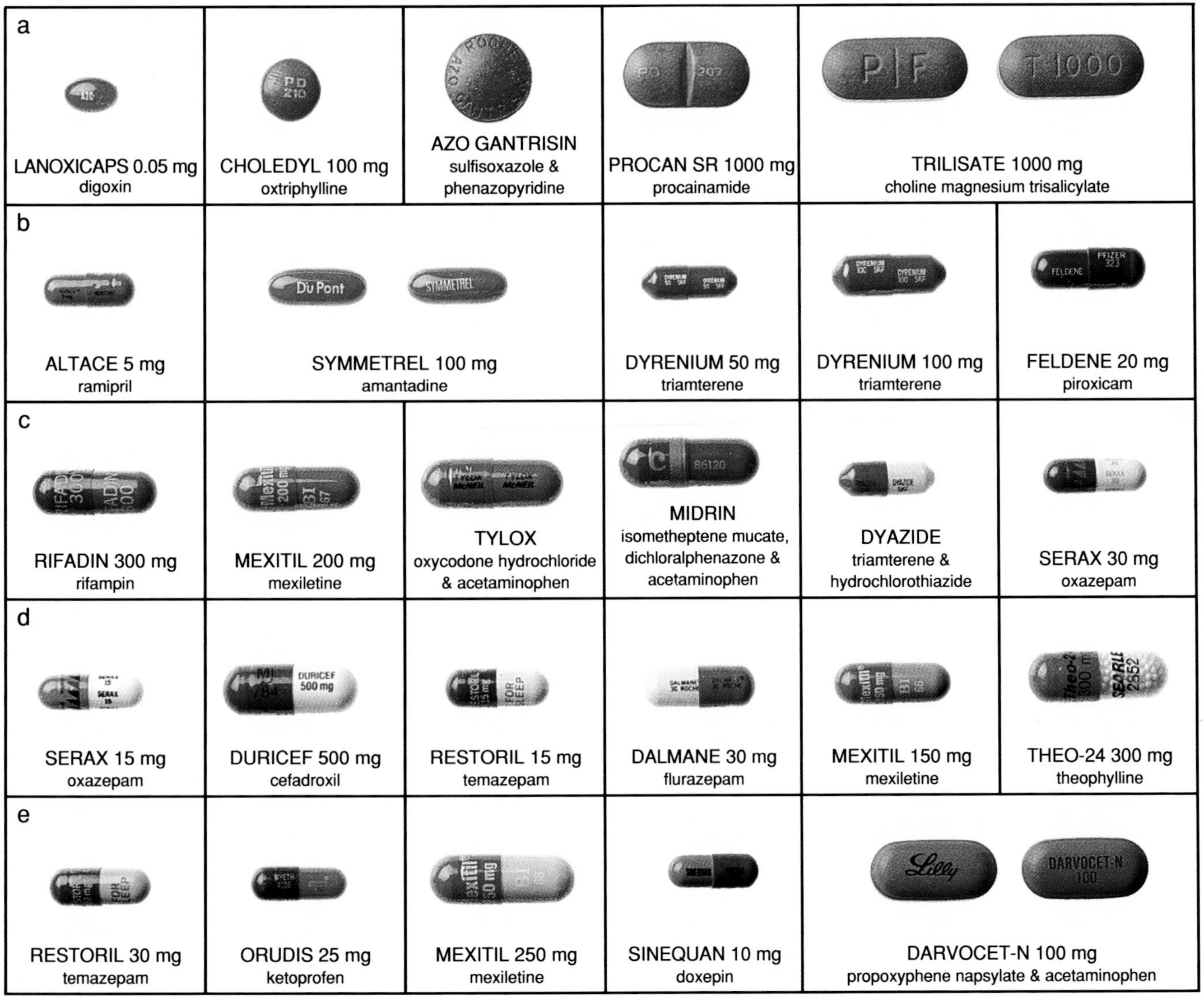

a

LANOXICAPS 0.05 mg
digoxin

CHOLEDYL 100 mg
oxtriphylline

AZO GANTRISIN
sulfisoxazole &
phenazopyridine

PROCAN SR 1000 mg
procainamide

TRILISATE 1000 mg
choline magnesium trisalicylate

b

ALTACE 5 mg
ramipril

SYMMETREL 100 mg
amantadine

DYRENIUM 50 mg
triamterene

DYRENIUM 100 mg
triamterene

FELDENE 20 mg
piroxicam

c

RIFADIN 300 mg
rifampin

MEXITIL 200 mg
mexiletine

TYLOX
oxycodone hydrochloride
& acetaminophen

MIDRIN
isometheptene mucate,
dichloralphenazone &
acetaminophen

DYAZIDE
triamterene &
hydrochlorothiazide

SERAX 30 mg
oxazepam

d

SERAX 15 mg
oxazepam

DURICEF 500 mg
cefadroxil

RESTORIL 15 mg
temazepam

DALMANE 30 mg
flurazepam

MEXITIL 150 mg
mexiletine

THEO-24 300 mg
theophylline

e

RESTORIL 30 mg
temazepam

ORUDIS 25 mg
ketoprofen

MEXITIL 250 mg
mexiletine

SINEQUAN 10 mg
doxepin

DARVOCET-N 100 mg
propoxyphene napsylate & acetaminophen

Color Identification Guide

a

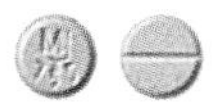

ESTRACE 1 mg
estradiol

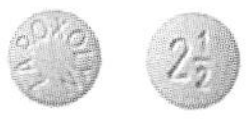

ZAROXOLYN 2.5 mg
metolazone

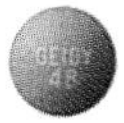

PBZ-SR 100 mg
tripelennamine

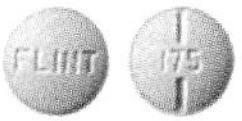

SYNTHROID
0.175 mg
levothyroxine

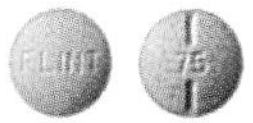

SYNTHROID
0.075 mg
levothyroxine

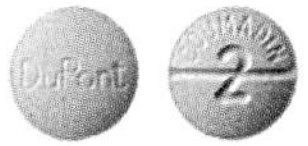

COUMADIN 2 mg
warfarin

b

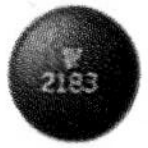

URISED
methenamine, methylene
blue, phenyl salicylate,
benzoic acid, atropine &
hyoscyamine

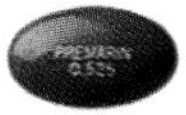

PREMARIN .625 mg
conjugated estrogens

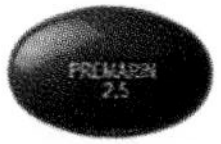

PREMARIN 2.5 mg
conjugated estrogens

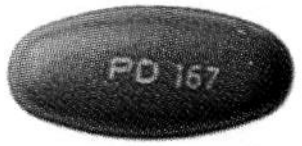

MANDELAMINE 1 g
methenamine mandelate

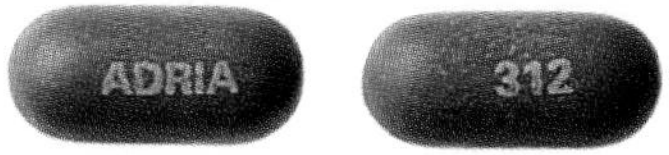

KAON   5 mEq
potassium gluconate

c

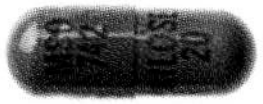

PRILOSEC 20 mg
omeprazole

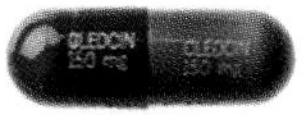

CLEOCIN HCl 150 mg
clindamycin

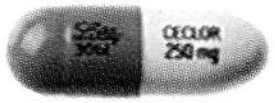

CECLOR 250 mg
cefaclor

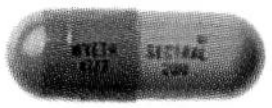

SECTRAL 200 mg
acebutolol

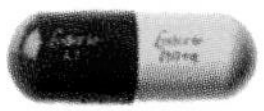

ACHROMYCIN V
250 mg
tetracycline

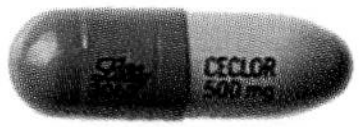

CECLOR 500 mg
cefaclor

d

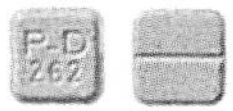

EUTHROID-2
liotrix

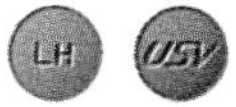

LEVOTHROID
0.125 mg
levothyroxine

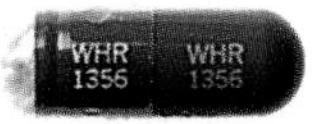

SLO-PHYLLIN
GYROCAPS 250 mg
theophylline

e

Color Identification Guide

a

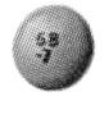

- NORPRAMIN 10 mg — desipramine
- ELAVIL 10 mg — amitriptyline
- STELAZINE 1 mg — trifluoperazine

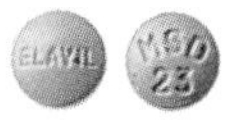

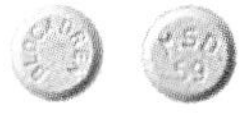

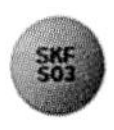

b

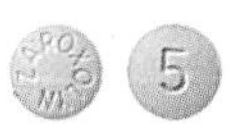

- ZAROXOLYN 5 mg — metolazone
- ESTROVIS 100 mcg — quinestrol
- BLOCADREN 5 mg — timolol maleate
- DIULO 5 mg — metolazone
- KLONOPIN 1 mg — clonazepam

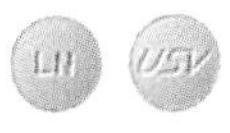

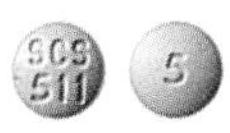

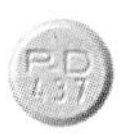

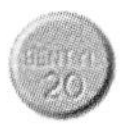

c

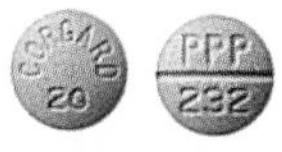

- CORGARD 20 mg — nadolol
- DITROPAN 5 mg — oxybutynin
- BENTYL 20 mg — dicyclomine
- SYNTHROID 0.15 mg — levothyroxine
- LEVOTHROID 0.15 mg — levothyroxine
- STELAZINE 2 mg — trifluoperazine
- APRESOLINE 25 mg — hydralazine

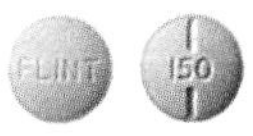

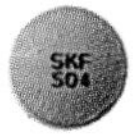

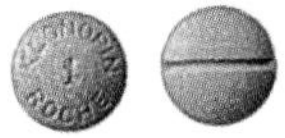

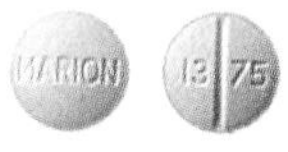

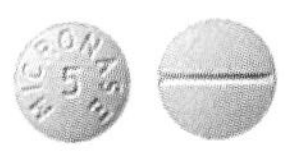

d

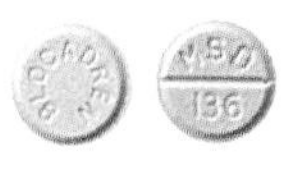

- BLOCADREN 10 mg — timolol maleate
- FLAGYL 250 mg — metronidazole
- APRESOLINE 50 mg — hydralazine
- MICRONASE 5 mg — glyburide
- MEGACE 20 mg — megestrol
- LIMBITROL — chlordiazepoxide & amitriptyline
- ISORDIL Oral Titradose 30 mg — isosorbide dinitrate
- METAHYDRIN 4 mg — trichlormethazide
- CORGARD 40 mg — nadolol

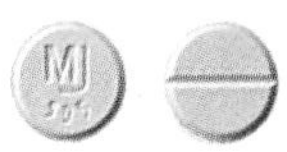

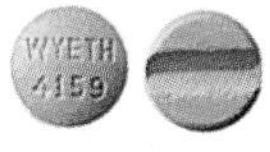

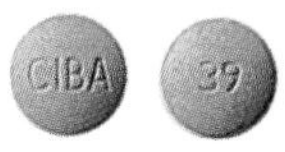

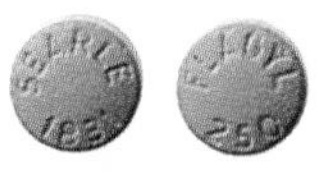

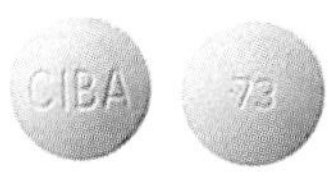

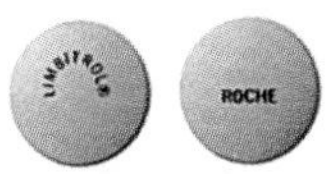

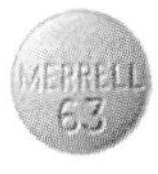

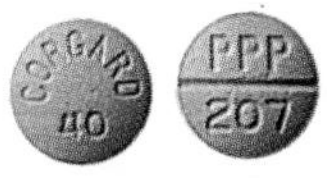

e

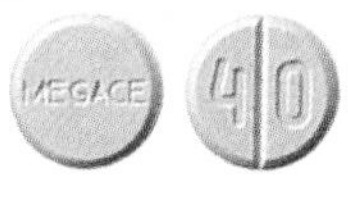

- MEGACE 40 mg — megestrol
- CORGARD 80 mg — nadolol
- NORMODYNE 300 mg — labetalol
- STELAZINE 10 mg — trifluoperazine
- COMBIPRES 0.2 mg — clonidine hydrochloride & chlorthalidone
- HALCION 0.25 mg — triazolam

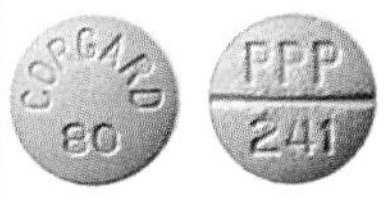

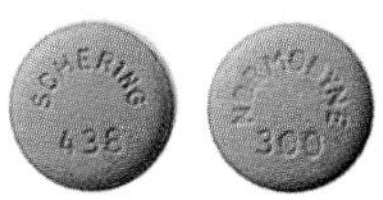

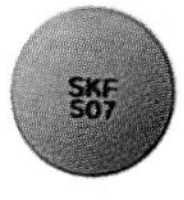

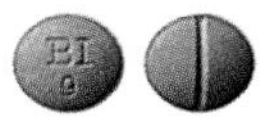

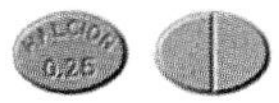

Color Identification Guide

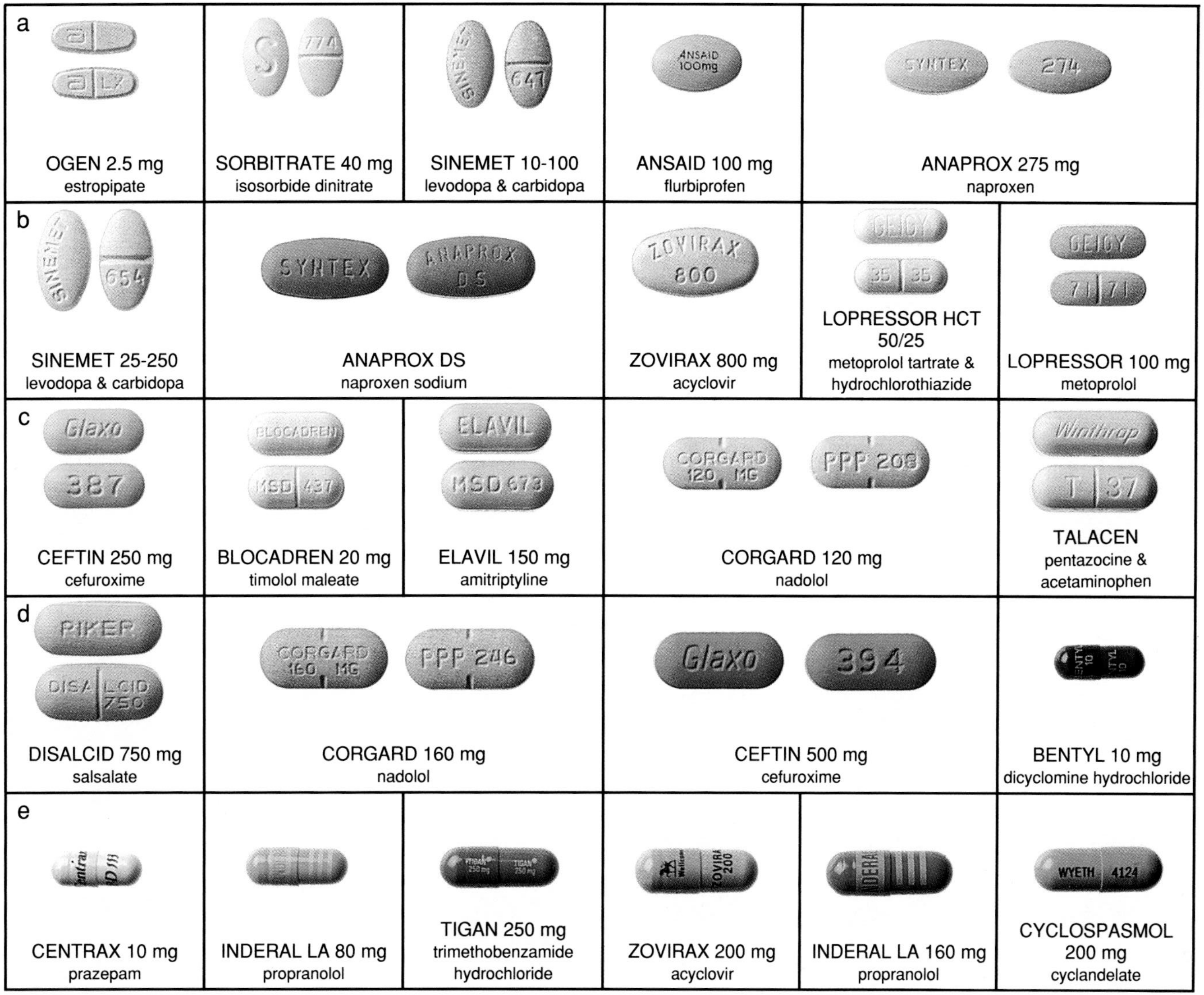

a

OGEN 2.5 mg
estropipate

SORBITRATE 40 mg
isosorbide dinitrate

SINEMET 10-100
levodopa & carbidopa

ANAPROX 275 mg
naproxen

b

SINEMET 25-250
levodopa & carbidopa

ANAPROX DS
naproxen sodium

ZOVIRAX 800 mg
acyclovir

LOPRESSOR HCT
50/25
metoprolol tartrate &
hydrochlorothiazide

LOPRESSOR 100 mg
metoprolol

c

CEFTIN 250 mg
cefuroxime

BLOCADREN 20 mg
timolol maleate

ELAVIL 150 mg
amitriptyline

CORGARD 120 mg
nadolol

TALACEN
pentazocine &
acetaminophen

d

DISALCID 750 mg
salsalate

CORGARD 160 mg
nadolol

CORGARD 160 mg
nadolol

CEFTIN 500 mg
cefuroxime

BENTYL 10 mg
dicyclomine hydrochloride

e

CENTRAX 10 mg
prazepam

INDERAL LA 80 mg
propranolol

TIGAN 250 mg
trimethobenzamide
hydrochloride

ZOVIRAX 200 mg
acyclovir

INDERAL LA 160 mg
propranolol

CYCLOSPASMOL
200 mg
cyclandelate

Color Identification Guide

a	VIBRAMYCIN 100 mg doxycycline	VELOSEF '500' cephradine	SINEQUAN 150 mg doxepin	CARDENE 30 mg nicardipine	INDERAL LA 120 mg propranolol	INDOCIN 25 mg indomethacin
b	INDERAL LA 60 mg propranolol	APRESAZIDE 25/25 hydralazine & hydrochlorothiazide	SURMONTIL 100 mg trimipramine	INDOCIN SR 75 mg indomethacin	INDOCIN 50 mg indomethacin	ISORDIL SA Tembids 40 mg isosorbide dinitrate
c	MINIPRESS 5 mg prazosin	SURMONTIL 25 mg trimipramine	VALRELEASE 15 mg diazepam	ANAFRANIL 50 mg clomipramine hydrochloride	VERELAN 240 mg verapamil hydrochloride	FIORINAL with Codeine No. 3 butalbital, aspirin, caffeine & codeine
d	SINEQUAN 100 mg doxepin	SINEQUAN 25 mg doxepin	SURMONTIL 50 mg trimipramine	VELOSEF '250' cephradine	SYNALGOS DC dihydrocodeine bitartrate & caffeine	FELDENE 10 mg piroxicam
e	CYCLOSPASMOL 400 mg cyclandelate	INDERAL 20 mg propranolol	DECADRON 0.75 mg dexamethasone	MEVACOR 20 mg lovastatin	VALIUM 10 mg diazepam	ASENDIN 100 mg amoxapine

Color Identification Guide

a LEVSIN SL 0.125 mg hyoscyamine sulfate	DIABINESE 100 mg chlorpropamide	HYGROTON 50 mg chlorthalidone	DIABINESE 250 mg chlorpropamide	TRANXENE T-TAB 3.75 mg clorazepate	TRIAVIL 2-10 perphenazine & amitriptyline
b XANAX 1 mg alprazolam				
c				
d				
e				

Color Identification Guide

a

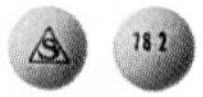

MELLARIL 10 mg
thioridazine

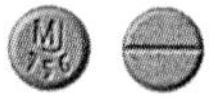

ESTRACE 2 mg
estradiol

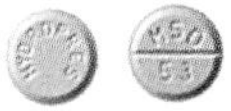

HYDROPRES 25
reserpine &
hydrochlorothiazide

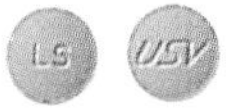

LEVOTHROID 0.3 mg
levothyroxine

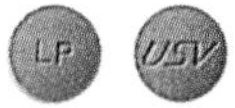

LEVOTHROID
0.175 mg
levothyroxine

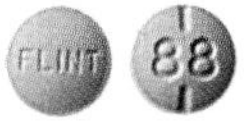

SYNTHROID
0.088 mg
levothyroxine

b

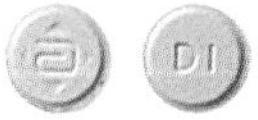

HYTRIN 10 mg
terazosin hydrocloride

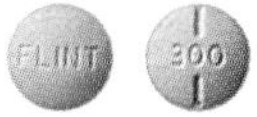

SYNTHROID 0.3 mg
levothyroxine

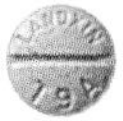

LANOXIN 0.5 mg
digoxin

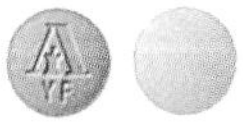

THYROLAR-2
liotrix

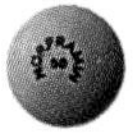

NORPRAMIN 50 mg
desipramine

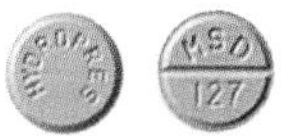

HYDROPRES 50
reserpine &
hydrochlorothiazide

c

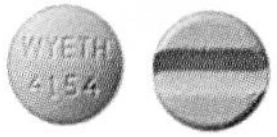

ISORDIL Oral
Titradose 20 mg
isosorbide dinitrate

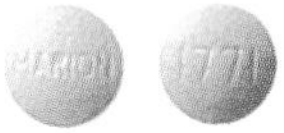

CARDIZEM 30 mg
diltiazem

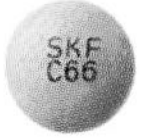

COMPAZINE 5 mg
prochlorperazine

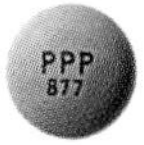

PROLIXIN 5 mg
fluphenazine

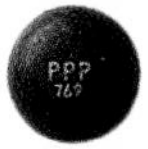

RAUZIDE
rauwolfia &
bendroflumethiazide

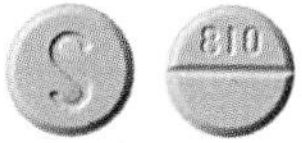

SORBITRATE
Chewable 5 mg
isosorbide dinitrate

d

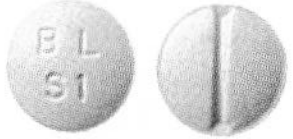

SALUTENSIN
reserpine &
hydroflumethiazide

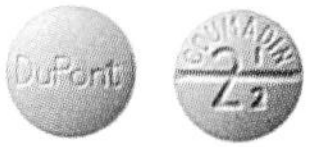

COUMADIN 2.5 mg
warfarin

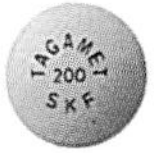

TAGAMET 200 mg
cimetidine

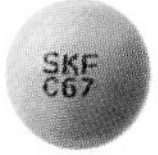

COMPAZINE 10 mg
prochlorperazine

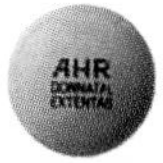

DONNATAL
Extentabs
belladonna alkaloids &
phenobarbital

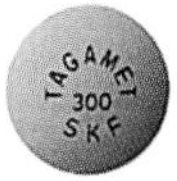

TAGAMET 300 mg
cimetidine

e

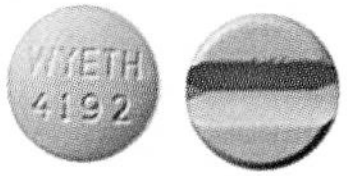

ISORDIL Oral
Titradose 40 mg
isosorbide dinitrate

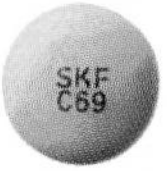

COMPAZINE 25 mg
prochlorperazine

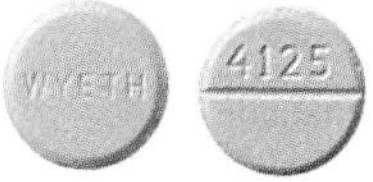

ISORDIL Tembids
40 mg
isosorbide dinitrate

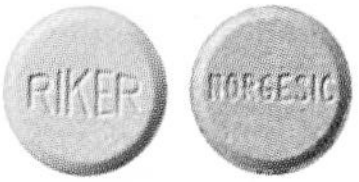

NORGESIC
orphenadrine, aspirin &
caffeine

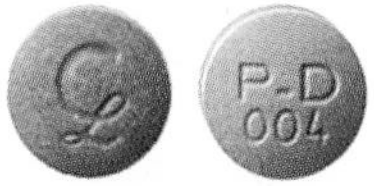

PERITRATE SA
80 mg
pentaerythritol tetranitrate

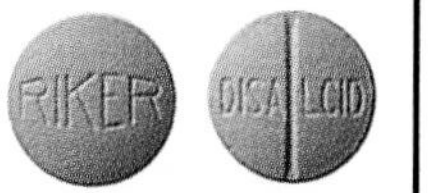

DISALCID 500 mg
salsalate

Color Identification Guide

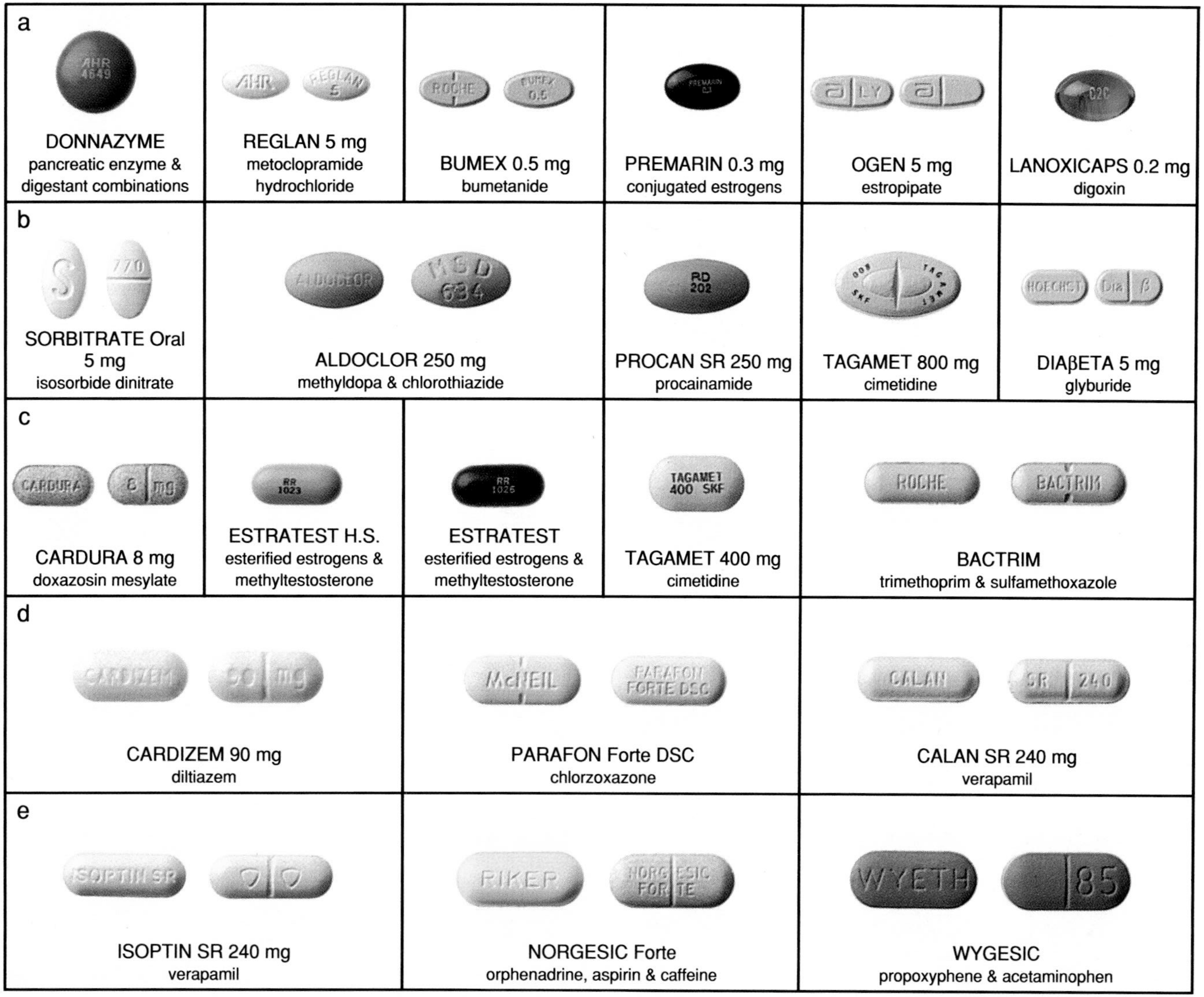

a

DONNAZYME
pancreatic enzyme & digestant combinations

REGLAN 5 mg
metoclopramide hydrochloride

BUMEX 0.5 mg
bumetanide

PREMARIN 0.3 mg
conjugated estrogens

OGEN 5 mg
estropipate

LANOXICAPS 0.2 mg
digoxin

b

SORBITRATE Oral 5 mg
isosorbide dinitrate

ALDOCLOR 250 mg
methyldopa & chlorothiazide

PROCAN SR 250 mg
procainamide

TAGAMET 800 mg
cimetidine

DIAβETA 5 mg
glyburide

c

CARDURA 8 mg
doxazosin mesylate

ESTRATEST H.S.
esterified estrogens & methyltestosterone

ESTRATEST
esterified estrogens & methyltestosterone

TAGAMET 400 mg
cimetidine

BACTRIM
trimethoprim & sulfamethoxazole

d

CARDIZEM 90 mg
diltiazem

PARAFON Forte DSC
chlorzoxazone

CALAN SR 240 mg
verapamil

e

ISOPTIN SR 240 mg
verapamil

NORGESIC Forte
orphenadrine, aspirin & caffeine

WYGESIC
propoxyphene & acetaminophen

Color Identification Guide

a

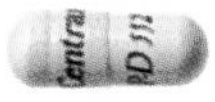

CENTRAX 5 mg
prazepam

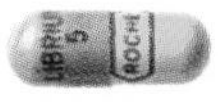

LIBRIUM 5 mg
chlordiazepoxide

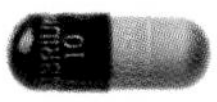

LIBRIUM 10 mg
chlordiazepoxide

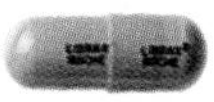

LIBRAX
chlordiazepoxide &
clidinium bromide

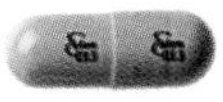

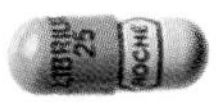

LIBRIUM 25 mg
chlordiazepoxide

b

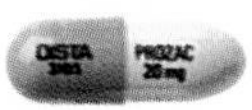

PROZAC 20 mg
fluoxetine hydrochloride

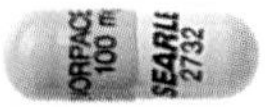

NORPACE CR
100 mg
disopyramide

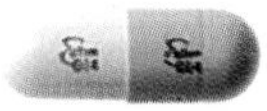

DOPAR 250 mg
levodopa

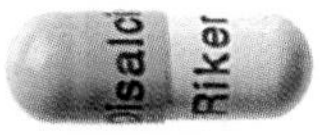

DISALCID 500 mg
salsalate

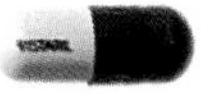

DOPAR 100 mg
levodopa

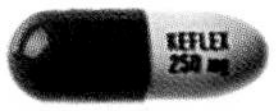

KEFLEX 250 mg
cephalexin

c

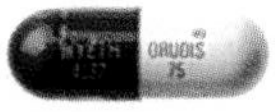

ORUDIS 75 mg
ketoprofen

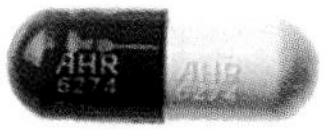

PHENAPHEN with
Codeine No. 4
codeine & acetaminophen

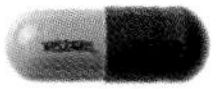

VISTARIL 25 mg
hydroxyzine pamoate

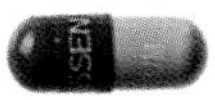

IMODIUM 2 mg
loperamide

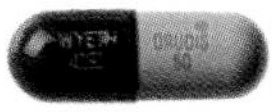

VISTARIL 50 mg
hydroxyzine pamoate

ORUDIS 50 mg
ketoprofen

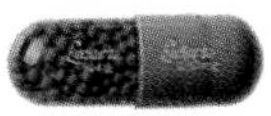

MINOCIN Pellet
100 mg
minocycline hydrochloride

d

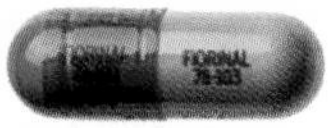

FIORINAL
butalbital, aspirin &
caffeine

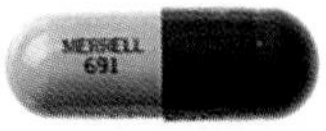

TACE 25 mg
chlorotrianisene

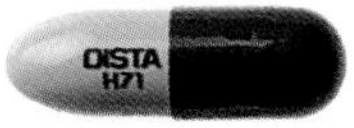

KEFLEX 500 mg
cephalexin

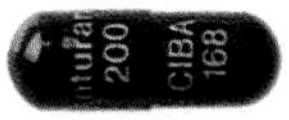

ANTURANE 200 mg
sulfinpyrazone

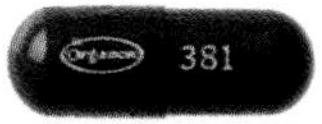

COTAZYM
pancrelipase

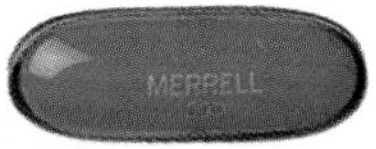

TACE 12 mg
chlorotrianisene

e

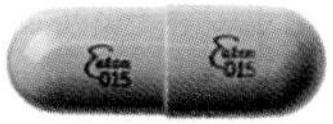

DOPAR 500 mg
levodopa

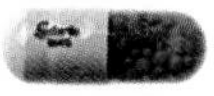

MINOCIN Pellet
50 mg
minocycline hydrochloride

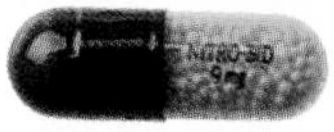

NITRO-BID 9 mg
nitroglycerin

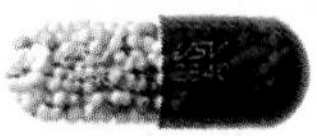

NICOBID 250 mg
niacin

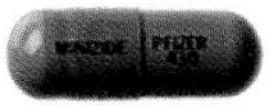

MINIZIDE 1
prazosin & polythiazide

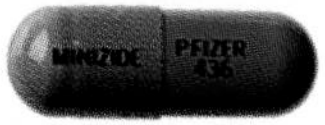

MINIZIDE 5
prazosin & polythiazide

Color Identification Guide

a 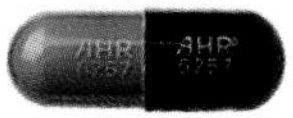 PHENAPHEN with Codeine No. 3 codeine & acetaminophen	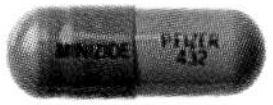 MINIZIDE 2 prazosin & polythiazide	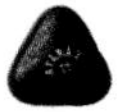 ATARAX 25 mg hydroxyzine hydrochloride	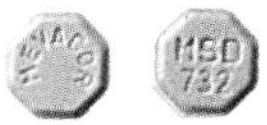 MEVACOR 40 mg lovastatin	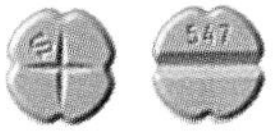 NAQUA 4 mg trichlormethiazide	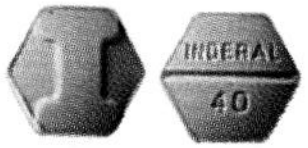 INDERAL 40 mg propranolol
b 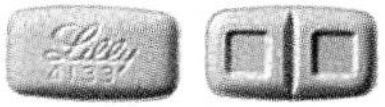 PERMAX 0.25 mg pergolide mesylate	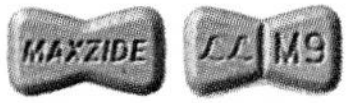 MAXZIDE 25 mg triamterene & hydrochlorothiazide	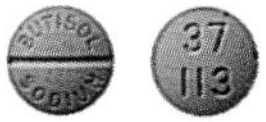 BUTISOL SODIUM 30 mg butabarbital			
c					
d					
e					

Color Identification Guide

a				
ISORDIL Sublingual 2.5 mg isosorbide dinitrate	SANSERT 2 mg methysergide	DIULO 10 mg metolazone	MEPHYTON 5 mg phytonadione (vitamin K)	LANOXIN 0.125 mg digoxin	DARANIDE 50 mg dichlorphenamide

b				
LEVOTHROID 0.1 mg levothyroxine	ELAVIL 25 mg amitriptyline	METHOTREXATE 2.5 mg methotrexate	TORECAN 10 mg thiethylperazine	ZAROXOLYN 10 mg metolazone	SYNTHROID 0.1 mg levothyroxine

c				
VOLTAREN 25 mg diclofenac sodium	THYROLAR-3 liotrix	APRESOLINE 10 mg hydralazine	ALDOMET 125 mg methyldopa	ZESTRIL 40 mg lisinopril	ETRAFON 2-10 perphenazine & amitriptyline

d				
NORPRAMIN 25 mg desipramine	COUMADIN 7.5 mg warfarin	RENESE 2 mg polythiazide	SALUTENSIN-Demi reserpine & hydroflumethiazide	SORBITRATE Chewable 10 mg isosorbide dinitrate	ESIDRIX 50 mg hydrochlorothiazide

e				
ISOPTIN 80 mg verapamil	ISMELIN 10 mg guanethidine	PURINETHOL 50 mg mercaptopurine	MELLARIL 100 mg thioridazine	ESTRATAB 0.625 mg esterified estrogens	ALDOMET 250 mg methyldopa

Color Identification Guide

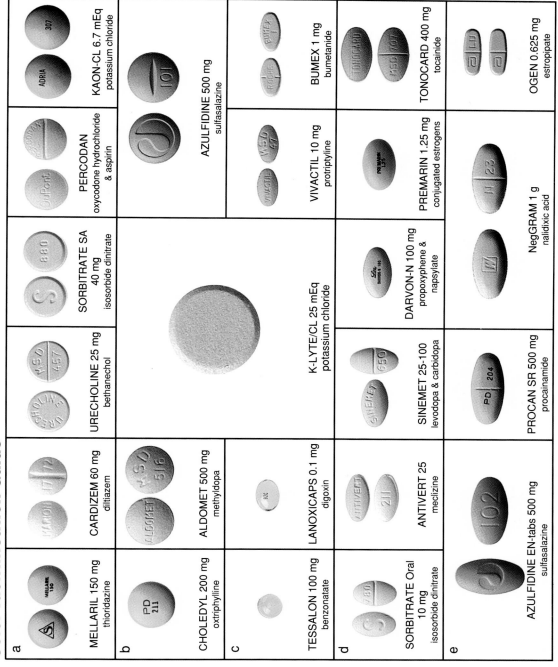

a

MELLARIL 150 mg
thioridazine

CARDIZEM 60 mg
diltiazem

URECHOLINE 25 mg
bethanechol

SORBITRATE SA
40 mg
isosorbide dinitrate

PERCODAN
oxycodone hydrochloride
& aspirin

KAON-CL 6.7 mEq
potassium chloride

b

CHOLEDYL 200 mg
oxtriphylline

ALDOMET 500 mg
methyldopa

AZULFIDINE 500 mg
sulfasalazine

c

TESSALON 100 mg
benzonatate

LANOXICAPS 0.1 mg
digoxin

K-LYTE/CL 25 mEq
potassium chloride

VIVACTIL 10 mg
protriptyline

BUMEX 1 mg
bumetanide

d

SORBITRATE Oral
10 mg
isosorbide dinitrate

ANTIVERT 25
meclizine

SINEMET 25-100
levodopa & carbidopa

DARVON-N 100 mg
propoxyphene &
napsylate

PREMARIN 1.25 mg
conjugated estrogens

TONOCARD 400 mg
tocainide

e

AZULFIDINE EN-tabs 500 mg
sulfasalazine

PROCAN SR 500 mg
procainamide

NegGRAM 1 g
nalidixic acid

OGEN 0.625 mg
estropipate

Color Identification Guide

a				
TALWIN NX pentazocine	LEVATOL 20 mg penbutolol sulfate	ZANTAC 300 mg ranitidine	K-TAB 10 mEq potassium chloride	LOPRESSOR HCT 100/50 metoprolol tartrate & hydrochlorothiazide
b GEOCILLIN 382 mg carbenicillin		DYMELOR 500 mg acetohexamide		BEROCCA Plus vitamins A, B₁, B₂, B₆, B₁₂; niacin; pantothenic acid; biotin; folic acid; iron; chromium; magnesium; manganese; copper & zinc
c BENEMID 0.5 g probenecid		HIPREX 1 g methenamine hippurate		NEMBUTAL Sodium 100 mg sodium pentobarbital / CENTRAX 20 mg prazepam
d PRONESTYL 250 mg procainamide	VERELAN 120 mg verapamil	CUPRIMINE 250 mg penicillamine	ANAFRANIL 75 mg clomipramine	GRISACTIN 250 mg griseofulvin / PANCREASE MT-4 pancrelipase
e AXID 150 mg nizatidine	ANAFRANIL 25 mg clomipramine	NALFON 300 mg fenoprofen	AVENTYL HCl 10 mg nortriptyline	AVENTYL HCl 25 mg nortriptyline / COMPAZINE 15 mg prochlorperazine

Color Identification Guide

a

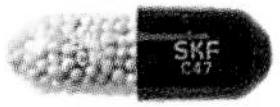

COMPAZINE 30 mg
prochlorperazine

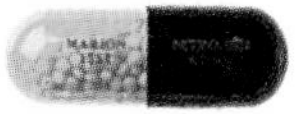

NITRO-BID 6.5 mg
nitroglycerin

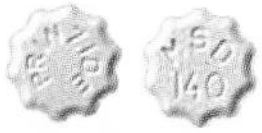

PRINZIDE 12.5 mg
lisinopril &
hydrochlorothiazide

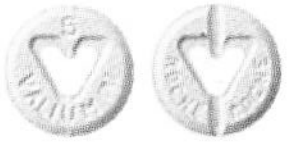

VALIUM 5 mg
diazepam

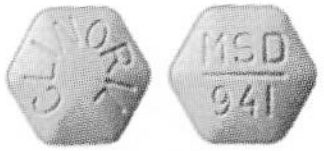

CLINORIL 150 mg
sulindac

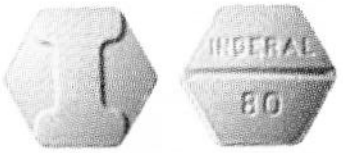

INDERAL 80 mg
propranolol

b

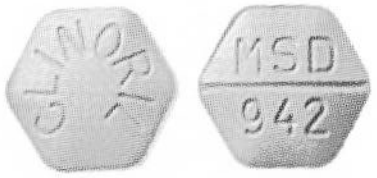

CLINORIL 200 mg
sulindac

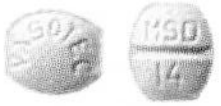

VASOTEC 2.5 mg
enalapril maleate

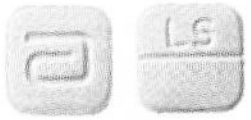

ENDURONYL
deserpidine &
methyclothiazide

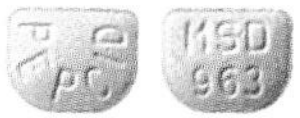

PEPCID 20 mg
famotidine

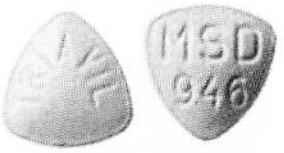

TRIAVIL 4-25
perphenazine &
amitriptyline

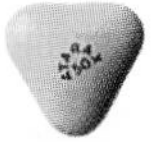

ATARAX 50 mg
hydroxyzine hydrochloride

c

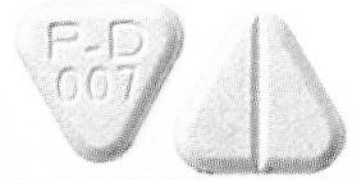

DILANTIN Infatabs
50 mg
phenytoin

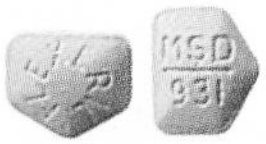

FLEXERIL 10 mg
cyclobenzaprine

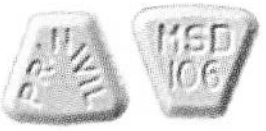

PRINIVIL 10 mg
lisinopril

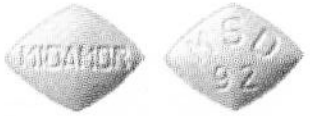

MIDAMOR 5 mg
amiloride

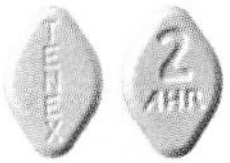

TENEX 2 mg
guanfacine

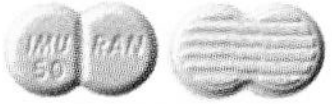

IMURAN 50 mg
azathioprine

d

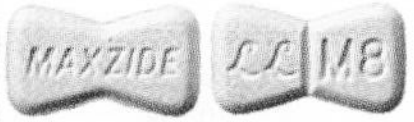

MAXZIDE
triamterene &
hydrochlorothiazide

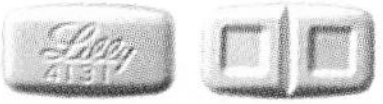

PERMAX 0.05 mg
pergolide mesylate

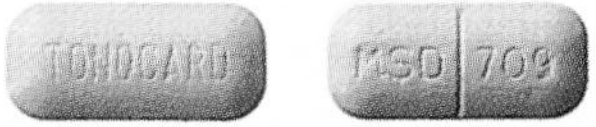

TONOCARD 600 mg
tocainide

e

Color Identification Guide

a

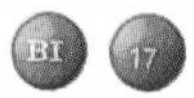

PERSANTINE 25 mg
dipyridamole

ERGOSTAT
Sublingual 2 mg
ergotamine tartrate

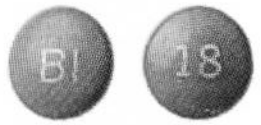

PERSANTINE 50 mg
dipyridamole

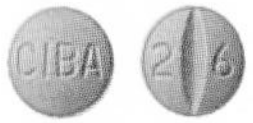

LUDIOMIL 50 mg
maprotiline

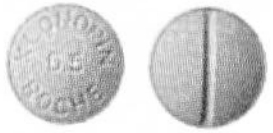

KLONOPIN 0.5 mg
clonazepam

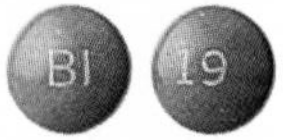

PERSANTINE 75 mg
dipyridamole

b

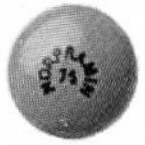

NORPRAMIN 75 mg
desipramine

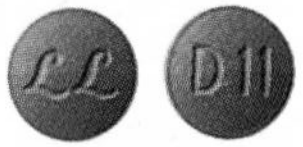

DECLOMYCIN
150 mg
demeclocycline

c

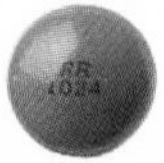

ESTRATAB 1.25 mg
esterified estrogens

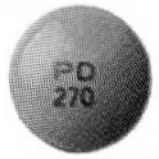

K-LYTE 25 mEq
potassium bicarbonate

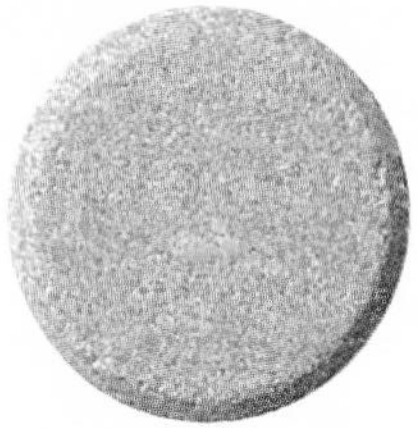

K-LYTE DS 50 mEq
potassium bicarbonate

NARDIL 15 mg
phenelzine

d

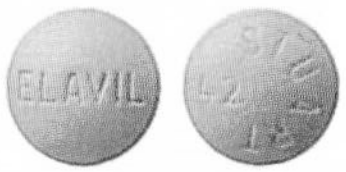

ELAVIL 75 mg
amitriptyline

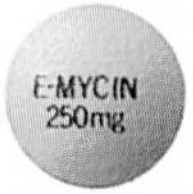

E-MYCIN 250 mg
erythromycin

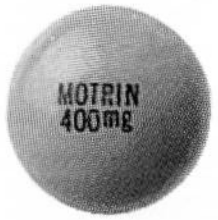

MOTRIN 400 mg
ibuprofen

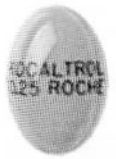

ROCALTROL
0.25 mcg
calcitriol (vitamin D)

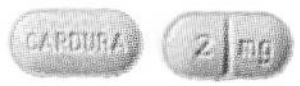

CARDURA 2 mg
doxazosin

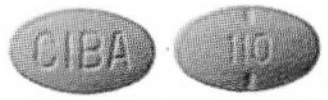

LUDIOMIL 25 mg
maprotiline

e

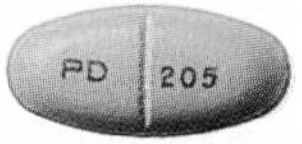

PROCAN SR 750 mg
procainamide

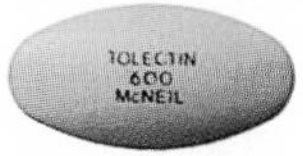

TOLECTIN 600 mg
tolmetin

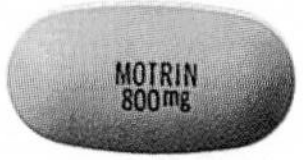

MOTRIN 800 mg
ibuprofen

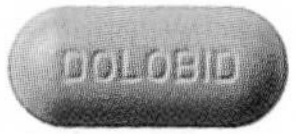

DOLOBID 500 mg
diflunisal

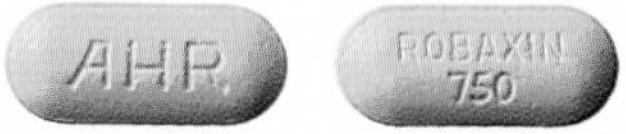

ROBAXIN 750 mg
methocarbamol

Color Identification Guide

a				
NALFON 600 mg fenoprofen	ROCALTROL 0.5 mcg calcitriol (vitamin D)	ADALAT 10 mg nifedipine	PROCARDIA 10 mg nifedipine	ADALAT 20 mg nifedipine

b				
PROCARDIA 20 mg nifedipine	ATROMID-S 500 mg clofibrate	DEPAKENE 250 mg valproic acid	ALTACE 2.5 mg ramipril	MECLOMEN 50 mg meclofenamate

c				
SECONAL Sodium 100 mg secobarbital	PAMELOR 75 mg nortriptyline	GRISACTIN 125 mg griseofulvin	TOLECTIN DS 400 mg tolmetin	ADAPIN 10 mg doxepin	MECLOMEN 100 mg meclofenamate

d				
PAMELOR 25 mg nortriptyline	NORPACE 100 mg disopyramide	THEO-24 100 mg theophylline	THEO-24 200 mg theophylline	PAMELOR 10 mg nortriptyline	THORAZINE 30 mg chlorpromazine	THORAZINE 75 mg chlorpromazine

e				
ERYC 250 mg erythromycin	DALMANE 15 mg flurazepam	VICON Forte multivitamin with minerals	ASENDIN 50 mg amoxapine	ENDURON 2.5 mg methyclothiazide	ATARAX 10 mg hydroxyzine hydrochloride

Color Identification Guide

a	PRO-BANTHINE 15 mg propantheline	HydroDIURIL 25 mg hydrochlorothiazide	PROVERA 2.5 mg medroxyprogesterone acetate	ESIDRIX 25 mg hydrochlorothiazide
				SYNTHROID 0.025 mg levothyroxine
				HYTRIN 2 mg terazosin
b	THYROLAR-1 liotrix	THYROLAR-1/2 liotrix	SYNTHROID 0.125 mg levothyroxine	NORMODYNE 100 mg labetalol
				HydroDIURIL 50 mg hydrochlorothiazide
				TRANDATE 100 mg labetalol
c	MARPLAN 10 mg isocarboxazid	PHENERGAN 12.5 mg promethazine	ESTINYL 0.5 mg ethinyl estradiol	COUMADIN 5 mg warfarin
				DESYREL 50 mg trazodone
				VIBRA-TABS 100 mg doxycycline
d	LITHOBID 300 mg lithium carbonate	NORPRAMIN 100 mg desipramine	TOFRANIL 50 mg imipramine	ALDORIL-15 methyldopa & hydrochlorothiazide
				PLENDIL 10 mg felodipine
				PLENDIL 5 mg felodipine
e	ZYLOPRIM 300 mg allopurinol	BRONDECON oxtriphylline & guaifenesin	LOPURIN 300 mg allopurinol	TRANDATE 300 mg labetalol
				GRISACTIN 500 mg griseofulvin
				KLOTRIX 10 mEq potassium chloride

Color Identification Guide

a

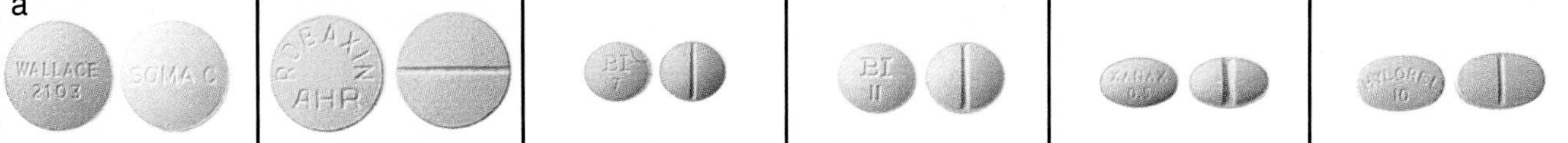

SOMA COMPOUND
carisoprodol & aspirin

ROBAXIN 500 mg
methocarbamol

CATAPRES 0.2 mg
clonidine

CATAPRES 0.3 mg
clonidine

XANAX 0.5 mg
alprazolam

HYLOREL 10 mg
guanadrel sulfate

b

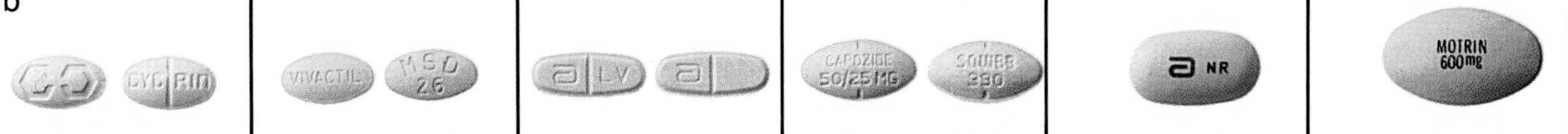

CYCRIN 10 mg
medroxyprogesterone
acetate

VIVACTIL 5 mg
protriptyline hydrochloride

OGEN 1.25 mg
estropipate

CAPOZIDE 50/25
captopril &
hydrochlorothiazide

DEPAKOTE 250 mg
divalproex sodium

MOTRIN 600 mg
ibuprofen

c

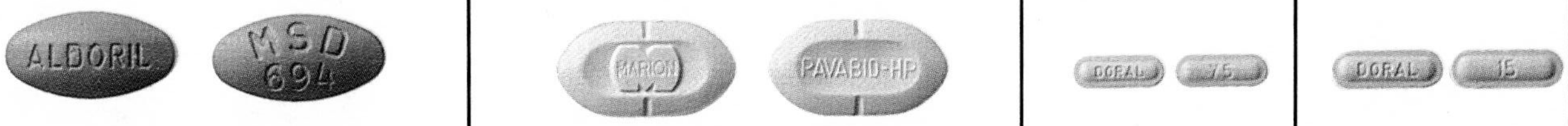

ALDORIL D30
methyldopa & hydrochlorothiazide

PAVABID HP 300 mg
papaverine

DORAL 7.5 mg
quazepam

DORAL 15 mg
quazepam

d

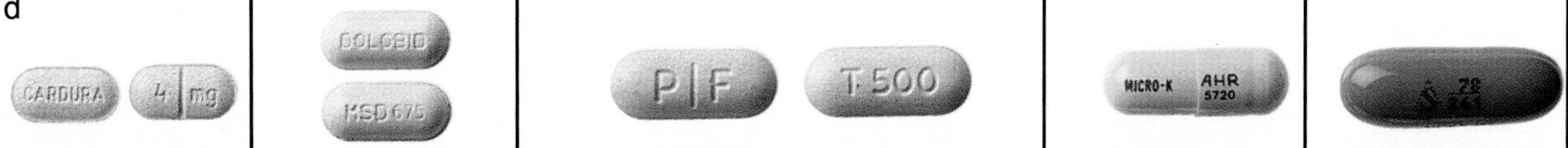

CARDURA 4 mg
doxazosin

DOLOBID 250 mg
diflunisal

TRILISATE 500 mg
choline & magnesium salicylate

INDERAL 10 mg
propranolol

MICRO-K Extencaps
8 mEq
potassium chloride

SANDIMMUNE
100 mg
cyclosporine

e

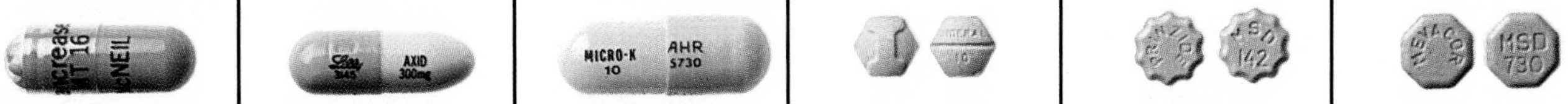

PANCREASE MT-16
pancrelipase

AXID 300 mg
nizatidine

MICRO-K 10
Extencaps 10 mEq
potassium chloride

PRINZIDE 25 mg
lisinopril &
hydrochlorothiazide

MEVACOR 10 mg
lovastatin

Color Identification Guide

a				
WYTENSIN 4 mg guanabenz acetate	VASOTEC 10 mg enalapril	VASOTEC 20 mg enalapril	ENDURON 2.5 mg methyclothiazide	ENDURON 5 mg methyclothiazide
b				
CAPOZIDE 25/25 captopril & hydrochlorothiazide	PRINIVIL 20 mg lisinopril	PRINIVIL 40 mg lisinopril	HYGROTON 25 mg chlorthalidone	TRIAVIL 2-25 perphenazine & amitriptyline
c				
MODURETIC amiloride & hydrochlorothiazide	PERMAX 1 mg pergolide mesylate	DESYREL 150 mg trazodone	TRANXENE T-TAB 7.5 MG chlorazepate	TRIAVIL 4-10 perphenazine & amitriptyline
d				
e				

Color Identification Guide

a
- HYTRIN 5 mg — terazosin
- MELLARIL 25 mg — thioridazine
- LOTENSIN 10 mg — benazepril
- VOLTAREN 50 mg — diclofenac
- ESTINYL 0.02 mg — ethinyl estradiol
- ZESTORETIC 20-25 — lisinopril & hydrochlorothiazide

b
- ALDACTONE 25 mg — spironolactone
- ALDACTAZIDE 25/25 — spironolactone & hydrochlorothiazide
- NAPROSYN 250 mg — naproxen
- CAFERGOT — ergotamine & caffeine
- VIOKASE — pancrelipase
- ALDACTONE 100 mg — spironolactone

c
- ESKALITH CR 450 mg — lithium carbonate
- SLOW-K 600 mg — potassium chloride
- CATAPRES 0.1 mg — clonidine
- CALAN 80 mg — verapamil
- ISOPTIN SR 120 mg — verapamil
- CALAN SR 120 mg — verapamil

d
- SINEMET CR 50/200 — carbidopa & levodopa
- ALDACTONE 50 mg — spironolactone
- ALDACTAZIDE 50/50 — spironolactone & hydrochlorothiazide
- NAPROSYN 500 mg — naproxen
- MESTINON Timespan 180 mg — pyridostigmine
- NALFON 200 mg — fenoprofen

e
- INDERIDE LA 80/50 — propranolol hydrochloride & hydrochlorothiazide
- HYDERGINE LC 1 mg — ergoloid mesylates
- EUTHROID-1 — liotrix
- NICORETTE 2 mg — nicotine polacrilex

Color Identification Guide

a	THORAZINE 10 mg chlorpromazine	THORAZINE 25 mg chlorpromazine	TOFRANIL 25 mg imipramine	ELAVIL 50 mg amitriptyline	THORAZINE 50 mg chlorpromazine
					TOFRANIL 50 mg imipramine
b	CALAN 120 mg verapamil	CHOLEDYL SA 600 mg oxtriphylline	RIDAURA 3 mg auranofin	PARLODEL 5 mg bromocriptine	INDERIDE LA 120/50 propranolol hydrochloride & hydrochlorothiazide
					EULEXIN 125 mg flutamide
c	SLO-PHYLLIN GYROCAPS 125 mg theophylline	PAVABID 150 mg papaverine	CARDIZEM SR 120 mg diltiazem	INDERIDE LA 160/50 propranolol hydrochloride & hydrochlorothiazide	CARDIZEM SR 60 mg diltiazem
					CARDIZEM SR 90 mg diltiazem
d	CREON pancreatin	NORPACE 150 mg disopyramide	SECTRAL 400 mg acebutolol	NORPACE CR 150 mg disopyramide	TOFRANIL 10 mg imipramine
					PEPCID 40 mg famotidine
e					

Color Identification Guide

a

PROLOID 30 mg
thyroglobulin

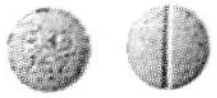

PROLOID 60 mg
thyroglobulin

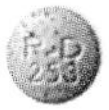

PROLOID 90 mg
thyroglobulin

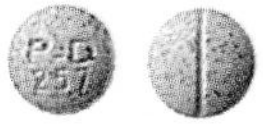

PROLOID 120 mg
thyroglobulin

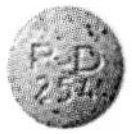

PROLOID 180 mg
thyroglobulin

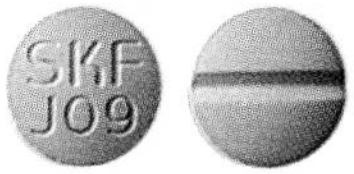

ESKALITH 300 mg
lithium carbonate

b

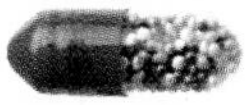

TEMARIL 5 mg
trimeprazine

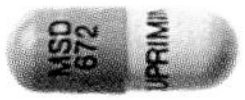

CUPRIMINE 125 mg
penicillamine

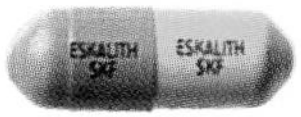

ESKALITH 300 mg
lithium carbonate

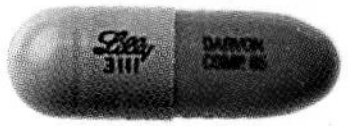

DARVON
Compound-65
propoxyphene, aspirin,
and caffeine

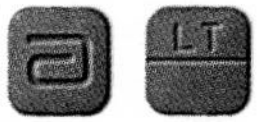

ENDURONYL Forte
deserpidine &
methyclothiazide

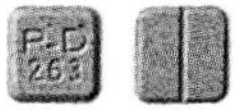

EUTHROID-3
liotrix

c

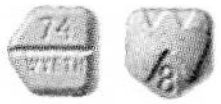

WYTENSIN 8 mg
guanabenz acetate

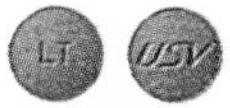

LEVOTHROID
0.075 mg
levothyroxine

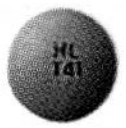

TEMARIL 2.5 mg
trimeprazine

d

e

Color Identification Guide

a
- ISORDIL SL 5 mg — isosorbide dinitrate
- SORBITRATE SL 2.5 mg — isosorbide dinitrate
- NITROSTAT 0.15 mg — nitroglycerin
- NITROSTAT 0.3 mg — nitroglycerin
- NITROSTAT 0.4 mg — nitroglycerin
- ARMOUR Thyroid 15 mg — thyroid, desiccated

b
- LOMOTIL — diphenoxylate & atropine
- CYTOMEL 5 mcg — liothyronine
- ARMOUR Thyroid 30 mg — thyroid, desiccated
- TENORMIN 25 mg — atenolol
- D.E.S. 1 mg — diethylstilbestrol
- PRO-BANTHINE 7.5 mg — propantheline

c
- COGENTIN 0.5 mg — benztropine mesylate
- MYLERAN 2 mg — busulfan
- TAMBOCOR 50 mg — flecainide acetate
- PROVENTIL 2 mg — albuterol
- LEVOTHROID 0.05 mg — levothyroxine
- ARLIDIN 6 mg — nylidrin

d
- DELTASONE 5 mg — prednisone
- VENTOLIN 2 mg — albuterol sulfate
- MEBARAL 32 mg — mephobarbital
- LANOXIN 0.25 mg — digoxin
- SYNTHROID 0.05 mg — levothyroxine
- LEUKERAN 2 mg — chlorambucil

e
- TAVIST 2.68 mg — clemastine fumarate
- ELDEPRYL 5 mg — selegiline hydrochloride
- CYTOTEC 100 mcg — misoprostol
- HISMANAL 10 mg — astemizole
- TENORMIN 50 mg — atenolol
- PROVERA 10 mg — medroxyprogesterone acetate

Color Identification Guide

a

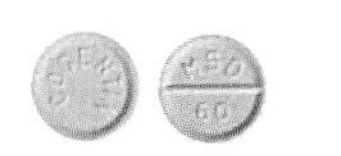

COGENTIN 2 mg
benztropine mesylate

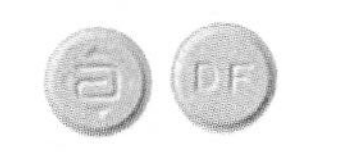

HYTRIN 1 mg
terazosin hydrochloride

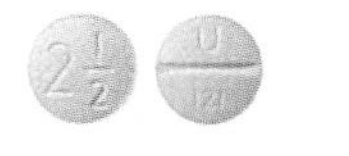

LONITEN 2.5 mg
minoxidil

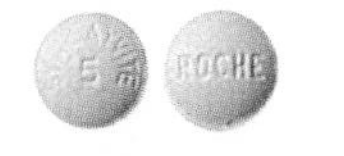

SYNKAYVITE 5 mg
vitamin K₃ or menadiol
sodium diphosphate

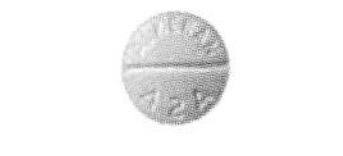

ALKERAN 2 mg
melphalan

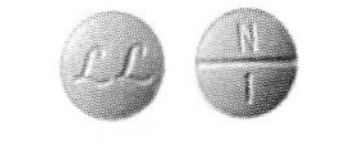

NEPTAZANE 50 mg
methazolamide

b

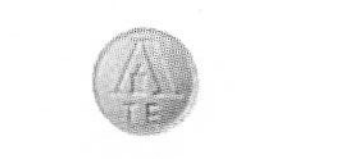

ARMOUR Thyroid
60 mg
thyroid, desiccated

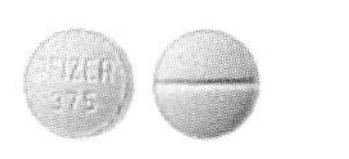

RENESE 1 mg
polythiazide

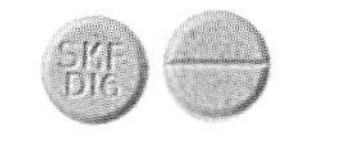

CYTOMEL 25 mcg
liothyronine

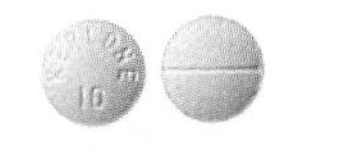

KERLONE 10 mg
betaxolol hydrochloride

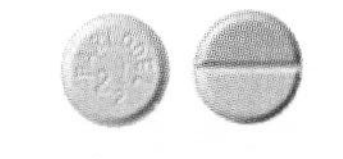

PARLODEL Snaptabs
2.5 mg
bromocriptine mesylate

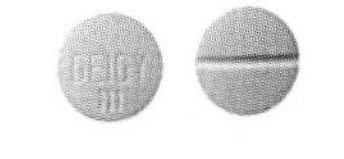

PBZ 25 mg
tripelennamine

c

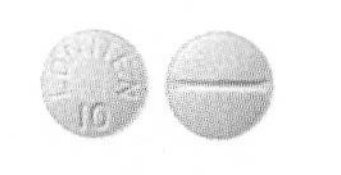

LONITEN 10 mg
minoxidil

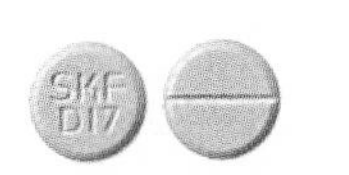

CYTOMEL 50 mcg
liothyronine

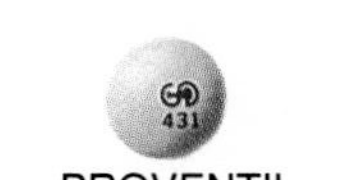

PROVENTIL
REPETABS 4 mg
albuterol

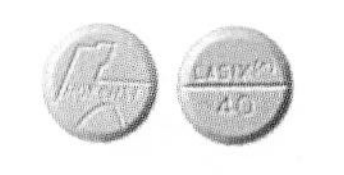

LASIX 40 mg
furosemide

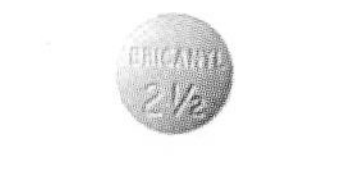

BRICANYL 2.5 mg
terbutaline

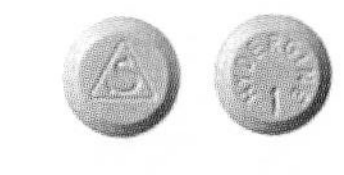

HYDERGINE 1 mg
ergoloid mesylates

d

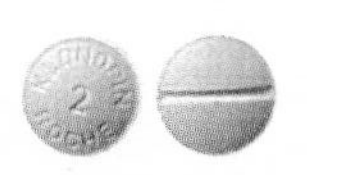

KLONOPIN 2 mg
clonazepam

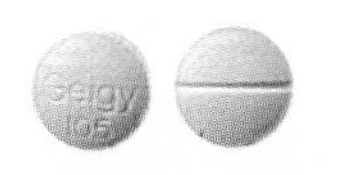

BRETHINE 5 mg
terbutaline

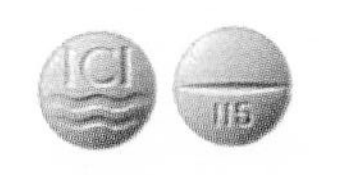

TENORETIC 50
atenolol & chlorthalidone

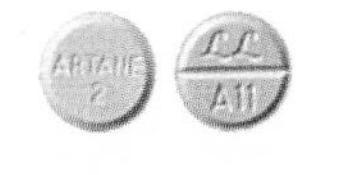

ARTANE 2 mg
trihexyphenidyl

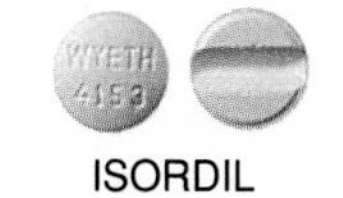

ISORDIL
Oral Titradose 10 mg
isosorbide dinitrate

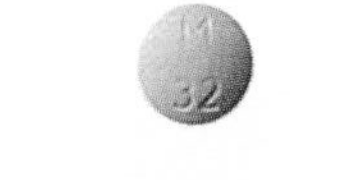

MEBARAL 50 mg
mephobarbital

e

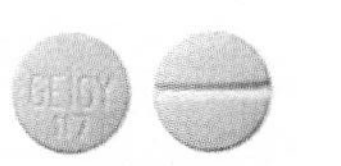

PBZ 50 mg
tripelennamine

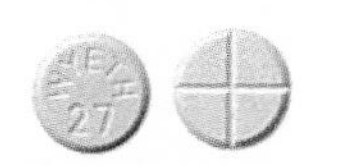

PHENERGAN 25 mg
promethazine

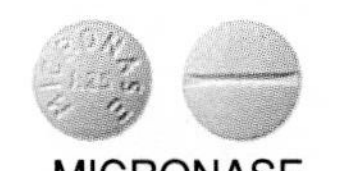

MICRONASE
1.25 mg
glyburide

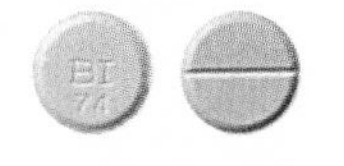

ALUPENT 10 mg
metaproterenol

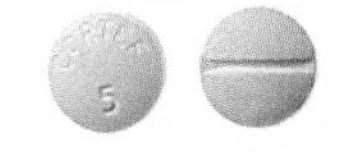

CORTEF 5 mg
hydrocortisone

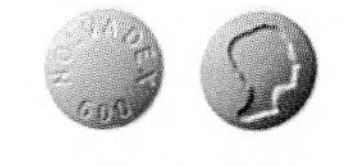

NOLVADEX 10 mg
tamoxifen

Color Identification Guide

a

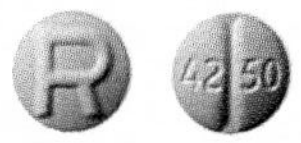

DONNATAL
belladonna alkaloids

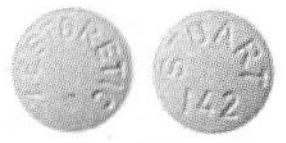

ZESTORETIC 20-12.5
lisinopril &
hydrochlorothiazide

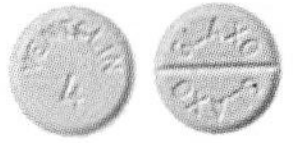

VENTOLIN 4 mg
albuterol sulfate

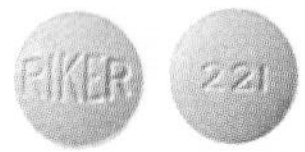

NORFLEX 100 mg
orphenadrine citrate

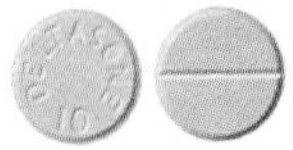

DELTASONE 10 mg
prednisone

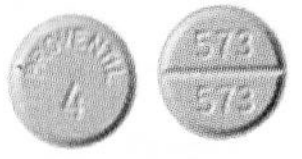

PROVENTIL 4 mg
albuterol

b

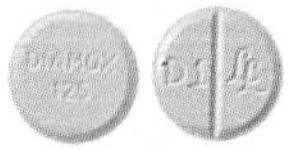

DIAMOX 125 mg
acetazolamide

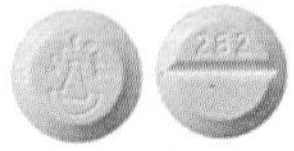

OPTIMINE 1 mg
azatadine

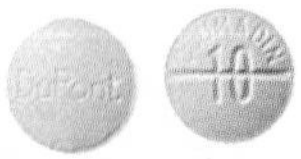

COUMADIN 10 mg
warfarin

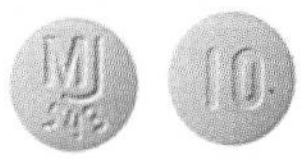

VASODILAN 10 mg
isoxsuprine

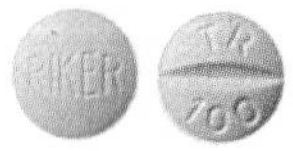

TAMBOCOR 100 mg
flecainide acetate

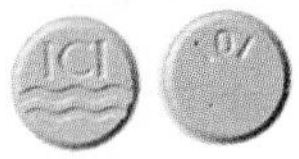

TENORMIN 100 mg
atenolol

c

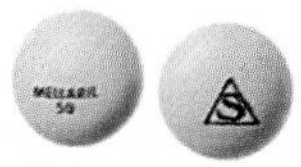

MELLARIL 50 mg
thioridazine

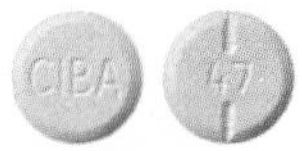

ESIMIL
guanethidine &
hydrochlorothiazide

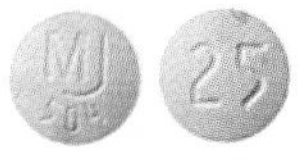

CYTOXAN 25 mg
cyclophosphamide

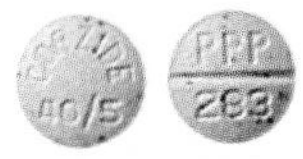

CORZIDE 40
nadolol &
bendroflumethiazide

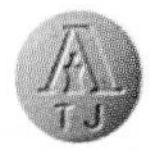

ARMOUR Thyroid
90 mg
thyroid, desiccated

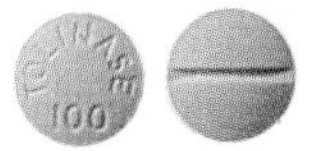

TOLINASE 100 mg
tolazamide

d

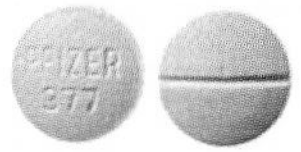

RENESE 4 mg
polythiazide

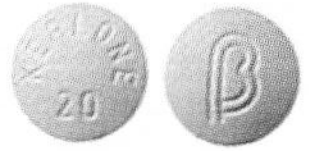

KERLONE 20 mg
betaxolol hydrochloride

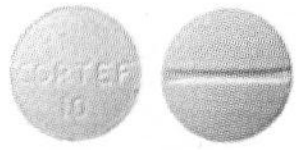

CORTEF 10 mg
hydrocortisone

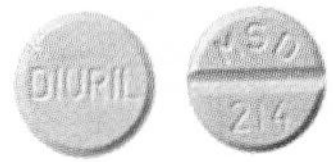

DIURIL 250 mg
chlorothiazide

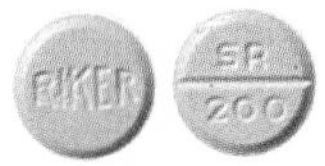

THEOLAIR-SR
200 mg
theophylline

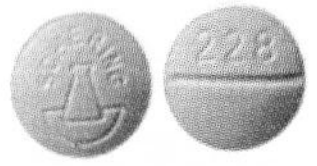

FULVICIN P/G
125 mg
griseofulvin

e

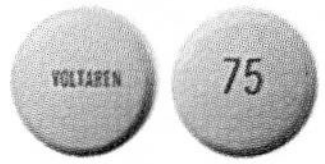

VOLTAREN 75 mg
diclofenac

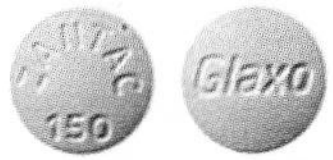

ZANTAC 150 mg
ranitidine

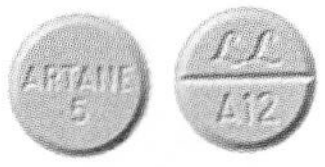

ARTANE 5 mg
trihexyphenidyl

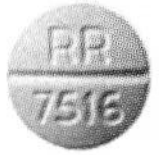

LITHOTABS 300 mg
lithium carbonate

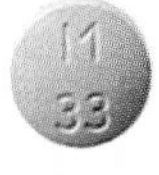

MEBARAL 100 mg
mephobarbital

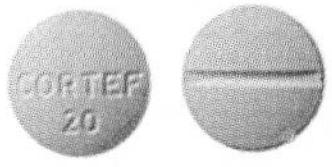

CORTEF 20 mg
hydrocortisone

Color Identification Guide

a	LIMBITROL DS chlordiazepoxide & amitriptyline	ISMELIN 25 mg guanethidine	ANTURANE 100 mg sulfinpyrazone	PEN-VEE K 250 mg penicillin V potassium	ALUPENT 20 mg metaproterenol	MESTINON 60 mg pyridostigmine bromide
b	CORZIDE 80 nadolol & bendroflumethiazide	THEO-DUR 100 mg theophylline	LASIX 80 mg furosemide	ARMOUR Thyroid 120 mg thyroid, desiccated	ORINASE 250 mg tolbutamide	TRANDATE 200 mg labetalol
c	ZYLOPRIM 100 mg allopurinol	TENORETIC 100 atenolol & chlorthalidone	NIZORAL 200 mg ketoconazole	GRIFULVIN V 250 mg griseofulvin	TYLENOL with Codeine No. 2 codeine & acetaminophen	NORMODYNE 200 mg labetalol
d	TEGRETOL Chewable 100 mg carbamazepine	NORPRAMIN 150 mg desipramine	ARMOUR Thyroid 180 mg thyroid, desiccated	TOLINASE 250 mg tolazamide	THEOLAIR 125 mg theophylline	UNIPHYL 400 mg theophylline
e	SELDANE 60 mg terfenadine	WIGRAINE ergotamine tartrate with caffeine	URISPAS 100 mg flavoxate	CYTOXAN 50 mg cyclophosphamide	LORELCO 250 mg probucol	EQUANIL 400 mg meprobamate

Color Identification Guide

a DESYREL 100 mg trazodone	TAVIST-D clemastine fumarate & phenylpropanolamine	ALDORIL 25 mg methyldopa & hydrochlorothiazide	TYLENOL with Codeine No. 4 codeine & acetaminophen	URECHOLINE 5 mg bethanechol
TYLENOL with Codeine No. 3 codeine & acetaminophen				
b ISOPTIN 120 mg verapamil	DIURIL 500 mg chlorothiazide	FIORINAL butalbital, aspirin & caffeine	DIAMOX 250 mg acetazolamide	ARMOUR Thyroid 240 mg thyroid, desiccated
CIPRO 250 mg ciprofloxacin				
c EMPIRIN with Codeine No. 4 codeine & aspirin	PERCOCET oxycodone hydrochloride & acetaminophen	TOLECTIN 200 mg tolmetin	FULVICIN U/F 250 mg griseofulvin	PEN-VEE K 500 mg penicillin V potassium
THEOLAIR-SR 250 mg theophylline				
d SOMA 350 mg carisoprodol	ORINASE 500 mg tolbutamide	EMPIRIN with Codeine No. 3 codeine & aspirin	GRIFULVIN V 500 mg griseofulvin	E-MYCIN 333 mg erythromycin
TOLINASE 500 mg tolazamide	MOTRIN 300 mg ibuprofen			
e QUINAGLUTE DURATAB 324 mg quinidine gluconate	QUINAMM 260 mg quinine	KAON-CL 10 mEq potassium chloride	MOTRIN 300 mg ibuprofen	QUINIDEX Extentabs 300 mg quinidine sulfate
FULVICIN U/F 500 mg griseofulvin				